IET HEALTHCARE TECHNOLOGIES SERIES 13

Handbook of Speckle Filtering and Tracking in Cardiovascular Ultrasound Imaging and Video

IET Book Series on e-Health Technologies – Call for Authors

Book Series Editor: Professor Joel P. C. Rodrigues, the National Institute of Telecommunications (Inatel), Brazil and Instituto de Telecomunicações, Portugal

While the demographic shifts in populations display significant socio-economic challenges, they trigger opportunities for innovations in e-Health, m-Health, precision and personalized medicine, robotics, sensing, the Internet of Things, cloud computing, Big Data, Software Defined Networks and network function virtualization. Their integration is however associated with many technological, ethical, legal, social and security issues. This new Book Series aims to disseminate recent advances for e-Health Technologies to improve healthcare and people's wellbeing.

Topics considered include Intelligent e-Health systems, electronic health records, ICT-enabled personal health systems, mobile and cloud computing for eHealth, health monitoring, precision and personalized health, robotics for e-Health, security and privacy in e-Health, ambient assisted living, telemedicine, Big Data and IoT for e-Health and more.

Proposals for coherently integrated International multi-authored edited or co-authored handbooks and research monographs will be considered for this Book Series. Each proposal will be reviewed by the Book Series Editor with additional external reviews from independent reviewers. Please email your book proposal for the IET Book Series on e-Health Technologies to: Professor Joel Rodrigues at joeljr@ieee.org or joeljr@inatel.br.

Handbook of Speckle Filtering and Tracking in Cardiovascular Ultrasound Imaging and Video

Edited by
Christos P. Loizou, Constantinos S. Pattichis and Jan D'hooge

The Institution of Engineering and Technology

Published by The Institution of Engineering and Technology, London, United Kingdom

The Institution of Engineering and Technology is registered as a Charity in England & Wales (no. 211014) and Scotland (no. SC038698).

First published 2018

The Institution of Engineering and Technology
Michael Faraday House
Six Hills Way, Stevenage
Herts, SG1 2AY, United Kingdom

www.theiet.org

British Library Cataloguing in Publication Data
A catalogue record for this product is available from the British Library

ISBN 978-1-78561-290-9 (hardback)
ISBN 978-1-78561-291-6 (PDF)

Typeset in India by MPS Limited
Printed in the UK by CPI Group (UK) Ltd, Croydon

The Lord said, “Do not be anxious, saying, ‘What shall we eat?’ or ‘What shall we drink?’ or ‘What shall we wear?’ For the Gentiles seek all these things; and your heavenly Father knows that you need them all. But seek first his kingdom and his righteousness, and all these things shall be yours as well. Therefore, do not be anxious about tomorrow, for tomorrow will be anxious for itself. Let the day’s own trouble be sufficient for the day. Or what man of you, if his son asks him for bread, will give him a stone? Or if he asks for a fish, will give him a serpent? If you then, who are evil, know how to give good gifts to your children, how much more will your Father who is in heaven give good things to those who ask him!”

Matthew 6:31–34; 7:9–11

Dedication

This book is dedicated

To my family.
Christos P. Loizou

To the patient and to my family.
Constantinos S. Pattichis

To Petra and my children, Linn and Elias.
Jan D'hooge

Contents

Preface

Medical imaging technology has experienced a dramatic change in the last 30 years. The use of ultrasound in the diagnosis and assessment of imaging organs and soft tissue structures as well as human blood is well established. Because of its non-invasive nature and continuing improvements in image quality, ultrasound imaging is progressively achieving an important role in the assessment and characterization of cardiovascular imaging.

Speckle is inherent in ultrasound imaging and according to Janjic and Soest,[1] it manifests itself as 'spotty' variations in image intensity, giving rise to a granular appearance instead of homogeneous, flat shades of grey, as is visible and as such, speckle can severely compromise interpretation of ultrasound images, particularly in discrimination of small structures. Moreover, it is argued by the same authors that it is fundamentally impossible to separate the 'true' image information from speckle corrupting it and for this reason, the common term 'speckle noise' is a misnomer, as there is no way to discriminate the speckle as a 'noise' source from the 'signal', that we are actually interested in. On the other hand, speckle can be used in the detection of time varying phenomena (i.e. blood vessels, for instance, can be identified based on their large speckle variance or short speckle decorrelation time), or tracking tissue motion.

The objective of this book is to provide a reference edited volume covering the whole spectrum of speckle phenomena, theoretical background and modelling, algorithms and selected applications in cardiovascular ultrasound imaging and video processing and analysis.

The book is organized under the following four parts, Part I: Introduction to Speckle Noise in Ultrasound Imaging and Video; Part II: Speckle Filtering; Part III: Speckle Tracking and Part IV: Selected Applications. Part I of this book begins with a brief review on ultrasound imaging and video techniques and provides in the second chapter the fundamental theory of speckle noise. The following chapter (Chapter 3) deals with the statistical modelling of speckle noise, while Chapter 4 provides a summary of Part I. Part II of the book presents a number of despeckle filtering techniques for imaging and video. It begins with an introduction (Chapter 5) and an overview of despeckle filtering techniques (Chapter 6). Linear and non-linear despeckle filtering is presented in Chapters 7 and 8, respectively, while Chapter 9 introduces wavelet despeckle filtering. A comparative evaluation of all filtering techniques is presented in Chapter 10, while Chapter 11 concludes Part II

[1]J. Janjic and G. Soest, *Speckle Physics*, this volume.

and provides future directions. Part III focuses on ultrasound speckle tracking techniques. It begins with an introduction to speckle tracking techniques in ultrasound video (Chapter 12) and provides in Chapter 13 the principles of speckle tracking. Block matching and image registration techniques for speckle tracking are presented in Chapters 14 and 15, respectively, while Chapter 16 deals with strain estimation in ultrasound video. Chapter 17 provides a summary on combined techniques for speckle filtering and tracking. Part III of the book concludes with summary and future directions on speckle tracking (Chapter 18).

Part IV begins with Chapter 19, which provides details on the segmentation of the carotid artery intima-media thickness (IMT) in ultrasound imaging. Chapter 20 presents an integrated system for the segmentation of ultrasound carotid plaques in video sequences. Chapter 21 illustrates examples on texture analysis of the carotid artery plaque for the prediction of the risk of stroke, while Chapter 22 provides details on the 3D segmentation and texture analysis of the carotid artery. In Chapters 23 and 24, carotid artery mechanics assessed by ultrasound and carotid artery wall motion and strain analysis using tracking are presented, respectively. Chapter 25 presents intravascular ultrasound (IVUS) tracking by discussing advantages and disadvantages of IVUS in the detection of artery geometrical features ad plaque type morphology. In Chapter 26, an introduction to speckle tracking in ultrasound imaging is provided, while Chapter 27 presents the assessment of systolic and diastolic heart failure. In Chapter 28 myocardial elastography and electromechanical wave imaging is discussed. Finally, Chapter 29 summarizes the contents of this book and provides future directions.

This book is intended for all those working in the field of image and video processing technologies and more specifically in medical imaging and in ultrasound image and video pre-processing and analysis. It provides different levels of material to researchers, biomedical engineers, computing engineers and medical imaging engineers interested in developing imaging and video systems with better quality by limiting the corruption of speckle in those systems as well as systems for flowing up the development of the disease. Moreover, application of speckle tracking in strain imaging is introduced which will enable the follow up of the video analysis of the carotid, the heart and other organs.

We wish to thank all the authors for their hard work, valuable time and efforts and for sharing their experiences so readily, and for their valuable comments in enhancing the content of this book. Furthermore, we would like to express our sincere thanks to the IET Books Team members, Jennifer Grace and Olivia Wilkins for their understanding, patience and support in materializing this project.

We hope that this book will be a useful reference for all the readers in the field of cardiovascular ultrasound imaging and video research and to contribute to the development and implementation of innovative imaging and video systems enabling the provision of better quality images and video for the delivery of a better service to the patient.

Christos P. Loizou
Constantinos S. Pattichis
Jan D'hooge

Guide to book contents

In this book, which consists of four different parts, we intent to provide a comprehensive overview of the theory and current practices of despeckle filtering and tracking techniques in ultrasound imaging and video.

Part I begins with an introduction to speckle noise in ultrasound imaging and video techniques and provides in the second chapter the fundamental theory and physics of speckle noise. Part I follows with Chapter 3, which deals with the statistical modelling of speckle noise and ends with a summary of the chapters presented in Part I.

In Part II, we provide an introduction to despeckle filtering (Chapter 5), while different state-of-the-art despeckle filtering techniques for ultrasound imaging and video are presented in Chapter 6. In Chapter 7, linear despeckle filtering is presented, while non-linear despeckle filtering is discussed in Chapter 8. Chapter 9 presents wavelet despeckle filtering, while a comparative evaluation of linear and non linear despeckle filtering techniques is presented and discussed in Chapter 10. Finally, in Chapter 11, we provide a summary of the different despeckle filtering techniques presented in Part II of this book and discuss future directions.

Part III deals with ultrasound speckle tracking techniques. It begins with an introduction to speckle tracking techniques in ultrasound video (Chapter 12) and provides in Chapter 13 the principles of speckle tracking. Block matching and image registration techniques for speckle tracking are presented in Chapters 14 and 15, respectively, while Chapter 16 deals with cardiac strain estimation in ultrasound video. Chapter 17 provides a summary of combined techniques for speckle filtering and speckle tracking. Part III of the book concludes with a 'summary and future directions' on speckle tracking in Chapter 18.

Part IV begins with Chapter 19, which provides details on the carotid artery segmentation of the intima-media complex (IMC) for ultrasound imaging. Segmentation of the ultrasound common carotid artery plaque in video is presented in Chapter 20. Chapter 21 introduces texture analysis of the carotid artery for the prediction of the risk of stroke in asymptomatic carotid plaque images. Chapter 22 presents 3D segmentation and texture analysis techniques of the carotid artery. In Chapters 23 and 24, carotid artery mechanics assessed by ultrasound and carotid artery wall motion and strain analysis using tracking are presented, respectively. Chapter 25 presents the intravascular ultrasound (IVUS) tracking and discusses its advantages and disadvantages in the detection of artery geometrical features and plaque type morphology. Chapter 26 provides an introduction to speckle tracking in cardiac ultrasound imaging, while Chapter 27 illustrates the assessment of systolic and diastolic heart failure. Chapter 28 presents myocardial elastography and electromechanical wave imaging. Finally, Chapter 29 summarizes the contents of Part IV of this book and provides future directions.

Part I

Introduction to speckle noise in ultrasound imaging and video

Chapter 1

A brief review of ultrasound imaging and video

Alfred C. H. Yu[1]

Since its introduction in the latter half of the twentieth century, ultrasound has emerged as a noninvasive imaging modality that can provide anatomical images in real time [1]. This imaging modality has been widely used in medical diagnoses of patients ranging from fetuses to the elderly [2]. It has distinct advantages over other medical imaging technologies like computed tomography and magnetic resonance imaging in terms of economic cost and bedside applicability [3,4]. In fact, it has championed itself as a unique imaging modality with point-of-care applicability [5].

Aside from its use in examining anatomical structures, ultrasound may also be used to examine blood-flow dynamics. In particular, through an imaging mode known as Doppler imaging (or color flow imaging), it is possible to use ultrasound to visualize the hemodynamics in various vessels and body organs. The flow information in Doppler imaging is shown in the form of color-coded pixels that are overlaid on top of a gray-scale image of the anatomical structure, and the flow pixels may either represent blood velocities or blood signal power [6]. Note that Doppler imaging has been used in a variety of cardiovascular diagnoses because of its real-time scanning capabilities [7]. For instance, it has been used to identify the presence of vascular stenoses, assess the development of aneurysms and tumors, study the patency of implanted shunts, and visualize blood regurgitations between heart chambers [8].

In this introductory chapter, a pedagogical overview on the technical foundations of ultrasound imaging will be provided to guide readers who are new to the biomedical ultrasound field. The intent here is to equip readers with fundamental principles that would serve well as background knowledge to understand the broad range of technical concepts covered in this book. Not only will the general physics of ultrasound and the key imaging considerations be outlined, engineering aspects such as system hardware will also be covered. In addition, commentary on the emerging trend toward high-frame-rate imaging will be included to highlight latest innovation thrusts in ultrasound imaging.

[1]Schlegel Research Institute for Aging and Department of Electrical and Computer Engineering, University of Waterloo, Canada

1.1 Revisiting the notion of ultrasound

As a prelude to describing what it means by ultrasound, it is worthwhile to briefly review the basics of sound. According to the dictionary, one definition of sound is "mechanical vibrations transmitted by an elastic medium." These mechanical (or acoustic) vibrations can come in various forms; the most common ones are compressional (longitudinal) and shear (transverse) waves, while other types such as torsional, Rayleigh, and Lamb waves also exist [9]. One important physical concept to be noted is that, for any type of mechanical wave, medium particles oscillate locally at some frequency, and it is the spatiotemporally synchronized particle motion that led to a net wavefront propagation. The speed at which the wavefront travels is known as the speed of sound c, and it is governed by the well-known relation $c = \lambda f$, where λ denotes the wavelength and f denotes the frequency at which medium particles are vibrating. Physically speaking, mechanical wave propagation is attributed to the spatiotemporal interaction between the local medium pressure and the particle velocity. More details on this physics aspect of acoustics can found in the tutorial article by Humphrey [10].

The key distinguishing characteristic between sound and ultrasound lies in the wave frequency f. For a mechanical wave to be considered as sound, its frequency must be within the frequency range that can be detected by the human ear, i.e., between 20 and 20,000 Hz. In contrast, ultrasound refers to mechanical waves that are beyond the human audible range—in other words, mechanical waves with frequency beyond 20,000 Hz. Note that ultrasound should not be confused with the notion of "supersonic," which refers to the phenomenon where objects move faster than the speed of sound. Also, ultrasound is fundamentally not the same as electromagnetic waves, whose energy propagation is attributed to the mutual induction between electric and magnetic fields.

Why is it worthwhile to use ultrasound instead of sound for imaging purpose? The reasons are 2-fold. First, the image resolution tends to be significantly finer at higher frequencies, because as will be described in Section 1.3, resolution is directly proportional to the wavelength, and based on the $c = \lambda f$ relation, it is apparent that higher frequencies would yield smaller wavelengths for the same speed of sound. As a brief example, for a speed of sound of 1,500 m/s in water, the wavelength at 20 kHz frequency is 7.5 cm, whereas it is 0.3 mm at 5 MHz frequency (i.e., resolution at 5 MHz is only 1/250th of the resolution at 20 kHz). The second reason for a strong preference toward using ultrasound (rather than sound) for imaging is out of practical considerations—devices can operate at much higher amplitudes without causing hearing pain. In reality, the sound pressure thresholds for the human ear to perceive pain and hearing damage are, respectively, 20 and 200 Pa [9]. These thresholds are in stark contrast with the megapascal-range pressure levels that are typically used in ultrasound imaging [10].

1.2 Basics of ultrasound imaging: the pulse-echo sensing principle

In terms of its data acquisition principles, ultrasound imaging works via the pulse-echo sensing principle in which an ultrasound transducer would first emit ultrasound pulses into the imaging medium and would then detect the returned echoes to obtain sensing data for image formation. The origin of pulse echoes is attributed to reflection and backscattering from echogenic structures within the medium. Note that the extent of echogenicity is physically dependent on (i) in the case of reflection, whether there is a mismatch in the local acoustic impedance (reflection is stronger if there is a strong impedance mismatch) [10]; (ii) in the case of backscattering, whether the scatterer radius is relatively large in proportion to the wavelength (stronger backscattering for larger scatter radii) [11]. As different body organs and tissues have slightly different medium properties (such as speed of sound, density, and medium size) [12], their corresponding ultrasound image signature may not be the same, and in turn it is often possible to distinguish between different body parts in ultrasound images.

Through the pulse-echo sensing principle, different ultrasound imaging modes have been proposed over the years. This chapter will give an overview of the technical principles for the most classical one (A-mode) and the ones commonly used in today's ultrasound scanners (M-mode and B-mode).

1.2.1 A-mode sensing (amplitude mode)

As the classical form of ultrasound pulse-echo sensing, A-mode ultrasound is a single-beam data acquisition process that works as follows. First, a single ultrasound scanline is used to monitor the imaging medium, and ultrasound pulses are emitted from the transducer periodically at a given pulse repetition frequency f_{PRF}. Second, in each pulse transmission event, the echoes returned from the medium are detected by the same transducer, and the signal envelope of the received echoes is derived after echo amplification and demodulation (achieved using electronic circuitry). As the output of this data acquisition process, a plot of envelope magnitude versus depth (or axial position) is rendered. An example of this display mode is shown in Figure 1.1.

For the pulse-echo sensing process, two salient points of interest should be noted. First, an ultrasound echo from an imaging depth z is the result of two propagation events: (i) the transmitted pulse traveling a distance z to reach the echogenic target at that depth; (ii) the echo traveling a distance z to reach the transducer. Second, the imaging depth z is directly proportional to the echo arrival time t because the relationship between speed, distance, and time is well governed by the well-known kinematics formula $v = d/t$. Accordingly, for a known speed of sound c (i.e., $v = c$) and noting that $d = 2z$ for two-way propagation, depth and time are correlated by the following formula:

$$z = \frac{ct}{2} \tag{1.1}$$

More details on related imaging considerations are given in Section 1.3.1.

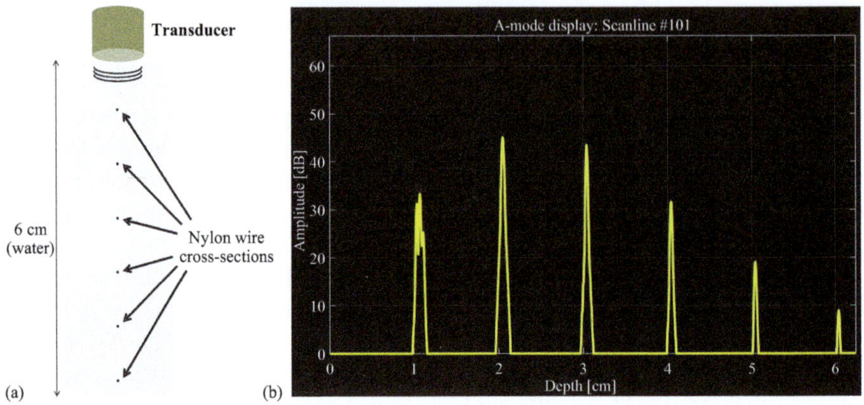

Figure 1.1 A-mode ultrasound sensing. (a) Imaging scenario showing a transducer (0.375″ diameter, 5 MHz frequency) sending pulses into an echolucent water bath with six echogenic nylon wire cross-sections. (b) The corresponding A-mode display of the detected pulse echoes from the six wires

1.2.2 M-mode mapping (motion mode)

M-mode ultrasound is an extension of A-mode in that the same transmission and reception operations apply (i.e., pulse-echo sensing at a single transducer position), but the output format is different. In particular, instead of displaying one-dimensional (1-D) graphs of envelope magnitude versus depth, M-mode ultrasound shows this information as a two-dimensional (2-D) image map. The two image axes respectively denote depth (information from the same pulse-echo event) and time (information from different pulse-echo events). The envelope magnitudes are rendered as gray-scale pixels in the M-mode ultrasound plot.

The key distinguishing factor between M-mode and A-mode ultrasound is that for M-mode, time-evolution mapping of echo magnitudes is enabled, whereas for A-mode, only the echo magnitudes from a single pulse-echo event are rendered. Accordingly, M-mode ultrasound has found its way into clinical use as a simple way of temporally tracking dynamic structures, such as assessing the motion of arterial pulsation and heart valves. Note that, in M-mode, motionless structures are typically rendered as a straight line of brightness along the time axis, while moving structure are depicted as curved traces in time. In the case of tracking arterial pulsation, the artery's proximal and distal walls are typically the two dynamic boundaries that are visualized in an M-mode map. An example of this scenario is shown in Figure 1.2(b). By measuring the instantaneous spatial separation between them, insight can be gained on how the arterial diameter evolves over the course of a cardiac cycle.

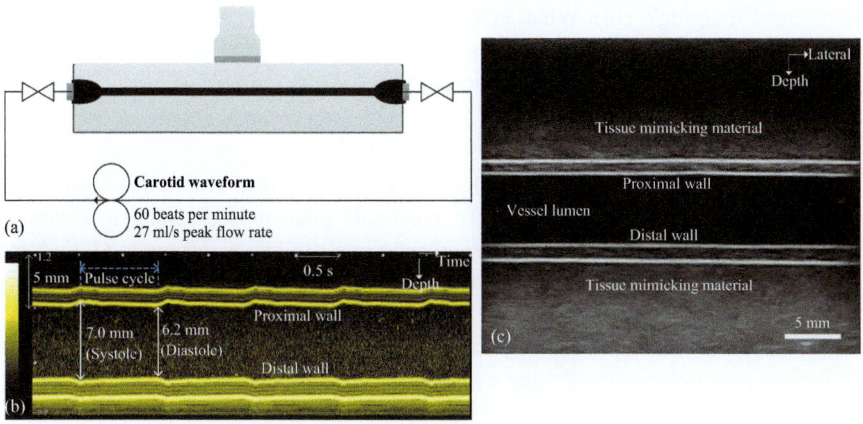

Figure 1.2 M-mode and B-mode imaging of an arterial phantom. (a) Imaging scenario showing a transducer (128-element linear array, 5 MHz imaging frequency) sending pulses into an echogenic tissue mimicking slab containing a pulsating vessel tube (60 beats per minute; 27 ml/s peak flow rate). (b) The corresponding M-mode map showing differences in systolic and diastolic vessel diameter. (c) A B-mode image of the long-axis view of the arterial phantom

1.2.3 B-mode imaging (brightness mode)

B-mode ultrasound, as the most common form of image information rendered in clinical ultrasound scanners, can be considered as a spatial extension of the image formation principles used in M-mode mapping. Specifically, rather than forming a depth versus time gray-scale pixel map like M-mode ultrasound, B-mode imaging seeks to form 2-D gray-scale maps based on echoes received from a 2-D spatial plane, whereby the vertical and horizontal axes respectively correspond to the depth (axial) and lateral dimensions of the image. For Figure 1.2(a) imaging scenario, Figure 1.2(c) shows the corresponding B-mode image of the long-axis view of the arterial phantom. It should be emphasized that, during data acquisition, a set of scanline positions along the lateral axis is defined, and pulse-echo sensing is performed once at each position, effectively forming one gray-scale pixel line of the B-mode image. Further discussion on this imaging paradigm is discussed in Section 1.6.

1.3 Imaging considerations: from frame rate to spatial resolution

While pulse-echo sensing has been well leveraged to develop a few different ultrasound imaging modes, there are a number of questions worth asking regarding the technical specifics of this process: (i) How much wait time should there be in between two transmission events? (ii) What is the general resolution range for ultrasound imaging? (iii) What is the frame rate achievable? (iv) What is the penetration depth of the pulse-echo sensing process? A brief explanation on each imaging consideration will be provided in this section.

1.3.1 Minimum pulse repetition interval

The overarching goal of the pulse-echo sensing process is to obtain distinguishable echoes from all depths of interest. To meet this goal, it is essential to establish a one-to-one mapping between depth and echo arrival time according to (1.1). Note that the maximum depth of interest $z_{\max}$ would need the longest time for the corresponding echoes to return to the transducer (i.e., $t_{\max} = 2z_{\max}/c$). Accordingly, this longest echo arrival time would correspond to the minimum wait time required before the next pulse-echo sensing event should be commenced. In other words, the pulse repetition interval T_{PRI} should be set to satisfy the relation

$$T_{\mathrm{PRI}} > \frac{2z_{\max}}{c} \tag{1.2a}$$

Because pulse repetition frequency f_{PRF} is simply the reciprocal of T_{PRI}, this frequency quantity should satisfy the following relation:

$$f_{\mathrm{PRF}} < \frac{c}{2z_{\max}} \tag{1.2b}$$

As a brief example, suppose we wish to perform pulse-echo sensing for up to 10 cm depth in tissues (whose speed of sound is 1,540 m/s), the minimum T_{PRI} and the maximum f_{PRF} would, respectively, be equal to 0.13 ms and 7.7 kHz.

As an illustration of this imaging consideration, Figure 1.3(a) shows a diagram for a case where there are two acoustic targets at two different depths of interest (Target B is situated deeper). The first row plots the timing of two pulse firings,

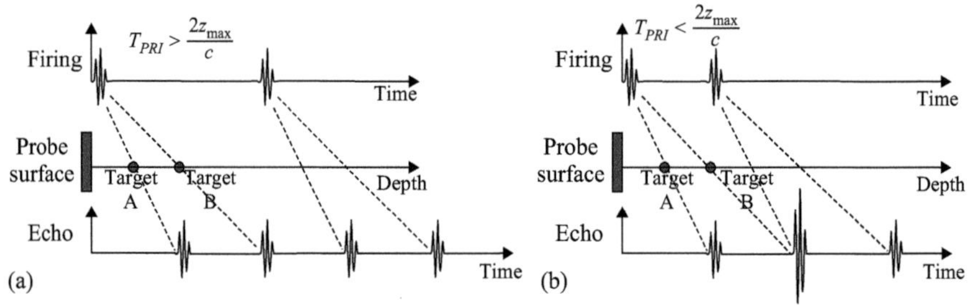

Figure 1.3 Illustration of the minimum pulse repetition interval (T_{PRI}) consideration in pulse-echo sensing, with the depth of Target B being regarded as the maximum sensing depth z_{max}. Two cases are illustrated: (a) T_{PRI} is greater than $2z_{max}/c$; (b) T_{PRI} is less than $2z_{max}/c$. Distinguishable pulse echoes from the two targets can be detected in the first case, but in the second case, the pulse echoes of Targets A and B may overlap temporally over two firings

while the third row plots the timing of the respective echoes from Targets A and B (each sloped line depicts the two-way propagation time of a pulse and its echo from a target at that depth). If the interval between the two transmit pulses is sufficiently long, they would collectively give rise to four distinct pulse-echo signatures at four different time points. Conversely, if the pulse repetition interval is not long enough, it is well possible for the second pulse-echo from Target A to overlap with the first pulse-echo from Target B, thereby making it difficult to provide useful diagnostic information. This problematic scenario is illustrated in Figure 1.3(b).

1.3.2 Frame rate

For B-mode imaging, the time required to form one image is dependent on the number of scanlines N and the pulse repetition interval between scanlines T_{PRI}. Specifically, the frame acquisition time T_{frame} is simply given by the relation $T_{\mathrm{frame}} = NT_{\mathrm{PRI}}$. In turn, the frame rate f_{frame}, which is simply the reciprocal of T_{frame}, is equal to

$$f_{\mathrm{frame}} = \frac{f_{\mathrm{PRF}}}{N} \tag{1.3}$$

Taken together with the notion of maximum pulse repetition frequency (which is influenced by the maximum imaging depth), it follows that the maximum frame rate can be found as

$$f_{\mathrm{frame(max)}} = \frac{c}{2z_{\mathrm{max}}N} \tag{1.4}$$

Using the same numerical example from the previous subsection, if there are 128 scanlines for a 10 cm imaging depth in tissue, $f_{\mathrm{frame(max)}}$ would be equal to 60 frames per second. It is worth emphasizing that this frame rate is well in the real-time display range. As such, B-mode ultrasound has long established itself as a real-time imaging modality.

1.3.3 Depth (or axial) resolution

To obtain distinguishable echoes from different acoustic targets, a key consideration to be considered is the resolvability of two targets from different depths. If the targets are axially too close, then the resulting pulse-echoes from the two targets may be blurred as a single pulse-echo signature. This scenario is illustrated in Figure 1.4(a). One salient point to be noted from this diagram is that the spatial correspondence of the transmit pulse duration is the key determining factor for the depth resolution. For a given pulse of duration T_p, its incidence upon two acoustic targets at different depths (A and B) would yield distinguishable echo signature if the spatial length of the transmitted pulse is shorter than the distance between the two targets. This latter scenario is shown in Figure 1.4(b).

Based on (1.1), the depth resolution z_{res} is essentially equal to $z_{\mathrm{res}} = cT_p/2$. For an M- cycle pulse of ultrasound frequency f_o, the pulse duration T_p is given by

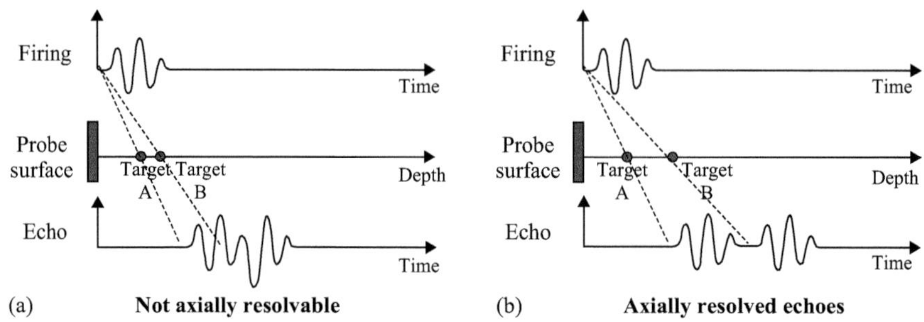

Figure 1.4 Axial resolvability of two acoustic targets in pulse-echo sensing. Two cases are illustrated: (a) when Targets A and B are too close to each other, their pulse echoes would be superimposed as a single echo signature; (b) when the two targets are further spaced apart, their pulse echoes are individually distinguishable

$T_p = M/f_o$. Accordingly, by recalling that $c = \lambda f$, z_{res} can be re-expressed as

$$z_{\text{res}} = \frac{M\lambda}{2} \tag{1.5}$$

In other words, the axial resolution is directly proportional to the ultrasound wavelength—a notion that has been pointed out in Section 1.1. As an example, suppose a 5-MHz, two-cycle ultrasound pulse is used for the pulse-echo sensing process in tissue. The corresponding axial resolution would equal to 0.308 mm (i.e., in the submillimeter range).

1.3.4 Lateral resolution

In addition to depth resolution, the lateral width of the ultrasound beam used for pulse-echo sensing is also an imaging consideration of interest. At a given imaging depth, a localized beam width would effectively avoid interference from nearby lateral targets. Correspondingly, the lateral resolution is governed by how localized the beam profile is. This notion is depicted in Figure 1.5, where the focal spot is at a given depth z_f for a transducer aperture diameter a. From acoustic field-profile analysis, it is known that, under Fraunhofer approximation conditions [13], the lateral field profile $l(x)$ at a given depth is directly proportional to a sinc function. In particular, it follows the relation

$$l(x) \propto \text{sinc}\left(\frac{x}{\lambda F_{\text{num}}}\right) \tag{1.6}$$

where F_{num} is known as the F-number and is given by the ratio between imaging depth and aperture width (i.e., $F_{\text{num}} = z_f/\text{a}$).

Insight into the lateral resolution can be gained by solving for the first zero-crossing points of the sinc function in $l(x)$. In particular, it is known that for a generic sinc function of the form $\text{sinc}(x/b)$, the first zero-crossing points appear

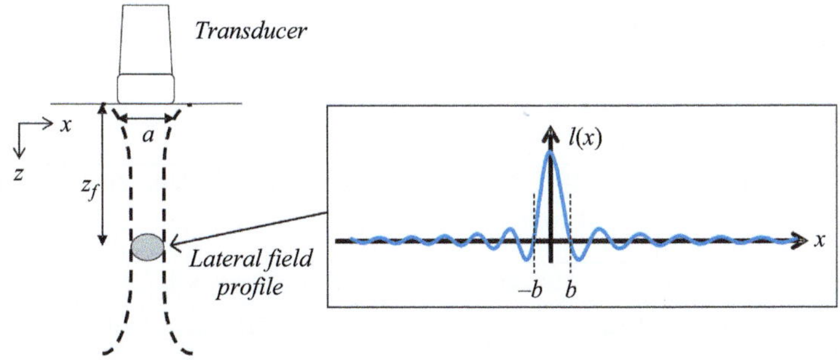

Figure 1.5 Lateral focusing of an ultrasound beam. For a given focal depth z_f and aperture size a, its corresponding lateral field profile l(x) at depth z_f is directly proportional to a sinc function sinc(x/b), whose first zero crossings appear at $x = \pm b$ (see inset)

at $x = \pm b$ (illustrated in the inset of Figure 1.5). If we assume the effective lateral width to be equal to the full width at half maximum, the lateral resolution l_{res} would be given by

$$l_{\text{res}} \approx 0.5[b - (-b)] = b = \lambda F_{\text{num}} \tag{1.7}$$

It should be noted that, as similar to axial resolution, the lateral resolution is also directly proportional to the ultrasound wavelength λ (in line with what has been pointed out in Section 1.1). As an example, suppose F_{num} is 4; the corresponding lateral resolution in tissue for 5-MHz ultrasound would be equal to 1.23 mm (i.e., on the order of millimeters).

1.3.5 Penetration depth

The ability for ultrasound to propagate into tissues is physically limited by the phenomenon of acoustic attenuation. Empirical measurements have generally found that attenuation linearly increases against ultrasound frequency in tissue [12]. As such, from an imaging standpoint, it is of practical interest to estimate the penetration depth that can be achieved. Note that this is a physical detection limit that is constrained by the nature of wave propagation, and it fundamentally differs from the maximum imaging depth specified in determining the minimum pulse repetition interval.

An exponential decay model is often used to derive the penetration depth. It is an empirical model that considers the intensity at a particular depth $I(z)$ as a fraction of the initial intensity emitted from the transducer:

$$I(z) = I_o\, e^{-2(\alpha f)z} \tag{1.8a}$$

where α is the attenuation coefficient and the factor of two is attributed to the fact that intensity is the squared form of ultrasound pressure. Reexpressing this equation in logarithmic form, we get

$$10 \log_{10}\left[\frac{I_o}{I(z)}\right] = \alpha_{\text{dB}} fz \tag{1.8b}$$

where α_{dB} is the decibel form of the attenuation coefficient and is equal to 20α ($\log_{10} e$). Accordingly, it follows that the penetration depth z_{pen} is given by

$$z_{\text{pen}} = \frac{\Delta I_{\text{dB(max)}}}{\alpha_{\text{dB}} f} \tag{1.9}$$

where $\Delta I_{\text{dB(max)}}$ is the maximum drop in intensity that can be detected by the imaging probe. In reality, α_{dB} is empirically measured to be 0.2–0.7 dB/(cm MHz) in tissues, while $\Delta I_{\text{dB(max)}}$ depends on the dynamic range of the ultrasound scanner (about 60 dB with current technology). As such, for the typical range of ultrasound frequencies used for imaging (between 2 and 15 MHz), the penetration depth ranges from a few centimeters to tens of centimeters.

1.4 Ultrasound imaging hardware

Leveraging the pulse-echo sensing principle and taking into account various imaging considerations, a number of ultrasound systems are commercially available nowadays. These systems can be considered as the integrative product of various engineering advances in transducer technology, scanner electronics, and human ergonomics. Typically, in each system, its console is consisted of a series of front-end electronics and the user interface, and it would support the connection of different transducers as peripherals to perform imaging operations. This section will provide a brief overview of various hardware components.

1.4.1 Array transducers

Transducers that are used in clinical scanning are often developed in the form of an array in which multiple transducer elements (e.g., 128) are present on the same device. Fabricated using ceramic composites that have piezoelectric properties (e.g., PZT—a mix of lead (Pb), zirconate (ZrO_3), and titanate (TiO_3)), transducer arrays can be designed to have submillimeter element sizes, and the array of elements collectively yield an overall aperture size of a few centimeters. Their geometries (i.e., how the array elements are aligned) may also be engineered to facilitate imaging operations of various types of field of views. The common array types include [14] (i) linear arrays, which provide rectangular imaging views and are suitable for imaging peripheral body parts (such as the carotid arteries); (ii) curvilinear arrays, which offer diverging imaging views and are frequently used in abdominal scans; (iii) phased arrays, which are used to generate a fan-shaped field of view and are essential to cardiac imaging. Linear arrays tend to work in the 5–15 MHz frequency range, while curvilinear and phased arrays are generally designed to work in 2–5 MHz range in order to achieve the penetration depth necessary to image deep organs. It should be noted that endoscope ultrasound probes and intravascular probes are also available [15]. As well, 2-D array probes that are intended for three-dimensional (3-D) imaging are becoming increasingly mature in technology [16]. Figure 1.6(a) shows a photo of the physical appearance of three types of commercially available array transducers. This photo shows that the physical aperture of a linear array transducer is wider than that of a phased array and a 2-D array.

The main rationale for using array transducers for imaging is that they can effectively facilitate the imaging of a 2-D scan plane (or 3-D scan volume) without mechanically moving the transducer. This technical functionality brings quite a few practical benefits. First, it effectively fosters real-time imaging, because mechanical movement of the transducer is after all not needed. Second, by electronically controlling the enabling and disabling of array elements, a subaperture can be created from a group of consecutive elements to form a local scanline, and its position can be updated between firings to sweep the scanline across the imaging view to acquire an image frame [14]. This principle is particularly applicable to linear and curvilinear arrays. Third, for a given array aperture, by adjusting the activation time of each element, it is possible to realize beam focusing (to improve the lateral localization of a pulse firing) and beam steering (to adjust the angle of sight of a pulse firing) [14,15]. Note that beam steering is particularly important

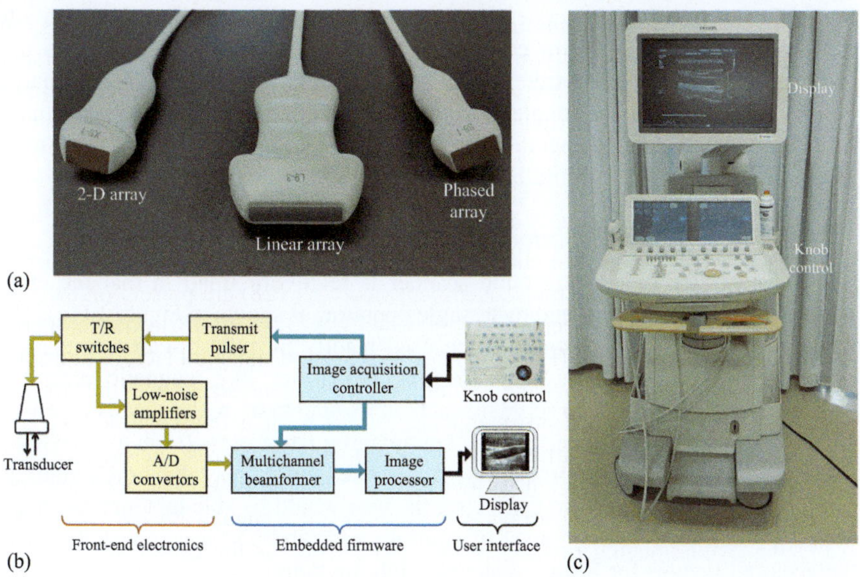

Figure 1.6 Overview of ultrasound imaging hardware. (a) Physical appearance of three types of arrays (linear, phased, and 2-D). (b) Generic block diagram of the system components involved in a typical ultrasound scanner. (c) Physical appearance of a clinical ultrasound scanner

in the case of phased arrays because this beam firing strategy is essential to generate a fan-shaped imaging view.

1.4.2 System electronics

To drive the operations of the array transducer, various front-end electronics are included in the ultrasound system, as illustrated in Figure 1.6(b). Some of the system components are responsible for controlling transmission (Tx) pulsing operations, and others are for generating image frames from the raw echo signals detected from the array elements [17]. Generically speaking, for the Tx pulsing operations, a set of pulser amplifiers is in place to send pulsed electrical signals to each array element, and the required voltage levels (can range greatly from a few volts to over 100 V) are generated by a power distribution module. These components usually come in the form of integrated circuit (IC) chips (dedicated chips for ultrasound systems development are commercially available nowadays) [18]. Also, a sequence controller is included to individually control each power amplifier, so as to coordinate the timing of pulse firing at each element to generate the required ultrasound beam pattern. This controller is usually implemented through programing the hardware fabric of a field programmable gate array (FPGA).

As the same transducer is used for both Tx and reception (Rx), a set of multiplexer switches is installed between the Tx and Rx electronics, so that the latter can be electrically isolated from the high-voltage electrical pulses that are sent from the Tx side. Behind these switches, the Rx electronics would have the following chain of components: (i) low-noise amplifiers and analog-to-digital convertors (IC chips) [19] to convert each element's detected echoes into data samples; (ii) receive beamformer (based on FPGA implementation) to form sharper images from the raw data samples; (iii) back-end digital signal processor for image filtering and fine-tuning operations. The end result (i.e., the generated B-mode image or M-mode map) would be displayed onto the screen.

1.4.3 Scanner appearance

The physical size of an ultrasound scanner is relatively small in that the entire system can be trolleyed around by a single operator, as shown in Figure 1.6(c). This makes it possible for ultrasound to be used readily in point-of-care settings [5]: an application domain that other imaging modalities like magnetic resonance imaging has not been able to serve. In each ultrasound system, the user can view the acquired images in real-time, and the key imaging parameters (such as ultrasound frequency, pulse repetition frequency, frame rate, and display dynamic range) are concurrently shown on the screen. Also, the user would be able to adjust the major imaging parameters through a set of control knobs and buttons, as well as saving the acquired images for further diagnostic interpretation.

1.4.4 Portable systems

One unique trend about ultrasound imaging is that some of the systems have been engineered to have a miniaturized physical size in the form of a laptop, thereby enabling them to be portable and be applied in remote out-hospital settings [20]. In the clinical literature, ultrasonography has been well regarded as a useful aid in emergency diagnoses during field medical operations [21], in on-site assessments of sport injuries [22], and in field missions to developing countries [23]. The design requirements for portable ultrasound devices are generally more stringent than the trolley-based scanners used in hospital-based diagnostics, because infrastructural resources are very limited in field situations. In particular, system transportability, physical compactness, and battery-driven powering are three important design considerations that must be taken into account given that the worksite may have limited space and may not be connected to mains power. These requirements are particularly essential when considering deployment in the developing world [24].

1.5 The Doppler mode

In many clinical ultrasound scanners, a flow modality called the Doppler mode is often included. The name of this modality originates from the fact that the Doppler effect is exploited for flow estimation purposes. In particular, it is known that echoes returned from moving targets, particularly the moving red blood cells in the case of blood flow, would exhibit a Doppler frequency shift f_D whose magnitude is given by [6]

$$f_D = \frac{2vf_o}{c}\cos\theta \tag{1.10}$$

where θ is the angle between the ultrasound scanline axis and the direction of motion. Since the extent of Doppler shift is directly proportional to the flow velocity v, it is possible to quantitatively assess the blood flow profile in the cardiovasculature by studying the Doppler shift pattern as a function of time. In clinical scanners, the Doppler mode is typically implemented in a pulsed form because its operation readily extends from pulse-echo sensing used in M-mode and B-mode imaging. Based on this principle, a few different Doppler display modes have been made available on clinical scanners, as described below.

1.5.1 Doppler spectrogram

The Doppler spectrogram (or spectral Doppler display) shows the time-varying flow velocity distribution derived from the measured Doppler frequencies. An example of this type of display is shown in Figure 1.7(b) for the case of pulsatile flow in the common carotid artery branch of a carotid bifurcation. It is worth noting that the spectrogram information is derived from a single-range gate position, whose size and position can both be adjusted by the user during a diagnostic procedure (often specified on top of a B-mode image of the field of view). In terms of the spectrogram's significance, clinicians often use this display mode to gain quantitative insights into the vascular flow dynamics within a certain range of interest inside the blood vessel. For instance, since vascular stenoses often give rise

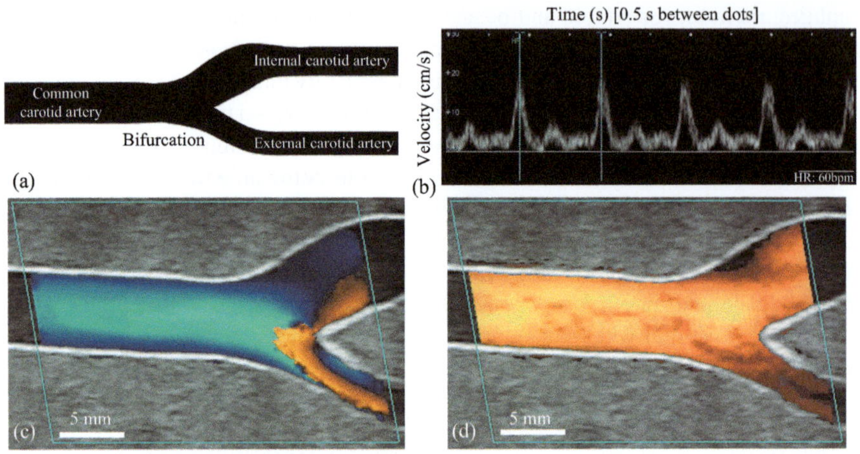

Figure 1.7 Doppler imaging mode for the case of a carotid bifurcation (co-planar phantom). (a) Illustration of the vascular geometry with key features as labeled. (b) Doppler spectrogram in the common carotid artery for pulsatile flow with pulse rate of 60 beats per minute. (c) Color flow image of the carotid bifurcation (blue box indicates the boundaries within which Doppler sensing was performed). (d) The corresponding power Doppler image of the carotid bifurcation

to disturbed flow conditions, clinicians can study the spectrogram to assess the healthiness of a patient's vasculature.

1.5.2 Color flow imaging

Another mode of display for Doppler ultrasound is a color flow image (or velocity map) that shows flow velocity estimates of different sample volumes within the transducer's field of view. An example of this type of display is illustrated in Figure 1.7(c). As shown in the figure, the velocity estimates are displayed in the form of color pixels, and they are superimposed onto a B-mode image of the anatomical structure. This duplex image display format allows clinicians to easily identify blood flow within an entire imaging view. In comparison to the spectrogram that shows the flow distribution, the color flow image only provides a single velocity estimate (usually the mean velocity) for each sample volume, although a red–blue bicolor hue is used to help highlight the detected flow direction (away or toward the transducer). As such, during a diagnostic procedure, the color flow image is usually used as a high-level flow visualization tool prior to conducting detailed diagnoses at specific parts of the vasculature through the Doppler spectrogram mode.

1.5.3 Power Doppler imaging

When rendering flow information in the form of maps, it is possible to display flow power estimates instead of showing the mean flow velocities. The resulting duplex images are often referred to as flow power maps (or Doppler power maps), and an example of this type of flow map is given in Figure 1.7(d). Note that, at large beam-flow angles, the flow power map has diagnostic advantage over the velocity map because the echo power returned from blood scatterers is less dependent of the beam-flow angle (while the Doppler shift magnitude is angle-dependent). On the other hand, the velocity map has the advantage of being able to provide directional flow information that can help identify arteries and veins (which tend to flow in different directions).

1.6 New trend toward high-frame-rate imaging

As discussed earlier in Section 1.3.2, B-mode ultrasound is a real-time imaging modality with video-range frame rates. Nevertheless, to properly assess cardiovascular dynamics (e.g., to obtain quantitative estimates of cardiac strain [25]), higher frame rates of over 100 Hz are essential. Deducing from (1.3) and Figure 1.8(a), it is technically possible to achieve a higher frame rate using the conventional scanline-based imaging by reducing the number of scanlines or increasing the pulse repetition frequency. Yet, this improvement in frame rate would be achieved at the expense of shrinking the imaging view (due to fewer scanlines, or shallower sensing depth due to the use of a higher f_{PRF}) or reducing the image quality (due to the use of fewer scanlines to cover the same lateral span). To increase the imaging frame rate substantially without concomitantly reducing the imaging view or image quality, it is necessary to exploit alternative imaging paradigms.

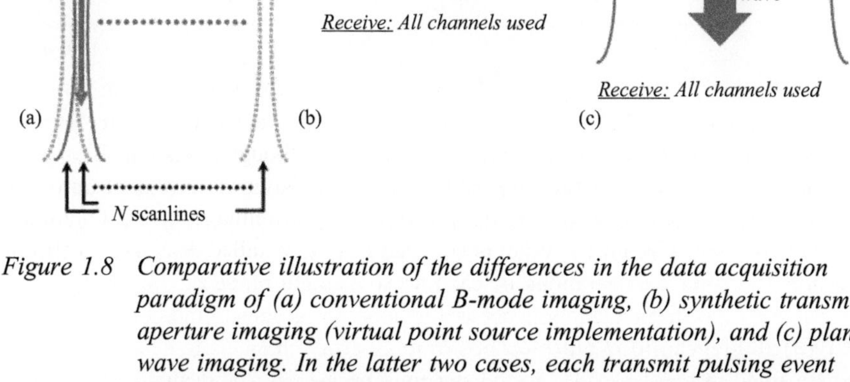

Figure 1.8 Comparative illustration of the differences in the data acquisition paradigm of (a) conventional B-mode imaging, (b) synthetic transmit aperture imaging (virtual point source implementation), and (c) plane wave imaging. In the latter two cases, each transmit pulsing event would insonate the entire imaging view, so it is possible to form one image for every firing

Similar issues are being faced by the Doppler imaging mode. In practice, the maximum frame rate achievable in color flow imaging can be about 30 Hz in arterial imaging applications. However, it can drop to as low as 4–5 Hz when examining low-velocity flow at greater depths [26]. Although such a frame rate can still be considered as real-time, it does not provide sufficient temporal resolution needed to visualize the hemodynamics of various phases in the cardiac cycle. For instance, even with a frame rate of 12 Hz, it is still insufficient for color flow imaging to accurately visualize mitral inflow patterns or flow jets inside the heart [27,28]. This limitation is even more apparent if 3-D color flow images are to be acquired [29]. Similar problems also arise when color flow imaging is used to examine tissue motion instead, where it has been shown that frame rates of over 100 Hz are required to properly assess myocardial functions in different cardiac phases [30].

1.6.1 Current progress in high-frame-rate imaging research

In recent years, various research labs have attempted to develop advanced ultrasound imaging paradigms with high-frame-rate potential. One representative example is the synthetic transmit aperture technique as shown in Figure 1.8(b) [31]. It is based upon the use of unfocused point-source firings for Tx and the sensing of echoes at all transducer channels for Rx. Since focused beam-lines are not formed physically, it is possible to form an image from each firing, thus realizing frame rates that approach the pulse repetition frequency (i.e., how frequent point-source firings are transmitted), which is usually in the kHz range in practice. Indeed, high-quality images with whole field-of-view focusing may be obtained computationally via recursive summation of a series of low-resolution synthetic aperture images [32].

Aside from the synthetic aperture technique, a few other novel methods exist to improve the ultrasound imaging frame rate without concomitantly reducing the quality. For instance, as shown in Figure 1.8(c), it is possible to use plane-wave excitation principles to simultaneously transmit all the beam-lines and then perform parallel receive beamforming on receive [33,34]. This approach should have potential in providing high-frame-rate, high-quality ultrasound images if it is combined with other image improvement strategies like limited-diffraction insonations [35] and adaptive beamforming [36].

1.6.2 Concurrent developments in new imaging hardware

It may be tempting to believe that high-frame-rate ultrasound imaging techniques can be readily implemented on currently available clinical ultrasound scanners. This notion is alas not true, because the front end of existing ultrasound scanners is seldom reconfigurable due to embedded system constraints [37,38]. New imaging hardware is after all required. What is required is a more software-centric platform that allows (i) the Tx operations of each array element to be flexibly programed according to the implementation needs for nonscanline-based imaging sequences [39]; (ii) all prebeamform pulse-echoes from all array channels to be acquired [40] and streamed in real-time [41] to the system's back-end. The design of these new platforms is under way. Some open-architecture scanner platforms have been developed by academic laboratories [42–44], while a few commercial prototyping systems have also been marketed. To facilitate fast processing of raw prebeamform data, high-speed software-based signal processing frameworks are concurrently being devised using parallel computing hardware such as graphics processing units [45]. Recent achievements on this topic include beamforming [46], speckle tracking [47], adaptive apodization [48], and eigen-processing [49].

1.6.3 Recent advances in high-frame-rate cardiovascular ultrasound

With new imaging paradigms and hardware, high-frame-rate ultrasound has demonstrated strong applicability in cardiovascular diagnostics. In particular, high-frame-rate ultrasound is highly useful in tracking physiological dynamics such as myocardial contraction and blood flow that naturally exist in the circulation system. Numerous labs are actively pursuing research on this topic. Briefly, in the cardiac application, some techniques have successfully captured myocardial contraction dynamics at high-frame rates [50,51], while others have shown the feasibility of tracking intraventricular flow patterns [52,53]. In the vascular application, it is now possible to achieve high-frame-rate visualization of flow speckle dynamics together with Doppler color coding [54]. Also, high-frame-rate imaging of flow vector fields in arteries is readily achievable [55–57], and their extension to 3-D flow imaging has shown promise [58,59]. Moreover, it now seems feasible to apply high-frame-rate imaging principles to track arterial wall pulsation [60] and pulse wave propagation through the artery wall [61].

1.7 Conclusion

Ultrasound imaging has enjoyed decades of success as a point-of-care imaging modality with widespread clinical use. Yet, such maturity in clinical applicability does not imply that ultrasound is verging upon a commodity business. With the ongoing wave of innovations in high-frame-rate imaging, ultrasound is now in the midst of a rapid surge in technological advancement. The clinical value of ultrasound imaging is poised for a further expansion as new achievements are made in developing new imaging principles, real-time hardware, computing frameworks, signal processing tools, and image processing algorithms. The rest of this book will particularly highlight on a variety of advances in speckle filtering and tracking, and how these algorithmic tools are being applied to cardiovascular ultrasound.

References

[1] P. N. T. Wells, “Ultrasound imaging”, *Physics in Medicine and Biology*, vol. 51, pp. R83–R98, 2006.

[2] A. B. Wolbarst and W. R. Hendee, “Evolving and experimental technologies in medical imaging”, *Radiology*, vol. 238, pp. 16–39, 2006.

[3] S. M. Erturk, C. Johnston, C. Tempany-Afdhal, and A. D. van den Abbeele, "Imaging tools in human research", in *Clinical and Translational Science*, D. Robertson and G. H. Williams (Ed). Amsterdam: Elsevier, 2009, pp. 87–104.

[4] P. L. Carson and A. Fenster, "Evolution of ultrasound physics", *Medical Physics*, vol. 36, pp. 411–428, 2009.

[5] C. L. Moore and J. A. Copel, "Point-of-care ultrasonography", *New England Journal of Medicine*, vol. 364, pp. 749–757, 2011.

[6] D. H. Evans, "Color flow and motion imaging", *Proceedings of the Institute of Mechanical Engineers, Part H: Journal of Engineering in Medicine*, vol. 224, no. 2, pp. 241–253, 2010.

[7] K. W. Beach, A. C. Keith, J. F. Primozich, et al., "Ultrasonic color flow mapping: the visualization of four-dimensional cardiac and vascular flow phenomena using two dimensions and 'real-time'", *Ultrasound in Medicine and Biology*, vol. 23, pp. 347–363, 1997.

[8] K. Ferrara and G. DeAngelis, "Color flow mapping", *Ultrasound in Medicine and Biology*, vol. 23, pp. 321–345, 1997.

[9] T. G. Leighton, "What is ultrasound?", *Progress in Biophysics and Molecular Biology*, vol. 93, pp. 3–83, 2007.

[10] V. F. Humphrey, "Ultrasound and matter—physical interactions", *Progress in Biophysics and Molecular Biology*, vol. 93, pp. 195–211, 2007.

[11] K. K. Shung and G. A. Thieme (Eds.), *Ultrasonic Scattering in Biological Tissues*, CRC Press: Boca Raton, Florida, 1993.

[12] J. C. Bamber, "Ultrasonic properties of tissues", in *Ultrasound in Medicine*, F. A. Duck, A. C. Baker, H. C. Starritt (Ed). Bristol: Institute of Physics, 1998, pp. 57–88.

[13] R. S. C. Cobbold. *Foundations of Biomedical Ultrasound*. Oxford University Press: Oxford, UK, 2007; Chapters 3 & 7.

[14] J. A. Jensen, "Medical ultrasound imaging", *Progress in Biophysics and Molecular Biology*, vol. 93, pp. 153–165, 2007.

[15] T.A. Whittingham, "Medical diagnostic applications and sources", *Progress in Biophysics and Molecular Biology*, vol. 93, pp. 84–110, 2007.

[16] E. Roux, A. Ramalli, H. Liebgott, C. Cachard, M. C. Robini, and P. Tortoli, "Wideband 2-D array design optimization with fabrication constraints for 3-D US imaging", *IEEE Transactions on Ultrasonics, Ferroelectrics, and Frequency Control*, vol. 64, pp. 108–125, 2017.

[17] K. E. Thomenius, "Miniaturization of ultrasound scanners", *Ultrasound in Clinics*, vol. 4, pp. 385–389, 2009.

[18] E. Brunner, "Ultrasound system considerations and their impact on front-end components," *Analog Dialogue*, vol. 36, no. 3, 2002.

[19] X. Xu, H. Venkataraman, S. Oswal, E. Bartolome, and K. Vasanth, "Challenges and considerations of analog front-ends design for portable ultrasound systems", *Proceedings of IEEE Ultrasonics Symposium*, pp. 310–313, 2010.

[20] B. P. Nelson, E. R. Melnick, and J. Li, "Portable ultrasound for remote environments, part I: feasibility of field deployment", *Journal of Emergency Medicine*, vol. 40, pp. 190–197, 2011.

[21] B. P. Nelson, E. R. Melnick, and J. Li, "Portable ultrasound for remote environments, part II: current indications", *Journal of Emergency Medicine*, vol. 40, pp. 313–321, 2011.

[22] C. Nofsinger and J. G. Konin, "Diagnostic ultrasound in sports medicine: current concepts and advances", *Sports Medicine and Arthroscopy Review*, vol. 17, pp. 25–30, 2009.

[23] J. K. Spencer and R. S. Adler, "Utility of portable ultrasound in a community in Ghana", *Journal of Ultrasound in Medicine*, vol. 27, pp. 1735–1743, 2008.

[24] P. Yager, G. J. Domingo, and J. Gerdes, "Point-of-care diagnostics for global health", *Annual Reviews in Biomedical Engineering*, vol. 10, pp. 107–144, 2008.

[25] T. H. Marwick, "Measurement of strain and strain rate by echocardiography", *Journal of the American College of Cardiology*, vol. 47, pp. 1313–1327, 2006.

[26] G. York and Y. Kim, "Ultrasound processing and computing: review and future directions", *Annual Reviews in Biomedical Engineering*, vol. 1, pp. 559–588, 1999.

[27] J. Pemberton, L. Hui, M. Young, X. Li, A. Kenny, and D. J. Sahn, "Accuracy of 3-dimensional color Doppler-derived flow volumes with increasing imaging depth", *Journal of Ultrasound in Medicine*, vol. 24, pp. 1109–1115, 2005.

[28] J. V. Chapman, "Semiquantitative and quantitative color flow mapping methods", *Journal of Diagnostic Medical Sonography*, vol. 22, pp. 167–179, 2006.

[29] L. Sugeng and R. M. Lang, "Current status of three-dimensional color flow Doppler", *Cardiology in Clinics*, vol. 25, pp. 297–303, 2007.

[30] H. Moladoust, M. Mokhtari-Dizaji, Z. Ojaghi-Haghighi, F. Noohi, and A. Khajavi, "Frame rate requirement for tissue Doppler imaging in different phases of cardiac cycle: radial and longitudinal functions", *International Journal of Cardiovascular Imaging*, vol. 24, pp. 377–387, 2008.

[31] J. A. Jensen, S. I. Nikolov, K. L. Gammelmark, and M. H. Pedersen, "Synthetic aperture ultrasound imaging", *Ultrasonics*, vol. 44, pp. e5–e15, 2006.

[32] S. I. Nikolov and J. A. Jensen, "In-vivo synthetic aperture flow imaging in medical ultrasound," *IEEE Transactions on Ultrasonics, Ferroelectrics, and Frequency Control*, vol. 50, pp. 848–856, 2003.

[33] G. Montaldo, M. Tanter, J. Bercoff, N. Benech, and M. Fink, "Coherent plane-wave compounding for very high frame rate ultrasonography and transient elastography", *IEEE Transactions on Ultrasonics, Ferroelectrics, and Frequency Control*, vol. 56, pp. 489–506, 2009.

[34] M. Tanter and M. Fink, "Ultrafast imaging in biomedical ultrasound", *IEEE Transactions on Ultrasonics, Ferroelectrics, and Frequency Control*, vol. 61, pp. 102–119, 2014.

[35] J. L. Lu, J. Cheng, and J. Wang, "High frame rate imaging system for limited diffraction array beam imaging with square-wave aperture weightings", *IEEE Transactions on Ultrasonics, Ferroelectrics, and Frequency Control*, vol. 53, pp. 1796–1812, 2006.

[36] J. F. Synnevag, A. Austeng, and S. Holm, "Adaptive beamforming applied to medical ultrasound imaging", *IEEE Transactions on Ultrasonics, Ferroelectrics, and Frequency Control*, vol. 54, pp. 1606–1613, 2007.

[37] National Cancer Institute, "Ultrasonic imaging: infrastructure for improved imaging methods", *Report of the OWH/NCI Sponsored Workshop*, 1999.

[38] P. Tortoli and J. A. Jensen, "Introduction to the special issue on novel equipment for ultrasound research", *IEEE Transactions on Ultrasonics, Ferroelectrics, and Frequency Control*, vol. 53, pp. 1705–1706, 2006.

[39] K. Dickie, C. Leung, R. Zahiri, and L. Pellisier, "A flexible research interface for collecting clinical ultrasound images", *Proceedings of SPIE*, vol. 7494, no. 749402, 2009.

[40] C. C. P. Cheung, A. C. H. Yu, N. Salimi, *et al.*, "Multi-channel pre-beamformed data acquisition system for research on advanced ultrasound imaging methods", *IEEE Transactions on Ultrasonics, Ferroelectrics, and Frequency Control*, vol. 59, pp. 243–253, 2012.

[41] M. Walczak, M. Lewandowski, and N. Żołek, "Optimization of real-time ultrasound PCIe data streaming and OpenCL processing for SAFT imaging", *Proceedings of IEEE Ultrasonics Symposium*, pp. 2064–2067, 2013.

[42] P. Tortoli, L. Bassi, E. Boni, A. Dallai, F. Guidi, and S. Ricci, "ULA-OP: an advanced open platform for ultrasound research", *IEEE Transactions on Ultrasonics, Ferroelectrics, and Frequency Control*, vol. 56, pp. 2207–2216, 2009.

[43] J. A. Jensen, H. Holten-Lund, R. T. Nilsson, *et al.*, "SARUS: a synthetic aperture real-time ultrasound system", *IEEE Transactions on Ultrasonics, Ferroelectrics, and Frequency Control*, vol. 60, pp. 1838–1852, 2013.

[44] P. Tortoli, L. Bassi, E. Boni, A. Dallai, F. Guidi, and S. Ricci, "ULA-OP 256: a 256-channel open scanner for development and real-time implementation of new ultrasound methods", *IEEE Transactions on Ultrasonics, Ferroelectrics, and Frequency Control*, vol. 63, pp. 1488–1495, 2016.

[45] H. So, J. Chen, B. Y. S. Yiu, and A. C. H. Yu, "Medical ultrasound imaging: to GPU or not to GPU?", *IEEE Micro*, vol. 31, no. 5, pp. 54–65, 2011.

[46] B. Y. S. Yiu, I. K. H. Tsang, and A. C. H. Yu, "GPU-based beamformer: fast realization of plane wave compounding and synthetic aperture imaging", *IEEE Transactions on Ultrasonics, Ferroelectrics, and Frequency Control*, vol. 58, pp. 1698–1705, 2011.

[47] B. Peng, Y. Wang, T. J. Hall, and J. Jiang, "A GPU-accelerated 3-D coupled subsample estimation algorithm for volumetric breast strain elastography", *IEEE Transactions on Ultrasonics, Ferroelectrics, and Frequency Control*, vol. 64, pp. 694–705, 2017.

[48] B. Y. S. Yiu and A. C. H. Yu, "GPU-based minimum variance beamformer for synthetic aperture imaging of the eye", *Ultrasound in Medicine and Biology*, vol. 41, pp. 871–883, 2015.

[49] A. J. Y. Chee, B. Y. S. Yiu, and A. C. H. Yu, "A GPU-parallelized eigen-based clutter filtering framework for ultrasound color flow imaging", *IEEE Transactions on Ultrasonics, Ferroelectrics, and Frequency Control*, vol. 64, pp. 150–163, 2017.

[50] M. Cikes, L. Tong, G. R. Sutherland, and J. D'Hooge, "Ultrafast cardiac ultrasound imaging: technical principles, applications, and clinical benefits", *Journal of the American College of Cardiology: Cardiovascular Imaging*, vol. 7, pp. 812–823, 2014.

[51] L. Tong, A. Ramalli, P. Tortoli, *et al.*, "Wide-angle tissue Doppler imaging at high frame rate using multi-line transmit beamforming: an experimental validation in vivo", *IEEE Transactions on Medical Imaging*, vol. 35, pp. 521–528, 2016.

[52] J. Faurie, M. Baudet, K. C. Assi, *et al.*, "Intracardiac vortex dynamics by high-frame-rate Doppler vortography–in vivo comparison with vector flow mapping and 4-D flow MRI", *IEEE Transactions on Ultrasonics, Ferroelectrics, and Frequency Control*, vol. 64, pp. 424–432, 2017.

[53] J. van Cauwenberge, L. Lovstakken, S. Fadnes, *et al.*, "Assessing the performance of ultrafast vector flow imaging in the neonatal heart via multiphysics modeling and in vitro experiments", *IEEE Transactions on Ultrasonics, Ferroelectrics, and Frequency Control*, vol. 64, pp. 1772–1785, 2016.

[54] B. Y. S. Yiu and A. C. H. Yu, "High-frame-rate ultrasound color-encoded speckle imaging of complex flow dynamics", *Ultrasound in Medicine and Biology*, vol. 39, pp. 1015–1025, 2013.

[55] B. Y. S. Yiu, S. S. M. Lai, and A. C. H. Yu, "Vector projectile imaging: time-resolved dynamic visualization of complex flow patterns", *Ultrasound in Medicine and Biology*, vol. 40, pp. 2295–2309, 2014.

[56] J. A. Jensen, S. I. Nikolov, A. C. H. Yu, and D. Garcia, "Ultrasound vector flow imaging. II: parallel systems", *IEEE Transactions on Ultrasonics, Ferroelectrics, and Frequency Control*, vol. 63, pp. 1722–1732, 2016.

[57] A. Goddi, C. Bortolotto, H. Fiorina, *et al.*, "High-frame rate vector flow imaging of the carotid bifurcation", *Insights Imaging*, vol. 8, pp. 319–328, 2017.

[58] M. J. Pihl, M. B. Stuart, B. G. Tomov, M. F. Rasmussen, and J. A. Jensen, "A transverse oscillation approach for estimation of three-dimensional velocity vectors. Part II: Experimental validation", *IEEE Transactions on Ultrasonics, Ferroelectrics, and Frequency Control*, vol. 61, pp. 1608–1618, 2014.

[59] M. Correia, J. Provost, M. Tanter, and M. Pernot, "4D ultrafast ultrasound flow imaging: in vivo quantification of arterial volumetric flow rate in a single heartbeat", *Physics in Medicine and Biology*, vol. 61, pp. L48–L61, 2016.

[60] S. Salles, A. J. Y. Chee, D. Garcia, A. C. H. Yu, D. Vray, and H. Liebgott, "2-D arterial wall motion imaging using ultrafast ultrasound and transverse oscillations", *IEEE Transactions on Ultrasonics, Ferroelectrics, and Frequency Control*, vol. 62, pp. 1047–1058, 2015.

[61] F. Li, Q. He, C. Huang, K. Liu, J. Shao, and J. Luo, "High frame rate and high line density ultrasound imaging for local pulse wave velocity estimation using motion matching: a feasibility study on vessel phantoms", *Ultrasonics*, vol. 67, pp. 41–51, 2016.

Chapter 2
Speckle physics

Jovana Janjic[1] *and Gijs van Soest*[1]

2.1 Introduction

Ultrasonic B-mode imaging is fundamentally gray-scale imaging: it forms an image based only on the amplitude of the detected echo. It processes the available information in the recorded echoes, which arise from scattering of the transmitted wave by acoustic discontinuities or heterogeneities in the imaged object. The translation from object features to image features is subject to the physics of the wave propagation, scattering and detection processes that carry the information from object to the imaging system. The imaging physics introduces familiar imaging concepts like image resolution, related to system bandwidth, imaging contrast and penetration depth, related to the acoustic properties of the medium, object and system parameters like sensitivity and noise. Image interpretation is principally an inversion of these steps: what can we infer about the object from the received echo, combined with some prior knowledge of the imaged object and the imaging system.

Speckle is one of the image features arising in the translation of object structure to an ultrasound image. It manifests itself as "spotty" variations in image intensity, giving rise to a granular appearance instead of homogeneous, flat shades of gray, as is visible in Figure 2.1. As such, speckle can severely compromise interpretation of ultrasound images, particularly in discrimination of small structures. As we will see in this chapter, it is fundamentally impossible to separate the "true" image information from speckle corrupting it. For this reason, the common term "speckle noise" is a misnomer, as there is no way to discriminate the speckle as a "noise" source from the "signal," that we are actually interested in. We will therefore not adopt the notion of "speckle as short-range correlated multiplicative noise" which is frequently applied but does not adequately represent the complex nature of the resulting scattered field, nor does it encapsulate the statistical properties of amplitude and phase of physical speckle. The concept of speckle as noise also forgoes its use in detection of time varying phenomena: blood vessels, for instance, can be identified by their large speckle variance or short speckle decorrelation time. Nevertheless, quoting the optical physicist Joseph Goodman, to

[1]Thorax Center, Erasmus University Medical Center, The Netherlands

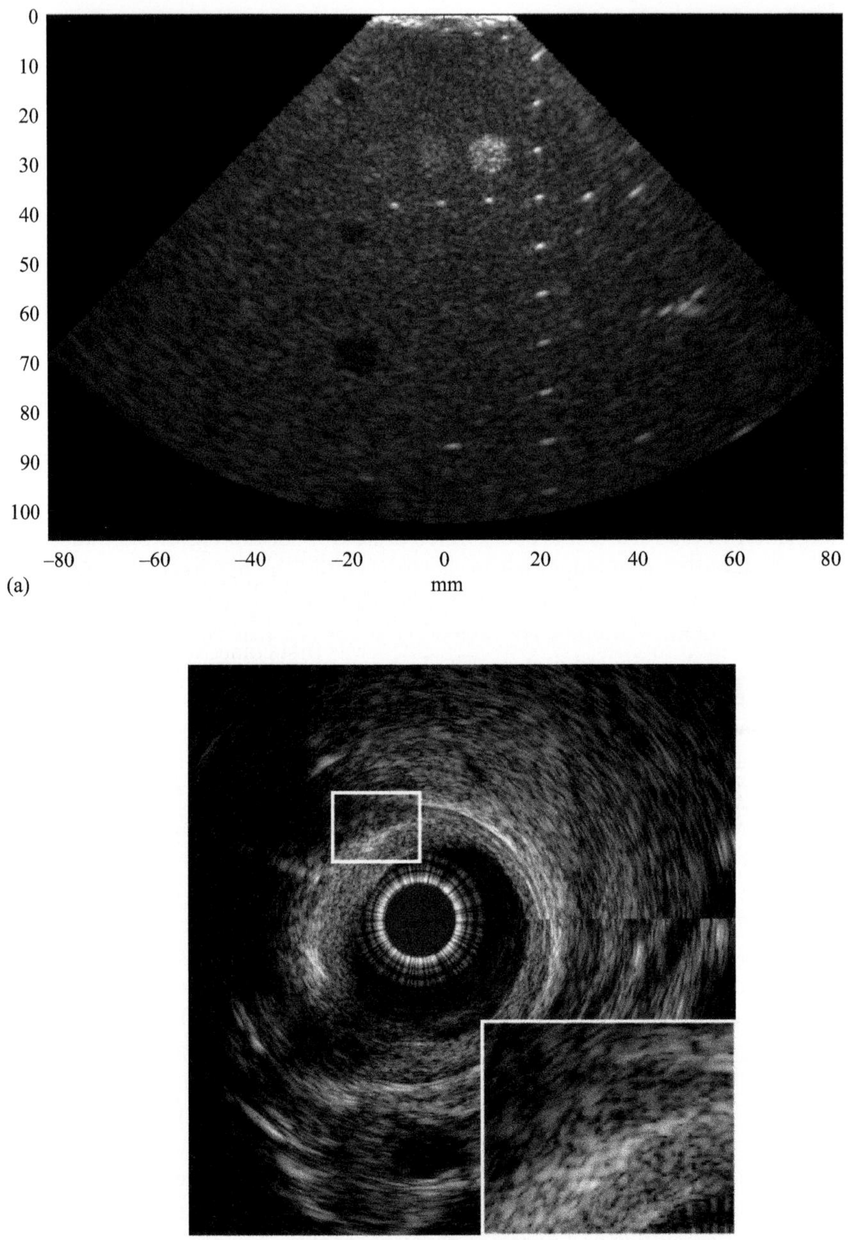

(a)

(b)

Figure 2.1 Ultrasound speckle. (a) Image of a CIRS ultrasound phantom, obtained with a phased array transducer with an element pitch of 295 μm and a frequency bandwidth of 1–4 MHz. It shows speckle instead of homogeneous gray areas. (b) IVUS image of a human coronary artery specimen ex vivo, rotating single element with a bandwidth of 20–38 MHz whom many of the concepts we present in this chapter are due, "Although a number of beneficial uses can be made of speckle, it usually is more of a hindrance than a help" [1].

In this chapter, we will discuss the basic physical origins of speckle and present different, but related, mathematical descriptions of speckle in simple model systems. We will start from a general description of scattered waves as phasors, deriving first-order statistics applicable to both laser speckle and ultrasound speckle. Subsequently, we discuss the correspondences and differences between laser speckle and ultrasound speckle, before presenting higher order statistics and imaging implications in an ultrasound context. We also introduce the impact of the imaging system characteristics on speckle appearance and statistics.

2.2 Speckle observations

2.2.1 Speckle in optics

Speckle arises from interference of many component waves with random phase, summed to a resultant vector with a stochastic distribution of amplitude and phase. This phenomenon was first described in the scintillation of stars in the late nineteenth century [2] caused by atmospheric disturbance of the planar wavefront arriving from point sources. The term "speckle" was first coined after the invention of the laser, where it is readily observable as the grainy appearance of laser light scattered off a rough surface [3], as shown in Figure 2.2.

These observations illustrate that optical speckle arises in two situations: the first is when coherent light illuminates an irregular surface, with a roughness on scale of the optical wavelength; the second situation is when coherent light travels through a medium with variable refractive index [3]. In both cases, the coherence of the illuminating source is a condition for the observation of speckle. A wave's degree of coherence expresses the degree of correlation in amplitude fluctuations

Figure 2.2 Speckle generated by a helium–neon laser transmitted through a diffuser

in space (spatial coherence) or time (temporal coherence) [4]: within the coherence time or coherence length, the phase relations between different points in the wave field are fixed. The coherence of a wave determines the ability to generate interference effects. Partial coherence refers to a situation where the observation time or area is larger than the coherence domain. By sampling multiple coherence windows in space or time, some of the interference is washed out.

When coherent light illuminates a rough surface, the returning optical wave is the result of the interference of coherent wavelets with random phase that are scattered from the microscopic structures of the surface. If the interference is constructive, a bright spot will characterize the image, whereas if the interference is destructive, the spot will appear dark [5]. The combination of constructive and destructive interferences leads to the speckle granularity in the image. Speckle appears from a set of many coherent wavelets with random phase. Random scattering of a coherent wavefront creates this system quite readily, as we will see. Complete randomization by heterogeneity in the propagation medium requires a long interaction length, such as occurs when starlight traverses a turbulent atmosphere. In practice, random scattering of coherent waves explains most observations of speckle in ultrasound, and we will focus our discussion on that situation. It is important to realize that, although the scattering randomizes the phase, this is a deterministic process: as long as the incident wave and the realization of the random scattering structure do not change, the observed speckle remains constant.

2.2.2 Mapping optical speckle concepts to ultrasonic imaging

Optical speckle is usually observed as intensity variations due to far-field interference in a wavefront with random spatial phase disturbances. Ultrasound transducers are sensitive to the amplitude of the incident wave and derive their contrast from temporal variations in the signal. Speckle manifests as amplitude variations due to temporal phase disturbances. These differences have to be accounted for in the application of speckle concepts from optics to ultrasonic imaging. Figure 2.3 illustrates that, both in the laser and in the acoustic case, speckle is caused by the superposition of wavelets having a random phase.

In classical laser speckle imaging, one can think of the wavelets as being positioned on a plane perpendicular to the direction of wave propagation. Invoking Huygens' principle, the resultant field on an observation screen is the sum of the propagated fields originating from wavelets within a coherence area of the incident field. For separations greater than the (transverse) coherence length of the field, the phase relations between the wavelets are not deterministic, and the interference pattern is washed out. In a ranging technique like ultrasonic imaging, the contributing wavelets are positioned at different, random, distance on the axis of propagation. The resultant amplitude now is the superposition of the waves along the time dimension, and interference results from waves separated in time by less than the coherence time of the field. In ultrasound, the coherence time is equal to the pulse duration: if the pulse spatial length is greater than the distance between

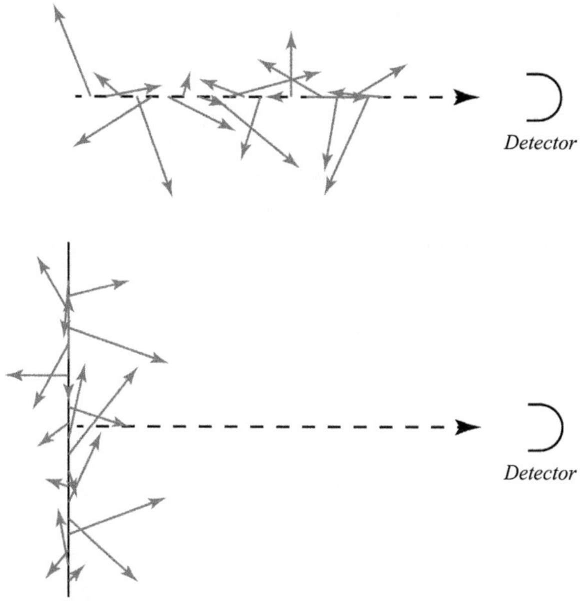

Figure 2.3 The detected field is the result of interference of Huygens wavelets with random amplitude and phase within one resolution. Top: the contributing wavelets are on the line of sight at slightly different delays, as in the case of ultrasound and OCT. Bottom: the contributing wavelets are distributed on a screen perpendicular to the wave propagation direction, as in the case of laser speckle

two scatterers, the phase is correlated and the pulse can be considered as coherent [5]. These two realizations of speckle are mathematically equivalent, and many results obtained in the rich literature on optical speckle can be applied to ultrasound imaging.

Optical detectors are sensitive to the energy of the incident field, which is proportional to the amplitude squared, unlike ultrasound transducers, which record the incident amplitude itself [6]. This means that in optical speckle, the phase is generally not available for analysis. It has to be inferred from auxiliary measurements, which are outside of the scope of this chapter; see [7] for an extensive review. The probability density functions and other statistics for the speckle field are identical for light and sound but need to be converted into intensity statistics to describe measurements of optical speckle.

Optical coherence tomography (OCT) [8] is often introduced as the "optical analog of ultrasonic imaging," and as such deserves special mention. In OCT, a depth-resolved image of scattering tissue is formed by interferometry. A light source with a short coherence time is used to achieve high axial resolution, much like short pulse in ultrasound imaging. Indeed, the speckle that manifests in OCT, shown in Figure 2.4, is very similar to that observed in ultrasound, and we have

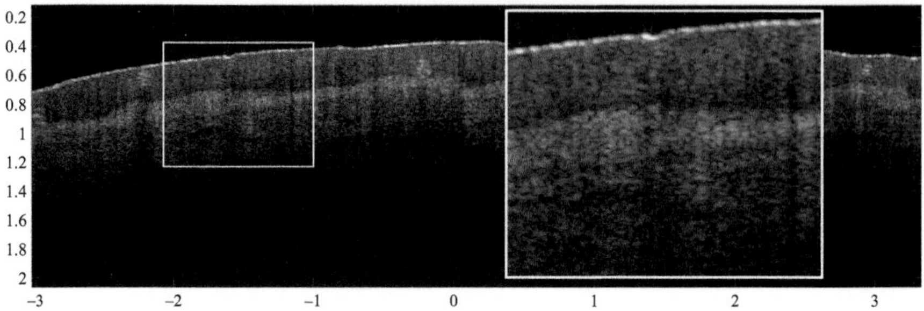

Figure 2.4 OCT image of a fingertip, showing speckle both the darker epidermis and bright dermis layer. Axes in mm

used concepts and results from the OCT literature in this chapter [9–11]. The main difference between OCT and ultrasound speckle is not in the physics, but in the beam "optics" (aperture, lenses) used to transmit and receive the sampling wave.

2.3 Speckle as a 2D random walk

The classical explanation for speckle is to conceive the sum of wavelets with random phase as a two-dimensional random walk [3]. For this discussion, we will adopt the conventional term of "phasor," which is a vector $\alpha_n e^{i(\omega_0 t + \varphi_n)}$ that rotates at an angular frequency ω_0, where $\omega_0 = 2\pi f_0$ and f_0 is the frequency of the incident wave. Its initial phase is φ_n a random variable, and t is the propagation delay from its origin to the detector. The amplitude φ_n is a positive random variable that reflects the scattering strength. In the simplest case, we assume that φ_n is uniformly distributed on $[-\pi, \pi\rangle$ and that there are sufficient contributing phasors to adequately sample the phase distribution [6]. The variation in t is only due to nonrandom, slowly varying geometric factors (we are not considering phase randomness due to variations in the medium, which affect t). Both α_n and φ_n are uncorrelated.

If there are N scatterers within a coherence volume of the incident wave, each projecting a wavelet, the resulting complex field S at the detector can be written as the sum of N phasors:

$$S = Ae^{i\Phi} = \frac{1}{\sqrt{N}} \sum_{n=1}^{N} a_n e^{i\varphi_n} \tag{2.1}$$

The random amplitudes $\alpha_n = a_n/\sqrt{N}$ have been normalized for energy conservation, and the propagation delay $e^{i\omega_0 t}$ has been suppressed. Figure 2.5 illustrates analogy between the vector sum of a few phasors and a 2D random walk in the complex plane. This representation of the field, combined with the simple assumptions on φ_n and α_n, allows us to derive some of its statistical properties. Note that in the following derivation, we do not need any information on the distribution of a_n, which makes the resulting speckle statistics robust in homogeneous random media and independent of the details of the scattering structure.

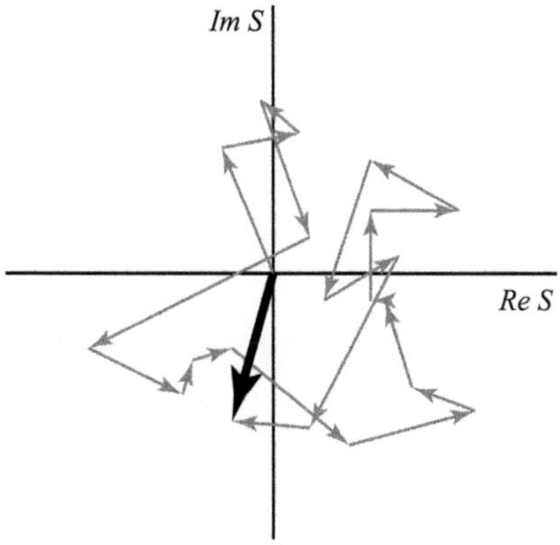

*Figure 2.5 Phasor sum as a random walk. The resultant field **S** (black arrow) is the sum of many phasors (smaller gray arrows), each with random amplitude α_n and uniformly distributed random phase φ_n*

2.3.1 First-order statistics

In order to compute statistics for amplitude and phase of the resultant vector, it is convenient to first decompose it into real and imaginary parts. These are given by

$$S_r = Re(S) = \frac{1}{\sqrt{N}} \sum_{n=1}^{N} a_n \cos\varphi_n \tag{2.2}$$

$$S_i = Im(S) = \frac{1}{\sqrt{N}} \sum_{n=1}^{N} a_n \sin\varphi_n \tag{2.3}$$

Since both the real and imaginary parts are the sum of independent random components, the central limit theorem enables us to conclude that they are, for large N, Gaussian random variables. The mean $\bar{S_r}$ and $\bar{S_i}$ are

$$\bar{S_r} = \frac{1}{\sqrt{N}} \sum_{n=1}^{N} \overline{a_n \cos\varphi_n} \tag{2.4}$$

$$\bar{S_i} = \frac{1}{N} \sum_{n=1}^{N} \overline{a_n \sin\varphi_n} \tag{2.5}$$

and, since the phases are uniformly distributed over $[-\pi, \pi\rangle$, $\bar{S_r} = \bar{S_i} = 0$. The variances σ_R^2 and σ_I^2 can be then calculated as the second moments $\bar{S_r^2}$ and $\bar{S_i^2}$, which are given by

$$\bar{S_r^2} = \frac{1}{N} \sum_{n=1}^{N} \sum_{k=1}^{N} \overline{a_n a_k \cos\varphi_n \cos\varphi_k} \tag{2.6}$$

$$\bar{S_i^2} = \frac{1}{N} \sum_{n=1}^{N} \sum_{k=1}^{N} \overline{a_n a_k \sin\varphi_n \sin\varphi_k} \tag{2.7}$$

and again due to the uniform distribution of the phases over $[-\pi, \pi\rangle$ we have

$$\overline{\cos\varphi_n \cos\varphi_k} = \overline{\sin\varphi_n \sin\varphi_k} = \begin{cases} 0 & k \neq n \\ \dfrac{1}{2} & k = n \end{cases} \tag{2.8}$$

Therefore,

$$\sigma_R^2 = \sigma_I^2 = \bar{S_r^2} = \bar{S_i^2} = \frac{1}{2N}\sum\nolimits_{n=1}^{N} a_n^2 = \frac{\bar{A}^2}{2} \tag{2.9}$$

The correlation between S_r and S_i is defined as

$$R_{S_rS_i} = \overline{S_rS_i} = \frac{1}{N}\sum_{k=1}^{N}\sum_{n=1}^{N}\overline{a_k a_n \cos\varphi_k \sin\varphi_n} \tag{2.10}$$

Terms with $k \neq n$ vanish because of the uncorrelated amplitudes and phases in the sum, while, since $\sin 2\varphi = 2\sin\varphi\cos\varphi$, we get

$$\overline{\cos\varphi_n \sin\varphi_n} = 0 \tag{2.11}$$

Therefore, S_r and S_i are uncorrelated.

To summarize, the real and imaginary parts of the resultant vector sum S are uncorrelated Gaussian random variables. They have identical variance and zero mean, as expected from the circular geometry of the problem.

To find the probability density function of the magnitude $A = |S| = \sqrt{S_r^2 + S_i^2}$ and phase Φ of the sum of the phasors, we need to define the joint probability density function of the real and imaginary parts $p_{S_rS_i}$. Again using the central limit theorem, and applying the first and second moments of S_r and S_i computed above, we can write for the joint probability density function

$$p_{S_rS_i}(S_r, S_i) = \frac{1}{2\pi\sigma^2}\exp\left(-\frac{S_r^2 + S_i^2}{2\sigma^2}\right) \tag{2.12}$$

with $\sigma^2 = \sigma_r^2 = \sigma_i^2$. The circular symmetry in $p_{S_rS_i}$, following from the uniform phase distribution, leads to the term "circular complex Gaussian" variate for the phasor sum S. From $p_{S_rS_i}$, we can indeed compute the joint probability function of the magnitude A and phase Φ by making the appropriate variable transformations [3]. We then derive the marginal distributions of A and Φ. First we define A and Φ as follows:

$$A = \sqrt{S_r^2 + S_i^2} \tag{2.13}$$

$$\Phi = \tan^{-1}\left(\frac{S_i}{S_r}\right) \tag{2.14}$$

S_r and S_i follow accordingly:

$$S_r = A\cos\Phi \tag{2.15}$$

$$S_i = A\sin\Phi \tag{2.16}$$

then we calculate the Jacobian of the transformation

$$\|J\| = \left\| \begin{matrix} \dfrac{\delta S_r}{\delta A} & \dfrac{\delta S_r}{\delta \Phi} \\ \dfrac{\delta S_i}{\delta A} & \dfrac{\delta S_i}{\delta \Phi} \end{matrix} \right\| = \left\| \begin{matrix} \cos\Phi & -A\sin\Phi \\ \sin\Phi & A\cos\Phi \end{matrix} \right\| = A \tag{2.17}$$

where $\|\ldots\|$ denotes the modulus of the determinant.

The joint density function for A and Φ is

$$p_{A,\Phi} = p_{S_r,S_i}(S_r = A\cos\Phi, S_i = A\sin\Phi)\cdot A \tag{2.18}$$

and if we use (2.12), we obtain

$$p_{A,\Phi} = \begin{cases} \dfrac{A}{2\pi\sigma^2}\exp\left(-\dfrac{A^2}{2\sigma^2}\right) & A \geq 0, -\pi \leq \Phi < \pi \\ 0 & \text{otherwise} \end{cases} \tag{2.19}$$

We compute the marginal density for the magnitude A by integration over Φ to get

$$p_A = \begin{cases} \dfrac{A}{\sigma^2}\exp\left(-\dfrac{A^2}{2\sigma^2}\right) & A \geq 0 \\ 0 & \text{otherwise} \end{cases} \tag{2.20}$$

This function is known as the Rayleigh density function, displayed in Figure 2.6. Note that the probability of $A = 0$ vanishes. Similarly, we can compute the marginal density for the phase Φ as follows:

$$p_\Phi = \begin{cases} \dfrac{1}{2\pi}\displaystyle\int_0^\infty \dfrac{A}{\sigma^2}\exp\left(-\dfrac{A^2}{2\sigma^2}\right)dA & -\pi \leq \Phi < \pi \\ 0 & \text{otherwise} \end{cases} \tag{2.21}$$

We can see that the integral argument is the Rayleigh probability density function. Therefore, the integral must be equal to 1. Thus, we obtain

$$p_\Phi = \begin{cases} \dfrac{1}{2\pi} & -\pi \leq \Phi < \pi \\ 0 & \text{otherwise} \end{cases} \tag{2.22}$$

Clearly, $p_{A,\Phi} = p_A p_\Phi$, as it should be for independent variables.

With these distributions at our disposal, we can compute the mean and variance of the scattered amplitude:

$$\bar{A} = \sqrt{\frac{\pi}{2}}\sigma \tag{2.23}$$

$$\sigma_A^2 = \left[2 - \frac{\pi}{2}\right]\sigma^2 \tag{2.24}$$

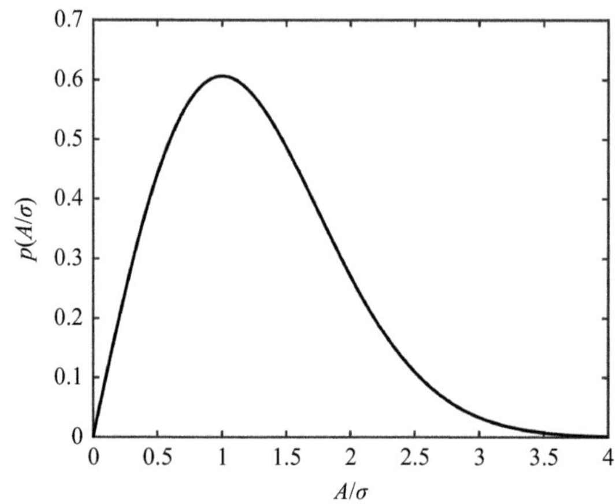

Figure 2.6 The Rayleigh distribution, describing the amplitude statistics of fully developed speckle

If we divide the standard deviation by the mean, we obtain the speckle contrast κ, the inverse of which is often loosely referred to as signal-to-noise ratio (SNR) [5,12]

$$\kappa = \frac{\sigma_A}{\bar{A}} = \sqrt{\frac{4-\pi}{\pi}} \approx 0.52; \mathrm{SNR} = \frac{1}{\kappa} \approx 1.91 \tag{2.25}$$

Figure 2.7 displays the result of an imaging experiment on a tissue-mimicking phantom, scanning a single element transducer along the phantom. The experiment was repeated 15 times, each at a slightly different location, to sample a different realization of the randomness that generates the speckle pattern. Each image has an SNR close to the theoretical value of 1.91. For ultrasound speckle, the statistics of the amplitude is the most relevant quantity.

For completeness, allowing the same approach used for the amplitude, we also compute the probability density function of the intensity $I = A^2$. First we relate the intensity and phase to the real and imaginary part by

$$S_r = \sqrt{I}\cos\Phi \tag{2.26}$$

$$S_i = \sqrt{I}\sin\Phi \tag{2.27}$$

The Jacobian of the transformation is

$$\|J\| = \left\| \begin{matrix} \dfrac{\delta S_r}{\delta I} & \dfrac{\delta S_r}{\delta \Phi} \\ \dfrac{\delta S_i}{\delta I} & \dfrac{\delta S_i}{\delta \Phi} \end{matrix} \right\| = \frac{1}{2} \tag{2.28}$$

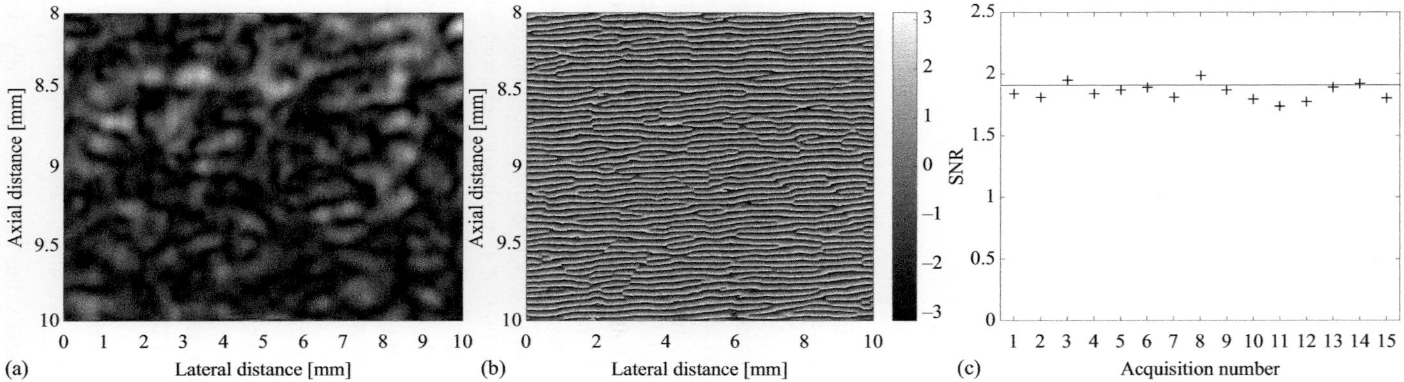

Figure 2.7 Scanning probe measurement: amplitude signal of one acquisition (a), corresponding phase (b) and SNR for all 15 acquisitions (c)

and the joint probability density function can be expressed as

$$p_{I,\Phi} = p_{S_r,S_i}\left(S_r = \sqrt{I}\cos\Phi, S_i = \sqrt{I}\sin\Phi\right)\cdot\frac{1}{2} \tag{2.29}$$

By substituting (2.19) in (2.29) we get

$$p_{I,\Phi} = \begin{cases} \frac{1}{4\pi\sigma^2}\exp\left(-\frac{I}{2\sigma^2}\right) & I \geq 0, -\pi \leq \Phi < \pi \\ 0 & \text{otherwise} \end{cases} \tag{2.30}$$

We can then integrate over the phase, obtaining

$$pI = \begin{cases} \frac{1}{2\sigma^2}\exp\left(-\frac{I}{2\sigma^2}\right) & I \geq 0, \\ 0 & \text{otherwise} \end{cases} \tag{2.31}$$

which is defined as the exponential probability density function, which has its maximum value at $I = 0$. The phase is obviously unaffected by the transformation and is still uniformly distributed on $[-\pi, \pi\rangle$. Note that for the intensity, $\bar{I} = \sigma^2 = 2\sigma^2$ and $\kappa = 1$, a result that seriously complicates imaging with coherent light! The physical interpretation of these results can be summarized as follows: if we have a medium that randomizes the phase of an incident wave to such a degree that the received signal can be represented as the sum of a large number of phasors, the amplitude of the complex scattered field follows a Rayleigh distribution, while the phase is uniformly distributed. The only assumptions we made are uncorrelated phasor amplitudes and phases, uniformly distributed phases; and large N, which allowed us to apply the central limit theorem that straightforwardly produces the Gaussian circular statistics for the field. Speckle fulfilling these criteria is called "fully-developed" and allows us to describe the underlying physics in a concise manner. A scattered field consisting of few phasors, phasors with nonuniformly distributed phases or correlated amplitudes, does not obey these simple statistics, as we will show later on in this chapter. Partially developed speckle is commonly encountered in ultrasound imaging. Its analysis is more complex and requires more knowledge about the scattering structure.

2.3.2 Sums of speckle patterns

We mentioned in Section 2.2.1 that speckle is a deterministic random process: the signal scattered by a random structure, probed by a wave of the same frequency content and directionality, will always yield the same speckle pattern. As will become clear in the remainder of this book, many strategies to mitigate the effects of speckle rely on some form of averaging, where one control variable is changed to produce different speckle patterns that can then be summed or compounded.

Consider two random phasor sums, $S_1 = \frac{1}{\sqrt{N}}\sum_{n=1}^{N} a_n e^{i\varphi_n}$ and $S_2 = \frac{1}{\sqrt{M}}\sum_{n=1}^{M} b_n e^{i\vartheta_n}$. If both satisfy the conditions for fully developed speckle,

a_n and b_n are uncorrelated random variables, as are the phases φ_n and ϑ_n. The sum of these two fields $S = S_1 + S_2 = \frac{1}{\sqrt{N}}\sum_{n=1}^{M} a_n e^{i\varphi n} + \frac{1}{\sqrt{M}}\sum_{n=1}^{M} b_n e^{i\vartheta_n}$ can be written as $S = \frac{1}{\sqrt{N+M}}\sum_{n=1}^{N+M} c_n e^{i\gamma_n}$, where $c = a \cup b$ and $\gamma = \varphi \cup \vartheta$. This again has the form of a random phasor sum: it represents a longer random walk. Addition of speckle patterns on a complex amplitude basis does *not* alter the statistics.

If we compute, on the other hand, the incoherent sum of the resultant field, based on the signal envelopes, $A_n = |S_n|$, the distribution does change. The sum of N speckle fields is

$$A_S = \sum_{n=1}^{N} A_n \tag{2.32}$$

Before going into mathematical detail, the net gain in SNR can be estimated from general results in probability theory. A sum A_S of N real-valued, identically distributed, uncorrelated random variates, each with a mean $\bar{A}$ and standard deviation σ_A, has an expected value $\bar{A_S} = N\bar{A}$ and standard deviation $\sigma_{A_S} = \sqrt{N}\sigma_A$. The SNR of the summed fields thus scales as $1/\sqrt{N}$, a well-known and commonly applied result.

If α and β are two random variables with probability density functions $p_\alpha(\alpha)$ and $p_\beta(\beta)$, the probability distribution of the sum $\alpha+\beta$ is given by the convolution of their individual distributions $p_{\alpha+\beta}(\alpha+\beta) = p_\alpha(\alpha) \otimes p_\beta(\beta)$. Hence, for a sum of $N = 2$ fully-developed speckles with identical magnitude (same σ), an exact result for the probability distribution of the resulting magnitude can be found from the convolution of a Rayleigh distribution with itself:

$$p_{S,N=2}(A_S) = \frac{A_S}{2\sigma^2}^{-\frac{A_S^2}{2\sigma^2}} + \frac{\sqrt{\pi}}{4\sigma} e^{-\frac{A_S^2}{4\sigma^2}} \left(\frac{A_S^2}{\sigma^2} - 2\right) \text{erf}\left(\frac{A_s}{2\sigma}\right) \tag{2.33}$$

where $\text{erf}(x) = \frac{2}{\sqrt{\pi}}\int_0^x e^{-t^2} dt$ is the error function, and the integration over the phase has been implicitly performed.

The distribution of the sum A_S can be computed for general N, in principle, using the characteristic function. The characteristic function $M_x(\omega)$ of a random variable x is the expectation value of $e^{i\omega x}$, or equivalently, the inverse Fourier transform of its probability density function. It can be found using symbolic manipulation software:

$$\begin{aligned} M_A(\omega) &= \int_0^\infty e^{i\omega A} p_A(A) dA = \frac{1}{2\pi}\int_0^\infty e^{i\omega A} \frac{A}{\sigma^2} e^{-\frac{A^2}{2\sigma^2}} dA \\ &= 1 - \sqrt{2}\sigma\omega D_+\left(\frac{\sigma\omega}{\sqrt{2}}\right) + i\sigma\omega\sqrt{\frac{\pi}{2}} e^{-\frac{\sigma^2\omega^2}{2}}. \end{aligned} \tag{2.34}$$

Here D_+ is the function known as Dawson's integral, defined as $D_+(x) = e^{-x^2} \int_0^x e^{t^2} dt$. The characteristic function of A_s then is

$$M_{A,S} = \prod_{n=1}^{N} M_{A,n} = [M_A(\omega)]^N. \tag{2.35}$$

The last equality holds if we assume that all contributing fields have the same mean amplitude (and thus, the same σ_n). We can write the probability distribution of A_S as the Fourier transform of M_S. It turns out, however, that for $N > 2$, the analytic form of $p_{S,N}$ cannot be straightforwardly computed, nor is it known in literature. The moments of the distribution can be found by serial differentiation of M_S (from which the probability distribution function itself can be approximated in principle by construction of a moments series). Again, by the central limit theorem, the distribution of magnitudes approaches a Gaussian for $N \to \infty$.

For some applications [13], the statistics of the signal power in a sum of speckles is of interest. The probability distribution function of a sum of intensities

$$I_S = \sum_{n=1}^{N} I_n = \sum_{n=1}^{N} |A_n|^2 \tag{2.36}$$

can be computed using the characteristic function of the exponentially distributed intensity [7]

$$M_I(\omega) = \frac{1}{1 - i\omega\bar{I}} \tag{2.37}$$

where $\bar{I} = 2\sigma^2$ is the average intensity as is defined in Section 2.3.1. As above, $M_{I,S} = \prod_{n=1}^{N} M_{I,n} = [M_I(\omega)]^N$, for an ensemble of N speckles with equal mean intensity, which can be Fourier transformed to yield

$$p_S(I_S) = \frac{I_S^{N-1}}{\Gamma(N)\bar{I}^N} e^{-I_S/\bar{I}} \tag{2.38}$$

where $\Gamma(N)$ is the gamma function and $\bar{I}$ is the mean intensity of each contributing field. For large N, the distribution again tends toward a Gaussian.

2.3.3 *Speckle pattern plus a nonrandom phasor*

The preceding sections discussed the case of fully developed speckle, arising when many wavelets with random phase interfere. In practical imaging situations, scattering media are often heterogeneous, containing strongly reflecting boundaries that can be resolved amidst a speckle generate by unresolved, microscopic scattering. The reflections generate a constant background field. The scattered field can now be described as the sum of a random walk and the constant, known phasor. The approach here follows [7]. Aligning the constant phasor A_0 with the real axis, we can add it to the real component of the field in (2.12) to yield

$$p_{S_r S_i}(S_r, S_i) = \frac{1}{2\pi\sigma^2} \exp\left(-\frac{(S_r + A_0)^2 + S_i^2}{2\sigma^2} \right) \tag{2.39}$$

We again perform the transformation of variables (2.15)–(2.17) and find

$$p_{A,\Phi}(A,\Phi) = \begin{cases} \dfrac{A}{2\pi\sigma^2}\exp\left(-\dfrac{A^2 + A_0^2 - 2AA_0\cos\Phi}{2\sigma^2}\right) & A > 0, -\pi < \Phi \leq \pi \\ 0 & \text{otherwise} \end{cases} \tag{2.40}$$

The probability distribution of the magnitude of the resultant phasor can be obtained by integration of above equation with respect to the phase Φ. Therefore,

$$p_A(A)=\begin{cases} \dfrac{A}{2\pi\sigma^2}e^{-\frac{A_0^2+A^2}{2\sigma^2}}\displaystyle\int_{-\pi}^{\pi} e^{-\frac{AA_0\cos\Phi}{\sigma^2}}d\Phi=\dfrac{A}{\sigma^2}e^{-\frac{A_0^2+A^2}{2\sigma^2}}I_0\left(\dfrac{A_0A}{\sigma^2}\right) & A>0 \\ 0 & \text{otherwise} \end{cases} \tag{2.41}$$

where I_0 is the modified Bessel function of the first kind and order zero. The above expression is known as the Rician density function; Figure 2.8 shows the distribution for a number of different background amplitudes $k = A_0/\sigma$. It reduces to the Rayleigh distribution for $A_0 = 0$, as expected. The mean and the variance can be calculated from the first two moments of the density function. Thus,

$$\bar{A} = \int_0^{\infty} \frac{A}{\sigma^2} e^{-\frac{A_0^2+A^2}{2\sigma^2}} I_0\left(\frac{A_0A}{\sigma^2}\right) dA = \sqrt{\frac{\pi}{2}}\sigma e^{-\frac{K^2}{4}}\left[\left(1+\frac{k^2}{2}\right)I_0\left(\frac{k^2}{4}\right)+\frac{k^2}{2}I_1\left(\frac{k^2}{4}\right)\right] \tag{2.42}$$

$$\bar{A^2} = \sigma^2\left[2 + k^2\right] \tag{2.43}$$

where I_1 is the modified Bessel function of the first kind and order one.

If k is large, then the density function of the magnitude approximates the Gaussian density function

$$p_A(A) \cong \frac{1}{\sqrt{2\pi}\sigma} e^{-\frac{(A-A_0)^2}{2\sigma^2}} \tag{2.44}$$

with $\bar{A} \cong A_0$ and $\bar{A}^2 \cong \sigma^2$.

To find the density function of the phase, we integrate with respect to the magnitude and we obtain

$$p_\Phi(\Phi) = \frac{e^{-\frac{k^2}{2}}}{2\pi} + \frac{k\cos\Phi}{\sqrt{2\pi}} e^{-\frac{k^2\sin^2\Phi}{2}} \left(\frac{1 + \operatorname{erf}\left(\frac{k\cos\Phi}{\sqrt{2}}\right)}{2}\right) \tag{2.45}$$

for $-\pi < \Phi \leq \pi$.

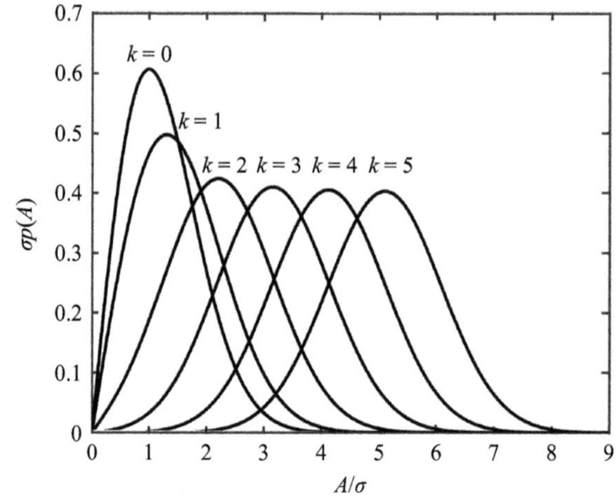

Figure 2.8 The Rician distribution, resulting from a random phasor sum and a constant background. The function is plotted for a number of different ratios $k = A_0/\sigma$ between background phasor amplitude and the standard deviation of the random scattered field. For $k = 0$, the Rayleigh distribution appears, while for $k \gg 1$, the curve tends toward a normal distribution

Note that for the $k = 0$ distribution is uniform, while for $k \to \infty$, the function converges to the delta function at $\Phi = 0$. If k is large, the density function of the phase approximates a Gaussian function [7]

$$p_\Phi(\Phi) \cong \frac{k}{\sqrt{2\pi}} e^{-\frac{k^2\Phi^2}{2}} \tag{2.46}$$

with $\bar{\Phi} \cong 0$ and $\bar{\Phi}^2 \cong \frac{1}{k^2}$ the first and second moment, respectively. The variance equals the second moment because $\bar{\Phi} \cong 0$.

2.3.4 Nonuniform phase distribution

Like the constant background phasor presented in the previous sections, deviations from uniform, uncorrelated, isotropic randomness in the scattering structure can give rise to nonuniformly distributed phases of the component phasors; one example in ultrasonic imaging is long-range correlation of scatterer position. If we relax the assumption of uniform phase distribution, there is no general closed form for the amplitude distribution, but maintaining the statistical independence of amplitudes and phases, we can still compute some properties of the scattered field (see [14]; Section 2.9 and Appendix B). We start from (2.4) and (2.5):

$$\bar{S}_r = \frac{1}{\sqrt{N}} \sum_{n=1}^{N} \overline{a_n} \, \overline{\cos\varphi_n} \tag{2.47}$$

$$\bar{S}_l = \frac{1}{\sqrt{N}} \sum_{n=1}^{N} \overline{a_n} \, \overline{\sin\varphi_n} \tag{2.48}$$

and recognize that the mean trigonometric functions can be expressed in terms of the characteristic function of the phase:

$$\overline{\cos\varphi_n} = \frac{1}{2}\left(\overline{e^{\iota\varphi}} + \overline{e^{-\iota\varphi}}\right) = \frac{1}{2}\left[M_\varphi(1) + M_\varphi(-1)\right] \tag{2.49}$$

$$\overline{\sin\varphi_n} = \frac{1}{2i}\left(\overline{e^{\iota\varphi}} - \overline{e^{-\iota\varphi}}\right) = \frac{1}{2i}\left[M_\varphi(1) - M_\varphi(-1)\right] \tag{2.50}$$

With this result, we can express the mean real and imaginary components of the resultant field as

$$\bar{S}_r = \frac{\sqrt{N}\bar{a}}{2}\left[M_\varphi(1) + M_\varphi(-1)\right] \tag{2.51}$$

$$\bar{S}_\iota = \frac{\sqrt{N}\bar{a}}{2i}\left[M_\varphi(1) - M_\varphi(-1)\right] \tag{2.52}$$

Again using Euler's formulas, the variances and covariance can be written in similar terms:

$$\begin{aligned}\sigma_r^2 = \bar{S_r^2} - \bar{S}_r^2 &= \frac{\bar{a^2}}{4}\left[2 + M_\varphi(2) + M_\varphi(-2)\right]\\ &- \frac{\bar{a}^2}{4}\left[2M_\varphi(1)M_\varphi(-1) + M_\varphi^2(1) + M_\varphi^2(-1)\right]\end{aligned} \tag{2.53}$$

$$\begin{aligned}\sigma_i^2 = \bar{S_\iota^2} - \bar{S}_\iota^2 &= \frac{\bar{a^2}}{4}\left[2 - M_\varphi(2) - M_\varphi(-2)\right]\\ &- \frac{\bar{a}^2}{4}\left[2M_\varphi(1)M_\varphi(-1) - M_\varphi^2(1) - M_\varphi^2(-1)\right]\end{aligned} \tag{2.54}$$

$$C_{ri} = \overline{S_r S_\iota} - \overline{S_r}\,\overline{S_\iota} = \frac{\bar{a^2}}{4i}\left[M_\varphi(2) - M_\varphi(-2)\right] - \frac{\bar{a}^2}{4i}\left[M_\varphi^2(1) - M_\varphi^2(-1)\right] \tag{2.55}$$

With a few extra assumptions, simpler expressions can be computed. First, in the important special case that $p_\varphi(\varphi)$ is symmetric around $\varphi = 0$ (and any probability distribution that is symmetric around a central value can be shifted to the origin by a rotation of the coordinate system), the characteristic function is even and real. As a result,

$$\begin{aligned}\bar{S}_r &= \sqrt{N}\bar{a}M_\varphi(1)\\ \bar{S}_\iota &= 0\\ \sigma_r^2 &= \frac{1}{2}\bar{a^2}\left[1 + M_\varphi(2)\right] - \bar{a}^2 M_\varphi^2(1)\\ \sigma_i^2 &= \frac{1}{2}\bar{a^2}\left[1 - M_\varphi(2)\right]\\ C_{ri} &= 0\end{aligned} \tag{2.56}$$

Inspection of these equations shows that the mean of the real part of the resultant field is now nonzero, and the variances of real and imaginary parts differ. Hence, the scattered field is no longer a circular complex random variable.

More specifically, if the phase is a zero-mean Gaussian variable with a probability density function $p_\varphi(\varphi) = \frac{1}{\sqrt{2\pi}\sigma_\varphi} \exp\left(-\frac{\varphi^2}{2\sigma_\varphi^2}\right)$, the characteristic function is

$$M_\varphi(\omega) = \exp\left(-\frac{\sigma_\varphi^2 \omega^2}{2}\right) \tag{2.57}$$

Substitution in the relations above yields

$$\begin{aligned} \bar{S}_r &= \sqrt{N}\bar{a}e^{-\frac{\sigma_\varphi^2}{2}} \\ \bar{S}_\iota &= 0 \\ \sigma_r^2 &= \frac{1}{2}\bar{a^2}\left[1 + e^{-2\sigma_\varphi^2}\right] - \bar{a}^2 e^{-\sigma_\varphi^2} \\ \sigma_i^2 &= \frac{1}{2}\bar{a^2}\left[1 - e^{-2\sigma_\varphi^2}\right] \\ C_{ri} &= 0 \end{aligned} \tag{2.58}$$

For $\sigma_\varphi^2 \to \infty$, the probability density function of the phase approaches a uniform distribution, and we retrieve the familiar means and variances of Section 2.3.1.

2.4 Speckle in ultrasonic imaging

In ultrasound imaging, the signal arises from backscattered waves inside the imaged object. Acoustic heterogeneity gives rise to scattering structures, which in biological tissue span a large range of characteristic length scales; micrometers at the subcellular level to centimeters or decimeters at the organ level. At length scales smaller than the acoustic wavelength, biological tissue can, to a degree, be modeled as a random acoustic medium with a spectrum of correlation lengths, and scattering coefficients that depend on tissue type. Larger structures reflect ultrasound, rather than scattering it, and present as readily recognizable structures (see, for instance, the wire reflections in Figure 2.1(a)). As these large structures do not exhibit randomness on the scale of a wavelength, they do not generate speckle.

In the treatment of speckle as an ultrasound scattering phenomenon, we will implicitly depend on the Born approximation, which states that the scattered field is small in comparison to the incident beam. This allows us to neglect multiple scattering and attenuation due to scattering, both reasonably accurate assumptions in most ultrasound imaging applications. Acoustic absorption of course exponentially attenuates the field amplitude but is not essential for understanding ultrasound speckle, since path length differences contributing to the random interference are small in the single scatter approximation.

2.4.1 Random ultrasound scattering in 1D

The phase randomness that is evident in the Rayleigh-distributed signal distribution arises because of the presence of many scatterers within a resolution cell, the scattered fields of which are added coherently to result in a random local phase. The random phasor sum (1) appears straightforwardly if we simplify the ultrasound scattering treatment to a one-dimensional linear systems description. In this framework, the field S emitted by a scattering potential Ψ that is insonified with a finite-length pulse can be written as the convolution

$$S = \Psi \otimes h \tag{2.59}$$

here h is the axial point spread function as determined by the temporal impulse response of the band-limited system, which we write as $h(t) = H(t)e^{i2\pi f_0 t}$, the product of a carrier wave of frequency f_0 and the envelope $H(t)$ that is the Fourier transform of the power spectral density of the pulse. For a single point-like scatterer located at position z_1, $\Psi = \Psi_1 \delta(z - z_1)$ and so

$$S_1(t) = \Psi_1 h(t - z_1/c) = \Psi_1 H(t - z_1/c)e^{i2\pi f_0 t}e^{-i2\pi f_0 z_1/c} \tag{2.60}$$

This expression shows that the amplitude response is limited in time by the extent of H, and that it incurs a phase $2\pi f_0 z_1/c$. Figure 2.9(a) shows a graph of the scattered field in response to a two-cycle Gaussian envelope excitation. If we now complicate the scattering structure by adding a few more point-like potentials at random positions, $\Psi = \frac{1}{\sqrt{N}}\sum_{n=1}^{N} \Psi_n \delta(z - z_n)$, then

$$S_N(t) = \frac{1}{\sqrt{N}}\sum_{n=1}^{N} \Psi_n H(t - z_n/c)e^{i2\pi f_0 t}e^{-i2\pi f_0 z_n/c} = \frac{1}{\sqrt{N}}\sum_{n=1}^{N} a_n e^{i\varphi_n} \tag{2.61}$$

The $a_n = \Psi_n H(t - z_n/c)$ form a set of random amplitudes at any given time t, and the phase $\varphi_n = 2\pi f_0\, z_n/c$. This expression has the exact form of (2.1) if the positions z_n are random. It follows that the scattered field from a random scattering potential is a speckle: it is a random zero-mean circular Gaussian variable. Its amplitude is a random variable that follows a Rayleigh distribution, and the phase is uniformly distributed on $|-\pi, \pi\rangle$, the random phase being a consequence of the random scatterer position. The one caveat is that the density of scatterers *per resolution cell* N needs to be large enough for the Rayleigh distribution to emerge, as illustrated by Figure 2.9(c) and (d). Sections of S that are separated in time by more than the width of $H(t)$ are uncoupled and have independent statistics. This argument can be expanded to two and three dimensions, as we will do to compute speckle spot size.

Returning to the linear systems formulation of scattering and Fourier transforming it (indicated by hats; $\mathscr{F}(\cdot) = \hat{\cdot}$) yields a product in spatial frequency space

$$\hat{S}(k) = \hat{\Psi}(k) \cdot \hat{h}(k) \tag{2.62}$$

The axial width of the point spread function is a consequence of the band limitation of the ultrasound imaging system, which appears here directly as $k_z = \frac{f}{c}$. For

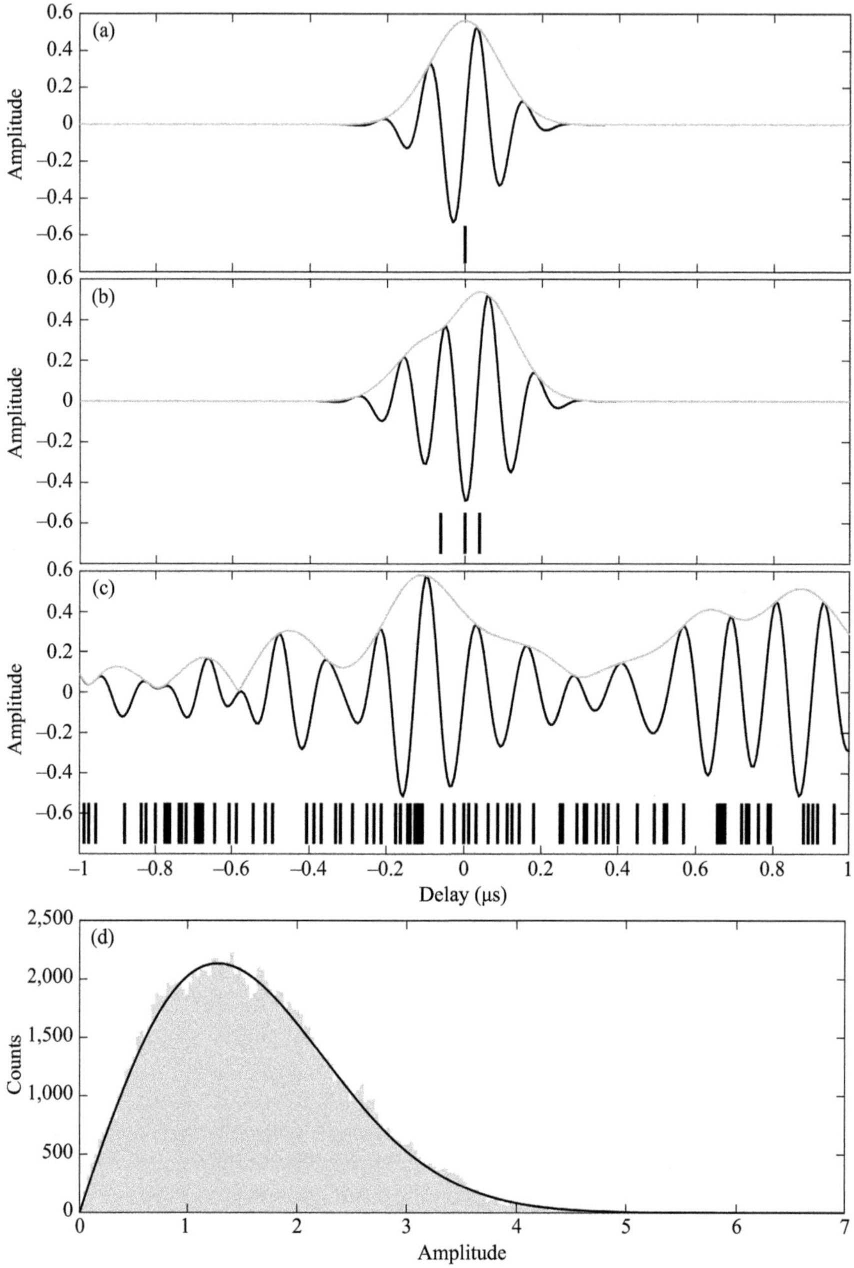

Figure 2.9 Response to a 2-cycle sine wave with a Gaussian envelope, simulated in a linear system as in (2.60). (a) Single scatterer (indicated by the vertical line). (b) Three randomly positioned scatterers within one resolution cell affect the amplitude and phase; note the shift of the trough over the center scatterer. (c) Many scatterers (N = 12 per resolution cell) exhibit speckle. (d) Increasing the number of scatterers and the length of the simulated trace yields a Rayleigh distribution of the envelope (simulation parameters are arbitrary)

frequencies outside the system bandwidth $f_0 \pm \Delta f/2$, the response of the system vanishes. This relation shows that the recorded scattered field only contains spatial frequencies within the band of $\hat{h}$. By the Wiener–Khinchine theorem, the frequency spectrum of S is the Fourier transform of the autocorrelation function $R_S = \langle S(z_1)S(z_2)\rangle = R_S(\Delta z)$. The scattered field only samples spatial frequencies of the scattering structure in a passband centered on $2/\lambda$, with a bandwidth of the order of $2\Delta f/c$, depending on the shape of the envelope of [15,16].

Tissues contain a range of randomly arranged scattering structures, ranging in size from vesicles and cells (large spatial frequency) to blood vessels (small spatial frequency). A range of tissue acoustic models exists that predict the frequency dependence of the scattered field, which is to some degree tissue specific. The equivalence of the linear scattering formulation in real space and k-space shows that the randomness of speckle obscuring features of the imaged structure, and the limited sampling of spatial frequency space, are in fact two sides of the same coin.

2.4.2 Second-order speckle statistics in ultrasound

The second-order statistics enables to describe the statistical relation between two different pixels in the image. Among many other speckle features, they allow the computation of the speckle spot size, which is an important parameter in determining the degree to which speckle affects the image. To derive the autocorrelation and autocovariance of the complex ultrasound field S, we again adopt the linear systems description of ultrasound scattering [12]. Therefore,

$$S = \int_{-\infty}^{+\infty} \Psi(\mathbf{x} - \mathbf{x}')h(\mathbf{x}')d\mathbf{x}' = \Psi(\mathbf{x}) \otimes h(\mathbf{x}) \tag{2.63}$$

where Ψ is the complex scattering amplitude and h is the point spread function.

The autocorrelation function R_s is

$$R_S = E[S(\mathbf{x}_1)S^*(\mathbf{x}_2)] = R_\Psi(\mathbf{x}_1, \mathbf{x}_2) \otimes h(\mathbf{x}_1) \otimes h^*(\mathbf{x}_2) \tag{2.64}$$

where $R_\Psi(\mathbf{x}_1, \mathbf{x}_2) = E[\Psi(\mathrm{x}_1)\Psi^*(\mathbf{x}_2)]$ and $E[\cdot]$ denotes the expectation operator. Since the real and imaginary parts of S are uncorrelated Gaussian random variables with zero mean, $C_s = R_s$, where C_s is the autocovariance of the speckle field.

As before, we assume weak interaction between the medium and the ultrasound field, discarding any multiple scattering. Furthermore, the coarse macroscopic scattering strength is slowly varying compared to the correlation of the microstructure. This diagonalizes the scattering amplitude autocovariance R_Ψ [12]:

$$R_\Psi(\mathbf{x}_1, \mathbf{x}_2) = |\Psi(\mathbf{x})|^2 \tag{2.65}$$

with $x_1 = x \cong x_2$ and $\Delta x = x_2 - x_1$.

If the imaging target is a homogenous distribution of scatterers, or, more generally, the macroscopic scattering structure is slowly varying compared to the width of the point spread function, we can write it as a constant locally: $|\Psi(\mathbf{x})|^2 = \Psi_0^2$. This allows us to rewrite

$$C_S(\Delta\mathbf{x}) = \Psi_0^2 h(-\Delta\mathbf{x}) \otimes h^*(\Delta\mathbf{x}) \tag{2.66}$$

From (2.66), we can conclude that, when imaging objects composed of randomly dispersed fine particles, speckle contains information only about the point spread function.

Assuming that we are in the focal region of the ultrasound transducer, the point spread function can be separated along two orthogonal directions: the insonification direction z (longitudinal) and the transverse direction x (lateral) [17]

$$h(x,z) = h_x h_z \tag{2.67}$$

and the covariance matrix can be written as follows

$$C_S(\Delta x, \Delta z) = C_{Sx}(\Delta x) C_{Sz}(\Delta z) \tag{2.68}$$

Therefore, it is possible to analyze the resulting two covariance functions separately.

For a rectangular transducer, the transverse point spread function in the focal plane is defined as

$$\begin{aligned} h(x) &= B\text{sinc}^2(\pi x \xi_0) \\ \xi_0 &= D/\lambda z_0 \end{aligned} \tag{2.69}$$

with B a normalization factor, D the width of the transducer, λ the wavelength and z_0 is the focal zone distance from the transducer. The expression in (2.69) is obtained assuming continuous wave approximation, which can be used as a first-order estimate of the spatial response in the focal zone.

The autocovariance matrix in the transverse direction is then

$$\begin{aligned} C_{S_x}(\Delta x) &= K_x \text{sinc}^2(\pi \Delta x \xi_0) \otimes \text{sinc}^2(\pi \Delta x \xi_0) \\ &= \left[K_x/(\pi \Delta x)^2\right] [1 - \text{sinc}\,(2\pi \Delta x \xi_0)] \end{aligned} \tag{2.70}$$

with K_x a normalization factor.

Regarding the autocovariance along the longitudinal direction, we should first define the longitudinal point spread function. If, for simplicity, we assume the shape of the pulse envelope to be Gaussian $\sim (0, \sigma_z^2)$, then

$$h(z) = \frac{1}{2\pi\sigma_z^2} \exp\left(-\frac{z^2}{2\sigma_z^2}\right) \tag{2.71}$$

and the autocovariance becomes

$$C_{Sz}(\Delta z) = K_z \exp\left[-\frac{\Delta z^2}{4\sigma_z^2}\right] \tag{2.72}$$

with K_z a normalization factor.

With the knowledge about the autocovariance matrix in the transverse and longitudinal direction, we can define the speckle spot size [12,17]. In fact, the speckle size along the transverse direction, δ_x, and along the longitudinal direction δ_z, are defined as follows

$$\delta_x = \int_{-\infty}^{+\infty} C_{S_x}(\Delta x)/C_x(0)d(\Delta x) \tag{2.73}$$

$$\delta_z = \int_{-\infty}^{+\infty} C_{S_z}(\Delta z)/C_z(0)d(\Delta z) \tag{2.74}$$

For a rectangular transducer, the lateral and axial correlation cell size are [18]

$$\delta_x = \frac{0.87}{\xi_0} \tag{2.75}$$

$$\delta_z = 0.91\frac{c}{\Delta f} \tag{2.76}$$

with c the speed of sound and Δf the frequency bandwidth. From (2.75) and (2.76), we can see that the speckle size in the transverse direction is proportional to the beam width, while in the longitudinal direction is inversely proportional to the bandwidth.

That means that the speckle size is comparable to the resolution cell size. The point spread function is not spatially invariant. Far from the focal region, the factorization in (2.67) does not hold, which complicates the detailed mathematical description of the speckle correlation, but not the approximate equality of speckle spot and resolution cell sizes as a result of (2.66).

2.4.3 *Partially developed speckle and speckle from few scatterers*

Thus far, we assumed that the density of microscopic scattering events was sufficiently high that the phase of the signal was randomized within one resolution cell. In practical ultrasonic imaging applications, this condition is often not met: the speckle is "partially developed." The assumptions of the central limit theorem are not fulfilled any longer, and the real and imaginary parts do not have a Gaussian distribution anymore. Different statistical models have to be applied to describe the signal [19]. One circumstance in which this occurs was discussed in the previous section: presence of strong, resolved reflectors or correlated scattering structures giving rise to a constant phasor background.

We briefly discuss here a few more special cases for which the speckle statistics can be computed, setting the stage for advanced speckle modeling in Chapter 3.

If we have a finite number of random scatterers, we can consider the problem as an N-dimensional random walk problem, with N a finite number. Assume again that the N phasors have independent phase and amplitude and that the phase is uniformly distributed. Recalling (2.1)–(2.3), and using the same definitions as before, we can write the complex field S as

$$S = \sum_{n=1}^{N} \alpha_n e^{i\varphi_n} = S_r + iS_i = Ae^{i\Phi} \tag{2.77}$$

The joint characteristic function of S_r and S_i is

$$M_{S_r,S_i}(\omega_1, \omega_2, N) = E\left[e^{i(\omega_1 S_r + \omega_2 S_i)}\right] = \int_0^\infty \int_{-\pi}^{\pi} e^{i(\omega_1 S_r + \omega_2 S_i)} p_{\alpha_n,\varphi_n} d\varphi_n d\alpha_n \tag{2.78}$$

where p_{α_n,φ_n} is the joint probability distribution of the amplitude and the phase of the individual scatterer; since S_r and S_i depend on α_n and φ_n only, the integration over S can be replaced by the phasor variables directly. Note that the characteristic function is a function of the number of scatterers N.

If we define the polar coordinates in the plane $(\omega_1\omega_2)$ through $\omega_1 = \Omega\cos\chi$ and $\omega_2 = \Omega\sin\chi$, we can rewrite (2.78) as

$$M_{S_r,S_i}(\omega_1\omega_2, N) = \int_0^\infty \prod_{n=1}^{N} J_0(\alpha_n\Omega) p_{\alpha_n} d\alpha_n \tag{2.79}$$

With J_0, the Bessel function of the first kind and order zero. Knowing that the scatterer amplitudes are independent and identically distributed, we obtain

$$M_{S_r,S_i}(\omega_1\omega_2, N) = \left[\int_0^\infty J_0(\alpha\Omega) p_\alpha d\alpha\right]^N \tag{2.80}$$

From (2.80), we can note that in order to compute the distributions of the phase and amplitude of the complex field, we need to define the probability density function p_α of the scatterer amplitude α. This dependence arises because for small N we cannot rely on the central limit theorem to produce Gaussian statistics. The interesting consequence of this complication is that for non-Rayleigh-distributed speckle, we can infer properties of the scattering medium from the speckle distribution. It is possible to demonstrate that the K distribution is a suitable model for p_α in many media. It is defined as follows

$$\begin{aligned} p_\alpha &= \frac{2b}{\Gamma(v+1)} \left(\frac{b\alpha}{2}\right)^{v+1} K_v(b\alpha) \quad \text{with } \alpha \geq 0, v \geq -1 \\ b &= 2\sqrt{\frac{N(v+1)}{E[\alpha^2]}} \end{aligned} \tag{2.81}$$

where $K_v(\cdot)$ is the modified Bessel function of the second kind and order v and $\Gamma(\cdot)$ is the Gamma function. By computing the characteristic function $M_{S_r,S_i}(\omega_1\omega_2, N)$

using the K distributed p_α and inverting to get the joint density function of the envelope A and phase $\mathbf{\Phi}$, we obtain

$$p_{A,\Phi} = \frac{1}{2\pi}\frac{2b}{\Gamma(Q)}\left(\frac{bA}{2}\right)^Q K_{Q-1}(bQ) \qquad \text{for } A > 0 \tag{2.82}$$

where we have substituted $Q = N(1+v)$, and so $b = 2\sqrt{\frac{Q}{E[A^2]}}$. Computing the marginal densities, we obtain

$$p_A = \frac{2b}{\Gamma(Q)}\left(\frac{bA}{2}\right)^Q K_{Q-1}(bA) \qquad \text{for } A > 0 \tag{2.83}$$

$$p_\pi = \frac{1}{2\pi} \qquad -\pi \leq 0 \leq \pi \tag{2.84}$$

Analysis of the parameters of the K distribution can provide information on the number of scatterers and on the scattering section. This is unlike the statistics of fully developed speckle, which only depends on the mean amplitude. The parameter υ represents the skewness of the distribution. For υ approaching infinity, p_α approaches a Rayleigh distribution while for υ approaching -1, p_α approaches a lognormal distribution. Therefore, we can appreciate the generality of the K distribution since it is possible to change the distribution of the scatterer amplitude by changing υ. Knowing the meaning of the parameter υ, it is possible to understand the physical significance of Q. For υ approaching -1, Q will be very small even if N is very large. Therefore, Q represents the effective number of scatterers per resolution cell. Thus, Q is a measure of both the number of scatterers and the variation in scattering cross section [19]. Figure 2.10 shows plots of the K-distribution for different effective numbers of scatterers Q, demonstrating that for $Q > 10$ the difference with the Rayleigh distribution becomes small.

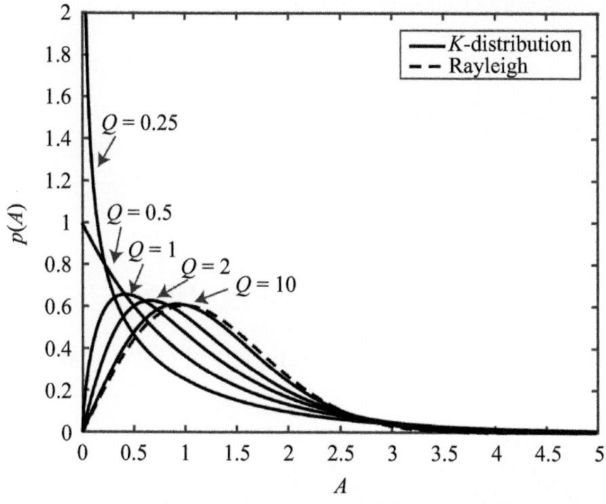

Figure 2.10 K-distribution for different effective number of scatterers Q

2.5 Effect of postprocessing on first- and second-order statistics

In standard B-mode imaging, the ultrasound signal detected by the transducer is usually processed nonlinearly in order to compress the incoming signal having wide range into a smaller signal with reduced range. This is done to overcome the problem of displaying a wide range signal using too many gray-scale levels that would not be distinguished by the observer [6]. Therefore, compression is needed in order to be able to display the images on the commercially available systems. This nonlinear postprocessing of the incoming signal will affect its statistics, leading to changes in the probability density functions. It is therefore important to study the effect of these compression mechanisms on the previously derived statistics. The most common way of compressing ultrasound data is to use a logarithmic amplifier. More in detail, the received signal amplitude A will be scaled and shifted according to the following expression:

$$A' = c \ln \mathrm{A} + d \tag{2.85}$$

where A' is the postprocessing amplitude and c and d are constants associated to the dynamic range and the gain setting respectively [20]. If $A_{\min}$ and $A_{\max}$ are the minimum and maximum respectively of the input A which lead to $A'_{\min}$ and $A'_{\max}$ of the output A', then

$$c = \frac{A'_{\max} - A'_{\min}}{\ln(A_{\max} - A_{\min})} \tag{2.86}$$

Knowing that the dynamic range is given by

$$DR = 20 \log\left(\frac{A_{\max}}{A_{\min}}\right) \tag{2.87}$$

We can rewrite (2.86) such that

$$c = \frac{20}{DR \ln(10)}\left(A'_{\max} - A'_{\min}\right) \tag{2.88}$$

Therefore, knowing the input and output dynamic range, it is possible to estimate the logarithmic amplifier parameter c.

To compute the probability density function of A', we can use the following expression [21]

$$p\left(A'\right) = p(A)\left(\frac{dA'}{dA}\right)^{-1} \tag{2.89}$$

with the probability density function of A given by (2.20). We then get

$$\frac{dA'}{dA} = \frac{c}{A} = \frac{c}{e^{\left(\frac{A'-d}{c}\right)}} \tag{2.90}$$

and $p(A')$ becomes

$$p\left(A'\right) = \frac{1}{\beta} e^{\left(-g-e^{-g}\right)} \tag{2.91}$$

with

$$g = \frac{\alpha - A'}{\beta} \quad \alpha = \frac{c \log(2\sigma^2)}{2} + d \quad \beta = \frac{c}{2} \tag{2.92}$$

Equation (2.91) is a double exponential (Fisher–Tippet) [20]. Note that α, c and d are functions of the standard deviation σ of the Rayleigh distribution. Therefore, we can compute the mean and variance of A' as

$$E\left[A'\right] = c\left(\frac{\ln 2}{2} + \ln \sigma - \frac{\gamma}{2}\right) + d \tag{2.93}$$

$$E\left[\left(A' - E\left[A'\right]\right)^2\right] = \frac{\pi^2 c^2}{24} \tag{2.94}$$

where γ is the Euler constant ($\gamma \approx 0.5772$). Figure 2.11 shows the effect of log-compression on the Rayleigh distribution.

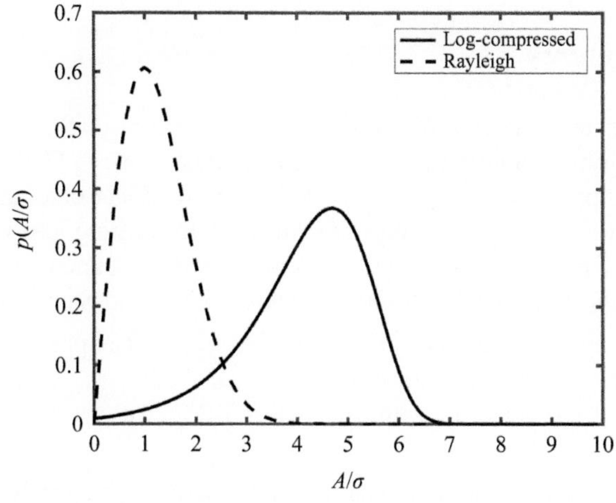

Figure 2.11 Rayleigh distribution and log-compressed distribution with c = 2 and d = 4

Knowing the variance of the log-compressed data, we can derive the values of the parameters c. Assuming the known variance is equal to v, we get

$$c = \frac{2\sqrt{6}}{\pi}\sqrt{v} \tag{2.95}$$

This means that, for fully developed speckle, we can derive the amplification parameter from the signal statistics (the variance).

2.6 Summary

Speckle is inherent to imaging with coherent waves. In this chapter, we have introduced the basic concepts of speckle as it appears in randomly scattered wave fields. Using concepts from laser speckle originating in optics, we have shown how the Rayleigh distributed magnitude appears as a very general and robust result from a random phasor sum, with minimal assumptions on the statistics of amplitude and phase of the contributing phasors. Subsequently, the statistics of a scattered field with a constant background and nonuniform phase distributions were demonstrated.

By writing ultrasound scattering in a linear systems formalism, the relations that govern speckle appear straightforwardly in the field scattered by a random structure. We have computed the second-order statistics to relate speckle spot size to ultrasound imaging parameters and found that the speckle size is similar, but not identical to the resolution cell dimensions. We have outlined the case of a small number of contributing waves, leading to the K-distribution, which is one of several heuristic models that will be elaborated on in subsequent chapters. Finally, we discussed the impact of dynamic range compression on speckle statistics, which is important to describe the signal distribution in practical imaging applications.

Acknowledgments

We would like to thank Prof. J.W. Goodman for discussions on the sum of Rayleigh distributed magnitudes and sharing his insights in this problem. GvS acknowledges Prof. D.D. Sampson and the School of Electrical, Electronic and Computer Engineering of the University of Western Australia for hosting him while working on this chapter, supported by a grant from the Raine Foundation. He enjoyed discussions on the finer details of OCT speckle with David Sampson and Andrea Curatolo.

References

[1] J. W. Goodman, "Some Fundamental Properties of Speckle," *Journal of the Optical Society of America*, vol. 66, pp. 1145–1150, 1976.

[2] K. Exner, "Ueber das Funkeln der Sterne und die Scintillation überhaupt," *Annalen der Physik*, vol. 253, pp. 305–322, 1882.

[3] J. W. Goodman, "Statistical properties of laser speckle patterns," in *Laser speckle and related phenomena*, ed: Berlin, Heidelberg: Springer, 1975, pp. 9–75.

[4] L. Mandel and E. Wolf, *Optical Coherence and Quantum Optics*. Cambridge: Cambridge University Press, 1995.

[5] C. B. Burckhardt, "Speckle in Ultrasound B-Mode Scans," *IEEE Transactions on Sonics and Ultrasonics*, vol. 25, pp. 1–6, 1978.

[6] R. S. C. Cobbold, *Foundations of Biomedical Ultrasound*. New York: Oxford University Press, Inc., 2007.

[7] J. W. Goodman, *Speckle Phenomena in Optics: Theory and Applications*: Greenwood Village, USA: Roberts and Company Publishers, 2006.

[8] D. Huang, E. A. Swanson, C. P. Lin, *et al.*, "Optical Coherence Tomography," *Science*, vol. 254, pp. 1178–1181, Nov 1991.

[9] J. M. Schmitt, S. H. Xiang, and K. M. Yung, "Speckle in Optical Coherence Tomography," *Journal of Biomedical Optics*, vol. 4, pp. 95–105, Jan 1999.

[10] B. Karamata, K. Hassler, M. Laubscher, and T. Lasser, "Speckle Statistics in Optical Coherence Tomography," *Journal of the Optical Society of America. A, Optics, Image Science, and Vision*, vol. 22, pp. 593–596, Apr 2005.

[11] A. Curatolo, B. F. Kennedy, D. D. Sampson, and T. R. Hillman, Speckle in Optical Coherence Tomography. R. K. Wang, V. V. Tuchin, eds. *Advanced Biophotonics*. Boca Raton: Taylor & Francis; 2014.

[12] R. F. Wagner, S. W. Smith, J. M. Sandrik, and H. Lopez, "Statistics of Speckle in Ultrasound B-Scans," *IEEE Transactions on Sonics and Ultrasonics*, vol. 30, pp. 156–163, 1983.

[13] F. L. Lizzi, S. K. Alam, S. Mikaelian, P. Lee, and E. J. Feleppa, "On the Statistics of Ultrasonic Spectral Parameters," *Ultrasound in Medicine & Biology*, vol. 32, pp. 1671–1685, Nov 2006.

[14] J. W. Goodman, *Statistical Optics*. New York, USA: John Wiley & Sons Inc.,1985.

[15] T. Hellmuth, "Contrast and Resolution in Optical Coherence Tomography," *Proceedings Of Optical Biopsies and Microscopic Techniques*, vol. 2926, pp. 228–237, 1996.

[16] F. L. Lizzi, M. Greenebaum, E. J. Feleppa, M. Elbaum, and D. J. Coleman, "Theoretical Framework for Spectrum Analysis in Ultrasonic Tissue Characterization," *Journal of the Acoustical Society of America*, vol. 73, pp. 1366–1373, 1983.

[17] R. F. Wagner, M. F. Insana, and S. W. Smith, "Fundamental Correlation Lengths of Coherent Speckle in Medical Ultrasonic Images," *IEEE Transactions on Ultrasonics Ferroelectrics and Frequency Control*, vol. 35, pp. 34–44, Jan 1988.

[18] T. L. Szabo, *Diagnostic Ultrasound Imaging: Inside Out.* Boston MA, USA: Academic Press, Boston University, 2004.

[19] P. M. Shankar, "A Model for Ultrasonic Scattering from Tissues Based on the K-Distribution," *Physics in Medicine and Biology*, vol. 40, pp. 1633–1649, Oct 1995.

[20] D. Kaplan and Q. G. Ma, "On the Statistical Characteristics of Log-Compressed Rayleigh Signals – Theoretical Formulation and Experimental Results," *IEEE 1993 Ultrasonics Symposium Proceedings*, Vols 1 and 2, pp. 961–964, 1993.

[21] J. M. Thijssen, B. J. Oosterveld, and R. F. Wagner, "Gray Level Transforms and Lesion Detectability in Echographic Images," *Ultrasonic Imaging*, vol. 10, pp. 171–195, Jul 1988.

Chapter 3

Statistical models for speckle noise and Bayesian deconvolution of ultrasound images

Ningning Zhao[1], *Adrian Basarab*[2], *Denis Kouamé*[2], *and Jean-Yves Tourneret*[3]

Ultrasound (US) pulse-echo imaging involves signals obtained by coherent summation of echoes backscattered from randomly located scatterers in the tissue under investigation. The scatterers are inhomogeneities (structures with sizes smaller than the US wavelengths) in the tissue that are not resolved by the imaging system [1]. On the other hand, speckle noise, shown as granular appearance, is the result of the constructive or destructive interference of a large number of randomly scattered waves [2,3] in a resolution cell. Speckle inherently exists not only in US images but also in optics, synthetic aperture radar, etc. Speckle heavily degrades the image readability and interferes with the detection and analysis of anatomical structures in US images.

Although the existence of speckle complicates the clinical diagnosis of US images, the speckle patterns are characteristics of specific tissues and organs. Specifically, speckle can be seen as a phenomenon carrying useful information about randomly distributed scatterers of a biological tissue. Speckle analysis has been a major subject under investigation in many applications ranging from speckle removal [4,5] to characterization of speckle patterns [6,7]. For instance, the changes of the speckle pattern can be used to measure tissue lesions [8], whereas the speckle features can be used for motion estimation or displacement detection of the imaged organs [9]. Bayesian methods were recently used to eliminate the speckle noise with a heavy-tailed probability distribution for the logarithm of US images [10]. Generalized Gaussian distributions (GGDs) were also investigated for the joint deconvolution and segmentation of US images [11]. Thus, the statistical analysis of speckle can facilitate the analysis and understanding of US images.

This chapter first summarizes existing results related to the statistical properties of US images based on both radio-frequency (RF) and envelope signals. In a second part of the chapter, we present a Bayesian deconvolution method that can be viewed as a general despeckling technique.

[1]Department of Radiation Oncology, University of California, USA
[2]IRIT, Université de Toulouse, CNRS, France
[3]IRIT-ENSEEIHT-TéSA, University of Toulouse, France

3.1 Statistical analysis of speckle noise

The backscattered RF signals or their envelope signals (magnitudes of complex in phase and quadrature (IQ) signals obtained from RF signals) have been widely explored regarding their statistical properties, see e.g., [12–14]. Figure 3.1 illustrates the relationship between the US RF signals, the corresponding envelope and B-mode axial profiles (logarithm-compressed envelope signals). Given an RF signal $Y(t)$, we denote its analytic signal by $Y(t) + jY_h(t)$. The complex IQ signal is defined as a frequency shift of the analytic signal, i.e.,

$$Y_I(t) + jY_Q(t) = [Y(t) + jY_h(t)]\exp(-j\omega_0 t) \tag{3.1}$$

where $Y_h(t)$ is the Hilbert transform of the RF signal $Y(t)$, $Y_I(t)$, and $Y_Q(t)$ are the *in-phase* (I) and *quadrature* (Q) components of the IQ signal and ω_0 is the central angular frequency of the transducer. The corresponding envelope signal at time instant t, denoted as $X(t)$ can then be obtained as

$$X(t) = \sqrt{Y_I^2(t) + Y_Q^2(t)}. \tag{3.2}$$

In this section, we introduce statistical models for RF signals, their envelopes and log-compressed (B-mode) representations through appropriate parametric probability density functions (pdfs). In order to simplify the notations, the time dependency will be omitted when there is no possible confusion, e.g., $Y(t)$ will be denoted as Y. Note that the analytical expressions of the pdfs associated with the backscattered signals are usually derived using the central limit theorem.

3.1.1 *Statistical models for radio-frequency signals*

RF signals are obtained after beamforming raw data/individual echo signals received by the transducers. Among the statistical distributions used to analyze RF signals, the most common one is the Gaussian distribution, see e.g., [12,15]. However, the Gaussian distribution assumption for RF signals may not be valid in many situations, see e.g., [16,17]. Thus, other non-Gaussian distributions have been investigated for RF signals, such as the K distribution [14,18], the GGD [19,20] and α-stable distributions [21,22]. These distributions have been obtained using partially and fully developed speckle assumptions. Note that the fully developed

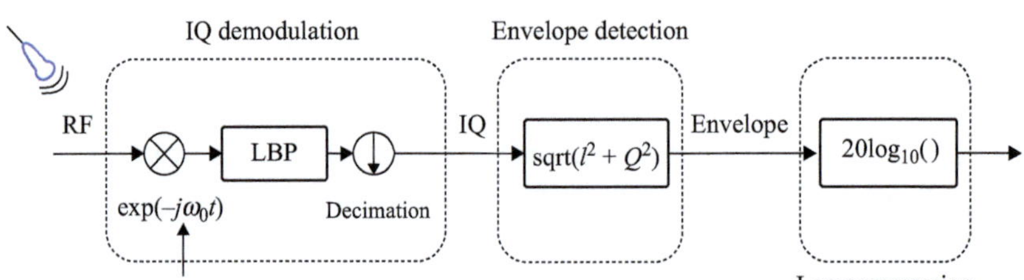

Figure 3.1 Relationship between different US image modes

speckle assumption implies a large number of scatterers and rough scatterer surfaces.

3.1.1.1 Gaussian distribution

Assuming that the speckle is fully developed in a backscattered resolution cell, the resulting number of independent scatterers is high per resolution cell. In these conditions, using the central limit theorem, the Gaussian distribution is well adapted to describe the statistical properties the RF signals leading to the following pdf

$$p_Y(y) = \frac{1}{\sqrt{2\pi\sigma^2}} \exp\left(-\frac{y^2}{2\sigma^2}\right), \quad y \in \mathbb{R} \tag{3.3}$$

where σ^2 is the variance, directly related to the scatterer concentrations defining the nature of the imaged tissues. The Gaussian assumption for the RF signal leads to a Rayleigh distribution for the corresponding envelopes, which is presented in the following section. However, the Gaussian distribution is not reliable in many situations such as in the presence of a specular biological target, partially developed speckle or when there are some dominant components present in the resolution cell. As a result, several non-Gaussian models have been explored in the literature for US images.

3.1.1.2 K_{RF} distribution

Assuming that the scatterers are uniformly distributed and that their amplitudes have a K distribution, the statistics of the RF signal is modeled using the K_{RF} distribution [14]. The K_{RF} distribution is described by the following pdf

$$p_Y(y) = \frac{b}{\sqrt{\pi}\Gamma(v)} \left(\frac{b|y|}{2}\right)^{v-0.5} K_{v-0.5}(b|y|) I_{\mathbb{R}^+}(y) \tag{3.4}$$

where v and b are shape and scale parameters, $\Gamma(\cdot)$ is the gamma function, $K_{v-0.5}(\cdot)$ is the modified Bessel function of the second kind of order $v - 0.5$[1] and $I_{\mathbb{R}^+}(x)$ denotes the indicator function on $\mathbb{R}^+$. Note that the K_{RF} distribution with parameter $v = 1$ reduces to the Laplace distribution and approaches the Gaussian distribution when $v \to \infty$. Methods allowing the parameters of the K_{RF} distribution to be estimated have been studied in [14]. Since there are no closed-form expressions for the maximum likelihood (ML) estimators of these parameters, the method of moments was investigated in [14]. Although the K_{RF} distribution has a well-established physical justification, the poor properties of its parameter estimators, especially when the shape parameter increases, have limited its practical use.

[1]The Bessel function of the first kind of order α is defined as $J_\alpha(x) = \sum_{m=0}^{\infty} \frac{(-1)^m}{m!\Gamma(m+\alpha+1)} \left(\frac{x}{2}\right)^{2m+\alpha}$. The modified Bessel function of the first kind of order α is defined by $I_\alpha(x) = i^{-\alpha} J_\alpha(x) = \sum_{m=0}^{\infty} \frac{1}{m!\Gamma(m+\alpha+1)} \left(\frac{x}{2}\right)^{2m+\alpha}$. The modified Bessel function of the second kind of order α is defined by $K_\alpha(x) = \frac{\pi}{2} \frac{I_{-\alpha}(x) - I_\alpha(x)}{\sin i(\alpha\pi)}$.

3.1.1.3 Generalized Gaussian distribution

In order to explore the statistics of the backscatterer signals in situations ranging from fully to partially-developed speckle, the GGD has been proposed for RF signals with applications in echocardiography, see e.g., [19,20]. As opposed to the K_{RF} distribution, the GGD has a simple pdf, which results to simpler expressions for the ML estimators of its parameters [23,24]. The pdf of the GGD is defined as

$$p_Y(y) = \frac{\beta}{2\alpha\Gamma(1/\beta)}\exp\left(-\frac{|y|^\beta}{\alpha^\beta}\right), \quad y \in \mathbb{R} \tag{3.5}$$

where α and β are scale and shape parameters. Note that the GGD reduces to the Laplace distribution for $\beta = 1$ and to the Gaussian distribution for $\beta = 2$. Note also that the relationship between the K_{RF} and GGDs was established in [19].

3.1.1.4 α-Stable distributions

Assuming that each scatterer contributes independently to the RF echo, the backscattered signal from a population of point scatterers can be expressed as

$$Y(t) = \sum_{i=0}^{M} a_i p(t - \tau_i) \tag{3.6}$$

where $a_i \in (0,1)$, τ_i is the relative position of the ith backscattered wave, M is the number of scatterers and $t \in T$ (T denotes the image region of interest). In many applications, we can assume that all scatterers in the region T interact with identical interrogating US pulses. Using the generalized central limit theorem, the limit distribution of $Y(t)$ is a symmetric α-stable ($S\alpha S$) distribution whose parameters do not depend on t, i.e.,

$$Y(t) = \sum_{i=0}^{M} a_i p(t - \tau_i) \overset{M\to\infty}{\sim} S\alpha S(\alpha, \gamma) \tag{3.7}$$

where $\overset{M\to\infty}{\sim}$ denotes the convergence in distribution when $M \to \infty$. The family of $S\alpha S$ distributions is fully characterized by the following characteristic function

$$E\{\exp[j\theta Y(t)]\} = e^{-\gamma^\alpha |\theta|^\alpha} \tag{3.8}$$

where $\alpha \in (0, 2]$ is the characteristic index and $\gamma \in \mathbb{R}^+$ is the spread of the $S\alpha S$ distribution. Note that (3.8) is the characteristic function of the Gaussian distribution when $\alpha = 2$ and that of the Cauchy distribution when $\alpha = 1$. Note also that γ is proportional to the number of scatterers and to the variability of the scattering cross sections [21,22,25].

3.1.2 *Statistical models for envelope signals*

Envelope signals are widely used in clinical imaging systems since they contain valuable information such as the location and amplitude of the backscattered US waves. The statistical models that have been proposed for envelope signals in the case of fully developed speckle include the Rayleigh and Rice models [26]. The probability distributions investigated for partially-developed speckle include the K distribution [27], the generalized-K [28] and homodyned-K distributions [29] and the Weibull distribution [30]. The Nakagami distribution [31] and the Rician inverse Gaussian distribution [17] have also been investigated to model varying scattering conditions. More details about the distributions used for envelope signals are presented below.

3.1.2.1 Rayleigh distribution

The received US signal is the superposition of the echoes resulting from different scatterers [14,32]. Using the phasor notation, the US signal can be expressed as the sum of random phasors, i.e.,

$$X = \frac{1}{\sqrt{N}} \sum_{i=1}^{N} S_i e^{j\theta_i} \tag{3.9}$$

where $s_i e^{j\theta_i}$ is the ith complex phasor component with length s_i and phase θ_i, N is the number of scatterers in the resolution cell, Y_I and Y_Q are the real and imaginary parts of X defined as

$$Y_I = \mathrm{Re}(X) = \frac{1}{\sqrt{N}} \sum_{i=1}^{N} s_i \cos\theta_i \quad \text{and} \quad Y_Q = \mathrm{Im}(X) = \frac{1}{\sqrt{N}} \sum_{i=1}^{N} s_i \sin\theta_i. \tag{3.10}$$

The following two assumptions are classical for US signals: (i) the phase term θ_i is uniformly distributed in $[-\pi, \pi]$ and independent of the amplitude; (ii) the amplitude/phase vector (s_i, θ_i) is statistically independent from (x_j, θ_j) for $i \neq j$. Applying the central limit theorem for a large number of scatterers ($N \to \infty$), the real and imaginary components Y_I and Y_Q are independent and have the same Gaussian distribution with zero mean and a variance denoted as σ^2. Thus, the joint pdf of (Y_I, Y_Q) can be written as

$$p_{Y_I,Y_Q}(y_I, y_Q) = \frac{1}{2\pi\sigma^2} \exp\left(-\frac{y_I^2 + y_Q^2}{2\sigma^2}\right), \quad (y_I, y_Q) \in \mathbb{R}^2. \tag{3.11}$$

Considering the following change of variables

$$X = \sqrt{Y_I^2 + Y_Q^2} \quad \text{and} \quad \theta = \arctan\left(\frac{Y_Q}{Y_I}\right) \tag{3.12}$$

it can be shown that the amplitude X has a Rayleigh distribution whose pdf is

$$p_X(x) = \frac{x}{\sigma^2} \exp\left(-\frac{x^2}{2\sigma^2}\right) I_{\mathbb{R}^+}(x). \tag{3.13}$$

The Rayleigh distribution (3.13) is parameterized by a the single parameter σ^2, which represents the total backscattered energy. This parameter can be estimated using the ML method [33].

3.1.2.2 Rice distribution

The scatterer condition used previously to obtain the Rayleigh distribution can be slightly modified in order to consider the presence of coherent component or strong reflector in the resolution cell (resulting from the strong specular scatterer model) [14,34]. In this case, a different distribution for the US envelope signal is obtained. More precisely, the coherent component can be considered by adding a constant amplitude x_0 to Y_I in (3.10) leading to

$$Y_I = x_0 + \frac{1}{\sqrt{N}} \sum_{i=1}^{N} s_i \cos \theta_i. \tag{3.14}$$

The pdf of the envelope signal X can then be expressed as

$$p_X(x) = \frac{x}{\sigma^2} \exp\left(-\frac{x^2 + x_0^2}{2\sigma^2} \right) K_0\left(\frac{x x_0}{\sigma^2} \right) I_{\mathbb{R}^+}(x) \tag{3.15}$$

where $K_0(\cdot)$ is the modified Bessel function of the first kind and order zero. The resulting pdf is known as the Rice distribution. When $x_0 \to 0$, it tends toward the Rayleigh distribution. We recall here that both Rayleigh and Rice models assume a large number of scatterers per resolution cell.

3.1.2.3 *K* distribution

If the number of scatterers in the resolution cell is reduced, a model characterized by the K distribution [18,27] is more relevant. The K distribution for envelope signals is based on the assumption that the scatterers are uniformly distributed in the region of interest [14,18,35]. The pdf of the K distribution is given by

$$p_X(x) = 2\left(\frac{x}{2} \right)^{\alpha} \frac{b^{\alpha+1}}{\Gamma(\alpha)} K_{\alpha-1}(bx) I_{\mathbb{R}^+}(x) \tag{3.16}$$

where α and b are the shape and scale parameters of this distribution, $K_{\alpha-1}(\cdot)$ is the modified Bessel function of the second kind and $b = \sqrt{4\alpha/E[X^2]}$, where E[.] is used for the mathematical expectation. Note that α modulates the number of scatterers associated with the echo envelope statistics. When $\alpha \to \infty$, the K distribution is known to converge toward the Rayleigh distribution. The ML estimators of the parameters of the K distribution can be determined using the method proposed in [1].

3.1.2.4 Homodyned-*K* distribution

Given the scenario of small scatterers density and a coherent component in the resolution, the corresponding model is characterized by the following homodyned-*K* distribution [14,29] whose pdf is

$$p_X(x) = \left(\int_0^\infty \frac{u}{1 + \frac{u^2\sigma^2}{2\alpha}} dJ_0(us) J_0(uA) du \right) x I_{\mathbb{R}^+}(x) \tag{3.17}$$

where J_0 is the Bessel function of the first kind of order zero, σ^2 is related with the diffuse signal energy and α corresponds to the effective number of scatterers. Note that the homodyned-K distribution converges to the Rice distribution as $\alpha \to \infty$ and that the K distribution is a specific case of the homodyned-K distribution [14]. Thus, the homodyned-K distribution can model a wide range of scattering conditions including the ones associated with the Rice, Rayleigh and K distributions. Finally, it is interesting to note that the parameters of the homodyned-K distribution can be computed using the methods of moments [36].

3.1.2.5 Nakagami distribution

Compared to the previous statistical models used for the envelope signals, the Nakagami distribution allows various speckle scenarios to be described, e.g., a large number of scatterers with or without constant phasor as well as a small number of scatterers with varying scatterer cross sections [14]. Due to its inherent simplicity and versatility, the Nakagami distribution is commonly adopted for the US envelope signals. The pdf of the Nakagami distribution is defined as

$$p_X(x) = \frac{2m^m x^{2m-1}}{\Gamma(m)\omega^m} \exp\left(-\frac{mx^2}{\omega} \right) I_{\mathbb{R}^+}(x) \tag{3.18}$$

where m and ω are the shape and scale parameters, m is related to the tissue property, whereas ω is associated with the US signal energy. Note that (3.18) reduces to the Rayleigh distribution for $m = 1$. The Nakagami parameters can be estimated either by using the method of moments [37] or by an iterative ML approach [38].

3.1.2.6 α-Rayleigh distribution

The envelop signal is distributed according to a generalized heavy-tailed Rayleigh distribution when the real and imaginary components of the complex envelope signal are identically and independently distributed according to $S\alpha S$ distributions [22], i.e.,

$$Y_I \sim S\alpha S(\alpha, \gamma) \quad \text{and} \quad Y_Q \sim S\alpha S(\alpha, \gamma). \tag{3.19}$$

The heavy-tailed Rayleigh distribution, denoted as α-Rayleigh has the following pdf

$$p_X(x) = \left(\int_0^\infty x\lambda \exp[-(\gamma\lambda)^\alpha] J_0(x\lambda) d\lambda \right) I_{\mathbb{R}^+}(x) \tag{3.20}$$

where $J_0(\cdot)$ is the 0th order Bessel function of the first kind. More details about this distribution and the estimation method for the parameter vector (α, γ) can be found in [22].

To finish this part, it is interesting to mention that other distributions have been considered to describe the statistical properties of the US image envelop such as the gamma, the generalized gamma or the Weibull distributions, e.g., [39].

3.1.3 Statistical models for B-mode image

The statistical models considered in the previous section only apply to envelope signals. However, B-mode images are more commonly considered in clinical applications. B-mode images are obtained by applying a logarithmic compression to the envelope signals, i.e.,

$$R = d\log(X) + g \tag{3.21}$$

where X is the envelope signal, d and g are related with the dynamic range and the linear gain of the output B-mode images. Many models have been considered for B-mode images [1,40–42]. For instance, in [1,43], the statistics of the B-mode images is modeled by a Fisher–Tippet distribution under the assumption of a Rayleigh distribution for the envelope signals (i.e., fully developed speckle assumption). The pdf of the Fisher–Tippett distribution is defined by

$$p_R(r) = \frac{2}{a}\exp\left[-\log(2\sigma^2) - 2\frac{r-b}{a} - \exp\left(-\log(2\sigma^2) - 2\frac{r-b}{a}\right)\right] I_{\mathbb{R}^+}(r). \tag{3.22}$$

3.1.4 Brief review of statistical despeckling techniques

This part presents a brief review of statistical despeckle techniques (see [44,45] for more details), whereas an explicit explanation of the speckle reduction methods will be presented in the following chapters. The existing methods for speckle reduction in US images can be roughly categorized into image filtering and compounding techniques.

3.1.4.1 Image filtering

A variety of speckle reduction filters have been developed for US images, which can be broadly divided into the following categories.

Adaptive local statistics filters

The regions containing speckle are identified by using *a priori* information about speckle statistics. Regions containing fully developed speckle are then smoothed using a low-pass (local mean) filter, see e.g., [46,47]. The parameters of this filter are adjusted differently in different image regions. Although these filters are able to effectively suppress speckle, they also remove the fine details due to their low-pass characteristic.

Wavelet filters

Speckle reduction in the wavelet domain has been receiving an increasing interest since wavelet filters attempt to remove noise while maintaining the anatomic structure boundaries. For instance, the distribution of US images in the wavelet domain has been exploited for speckle reduction in [10].

Anisotropic diffusion filters
Image diffusion leading to speckle reduction is generally controlled by a partial differential equation. Anisotropic diffusion is required for suppressing speckle while preserving image edges, see e.g., [48,49].

Nonlocal mean-based filters
In [50], a nonlocal (NL) means filter is used for US speckle reduction. Filters based on NL means link the intensity of each pixel to the pixel intensities of different parts of the image, leading to better resolved despeckled images.

Finally, it is interesting to note that a comparison between different speckle reduction methods can be found in [51].

3.1.4.2 Compounding

Compounding methods involve the fusion of multiple images obtained by varying one or more system parameters during data acquisition [44]. These methods are not considered in this chapter. The readers are invited to consult [44] and the references therein for more details.

3.2 Bayesian method for US image deconvolution

This section studies a US image deconvolution method, which can be used for image despeckling. US image deconvolution, aiming at estimating the tissue reflectivity function (TRF) $\mathbf{x}$ from the RF image $\mathbf{y}$, is a typical ill-posed problem. Imposing a regularization term is a traditional way to cope with this problem. The regularization term usually reflects the prior knowledge about $\mathbf{x}$, e.g., the statistics of the US TRF. Moreover, due to the tight relationship between image deconvolution and segmentation, it is interesting to consider them jointly. This idea has been recently exploited for piecewise constant images using the Mumford–Shah model, the Potts model or the generalized linear models in Bayesian or variational frameworks [52–54]. Moreover, segmentation-based regularizations have shown to improve the performance of image reconstruction. However, due to the existence of speckle, these methods are not efficient to simultaneously restore and segment US images [11].

In order to develop US image deconvolution and segmentation methods, it is common to take advantage of the statistical properties of the TRF. Alessandrini *et al.* recently investigated a deconvolution method for US images based on GGDs using the expectation maximization algorithm [55]. This method assumed that the US image can be divided into different regions characterized by GDDs with different parameters. A US image deconvolution method using Markov chain Monte Carlo (MCMC) methods was investigated in [56]. This method was based on a GGD for the US image and an *a priori* label map for different image regions. More recently, a joint Bayesian deconvolution and segmentation method was investigated for US images [11]. The method studied in [11] generalizes the results of [56] to situations where the label map is unknown. It is summarized in the rest of this section[2].

Under the first order Born approximation and the assumption of weak scattering classically assumed for soft tissues, the linear image formation model (3.23) is widely considered for US RF images [6], i.e.,

$$\mathbf{y} = \mathbf{H}\mathbf{x} + \mathbf{n} \tag{3.23}$$

where the vectors ($\in \mathbb{R}^{N\times 1}$) $\mathbf{y}$, $\mathbf{x}$ and $\mathbf{n}$ are the observed RF image, the TRF to be estimated and the measurement noise, and where the matrix $\mathbf{H} \in \mathbb{R}^{N\times N}$ is associated with the point spread function (PSF). Note that the PSF is usually unknown in practical applications. Hereinafter, the PSF is estimated in a pre-processing step and assumed to be shift-invariant.

3.2.1 Bayesian model for joint deconvolution and segmentation

We assume that the US TRF $\mathbf{x} = (x_1, \ldots, x_N)^T$ can be divided into K statistical homogeneous regions, denoted as $\{\mathcal{R}_1, \ldots, \mathcal{R}_K\}$ and we introduce a hidden label field $\mathbf{z} = (z_1, \ldots, z_N)^T \in \mathbb{R}^N$ mapping the image into these K regions. Precisely, $z_i = k$ if and only if the corresponding pixel x_i belongs to the region $\mathcal{R}_k$, where $k \in \{1, \ldots, K\}$ and $i \in \{1, \ldots, N\}$. The conditional distribution of pixel x_i is then defined as

$$x_i | z_i = k \sim \mathrm{GGD}(\xi_k, \gamma_k) \tag{3.24}$$

where ξ_k and γ_k are the shape and scale parameters of the GGD associated with the region $\mathcal{R}_k$. We remind that a univariate GGD with shape parameter ξ and scale parameter γ denoted as $\mathrm{GGD}(\xi, \gamma)$ has the following pdf

$$p(x) = \frac{1}{2\gamma^{1/\xi}\Gamma(1+1/\xi)} \exp\left(-\frac{|x|^{\xi}}{\gamma}\right), \qquad x \in \mathbb{R}. \tag{3.25}$$

Assuming that the pixels are independent conditionally to the knowledge of their classes, the TRF is distributed according to a mixture of GGDs given by

$$p(x_i) = \sum_{k=1}^{K} w_k \mathrm{GGD}(\xi_k, \gamma_k) \text{ with } w_k = P(z_i = k). \tag{3.26}$$

In addition, we assign a Potts model to the hidden field $\mathbf{z}$ to exploit the dependencies between pixels that are nearby in the image, see, e.g., [8]. The resulting model is referred to as GGD-Potts model. In the following, we define a hierarchical Bayesian model based on this GGD-Potts model for the joint segmentation and

[2]The material presented below has been partly presented in the journal paper [11].

deconvolution of US images. The joint posterior of the unknown parameters can be determined using the Bayes rule. The following result can be obtained

$$p(\mathbf{x}, \mathbf{z}, \theta|\mathbf{y}) \propto p(\mathbf{y}|\mathbf{x}, \theta)p(\mathbf{x}|\mathbf{z}, \theta)p(\mathbf{z}|\theta)p(\theta) \tag{3.27}$$

where $\propto$ means "proportional to," θ is a parameter vector containing all the model parameters and hyperparameters except $\mathbf{x}$ and $\mathbf{z}$, i.e., the noise variance, the shape and scale parameters of the different GGDs. The likelihood $p(\mathbf{y}|\mathbf{x}, \theta)$ depending on the noise model and the prior distributions $p(\mathbf{x}|\mathbf{z}, \theta), p(\mathbf{z}|\theta)$ based on the GGD-Potts model are detailed hereinafter.

3.2.1.1 Likelihood

Assuming an additive white Gaussian noise (AWGN) with a constant variance σ_n^2, the likelihood function associated with the linear model (3.23) is

$$p(\mathbf{y}|\mathbf{x}, \sigma_n^2) = \frac{1}{(2\pi\sigma_n^2)^{N/2}} \exp\left(-\frac{1}{2\sigma_n^2}\|\mathbf{y} - \mathbf{H}\mathbf{x}\|_2^2\right) \tag{3.28}$$

where $\|\cdot\|_2$ is the Euclidean ℓ_2-norm.

3.2.1.2 Prior distributions

Tissue reflectivity function $\mathbf{x}$

As explained beforehand, a mixture of GGD priors is assigned to the TRF. Assuming that the pixels are independent conditionally to the knowledge of their classes, we obtain the following prior to the target image

$$\begin{aligned} p(\mathbf{x}|\mathbf{z}, \xi, \gamma) &= \prod_{k=1}^{K}\prod_{i=1}^{N_k} \frac{1}{2\gamma_k^{1/\xi_k}\Gamma(1 + 1/\xi_k)} \exp\left(-\frac{|x_i|^{\xi_k}}{\gamma_k}\right) \\ &= \prod_{k=1}^{K} \frac{1}{\left[2\gamma_k^{1/\xi_k}\Gamma(1 + 1/\xi_k)\right]^{N_k}} \exp\left(-\frac{\sum_{i=1}^{N_k}|x_i|^{\xi_k}}{\gamma_k}\right) \\ &= \prod_{k=1}^{K} \frac{1}{\left[2\gamma_k^{1/\xi_k}\Gamma(1 + 1/\xi_k)\right]^{N_k}} \exp\left(-\frac{\|\mathbf{x}_k\|_{\xi_k}^{\xi_k}}{\gamma_k}\right) \end{aligned} \tag{3.29}$$

where $\xi = (\xi_1, \ldots, \xi_K)^T$ and $\gamma = (\gamma_1, \ldots, \gamma_K)^T$, ξ_k and γ_k are the shape and scale parameters of the kth region $\mathcal{R}_k$, N_k is the number of pixels in $\mathcal{R}_k$, x_k contains all the pixels assigned to $\mathcal{R}_k$, $\Gamma(\cdot)$ is the gamma function and $\|\mathbf{x}_k\|_\xi = \left(\sum_{i=1}^{N_k} |x_i|^\xi\right)^{1/\xi}$ denotes the ℓ_ξ-norm.

Noise variance σ_n^2

In the presence of an AWGN, it is standard to assign a conjugate inverse gamma prior to the noise variance, i.e.,

$$\begin{aligned} p(\sigma_n^2) &\sim \mathrm{IG}(\alpha, \nu) \\ &= \frac{\nu^\alpha}{\Gamma(\alpha)} \frac{1}{\sigma_n^{2\alpha+2}} \exp\left(-\frac{\nu}{\sigma_n^2}\right) I_{\mathbb{R}^+}(\sigma_n^2). \end{aligned} \tag{3.30}$$

Labels $\mathbf{z}$

A Potts model is considered as prior for the hidden image label field, which establishes dependencies between pixels that are nearby in an image [8,57]. Specifically, adjacent labels of the image are dependent and tend to belong to the same class. The conditional distribution of z_n (associated with pixel x_n) for the Potts Markov random field (MRF) is

$$P(z_n|\mathbf{z}_{-n}) = p\left(z_n|\mathbf{z}_{\mathcal{V}(n)}\right) \tag{3.31}$$

where $\mathbf{z}_{-n} = (z_1, \ldots, z_{n-1}, z_{n+1}, \ldots, z_N)$ and $\mathcal{V}(n)$ contains the neighbors of label z_n. In this chapter, a first order neighborhood structure (i.e., four nearest pixels) is considered. The whole set of random variables $\mathbf{z}$ forms a random field. Using the Hammersley–Clifford theorem, the prior of $\mathbf{z}$ can be expressed as a Gibbs distribution, i.e.,

$$p(\mathbf{z}) = \frac{1}{C(\beta)} \exp\left[\sum_{n=1}^{N} \sum_{n' \in \mathcal{V}(n)} \beta\delta\left(z_n - z_{n'}\right)\right] \tag{3.32}$$

where β is the granularity coefficient or smooth parameter, $\delta(\cdot)$ is the Kronecker function and $C(\beta)$ is the normalizing constant.

Shape and scale parameters

The prior used for the US TRF defined in (3.29) depends on the shape and scale parameters of the GGD, which are usually referred to as hyperparameters. The following priors can be used for these hyperparameters

$$p(\xi) = \prod_{k=1}^{K} p(\xi_k) = \prod_{k=1}^{K} \frac{1}{3} I_{[0,3]}(\xi_k) \tag{3.33}$$

$$p(\gamma) = \prod_{k=1}^{K} p(\gamma_k) = \prod_{k=1}^{K} \frac{1}{\gamma_k} I_{\mathbb{R}^+}(\gamma_k) \tag{3.34}$$

where $k \in \{1, \ldots, K\}$. Note that the range $[0, 3]$ covers all the possible values of ξ_k and that $p(\gamma_k)$ is the uninformative Jeffreys prior for γ_k.

3.2.1.3 Joint posterior distribution

The joint posterior distribution of the unknown parameters $\mathbf{x}, \sigma_n^2, \xi, \gamma, \mathbf{z}$ can be determined as follows

$$\begin{aligned}
&p\left(\mathbf{x}, \sigma_n^2, \xi, \gamma, \mathbf{z} | \mathbf{y}\right) \\
&\quad \propto p\left(\mathbf{y} | \mathbf{x}, \sigma_n^2, \xi, \gamma, \mathbf{z}\right) p\left(\mathbf{x}, \sigma_n^2, \xi, \gamma, \mathbf{z}\right) \\
&\quad \propto p\left(\mathbf{y} | \mathbf{x}, \sigma_n^2, \xi, \gamma, \mathbf{z}\right) p(\mathbf{x} | \xi, \gamma, \mathbf{z}) p\left(\sigma_n^2\right) p(\xi) p(\gamma) p(\mathbf{z}) \\
&\quad \propto \frac{1}{\left(2\pi\sigma_n^2\right)^{N/2}} \exp\left(-\frac{1}{2\sigma_n^2} \|\mathbf{y} - \mathbf{H}\mathbf{x}\|_2^2\right) \times \frac{1}{\sigma_n^{2\alpha+2}} \exp\left(-\frac{\nu}{\sigma_n^2}\right) \\
&\quad \times \prod_{k=1}^{K} \left\{ a_k^{N_k} \exp\left(-\frac{\|\mathbf{x}_k\|_{\xi_k}^{\xi_k}}{\gamma_k}\right) \times \exp\left[\sum_{n=1}^{N} \sum_{n' \in \mathscr{V}(n)} \beta\delta\left(z_n - z_{n'}\right)\right] \right. \\
&\quad \left. \times \frac{1}{3} I_{[0,3]}(\xi_k) \frac{1}{\gamma_k} I_{\mathbb{R}^+}(\gamma_k) \right\}
\end{aligned} \tag{3.35}$$

where $a_k = \frac{1}{2\gamma_k^{1/\xi_n}\Gamma(1+1/\xi_k)}$ and where the hyperparameters are supposed to be *a priori* independent.

3.2.2 *Sampling the posterior and computing Bayesian estimators*

Computing closed-form expressions of the minimum mean square error (MMSE) or maximum a posteriori (MAP) estimators for the unknown parameters $\mathbf{x}, \sigma_n^2, \xi, \gamma, \mathbf{z}$ from (3.35) is clearly complicated. In this case, a possible solution is to consider MCMC methods in order to generate samples asymptotically distributed according to (3.35) and to use the generated samples to build estimators of the unknown parameters. This section investigates a hybrid Gibbs sampler generating samples of $\mathbf{x}, \sigma_n^2, \xi, \gamma, \mathbf{z}$ according to their conditional distributions. These generated samples are then used to compute the Bayesian estimators of the variables of interest.

3.2.2.1 Hybrid Gibbs sampler

The hybrid Gibbs sampler considered in this work is summarized in Algorithm 1, whereas the corresponding conditional distributions are provided below.

Algorithm 1 Hybrid Gibbs Sampler

---

1. Sampling the noise variance σ_n^2 with its conditional distribution
2. Sampling the shape parameter ξ with its conditional distribution
3. Sampling the scale parameter γ
4. Sampling the labels $\mathbf{z}$ with its normalized conditional distribution
5. Sampling the TRF $\mathbf{x}$

3.2.2.2 Parameter estimation

Bayesian estimators of the unknown parameters are computed using the generated samples obtained by the hybrid Gibbs sampler. Since the labels are discrete variables, marginal MAP estimators are chosen for the labels. The MMSE estimators for the other variables (the TRF $\mathbf{x}$, noise variance σ_n^2 and GGD parameters ξ, γ) are calculated. For example, the MMSE estimator of the TRF $\mathbf{x}$ is computed by

$$\hat{\mathbf{x}}_{\text{MMSE}}|\hat{\mathbf{z}}_{\text{MAP}} \triangleq E\{\mathbf{x}|\mathbf{z} = \hat{\mathbf{z}}_{\text{MAP}}\} = \int p(\mathbf{x}|\mathbf{z} = \hat{\mathbf{z}}_{\text{MAP}})d\mathbf{x}. \tag{3.36}$$

For each pixel, we can approximate this estimator as follows

$$\hat{x}_{n,\text{MMSE}}|\hat{z}_{n,\text{MAP}} \simeq \frac{1}{M}\sum_{i=1}^{M} x_n^{(i)}|z_n^{(i)} = \hat{z}_{n,\text{MAP}} \tag{3.37}$$

where M is the number of iterations after the so-called burn-in period that satisfy $z_n^{(i)} = \hat{z}_{n,\text{MAP}}$, the superscript i represents the ith generated sample and the subscript n is used for the nth pixel. Note that $\hat{\mathbf{z}}_{\text{MAP}}$ is the marginal MAP estimator of the label map and that $\hat{\mathbf{x}}_{\text{MMSE}}$ is the MMSE estimator of the reflectivity.

3.2.3 *Experimental results*

This section presents several experiments conducted on real US data using the algorithm summarized in Section 3.2.2.1 and initially introduced in [11]. The *in vivo* images used in these experiments were acquired with a 20 MHz single-element US probe. The first results correspond to a mouse bladder image with $K = 3$, and the other results have been obtained with a skin melanoma image with $K = 4$. The restored images are displayed in Figure 3.2 whereas all quantitative results are reported in Table 3.1.

Evaluation metrics

Since the ground truth of the TRF and the label map are not available for *in vivo* US data, the quality of the deconvolution results is evaluated using two other metrics commonly used in US imaging: the resolution gain (RG) [58] and the contrast-to-noise ratio (CNR) [59]. The RG is the ratio of the normalized autocorrelation (higher than −3 dB) of the original RF US image to the normalized autocorrelation (higher than −3 dB) of the deconvolved image/restored TRF. The definition of the CNR is given by

$$\text{CNR} = \frac{|\mu_1 - \mu_2|}{\sqrt{\sigma_1^2 + \sigma_2^2}} \tag{3.38}$$

where μ_1, μ_2, σ_1 and σ_2 are the means and standard deviations of pixels located in two regions extracted from the image. Note that the regions selected for the computation of CNR are shown in the red rectangles in Figure 3.2.

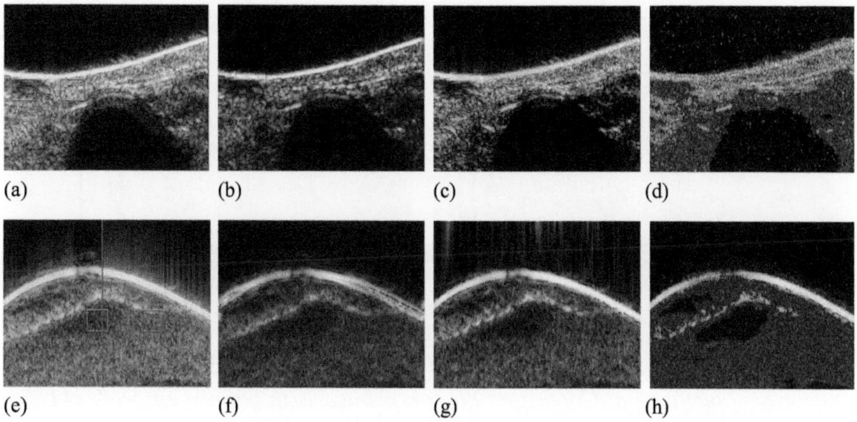

Figure 3.2 From up to down: 1st row corresponds to the mouse bladder; 2nd row is for the skin melanoma. From left to right: 1st column corresponds to the observed B-mode image; 2nd to 4th columns are the restored B-mode images with ℓ_2-norm prior, ℓ_1 norm prior and the proposed method respectively. The regions selected for computing CNR are shown in the red boxes displayed in (a), (e). Copyright 2017, reprinted from [11]

Table 3.1 Deconvolution quality for the real US data

Group	**Group 1—mouse bladder**			**Group 2—skin melanoma**		
Metrics	**RG**	**CNR**	**Time (s)**	**RG**	**CNR**	**Time (s)**
Observation	–	1.08	–	–	1.17	–
ℓ_2	3.82	1.00	0.006	3.01	1.09	0.007
ℓ_1	3.29	**1.11**	5.07	4.63	1.19	3.53
Proposed	**3.94**	0.94	3904.8	**10.01**	**1.35**	1303.4

The bold values indicate the best results

Mouse bladder

The number of homogeneous regions was set to $K=3$ in this experiment, which is sufficient to represent the anatomical structures of the image. Figure 3.2(b)–(d) display the restored TRFs obtained with the ℓ_2 and ℓ_1 optimization algorithms and the proposed method. The proposed method provides good restoration results, especially with clearer boundaries. These results are confirmed in Table 3.1 showing more quantitative results. Finally, Figure 3.3(a) shows the marginal MAP estimates of the labels, which segment the estimated image into several statistically homogeneous regions.

Skin melanoma

The number of homogeneous regions was fixed to $K=4$. Figure 3.2(f)–(h) display the restored TRFs with the different methods (ℓ_2, ℓ_1 optimization algorithms and

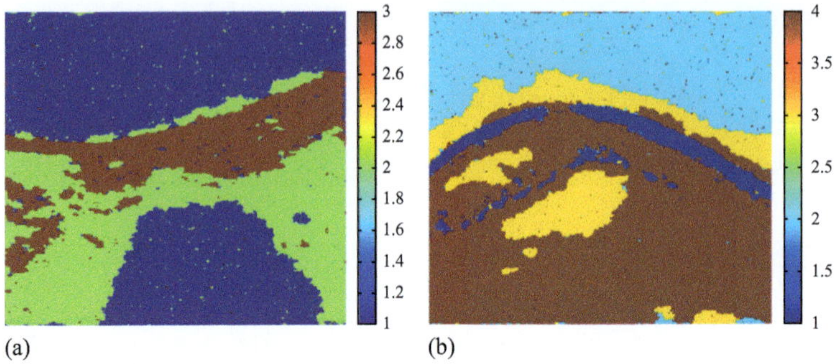

Figure 3.3 Marginal MAP estimates of labels: (a) mouse bladder and (b) skin melanoma. Copyright 2017, reprinted with permission from [11]

proposed method). Note that Figure 3.2(h) shows an improved contrast between the tumor and the healthy skin tissue when compared to the observed B-mode image in Figure 3.2(a). The boundaries are also better defined for the image obtained with the proposed method, when compared to the observed B-mode image. These observations are confirmed by more quantitative results available in Table 3.1. Finally, the marginal MAP estimates of the image labels are shown in Figure 3.3(b). The four estimated labels correspond to the water-gel (light blue), tumor (yellow) and skin tissues (the two shades of red).

3.3 Conclusions

Determining the distribution of speckle in US images has received a considerable attention in the literature, with a wide range of applications including image segmentation, tissue characterization and image enhancement. While the most common assumption motivated by the central limit theorem consists of choosing a Gaussian distribution for RF images, leading to a Rayleigh distribution for the envelope images, a large variety of statistical models has been explored in the context of US imaging. The first part of this chapter reviewed the most significant distributions used to describe the statistical properties of speckle, both in the RF and envelope domains.

As an illustration of the proposed speckle models, the second part of the chapter introduced a Bayesian framework dedicated to the restoration of US images. Assuming a linear image formation model and a GGD for speckle, a method was proposed to both deconvolve RF images, i.e., estimate the TRF by removing the blurring effect of the PSF, and segment the images into statistically homogeneous regions. The segmentation part of the algorithm provided a label map dividing the image into piecewise constant regions that can be associated with the concept of US despeckling. The interest of the method was shown through two *in vivo* images acquired with a high frequency scanner on a mouse and on a patient with a malignant skin tumor.

References

[1] V. Dutt, "Statistical analysis of ultrasound echo envelope," *Ph.D. dissertation*, Mayo Graduate School, 1995.

[2] J. M. Sanches, A. F. Laine, and J. S. Suri, Eds., *Ultrasound imaging: advances and applications*. New York: Springer, 2011.

[3] R. S. C. Cobbold, Ed., *Foundations of biomedical ultrasound*. New York: Oxford University Press, 2007.

[4] O. Michailovich and A. Tannenbaum, "Despeckling of medical ultrasound images," *IEEE Trans. Ultrason. Ferroelectr. Freq. Control*, vol. 53, no. 1, pp. 64–78, 2006.

[5] C. P. Loizou, C. S. Pattichis, C. I. Christodoulou, R. S. H. Istepanian, M. Pantziaris, and A. Nicolaides, "Comparative evaluation of despeckle filtering in ultrasound imaging of the carotid artery," *IEEE Trans. Ultrason. Ferroelectr. Freq. Control*, vol. 52, no. 10, pp. 1653–1669, 2005.

[6] M. Alessandrini, S. Maggio, J. Poree, L. D. Marchi, N. Speciale, E. Franceschini, O. Bernard, and O. Basset, "A restoration framework for ultrasonic tissue characterization," *IEEE Trans. Ultrason. Ferroelectr. Freq. Control*, vol. 58, no. 11, pp. 2344–2360, 2011.

[7] J.-M. Girault, F. Ossant, A. Ouahabi, D. Kouamé, and F. Patat, "Time-varying autoregressive spectral estimation for ultrasound attenuation in tissue characterization," *IEEE Trans. Ultrason. Ferroelectr. Freq. Control*, vol. 45, no. 3, pp. 650–659, 1998.

[8] M. Pereyra, N. Dobigeon, H. Batatia, and J.-Y. Tourneret, "Segmentation of skin lesions in 2-D and 3-D ultrasound images using a spatially coherent generalized Rayleigh mixture model," *IEEE Trans. Med. Imag.*, vol. 31, no. 8, pp. 1509–1520, 2012.

[9] A. Basarab, H. Liebgott, F. Morestin, A. Lyshchik, T. Higashi, R. Asato, and P. Delacharte, "A method for vector displacement estimation with ultrasound images and its application for thyroid nodular disease," *Med. Image Anal.*, vol. 12, no. 3, pp. 259–274, 2008.

[10] A. Achim, A. Bezerianos, and P. Tsakalides, "Novel Bayesian multiscale method for speckle removal in medical ultrasound images," *IEEE Trans. Med. Imag.*, vol. 20, no. 8, pp. 772–783, 2001.

[11] N. Zhao, A. Basarab, D. Kouamé, and J.-Y. Tourneret, "Joint segmentation and deconvolution of ultrasound images using a hierarchical Bayesian model based on generalized Gaussian priors," *IEEE Trans. Image Process.*, vol. 25, no. 8, pp. 3736–3750, 2016.

[12] R. F. Wagner, M. F. Insana, and D. G. Brown, "Statistical properties of radio-frequency and envelope-detected signals with applications to medical ultrasound," *J. Opt. Soc. Am. A*, vol. 4, no. 5, pp. 910–922, 1987.

[13] O. Bernard, J. D'hooge, and D. Friboulet, "Statistics of the radio-frequency signal based on K distribution with application to echocardiography," *IEEE*

Trans. Ultrason. Ferroelectr. Freq. Control, vol. 53, no. 9, pp. 1689–1694, 2006.

[14] T. J. Klein, "Statistical image processing of medical ultrasound radio frequency data," Ph.D. dissertation, Technische Universitat München, 2012.

[15] J. W. Goodman, "Some fundamental properties of speckle," *J. Opt. Soc. Am.*, vol. 66, pp. 1145–1150, 1976.

[16] L. C. Gilman, "First-order statistics of pulsed-sinusoid backscatter from random media: basic elements of an exact treatment," *IEEE Trans. Ultrason. Ferroelectr. Freq. Control*, vol. 44, no. 4, pp. 798–804, 1997.

[17] T. Eltoft, "The Rician inverse Gaussian distribution: a new model for non-Rayleigh signal amplitude statistics," *IEEE Trans. Image Process.*, vol. 14, no. 11, 2005.

[18] P. M. Shankar, "A model for ultrasonic scattering from tissues based on the K distribution," *Phys. Med. Biol.*, vol. 40, no. 10, pp. 1633–1649, 1995.

[19] O. Bernard, B. Touil, J. Dhooge, and D. Friboulet, "Statistical modeling of the radio-frequency signal for partially- and fully-developed speckle based on a generalized Gaussian model with application to echocardiography," *IEEE Trans. Ultrason. Ferroelectr. Freq. Control*, vol. 54, no. 10, pp. 2189–2194, 2007.

[20] G. Moser, J. Zerubia, and S. B. Serpico, "SAR amplitude probability density function estimation based on a generalized Gaussian model," *IEEE Trans. Image Process.*, vol. 15, no. 6, pp. 1429–1442, 2006.

[21] M. A. Kutay, A. P. Petropulu, and C. W. Piccoli, "On modeling biomedical ultrasound RF echoes using a power-law shot-noise model," *IEEE Trans. Ultrason. Ferroelectr. Freq. Control*, vol. 48, no. 4, pp. 953–968, 2001.

[22] M. A. Pereyra and H. Batatia, "Modeling ultrasound echoes in skin tissues using symmetric α-stable processes," *IEEE Trans. Ultrason. Ferroelectr. Freq. Control*, vol. 59, pp. 60–72, 2012.

[23] M. N. Do and M. Vetterli, "Wavelet-based texture retrieval using generalized Gaussian density and Kullback–Leibler distance," *IEEE Trans. Image Process.*, vol. 11, no. 2, pp. 146–158, 2002.

[24] S. Meignen and H. Meignen, "On the modeling of small sample distributions with generalized Gaussian density in a maximum likelihood framework," *IEEE Trans. Image Process.*, vol. 15, no. 6, pp. 1647–1652, 2006.

[25] M. Pereyra, "Statistical modeling and processing of high frequency ultrasound images: application to determatologic oncology," *Ph.D. dissertation*, Institut National Polytechnique de Toulouse (INP Toulouse), 2012.

[26] R. Wagner, S. Smith, J. Sandrik, and H. Lopez, "Statistics of speckle in ultrasound B-scans," *IEEE Trans. Sonics and Ultrason.*, vol. 30, no. 5, pp. 156–163, 1983.

[27] P. M. Shankar, J. M. Reid, H. Ortega, C. W. Piccoli, and B. B. Goldberg, "Use of non-Rayleigh statistics for the identification of tumors in ultrasonic

B-scans of the breast," *IEEE Trans. Med. Imag.*, vol. 12, no. 4, pp. 687–692, 1993.

[28] R. Barakat, "Weak-scatterer generalization of the k-density function with application to laser scattering in atmospheric turbulence," *J. Opt. Soc. Am. A*, vol. 3, no. 4, pp. 401–409, 1986.

[29] V. Dutt and J. F. Greenleaf, "Ultrasound echo envelope analysis using a homodyned K distribution signal model," *Ultrasonic Imaging*, vol. 16, no. 4, pp. 265–287, 1994.

[30] B. I. Raju and M. A. Srinivasan, "Statistics of envelope of high-frequency ultrasonic backscatter from human skin in vivo," *IEEE Trans. Ultrason. Ferroelectr. Freq. Control*, vol. 49, no. 7, pp. 871–882, 2002.

[31] P. Shankar, "A general statistical model for ultrasonic backscatter from tissues," *IEEE Trans. Ultrason. Ferroelectr. Freq. Control*, vol. 47, no. 3, pp. 727–736, 2000.

[32] J. W. Goodman, Ed., *Speckle phenomena in optics: theory and applications*. Roberts and Company Publishers, 2007.

[33] A. Sarti, C. Corsi, E. Mazzini, and C. Lamberti, "Maximum likelihood segmentation of ultrasound images with Rayleigh distribution," *IEEE Trans. Ultrason. Ferroelectr. Freq. Control*, vol. 52, no. 6, pp. 947–960, 2005.

[34] T. A. Tuthill, R. H. Sperry, and K. J. Parker, "Deviation from Rayleigh statistics in ultrasonic speckle," *Ultrasonic Imaging*, vol. 10, no. 2, pp. 81–90, 1988.

[35] E. Jakeman, "On the statistics of *K*-distribution noise," *J. Phys. A.: Math. Gen.*, vol. 13, no. 1, pp. 31–48, 1980.

[36] D. P. Hruska and M. L. Oelze, "Improved parameter estimates based on the homodyned K distribution," *IEEE Trans. Ultrason. Ferroelectr. Freq. Control*, vol. 56, no. 11, pp. 2471–2481, 2009.

[37] J. Cheng and N. Beaulieu, "Generalized moment estimators for the Nakagami fading parameters," *IEEE Commun. Lett.*, vol. 6, no. 4, pp. 144–146, 2002.

[38] J. Cheng and N. Beaulieu, "Maximum-likelihood based estimation of the Nakagami-m parameter," *IEEE Commun. Lett.*, vol. 5, no. 3, pp. 101–103, 2001.

[39] T. Z, T. H.D, and D. Beaty, "Evaluation of four probability distribution models for speckle in clinical cardiac ultrasound images," *IEEE Trans. Med. Imaging*, vol. 25, no. 11, p. 1483–1491, 2006.

[40] R. F. Wagner, S. W. Smith, M. Sandrik, and H. Lopez, "Statistics of speckle in ultrasound b-scans," *IEEE Trans. Son. Ultrason*, vol. 30, pp. 156–163, 1983.

[41] D. V and G. J. F, "Adaptive speckle reduction filter for log-compressed b-scan images," *IEEE Trans. Med. Imaging*, vol. 15, no. 6, pp. 802–813, 1996.

[42] J. Seabra and J. Sanches, "Modeling log-compressed ultrasound images for radio frequency signal recovery," in *Proc. IEEE Eng. Med. Biol. Conf. (EMBC)*, Vancouver, BC, Canada, 2008, pp. 426–429.

[43] D. Kaplan and Q. Ma, "On the statistical characteristics of log-compressed Rayleigh signals," in *Proc. IEEE Ultrasonics Symposium (IUS)*, New York, 1993, pp. 961–964.

[44] A. Perperidis, "Postprocessing approach for the improvement of cardiac ultrasound B-mode images: a review," *IEEE Trans. Ultrason. Ferroelectr. Freq. Control*, vol. 63, no. 3, pp. 470–485, 2016.

[45] R. Touzi, "A review of speckle filtering in the context of estimation theory," *IEEE Trans. Geosci. Remote Sens.*, vol. 40, no. 11, pp. 2392–2404, 2002.

[46] J. C. Bamber and C. Daft, "Adaptive filtering for reduction of speckle in ultrasonic pulse-echo images," *Ultrasonics*, vol. 24, no. 1, pp. 41–44, 1986.

[47] Y. Chen, R. Yin, P. Flynn, and S. Broschat, "Aggressive region growing for speckle reduction in ultrasound images," *Pattern Recogn. Lett.*, vol. 24, no. 4–5, pp. 677–691, Feb. 2003.

[48] Y. Yu and S. T. Acton, "Speckle reducing anisotropic diffusion," *IEEE Trans. Image Process.*, vol. 11, no. 11, pp. 1260–1270, 2002.

[49] K. Krissian, C. F. Westin, R. Kikinis, and K. G. Vosburgh, "Oriented speckle reducing anisotropic diffusion," *IEEE Trans. Image Process.*, vol. 16, no. 5, pp. 1412–1424, 2007.

[50] P. Coupé, P. Hellier, C. Kervrann, and C. Barillot, "Nonlocal means-based speckle filtering for ultrasound images," *IEEE Trans. Image Process.*, vol. 18, no. 10, pp. 2221–2229, 2009.

[51] S. Finn, M. Glavin, and E. Jones, "Echocardiographic speckle reduction comparison," *IEEE Trans. Ultrason. Ferroelectr. Freq. Control*, vol. 58, no. 1, pp. 82–101, 2011.

[52] R. Chan, H. Yang, and T. Zeng, "A two-stage image segmentation method for blurry images with Poisson or multiplicative gamma noise," *SIAM J. Imag. Sci.*, vol. 7, no. 1, pp. 98–127, 2014.

[53] M. Storath, A. Weinmann, J. Frikel, and M. Unser, "Joint image reconstruction and segmentation using the Potts model," *Inv. Prob.*, no. 2, pp. 1–29, 2015.

[54] G. Paul, J. Cardinale, and I. F. Sbalzarini, "Coupling image restoration and segmentation: A generalized linear model/Bregman perspective," *Int. J. Comput. Vis.*, vol. 104, no. 1, pp. 69–93, 2013.

[55] M. Alessandrini, A. Palladini, L. D. Marchi, and N. Speciale, "Expectation maximization for joint deconvolution and statistics estimation," *Acoust. Imag.*, vol. 30, no. 11, pp. 335–343, 2011.

[56] N. Zhao, A. Basarab, D. Kouamé, and J.-Y. Tourneret, "Restoration of ultrasound images using a hierarchical Bayesian model with a generalized Gaussian prior," in *Proc. IEEE Int. Conf. Image Process. (ICIP)*, Paris, France, 2014.

[57] M. Pereyra, N. Dobigeon, H. Batatia, and J.-Y. Tourneret, "Estimating the granularity coefficient of a Potts-Markov random field within a Markov chain Monte Carlo algorithm," *IEEE Trans. Image Process.*, vol. 22, no. 6, pp. 2385–2397, 2013.

[58] C. Yu, C. Zhang, and L. Xie, "A blind deconvolution approach to ultrasound imaging," *IEEE Trans. Ultrason. Ferroelectr. Freq. Control*, vol. 59, no. 2, pp. 271–280, 2012.
[59] B. M. Asl and A. Mahloojifar, "Eigenspace-based minimum variance beamforming applied to medical ultrasound imaging," *IEEE Trans. Ultrason. Ferroelectr. Freq. Control*, vol. 57, no. 11, pp. 2381–2390, 2010.

Chapter 4

Summary

Christos P. Loizou[1]

In this final chapter of Part I (Introduction to speckle noise in ultrasound imaging and video), we present the summary findings of the chapters presented.

After the foreword and the guide to the books contents, we presented in Chapter 1 a brief review on ultrasound imaging and video where a pedagogical overview on the technical foundations of ultrasound imaging was provided. It was intended to equip readers with fundamental principles that would serve well as background knowledge to understand the broad range of technical concepts covered in this book. The key imaging considerations as well as the engineering aspects such as system hardware were covered. A commentary on the emerging trend toward high-frame-rate imaging was included to highlight latest innovation thrusts in ultrasound imaging.

In Chapter 2, the basic physical origins of speckle and different, but related, mathematical descriptions of speckle in simple model systems were discussed. The chapter started with a general description of scattered waves as phasors, deriving first-order statistics applicable to both laser speckle and ultrasound speckle. It then discussed the correspondences and differences between laser speckle and ultrasound speckle, before presenting higher order statistics and imaging implications in an ultrasound context. The impact of the imaging system characteristics on speckle appearance and statistics was then at the end introduced and outlined.

Chapter 3 summarizes existing results related to the statistical properties of ultrasound images based on both radio-frequency and envelope signals. In a second part of the chapter, a Bayesian deconvolution method that can be viewed as a general despeckling technique was presented.

Part I concludes with a summary of the chapters presented.

The rest of this book will particularly highlight on a variety of advances in speckle filtering and tracking, and how these algorithmic tools are being applied to cardiovascular ultrasound.

[1]University of Cyprus, Department of Electrical and Computer Engineering, Cyprus

Part II

Speckle filtering

Chapter 5
Introduction to speckle filtering

Gabriel Ramos-Llordén[1], Santiago Aja-Fernández[2], and Gonzalo Vegas-Sánchez-Ferrero[3,4]

This chapter aims to introduce the reader into the field of speckle filtering, by emphasizing its particular characteristics that are relevant for every practitioner in the field. We begin with an introduction to filtering in medical imaging where we stress the importance of information preservation over complete filtering. This broad view motivates the following discussion on the main issues concerning speckle filtering and provides a reasonable framework to approach it. We elaborate on topics that we believe are rather specific to speckle and should be taken into account whenever the different filters described in following chapters are utilized.

5.1 The problem of filtering in medical imaging

It is important to have in mind when dealing with medical imaging that the data under consideration usually incorporates sensitive information. The knowledge contained into the intensity pattern that conforms the image has not been acquired with esthetic purposes but with a clinical or research aim. Therefore, special care must be taken not to eliminate or modified that information: no filtering procedure should be done with simple esthetic purposes. Although this premise is clearly shared by most medical imaging researchers, it is sometimes left aside when validating new filtering schemes using *visual comparison*.

From a practical point of view, filtering in medical imaging (particularly in ultrasound imaging) must be **conservative** under the following terms [1]:

1. No significant information present in the image must be removed of modified. In ultrasound imaging, important structures can be interleaved with speckle and thus aggressive filtering can eliminate small regions of interest or texture information, which could be a risk for diagnosis. In addition, some filtering

[1]Imec-Vision Lab, Department of Physics, University of Antwerp, Belgium
[2]ETSI Telecomunicación, Universidad de Valladolid, Spain
[3]Applied Chest Imaging Laboratory (ACIL), Brigham and Women's Hospital, Harvard Medical School, USA
[4]Biomedical Image Technologies Laboratory (BIT), ETSI Telecomunicación, Universidad Politécnica de Madrid, and CIBER-BBN, Spain

methodologies can alter the edges on the image causing a distortion of objects' sizes, introducing errors and bias in the measure of volume or distances.
2. Keep intact all information relevant to the physicians. The speckle pattern, that usually is seen as *noise* by engineers, has texture information that is useful for the expert. Before *cleaning* or smoothing a specific area of the image, its visual role of noise in diagnosis must be checked. Note that sometimes the removal of all the speckle patterns can also remove valuable information about the mobility of certain structures.
3. Do not add information. Filtering artifacts can appear as a side effect of certain denoising techniques. Sometimes, these artifacts can be interpreted as anatomical features, and a false diagnosis can be derived.

Thus, the rule of thumb for filtering any medical imaging modality would be "if you cannot keep all the important information, do not filter." Most of the approaches in literature are usually validated via spectacular visual results. However, the main quality of medical imaging filter is not its ability to produce good-looking pictures but to ensure that no relevant information is removed. In [2], for instance, the visual subject evaluation of several speckle filters over ultrasound data that was carried out by clinical experts produced some paradoxical results: the image with the highest score was that without filtering. The output of any filter was perceived by clinical experts as a loss of quality.

With this requirement in mind, the first step before utilizing any speckle reduction filter is to consider the final purpose of the specific filtering process. Every method in literature presents some advantages and disadvantages, and there is no multipurpose universal method. Thus, the removal or reduction of speckle in ultrasound data has to be done attending the utterly use of the filtered image. The most common scenarios are the following:

1. **Visual quality:** Ultrasound data is filtered in order to improve its visual quality. No further processing is going to be made, or numerical markers obtained from the data; the purpose is just to reduce the speckle in order to help a visual inspection. Although many of the filters proposed in literature can be used, it is important to notice that the total elimination of the speckle pattern does not help an expert to better understand the image. On the contrary, the total removal of speckle makes the image looks *fake* or *artificial*, and the expert will discard it as not suitable for diagnosis. It is important, then, to keep the speckle in those areas that can have important structural information.

   Once more, we must keep in mind that the processing to achieve better visual results must not only seek *good-looking* pictures, but to ease the visual understanding of the data by an expert. Note that noise is an acceptable artifact for the human eye, which is used to work with it. Thus, noise must be erased only if it hinders the expert from properly understanding the data, or if it hides important information. Thus, overfiltering to achieve better visual results is not advisable.
2. **Further processing:** Most of the times, the purpose of filtering ultrasound data is not to simply improve its visual quality, but to improve the response of

different algorithms that will be used to extract information from the data. Note that, this time, the quality of a filtering method is no longer related to the nice appearance of the images, but to the improvement in the accuracy of the algorithms. Some significant applications are:

(i) **Segmentation:** One of the purposes of noise reduction in an image is to improve the accuracy of different segmentation procedures. Note that, for this specific application, there is no need of maintaining the original levels or even to keep all the small details in the image. On the contrary, we are interested in enhancing the borders and transitions between structures and smoothing homogeneous regions.

(ii) **Measure of geometrical distances:** Similar to the previous application, measuring distances, areas or volumes inside the image do not require to keep the original values, but to enhance the structures to be measured. There is no need to obtain a realistic image. However, note that this application is very sensitive to border effects and to dilation and contraction of edges resulting from the processing. A median filter, for instance, could provide good-looking images, but the risk of modifying the area of different regions is high.

We want to recall the importance of selecting filtering and validation methods totally adapted to the specific needs of the problem. There is no all-purpose filter that, with the same configuration parameters, could perform excellent in all situations. Sometimes, very simple filtering techniques are enough for the requirements of the application.

5.2 Important issues about speckle filtering

Following the premises set in the previous section, let us now go deeper into the particular topics of speckle filtering that are not necessarily shared by other medical imaging modalities and hence are of notable interest.

5.2.1 On the ultimate goal of speckle filtering

In Section 5.1, we have already stated that the filter of speckle patterns must follow a specific purpose. Furthermore, even with that purpose in mind, there is no definite consensus about the ultimate goal of speckle filtering. This apparently bold statement stems from the recognized debate on the meaning of speckle in terms of information theory: any kind of speckle removal will depend on what speckle means from a signal processing perspective [3–5]. *Is speckle useful information that should be maintained?* Instead, *should it be considered as noise, and therefore it must be totally removed? Are there situations where may be beneficial to preserve speckle in some regions while suppress it in others?* All of these questions are yet at the heart of the ultrasound speckle filtering field. There is no perfect answer for all them. We instead believe that those questions are better responded if the final target of the processing pipeline is considered. In other words, the final application must determine what kind of filtering approach should be accomplished. In the following, we consider two different scenarios.

5.2.1.1 Complete speckle elimination

Let us assume that the purpose of the processing pipeline is the segmentation of regions or organs from the ultrasound data. Broadly speaking, image segmentation is the process of partitioning an image into multiple segments or regions to ease the final understanding of the information. Segmentation of medical imaging is known to be a complicated task, specially hard when dealing with ultrasound imaging, where many sophisticated segmentation methods are constantly been proposed [6]. The separation of regions relies on the ability to distinguish features that are different between regions. The simplest feature to take into account is the intensity value of each region. However, most general purpose segmentation methods are known to fail when directly applied over ultrasound data, due precisely to the variability of the speckle pattern. Consequently, in this situation, the removal of the whole speckle pattern is notably recommendable. Most of the classical speckle filters [7,8] as well as the initial contributions in diffusion-based filters [9–12] are examples of techniques that aim to remove speckle for segmentation purposes. All these filters are based on a multiplicative model that considers the speckle to be *noise* that must be removed. As a consequence, the output images are nearly piecewise constant inside each tissue. Though cartoon-like images may not be visually pleasant, they can be convenient for segmentation-based goals.

5.2.1.2 Selective speckle elimination

Opposite to the previous example, there are many cases in which a total removal of the speckle is not advisable. It is well known that speckle may contain clinical relevant information [3,4], with applications to tissue characterization [13,14] or to the derivation of biomarkers, which are mainly based on geometrical distances and volumes. In those cases, total elimination of the speckle pattern may remove sensitive information for diagnosis. On the other hand, in some automatic processing applications, like *speckle tracking*, the presence of speckle is also relevant. Speckle tracking algorithms follow the motion of the tissues precisely using the features present in speckle [15]. Finally, if final purpose of the image is to be used by a clinical expert, the image can be *enhanced* but, for a better visual understanding, it is preferable to keep some of the speckle.

In those situations, the design of the filtering process should be aware of the necessity of maintaining salient features that are crucial for subsequent steps. In this regard, speckle filters should not only maintain the edges definition but also to retain the texture and the structural details, that is, the speckle pattern, inside regions that are clinically relevant in further analysis steps. In common highly detail preservation speckle filters, such as nonlocal means based [16] or other sophisticated diffusion filters [17], there is a trade-off between detail preservation and speckle removal. Allowing subtle details definitions may lead to maintain speckle in areas with relatively low clinical relevance, such as regions containing blood. That trade-off can be substantially reduced by using tissue-selective speckle filters, such as the probabilistically memory-driven diffusion filter technique proposed in [18]. Such techniques often rely on a good classification mechanism to separate between clinical regions and nuisance areas. Indeed, that kind of filtering can be seen as joint segmentation-filtering process, where both techniques benefit from each other to yield highly detailed denoised ultrasound images.

5.2.2 On the necessity of an accurate speckle model

As we mentioned in the introduction, we really stick to the idea that information preservation should be given priority in comparison to purely spurious fluctuation denoising when an ultrasound speckle filter is assessed. From an information theory point of view, one needs to distinguish what is information from what is considered noise. To do such a distinction, one necessitates of a physical model which characterizes the complete physical process, from the US echoes generated in the tissue interfaces to the voltage signal conversion in the transducer. A physical model which characterizes such a process is called a speckle model. That speckle model should be taken into account when the despeckling filter is designed. Thereby, the quality of the speckle model has a crucial effect on the filter's performance. Yet, a wide variety of speckle filters rely on the simple but popular so-called multiplicative speckle model [10].

More accurate and elaborated speckle models rely on a probabilistic description of the ultrasound signals. For this purpose, and due to the random nature of the speckle, several statistical models have been proposed in the literature. The parameters of the statistical models allow identifying the features of these tissues and provide important descriptors for classification. Probably the most well-known models are the Rayleigh model or the Rician model [19]. These probabilistic distributions arise when the effective number of scatterers that are present in the resolution cell are considered [14,18]. Although those models are based on physical assumptions of the backscattering process, some other distributions have proved to result in a good performance on real images. This is the case of Nakagami [20] and especially the Gamma distribution [14]. Note that every signal processing step applied to the received US voltage signal will make the statistics deviate from the ideal conditions that give rise to Rayleigh or Rician model. This is the case of simple but ubiquitous operations such as interpolation or filtering [14].

5.2.3 Practical implementation, filter parameters and noise estimation

One important issue that must also be considered is the practical implementation of the proposed methods. The implementation involves important steps such as the discretization of the proposed algorithm, numerical approximation or the specifics of the available data. The final performance of a filtering process many times lays on the way it is implemented, rather than on the correctness of the theoretical developments.

In addition to the election of proper numerical implementation, some of the methods have some input parameters that must be tuned in order to achieve an optimal estimation. Some of these parameters are more sensitive to variations than others. A robust method would be that that allows variations in the parameters without great variations in the result. For instance, the so-called speckle diffusion filters in [10,11] avoids the manual tuning of the diffusion parameters by automatically estimated them from the level of noise. On the other hand, hose methods that use a neighborhood around each pixel, like the classical filters in [7,8,21,22], highly depend on the size and shape of this neighborhood. The larger the window, the larger the number of points and the better the estimation of the parameters inside that window. However, a larger size may imply some edge blurring and an augmentation of the partial volume effect when different signal regions lie in the neighborhood of the pixel.

5.2.3.1 Some practical implementation issues

Probably, the most important advantage of ultrasound imaging in comparison to other medical imaging modalities is that images can be acquired on real time. Movement of anatomical structures can be observed at the time it really occurs. Thereby, if speckle filter is included as part of the image processing pipeline in a real-time application, time constraints should be taken into account when the filter is constructed. In particular, it should be assured that the computation time required for the filtering process does not prevent from being able to get images with enough temporal resolution. Time constraints are normally not an issue for simple filters but can be a serious concern for speckle filters based on iterative algorithms, such as diffusion filters. As it will be described in other chapters, diffusion filters rely on the discretization of partial differential equation, thus leading to iterative schemes that could be time consuming. Though effort in better discretization scheme have been done during the last decades, yet computational speed remains as one of the main handicaps of those approaches, which in turn limits their applicability on real time scenarios. Though not directly related, memory requirements are other aspect that speckle filter designer may consider to reduce the computational burden. Such memory conditions often appear in speckle filters that can be cast as an optimization framework. In large-scale optimization problems is often necessary to store data with high dimensionality. Hence, portable US devices may have difficulties in incorporating hardware requirements to accommodate such load of information.

Other criterion that may be assessed is the automation of the filter, in the sense that it can work without any user intervention. An unsupervised functioning is relevant for real-time applications but also for an off-line analysis of US images since manual preprocessing of every US image could be highly time consuming. It should be noted that some filter requires the delineation of several regions in the image with the aim of estimating some parameters inherent to the filter. That is the case of the coefficient of variation, briefly described in next section, and which is often used in diffusion speckle filters. An automatic process instead would be of high interest and may enhance the applicability of the filtering method substantially.

5.2.3.2 Estimation of the coefficient of variation

As previously stated, some methods avoid the manual choice of the filter parameters by linking them to the level of noise in the image. The term *noise* in speckle may be ambiguous, since not all the speckle pattern can be strictly considered as noise. Let us focus on those filters that assume that the speckle is a kind of multiplicative noise. Some of the most common filtering methods in literature are based on the assumption of a Gaussian multiplicative model:

$$I(\mathbf{x}) = A(\mathbf{x})\eta_N\left(\mathbf{x};\mu,\sigma^2\right), \tag{5.1}$$

where $\mathbf{x}$ denotes the spatial position in a given set Ω, and where $A(\mathbf{x})$ is the underlying signal and $\eta_N(\mathbf{x};\mu,\sigma^2)$ is Gaussian noise with mean μ and variance σ^2. The (square) coefficient of variation of noise is then defined as

$$C_N^2 = \frac{\sigma^2}{\mu}. \tag{5.2}$$

This coefficient of variation of noise has been use as a measure of the *noise level* in some of the first statistical approaches, like the linear minimum mean square error approaches by Lee [21], Frost [7], and Kuan [22], in the anisotropic diffusion speckle filter proposed by Yu and Acton [10], and in many other filters like [11,12,23–27]. In Synthetic Aperture Radar (SAR) imaging, this coefficient is inversely related to the *effective number of looks*.

An accurate estimation of this parameter is key for the proper behavior of the filters. Many different methods have been proposed in order to estimate C_N^2. The most direct way, as done in [7,10,21], is the use of the mean and variance of the image intensity over a homogeneous area. In [28], authors propose a methodology that no longer needs the segmentation of a homogeneous area:

$$\hat{C}_N = \frac{1.4826}{\sqrt{2}}\mathrm{MAD}\{\nabla\log I(\mathbf{x})\} \tag{5.3}$$

where MAD is the absolute deviation of the median, a robust estimator defined as

$$\mathrm{MAD}\{S_N\} = \mathrm{median}\{\|S_N - \mathrm{median}\{S_N\}\|\}. \tag{5.4}$$

In [29], authors develop an estimator based on the maximum value of the distribution, i.e., the mode

$$\hat{C}_N^2 = \mathrm{mode}\left\{C_I^2(\mathbf{x})\right\}, \tag{5.5}$$

where $C_I^2(\mathbf{x})$ is the local sample (square) coefficient of variation of the noisy signal. The advantage of this estimator is that it does not require a segmentation of an area of interest. Nevertheless, it is sensitive to a proper estimation of the mode of the distribution, so it requires some robust method to do it. Further discussion about this issue can be found in [30].

Note that the use of this coefficient variation has sense only when the multiplicative Gaussian model is assumed. If we consider other common speckle model, such as the Rayleigh or Rayleigh, the coefficient of variation is no longer a valid measure of noise, since it will be a constant, regardless of the signal or noise value:

$$C_N^2 = \frac{4 - \pi}{\pi}. \tag{5.6}$$

5.2.4 Evaluation and validation of speckle filtering

As in other medical imaging modalities, the validation of speckle filters could be either quantitative or qualitative. While in the former case, the quality of the final result is assessed by using numerical metrics that aim to capture desirable properties that a "good" filtering should possess, within a qualitative assessment, a judgment about the filtering performance is carried out by a clinical specialist.

Probably, the most widespread approach in a medical imaging quantitative evaluation framework is that based on simulation-based experiments. In that approach, a synthetic image is created. This image, naturally, should resemble a real acquired image (an ultrasound image in the given case) as much as possible. To produce accurate and realistic simulation setups, an image formation model is needed. That image formation model is what we have described as speckle model before. Implicitly, in that model, there is a clear distinction between what is considered the true image, that is, the information to be preserved, and the noise, the part that may be suppressed. If that if so, the filtered synthetic image with a given filter, let's say $\hat{I}(\mathbf{x})$, can be compared to the *true* image (ground-truth image), $I_{\mathrm{GT}}(\mathbf{x})$. Large deviations from this ground-truth image suggest that the speckle filtering was inadequate. Conversely, the closest the filtered image becomes, the better the filtering process is. The dissimilarity between the ground-truth and the filtered image could be measured with, for example, the mean squared error, the absolute differences deviation or more complex metrics which incorporates aspects from visual perception, such as the structural similarity index metric (SSIM) [31]. Other used metrics are the geometric average error and peak signal-to-noise ratio. In Table 5.1, we report a complete list of metrics that are often use in speckle filtering validation based on ground-truth measures.

Unfortunately, being able to define a well-accepted ground-truth image in ultrasound denoising is a rather idealistic situation. In contrast to other medical modalities, there is no a *de facto* standard image formation model, as it was discussed on Section 5.2.2, where several speckle models were mentioned. We would like to make the reader aware of this point when attempting to validate a speckle filter and draw categorical conclusions. While with the simplistic multiplicative speckle noise, definition of the ground-truth image may be possible, more accurate statistical speckle models make this approach often impossible. Hence, other quantitative approaches may be pursued, and those can be made directly on actual ultrasound images and not necessarily synthetic ones. This approach is common practice in ultrasound denoising validation, and it may provide more informative

Table 5.1 The quantitative measures commonly employed in speckle filter assessment with a given ground-truth image

Metric	Mathematical expression	Ref.
Mean squared error (MSE)	$\mathrm{MSE} = \frac{1}{\lvert\Omega\rvert}\sum_{\mathbf{x}\in\Omega}\left(I_{\mathrm{GT}}(\mathbf{x}) - \hat{I}(\mathbf{x})\right)^2$	[32]
Average difference (AD)	$\mathrm{AD} = \frac{1}{\lvert\Omega\rvert}\sum_{\mathbf{x}\in\Omega}\lvert I_{\mathrm{GT}}(\mathbf{x}) - \hat{I}(\mathbf{x})\rvert$	[32]
Root mean square error (RMSE)	$\mathrm{RMSE} = \sqrt{\frac{1}{\lvert\Omega\rvert}\sum_{\mathbf{x}\in\Omega}\left(I_{\mathrm{GT}}(\mathbf{x}) - \hat{I}(\mathbf{x})\right)^2}$	[32]
Peak signal-to-noise ratio (PSNR)	$\mathrm{PSNR} = 10\log_{10}\left(\frac{(\max\{I_{\mathrm{GT}}(\mathbf{x})\})^2}{\mathrm{MSE}}\right)$	[32]
Geometric average error (GAE)	$\mathrm{GAE} = \left(\prod_{\mathbf{x}\in\Omega}\sqrt{I_{\mathrm{GT}}(\mathbf{x}) - \hat{I}(\mathbf{x})}\right)^{\frac{1}{\Omega}}$	[31]
Figure of merit (FOM)	$\mathrm{FOM} = \frac{1}{\max\{N, N_{\mathrm{GT}}\}}\sum_{i=1}^{N}\frac{1}{1+\alpha d_i^2}$	[10]
Structural similarity index (SSIM)	$\mathrm{SSIM} = \frac{\left(2\mu_{\hat{I}}\mu_{I_{\mathrm{GT}}} + C_1\right)\left(2\sigma_{\hat{I},I_{\mathrm{GT}}} + C_2\right)}{\left(\mu_{\hat{I}}^2 + \mu_{I_{\mathrm{GT}}}^2 + C_1\right)\left(\sigma_{\hat{I}}^2 + \sigma_{I_{\mathrm{GT}}}^2 + C_2\right)}$	[33]
Quantitative index based on local variance (QILV)	$\mathrm{QILV} = \frac{\left(2\mu_{Var\{\hat{I}\}}\mu_{\mathrm{Var}\{I_{\mathrm{GT}}\}}\right)\left(2\sigma_{\mathrm{Var}\{\hat{I}\}\,\mathrm{Var}\{I_{\mathrm{GT}}\}}\right)}{\left(\mu_{\mathrm{Var}\{\hat{I}\}}^2 + \mu_{\mathrm{Var}\{I_{\mathrm{GT}}\}}^2\right)\left(\sigma_{\mathrm{Var}\{\hat{I}\}}^2 + \sigma_{Var\{I_{\mathrm{GT}}\}}^2\right)}$	[34]

$\lvert\Omega\rvert$ denotes the cardinal of Ω. FOM: N and N_{GT} represents the number of detected edges in $\hat{I}(\mathbf{x})$ and the number of edges in $I_{\mathrm{GT}}(\mathbf{x})$, respectively; d_i is the Euclidean distance between the ith detected edge pixel and the nearest ideal edge pixel; α is a constant set typically to 1/9 [10]. SSIM: the local mean of filtered image $\hat{I}(\mathbf{x})$ and GT image $I_{\mathrm{GT}}(\mathbf{x})$ is represented by μ_I and μ_{IGT}, whereas the local standard deviation is written as σ_I and $\sigma_{I_{GT}}$; $\sigma_{I,I_{GT}}$ is the covariance between those two images; constants C_1 and C_2 are used for normalization and do not convey any structural information. QILV: $Var\{\hat{I}\}$ and $Var\{I_{\mathrm{GT}}\}$ represent the so-called variance image of $\hat{I}(\mathbf{x})$ and $I_{\mathrm{GT}}(\mathbf{x})$, respectively.

results than a simulation-based experiment. Some of the techniques that have been employed in this framework are based on texture analysis and k-nearest neighbors (k-NN) classifiers, to name just a few. The interested reader is referred to [31] for a more detailed description.

Last, we should not obviate the importance of qualitative assessment. Qualitative assessment of speckle denoising has the advantage of being able to take into account relevant aspects for physicians and clinical scientist which are left aside using quantitative metrics, or that simply are impossible to conceptualize with mathematical models. After all, as mentioned in the introduction, human observers have the ability of understanding image information under the presence of noise. In those cases, though, a rigorous protocol has inevitably to deal with the inter- and intra-observer variability [31].

A general conclusion that may be extracted from these words is that a prescribed validation framework for speckle filter is always inherently arguable. Perhaps, a more comprehensive approach should instead considering the ultimate goal of the filtering process within pipeline, and often this necessitates of a less constrained evaluation framework that incorporates both qualitative assessment and numerical metrics directly related to the purpose at hand.

5.2.5 On the similarity between SAR and ultrasound images

When one seeks for speckle denoising filters in ultrasound imaging it is often common to discover that those filters have already been utilized in a different image modality called SAR imaging. SAR imaging is a well-developed coherent remote sensing technique which provides large-scale 2D high spatial resolution images of the Earth's surface. As SAR imaging is also based on the coherent interference of many wave components which are reflected from different elements, speckle noise naturally appears as in ultrasound imaging. Therefore, speckle models that are valid in SAR imaging also hold in ultrasound imaging. The fact that speckle models are in principle equally applicable in both disciplines, explain why speckle filters conceived for SAR images are also often used for despeckling medical ultrasound images. For instance, many well-known filters like [7, 10, 21, 22] were derived for SAR images. In those images, the multiplicative model for speckle holds, and therefore many of the methods defined in literature for SAR can be easily extrapolated to ultrasound.

5.3 Some final remarks

With this chapter, we have attempted to cover relevant aspects of speckle filtering that are useful to bear in mind before analyzing each speckle filtering methodology in detailed. We have begun by elaborating on the importance of preserving information over drastic filtering. Being our personal point-of-view, we really believe that this philosophy can be strongly supported, independent of personal taste, in the case of medical imaging, where quantitative information is of uttermost importance. Ultrasound imaging is not, of course, an exception. As elaborated in the second section, about particular issues on speckle filtering, we stressed that the ultimate step of the image processing pipelines considerably shaped the speckle filtering design before. Different speckle filters may demonstrate a fantastic performance for one particular application but can miserably failed in other cases. The interested practitioner should be aware of this. Filtering assessment-based aspects and implementation issues are also addressed in last sections, as well as the influence of the SAR field on the developing of new medical US filters. Perhaps more importantly, we want to remark the relevance of speckle modeling alone. From our experience, speckle filtering should be accompanied with an accurate speckle model behind. Since speckle modeling is still a very hot-topic research with new speckle models continuously arising, we expect that the future of the speckle filtering field is going to evolve mainly stimulated by new findings on modeling rather than on implementation-based improvements.

Acknowledgments

This work was supported by Ministerio de Ciencia e Innovación (Spain) with research grant TEC2013-44194-P. Gonzalo Vegas-Sánchez-Ferrero acknowledges Consejería de Educación, Juventud y Deporte of Comunidad de Madrid and the People Programme (Marie Curie Actions) of the European Union's Seventh Framework Programme (FP7/2007–2013) for REA grant agreement no. 291820.

References

[1] Aja-Fernández S, Vegas-Sánchez-Ferrero G. Noise filtering in MRI. In: Statistical Analysis of Noise in MRI. AG Switzerland: Springer International Publishing; 2016. p. 89–119.

[2] Finn S. Speckle Reduction and Edge Detection in Ultrasound Imagery [PhD Thesis]. National University of Ireland Galway. Galway, Ireland; 2010.

[3] Wagner RF, Smith SW, Sandrik JM, Lopez H. Statistics of speckle in ultrasound B-scans. IEEE Trans Ultrason Ferroelectr Freq Control. 1983;30 (3): 156–163.

[4] Wagner RF, Insana MF, Brown DG. Unified approach to the detection and classification of speckle texture in diagnostic ultrasound. Opt Eng. 1986;25 (6): 738–742.

[5] Thijssen J, Oosterveld B. Texture in tissue echograms: speckle or information? J Ultrasound Med. 1990;9(4): 215–229.

[6] Noble JA, Boukerroui D. Ultrasound image segmentation: a survey. IEEE Trans Med Imaging. 2006;25(8): 987–1010.

[7] Frost VS, Stiles JA, Shanmugan KS, Holzman JC. A model for RADAR images and its application to adaptive digital filtering of multiplicative noise. IEEE Trans Pattern Anal Mach Intell. 1982;PAMI-4(2): 157–166.

[8] Kuan DT, Sawchuk AA, Strand TC, Chavel P. Adaptive restoration of images with speckle. IEEE Trans Acoust Speech Signal Process. 1987 Mar; ASSP-35(3): 373–383.

[9] Aja S, Alberola C, Ruiz A. Fuzzy anisotropic diffusion for speckle filtering. In: Acoustics, Speech, and Signal Processing, 2001. Proceedings (ICASSP'01). 2001 IEEE International Conference on. vol. 2. IEEE; 2001. p. 1261–1264.

[10] Yu Y, Acton ST. Speckle reducing anisotropic diffusion. IEEE Trans Image Process. 2002;11(11): 1260–1270.

[11] Aja-Fernández S, Alberola-López C. On the estimation of the coefficient of variation for anisotropic diffusion speckle filtering. IEEE Trans Image Process. 2006;15(9): 2694–2701.

[12] Krissian K, Westin CF, Kikinis R, Vosburgh KG. Oriented speckle reducing anisotropic diffusion. IEEE Trans Image Process. 2007;16(5): 1412–1424.

[13] Seabra JC, Ciompi F, Pujol O, Mauri J, Radeva P, Sanches J. Rayleigh mixture model for plaque characterization in intravascular ultrasound. IEEE Trans Biomed Eng. 2011;58(5): 1314–1324.

[14] Vegas-Sanchez-Ferrero G, Seabra J, Rodriguez-Leor O, *et al.* Gamma mixture classifier for plaque detection in intravascular ultrasonic images. IEEE Trans Ultrason Ferroelectr Freq Control. 2014;61(1): 44–61.

[15] Curiale AH, Vegas-Sánchez-Ferrero G, Aja-Fernández, S. Influence of ultrasound speckle tracking strategies for motion and strain estimation. Med Image Anal. 2016;32:184–200.

[16] Coupé P, Hellier P, Kervrann C, Barillot C. Nonlocal means-based speckle filtering for ultrasound images. IEEE Trans Image Process. 2009;18(10): 2221–2229.

[17] Vegas-Sanchez-Ferrero G, Aja-Fernaández S, Martín-Fernández M, Frangi AF, Palencia C. Probabilistic-driven oriented speckle reducing anisotropic diffusion with application to cardiac ultrasonic images. In: International Conference on Medical Image Computing and Computer-Assisted Intervention. Springer; 2010. p. 518–525.

[18] Ramos-Llordén G, Vegas-Sánchez-Ferrero G, Martin-Fernandez M, Alberola-López C, Aja-Fernández S. Anisotropic diffusion filter with memory based on speckle statistics for ultrasound Images. IEEE Trans Image Process. 2015;24(1): 345–358.

[19] Vegas-Sanchez-Ferrero G. Probabilistic Models for Tissue Characterization in Ultrasonic and Magnetic Resonance Medical Images and Applications [PhD Thesis]. University of Valladolid. Valladolid, Spain; 2012.

[20] Shankar PM, Dumane VA, Reid JM, *et al.* Classification of ultrasonic B-mode images of breast masses using Nakagami distribution. IEEE Trans Ultrason Ferroelectr Freq Control. 2001 Mar;48(2): 569–580.

[21] Lee JS. Speckle analysis and smoothing of synthetic aperture RADAR images. Comput Graph Image Process. 1981;17(1): 24–32.

[22] Kuan DT, Sawchuk AA, Strand TC, Chavel P. Adaptive noise smoothing filter for images with signal-dependent noise. IEEE Trans Pattern Anal Mach Intell. 1985 Mar;PAMI-7(2): 165–177.

[23] Kuan D, Sawchuk A, Strand T, Chavel P. Adaptive restoration of images with speckle. IEEE Trans Acoust Speech Signal Process. 1987;35(3): 373–383.

[24] Lopes A, Nezry E, Touzi R, Laur H. Structure detection and statistical adaptive speckle filtering in SAR images. Int J Remote Sens. 1993;14(9): 1735–1758.

[25] Lopes A, Touzi R, Nezry E. Adaptive speckle filters and scene heterogeneity. IEEE Trans Geosci Remote Sens. 1990 Nov;28(6): 992–1000.

[26] Argenti F, Alparone L. Speckle removal from SAR images in the undecimated wavelet domain. IEEE Trans Geosci Remote Sens. 2002 Nov;40(11): 2363–2374.

[27] Simard M, DeGrandi G, Thomson KPB, Benie GB. Analysis of speckle noise contribution on wavelet decomposition of SAR images. IEEE Trans Geosci Remote Sens. 1998 Nov;36(6): 1953–1962.

[28] Yu Y, Acton ST. Edge detection in ultrasound imagery using the instantaneous coefficient of variation. IEEE Trans Image Process. 2004;13(12): 1640–1655.

[29] Aja-Fernández S, Vegas-Sánchez-Ferrero G, Martín-Fernández M, Alberola-López C. Automatic noise estimation in images using local statistics. Additive and multiplicative cases. Image Vision Comput. 2009 May;27 (6): 756–770.

[30] Aja-Fernández S, Vegas-Sánchez-Ferrero G. Noise analysis in MRI: overview. In: Statistical Analysis of Noise in MRI. AG Switzerland: Springer International Publishing; 2016. p. 73–88.

[31] Loizou CP, Pattichis CS, Christodoulou CI, Istepanian RSH, Pantziaris M, Nicolaides A. Comparative evaluation of despeckle filtering in ultrasound imaging of the carotid artery. IEEE Trans Ultrason Ferroelectr Freq Control. 2005 Oct;52(10): 1653–1669.

[32] Eskicioglu AM, Fisher PS. Image quality measures and their performance. IEEE Trans Commun. 1995;43(12): 2959–2965.

[33] Wang Z, Bovik AC, Sheikh HR, Simoncelli EP. Image quality assessment: from error visibility to structural similarity. IEEE Trans Image Process. 2004 Apr;13(4): 600–612.

[34] Aja-Fernández S, San Jose-Estepar R, Alberola-Lopez C, Westin CF. Image quality assessment based on local variance. In: 2006 International Conference of the IEEE Engineering in Medicine and Biology Society; 2006. p. 4815–4818.

Chapter 6

An overview of despeckle-filtering techniques

Christos P. Loizou[1] *and Constantinos S. Pattichis*[2]

This chapter provides an introduction and a brief overview of selected despeckle-filtering techniques for ultrasound imaging and video expanded from [1]. A despeckle-filtering evaluation protocol is proposed, a brief literature review, as well as an image despeckle-filtering (IDF) toolbox [3] and a video despeckle filtering (VDF) [4] software toolbox are presented. Moreover, selected applications for ultrasound image and VDF techniques are illustrated. Speckle is a multiplicative noise [1–4], which degrades ultrasound images and videos and negatively influences the image and video interpretation, diagnosis and visual appearance [5]. Noise speckle reduction is therefore essential for improving the visual observation quality or as a preprocessing step for further automated analysis, such as image/video segmentation, texture analysis and encoding in ultrasound image and video. On the other hand, speckle can also be used as an information carrier on the underlying tissue properties. As illustrated in the previous chapters in Part I (see also Part IV), this implies it can be used, for example, for tissue classification. Alternatively, assuming that speckle moves in the image in the same way as the underlying tissue, it allows for tissue motion estimation using one of the many speckle tracking approaches presented in literature. A large number of despeckle-filtering techniques have been proposed in the past years for ultrasound images and very few for videos, which is usually applied for improving their visualization and interpretation or as a preprocessing step for further image/video analysis. This analysis includes segmentation, feature extraction, image and video compression, data transfer and registration. The present review study discusses, compares and evaluates ultrasound image and VDF techniques for the common carotid artery (CCA) introduced so far in the literature. Applications of the techniques are presented on simulated and real ultrasound images and videos (see also Chapters 7–10) of the CCA.

[1]University of Cyprus, Department of Electrical and Computer Engineering, Cyprus
[2]University of Cyprus, Department of Computer Science, Cyprus

6.1 An overview of despeckle-filtering techniques

In recent years, significant technological advancements and progress in image and video processing in a number of areas have been achieved; however, still a number of factors in the visual quality of images has hinder the automated analysis [5] and disease evaluation [6]. These include imperfections of image acquisition instrumentations, natural phenomena, transmission errors and coding artifacts, which all degrade the quality of an image in the form of induced noise [7–15]. Ultrasound imaging and video is a powerful noninvasive diagnostic tool in medicine, but it is degraded by a form of multiplicative noise (speckle), which makes visual observation difficult [1–4,16–28]. Speckle is mainly found in echogenic areas of the image in the form of a granular appearance that affects texture of the image [29–33], which may carry important information about the shape of tissues and organs. Texture [6,9,34] and morphology [35] may provide additional quantitative information of the area under investigation, which may complement the human evaluation and provide additional diagnostic details. It is therefore of interest for the image and video processing community to investigate and apply new IDF techniques that can increase the visual perception evaluation and further automate image and video analysis, thus improving the final result. These techniques are usually incorporated into integrated software for image processing applications.

Despeckle-filtering has been a rapidly emerging research area in recent years, and a significant number of representative studies have been published in numerous journals. The basic principles, the theoretical background and the algorithmic steps of a representative set of despeckle filters are covered in [1,2]. In addition, selected representative applications of image and video despeckling covering a variety of ultrasound image and video-processing tasks will be presented in this book.

Table 6.1 summarizes the different despeckle-filtering techniques for ultrasound imaging and video proposed in the literature [1]. These are grouped under the following categories: linear filtering, nonlinear filtering, diffusion filtering and wavelet filtering. Furthermore, in Table 6.1, the main characteristics, the references of the main investigators and the corresponding filter names for each filtering method are given.

Figure 6.1 illustrates an original longitudinal ultrasound asymptomatic (see Figure 6.1(a)) and symptomatic image of the CCA (see Figure 6.1(e)) and their despeckled images (see Figure 6.1(b) and (f)), respectively. Asymptomatic images were recorded from patients at risk of atherosclerosis in the absence of clinical symptoms, whereas symptomatic images were recorded from patients at risk of atherosclerosis, which have already developed clinical symptoms, such as a stroke episode. Figure 6.1(c)–(h) shows an enlarged window from the original and despeckled ultrasound images (shown in a rectangle in Figure 6.1(b) and (f)).

Figure 6.2 presents the 100th frame of an ultrasound video of the CCA from a symptomatic subject for the original and the despeckled ultrasound video frames with filters *DsFlsmv*, *DsFhmedian*, *DsFkuwahara* and *DsFsrad* when applied to the whole video frame (left column) and on a region of interest (ROI) selected by the user of the system (right column), respectively (see list of filters tabulated in Table 6.1). The automated plaque segmentations performed by an integrated

Table 6.1 An overview of despeckle-filtering techniques presented in this book

Speckle reduction technique	Method	Investigator	Filter name
Linear filtering	Moving window utilizing local statistics		
	(a) mean (m), variance (σ^2)	[7–20,19–38]	*DsFlsmv*
	(b) mean, variance, 3rd and 4th moments (higher statistical moments) and entropy	[7–20]	*DsFlsmvskld* *DsFlsmvsk2d*
	(c) Homogeneous mask area filters	[39]	*DsFlsminsc*
	(d) Wiener filtering	[20–22,28]	*DsFwiener*
Nonlinear filtering	Median filtering	[40]	*DsFmedian*
	Linear scaling of the gray level values	[41]	*DsFls* *DsFca* *DsFlecasort*
	Based on the most homogeneous neighborhood around each pixel	[27]	*DsFhomog*
	Nonlinear iterative algorithm (Geometric Filtering)	[16]	*DsFgf4d*
	The image is logarithmically transformed, the Fast Fourier transform (FFT) is computed, denoised, the inverse FFT is computed and finally exponentially transformed back	[22,42,43]	*DsFhomo*
	Hybrid median filtering	[44]	*DsFhmedian*
	Kuwahara filtering	[45]	*DsFKuwahara*
	Nonlocal filtering	[46]	*DsFnlocal*
Diffusion filtering	Nonlinear filtering technique for simultaneously performing contrast enhancement and noise reduction	[18,19,22, 25,47–51]	*DsFad*
	Exponential damp kernel filters utilizing diffusion	[25]	
	Speckle reducing anisotropic diffusion based on the coefficient of variation	[52]	*DsFsrad*
	Nonlinear anisotropic diffusion	[52]	*DsFnldif*
	Nonlinear complex diffusion	[53]	*DsFncdf*
Wavelet filtering	Threshold wavelet coefficients based on speckle noise at different levels	[38,54–59]	*DsFwaveltc*

system proposed in [14], are also shown in the images. The filters *DsFlsmv* and *DsFhmedian* smoothed the video frame without destroying subtle details.

A despeckle filtering and evaluation protocol was given in [2] which proposes the steps which are necessary to be taken when images will be processed for further image analysis. Two despeckle toolboxes supporting image and video processing respectively that were developed by our team and are companion to this book are also documented in [1,2]. These toolboxes are freeware and can be used to investigate the usefulness of despeckle filtering in different problems under investigation.

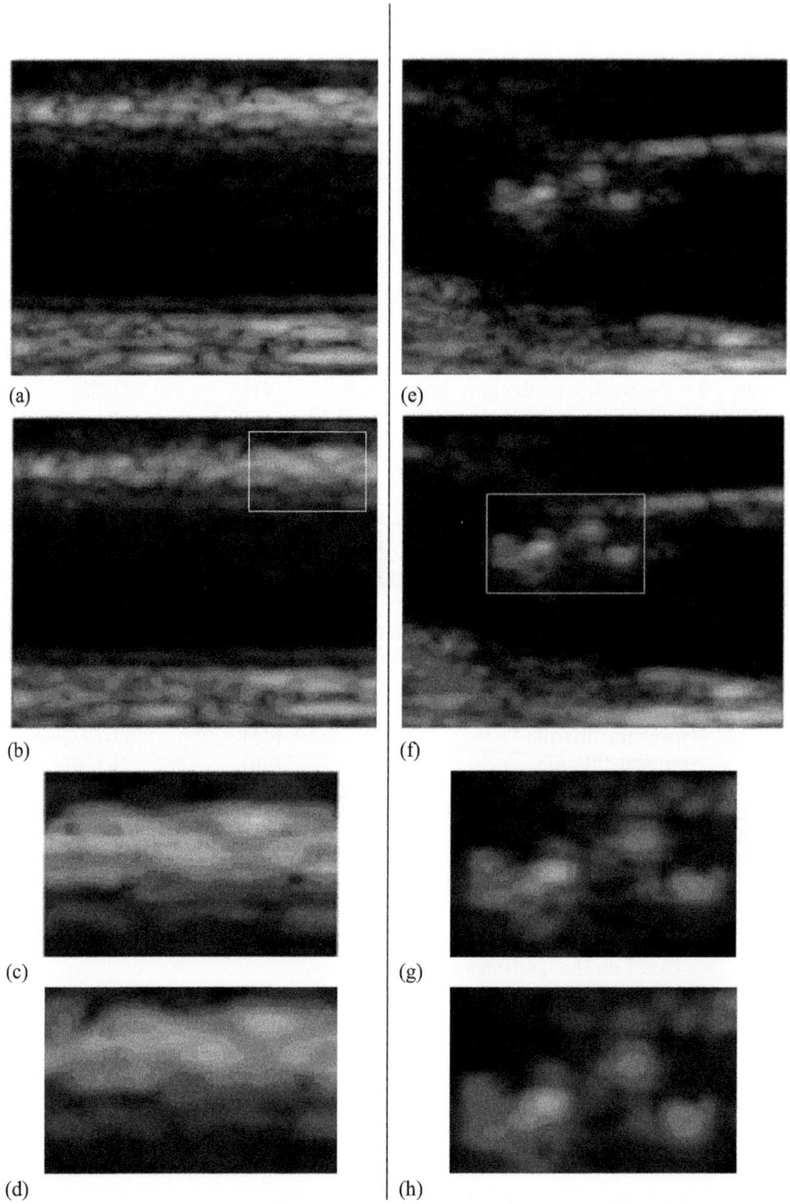

Figure 6.1 Results of image despeckle filtering based on linear filtering (first-order local statistics, DsFlsmv). Asymptomatic case: (a) original, (b) despeckled, (c) enlarged region marked in (b) of the original, (d) enlarged region marked in (b) of the despeckled image. Symptomatic case: (e) original, (f) despeckled, (e) enlarged region marked in (f) of the original, (h) enlarged region marked in (f) of the despeckled image. Regions were enlarged by a factor of three

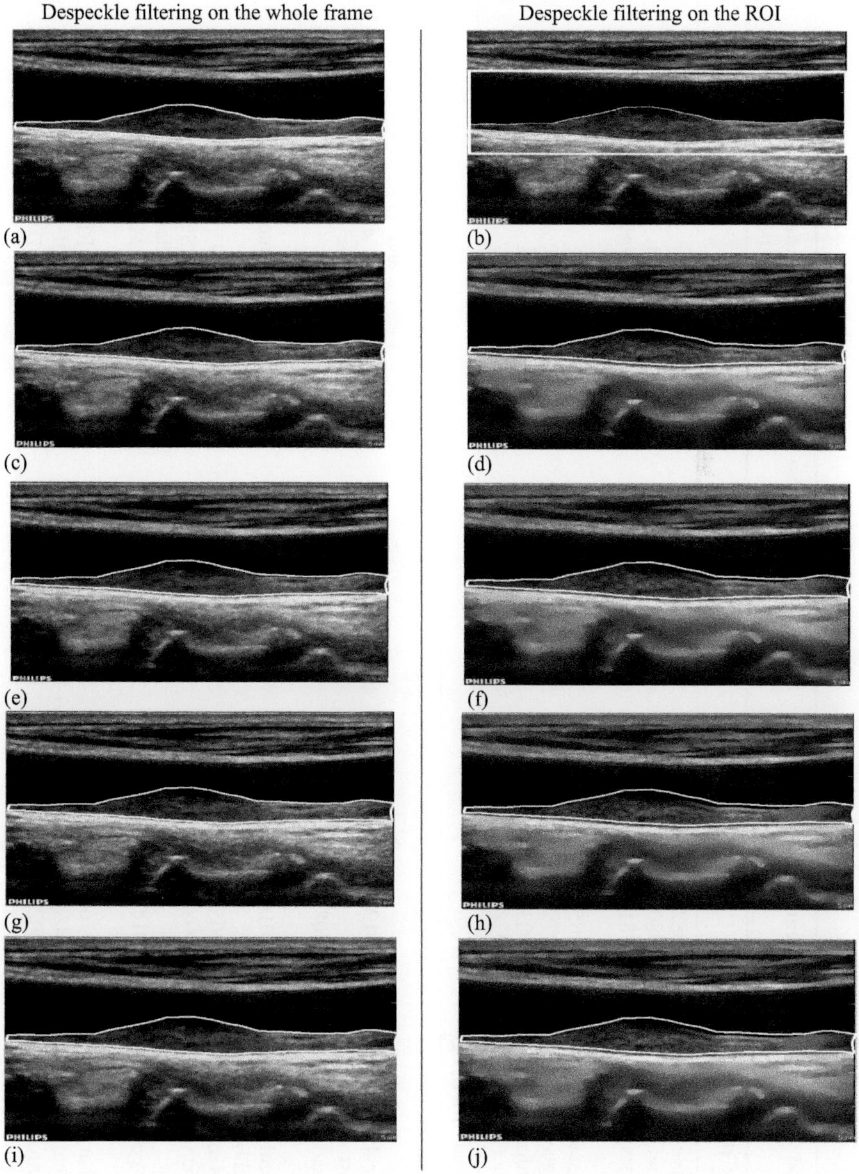

Figure 6.2 Examples of despeckle filtering on a video frame of a CCA video acquired from a male symptomatic subject at the age of 62 with 40% stenosis and a plaque at the far wall of the CCA, for the whole image frame in the left column, and on an ROI (including the plaque (shown in (b)), in the right column for: (a and b) original, (c and d) DsFlsmv, (e and f) DsFhmedian, (g and h) DsFkuwahara and (i and j) DsFsrad. The automated plaque segmentations were performed with the system proposed in [14] and are shown in all examples

Table 6.2 An overview of selected despeckle filtering applications

Principal investigator	Method	Year	Input	N	Software platform	Observers	Evaluation metrics and findings
	Linear filtering						
Frost [19]	Adaptive digital	1982	SAR, SIM	5	–	–	MSE = 121
Lee [20]	Local adaptive	1980	RWI	4	–	1	Mean, $\sigma^2 = 1.32$
Lee [7,20,28]	Local statistics	1981	PUI, RWI, UI, SAR	4	C++	–	$\sigma^2 = 0.82$. Line plots
Kuan [17,38]	Local statistics	1985	SAR	3	–	–	Mean, σ^2
Nagao [39]	Homogeneous mask area	1979	SAR	3	–	–	Mean = 1.25, $\sigma^2 = 1.27$
Pižurica [67]	Generalized likelihood	2003	MRI, PUI, UI	3	–	1	SNR = 13.6
Burckhardt [22]	Wiener filtering	1978	UI	1	–	–	Mean, σ^2
	Nonlinear filtering						
Zhan [68]	Nonlocal means	2014	LUI, PUI, CUI, SUI	10	M	1	MAE, COV, PSNR, SSIM Improved metrics and VI
Maggioni [69]	Nonlocal spatiotemporal transform (3D and 4D)	2012	RWV	8	M	1	PSNR = 41, MOVIE index = 0.94, VQA, a, VI,
Buades [46]	Nonlocal means	2008	RWI, RWV, Field II	6	C++	–	SSIN = 0.91
Lui [70]	Nonlocal means K-nearest neighbor	2010	RWV	5	M	1	$\sigma = 40$, VI Intensity graphs
Chan [71]	Spatiotemporal varying	2005	RWV	5	–	–	PSNR = 41.93
Varghese [72]	Gaussian scale mixture	2008	RWV	5	M	–	PSNR = 41, SSIM = 0.95 motion compensation
Biradar [73]	Fuzzy geometric Wiener	2014	CUI	5	M	2	PSNR = 23, MSE = 222, SSIM = 0.99, $\rho = 0.91$
Kuwahara [45]	Kuwahara filtering	1976	LUI	4	M	–	PSNR = 27, RMSE, MSE = 0.34
Coupé [74]	Nonlocal means	2009	LUI, MRI, PUI	4	–	–	SNR = 64, QI = 2.71
Zlokolica [75,76]	α-Trimmed mean filter	2002	UV	3	C++	1	PSNR, VI, 3D filtering
Busse [16]	Geometric filter	1995	UI	3	–	–	Mean = 122
Loupas [77]	Adaptive weighted median	1989	LUI	3	–	–	MSE = 22

Nieminen [44]	Hybrid median	1987	UI	3	–	1	PSNR = 24, RMSE = 0.043, MSE = 20
Solbo [42, 43]	Homomorphic	2004	UI	3	–	–	ENL = 22, mean = 121, median = 126, $\sigma = 1.4$
Huang [40]	Median filtering	1979	RWI	2	F	–	Window size = 5×5, 7×7, 9×9
	Diffusion filtering						
Cardoso [78]	Inference and anisotropic diffusion	2012	Filed II	4	M	–	ISFAD = 90%, SSIM = 0.95
Yongjian [25]	SRAD	2002	Field II, UCA	3	–	–	Mean = 122, $\sigma^2 = 1.19$, CV% = 1.14, FOM = 0.72
Narayanan [79]	Coupled PDE diffusion	2011	UI	2	–	–	CNR = 2.56, SSIM = 0.81, FOM = 0.91
Perona-Malik [51]	Anisotropic diffusion	1990	RWI	5	M	1	VI
Jin [47]	Nonlinear AD	2000	BUI, KUI	4	–	–	Histograms
Abd-Elmoniem [52]	Nonlinear coherent diffusion	2002	CUI, KUI, PUI, LUI	4	C++	–	Line plots, VI
Ullom [80]	Frequency compounding	2012	Field II	3	M	0	CNR = 348%
Weickert [48]	Nonlinear diffusion	1998	MRI, PUI	2	–	2	CPU time = 152 sec, %error = 0.27%
Bernardes [53]	Complex diffusion	2010	PUI, UI	2	M	3	MSE = 37, ENL = 46.3, CNR = 13.8, line plots
Tay [81]	Local adaptive anisotropic diffusion	2010	Field II, CU	1	C++	1	SSIM = 0.84
Ramos-Llorden [82]	Memory anisotropic diffusion	2015	KUI, IVUS	5	M	1	MS = 0.001/SSIM = 0.88/Q = 3.21
	Wavelet filtering						
Zong [56]	Multiscale wavelet	1998	CUI	10	–	–	MSE = 29, Line plots
Abrahim [83]	Wavelet thresholding	2012	LUI	2	–		MSE = 10, SNR = 25, PSNR = 45, SSIN = 0.99, Q = 0.85
Bioucas [84]	Variable splitting	2010	RWI	5	M	0	SNR = 24, MAE = 20, RE = 17
Dabov [85]	Hard thresholding and Wiener (3D)	2007	RWV	5	M	1	PSNR = 26

(Continues)

Table 6.2 (*Continued*)

Principal investigator	Method	Year	Input	N	Software platform	Observers	Evaluation metrics and findings
Rusanovskyy [86]	Block matching and hard-thresholding	2006	RWV	3	C++	–	PSNR = 34, VI
Gupta [87]	Multiscale (wavelet)	2004	KUI	3	–	–	MSE = 27, $\rho = 0.99$, $\beta = 0.92$ (shape parameter)
Yue [88]	Nonlinear multiscale	2006	LUI, UI	2	–	–	FOM = 0.91, p = 0.98, Line plots
	Review studies						
Loizou [8]	Review	2005	Field II, UI	440	M	2	61 texture features,16 quality metrics, 10 despeckle, *DsFIsmv* best performance
Sivakumar [89]	Review	2010	KUI, LUI	200	M	1	21 quality metrics, 12 despeckle filters SRAD best performance
Zhang [90]	Review	2015	Field II, BUI	200	M	2	4 quality metrics, 11 despeckle filters. NIQE best quality metric
Finn [60]	Review	2011	Field II, UV,	100	–	1	5 quality metrics, 15 despeckle filters OSRAD best performance
Loizou [15]	Comparison	2012	UV	10	M	1	4 despeckle filters. *DsFIsmv* best performance
Ortiz [91]	Review	2012	Field II, UI	2	M	–	3 quality metrics, 6 despeckle filters
Biradar [92]	Review	2015	CUI	200	M	1	15 quality metrics, 10 despeckle filters, improved segmentation after filtering

BUI: breast ultrasound imaging, CUI: cardiac ultrasound images, IVUS: intravascular ultrasound, KUI: Kidney ultrasound image, LUI: liver ultrasound images, PUI: phantom ultrasound images, RWI: real world images, RWV: real world videos, SAR: synthetic aperture radar images, SIM: simulated images, USC: ultrasound muscular arteries, SUI: spine ultrasound images, UCA: ultrasound carotid artery images, UV: ultrasound video, AD: anisotropic diffusion, β: shape parameter, CV%: coefficient of variation, CNR: contrast-to-noise ratio, ENL: effective number of looks, FOSSIM: structural similarity index, F: FORTRAN, M: Pratt's figure of merit, M: MATLAB®, MSE: mean square error, MAE: mean absolute error, N: number of subjects investigated, OSRAD: oriented speckle-reducing anisotropic diffusion, PSNR: peak-signal-to-noise ratio, QI: quality index, ρ: correlation coefficient, RE: relative error, SAR: synthetic aperture radar, SNR: signal-to-noise ratio, VI: visual inspection. © Reproduced, with permission, from [2].

6.2 Selected despeckle-filtering applications in ultrasound imaging and video

There is a significant number of studies reported in the literature for despeckling of ultrasound images of different imaging modalities using the different type of filters presented in Table 6.1. Table 6.2 tabulates selected despeckle-filtering applications in ultrasound image covering the liver, pancreas, carotid artery, heart and others. A rather limited number of studies have been reported for video despeckling [46,60]. The studies presented in Table 6.2 are grouped under the despeckle-filtering groups already presented in Table 6.1. In addition to the studies presented in Table 6.2, there is a plethora of studies published in the literature. A small number of these studies are discussed in this paragraph and will be further discussed and evaluated in Chapters 7–10. Zain *et al.* [61] reported the use of average, median and Weiner filtering for speckle removal in ultrasound images of the liver. Senel *et al.* [62] applied the topological median filter to improve conventional median filtering on ultrasound images of the pancreas. The topological median filters implemented some existing ideas and some new ideas on fuzzy connectedness to improve the extraction of edges in noise (versus the conventional use of a median filter). A speckle reduction technique for 3D liver ultrasound images was proposed by extending the 2D speckle reducing anisotropic diffusion (SRAD) algorithm to a 3D algorithm [63]. The anisotropic diffusion model was effectively used for identifying edges in an image in the analysis phase, researched by Kim *et al.* [64]. Nadernejad [65] used an anisotropic diffusion filter in artificial images where speckle noise was successfully removed. A comparative study between wavelet coefficient shrinkage filter and several standard despeckle filters showed that the discrete wavelet-based filtering gave the best results for speckle removal [66].

References

[1] C.P. Loizou, C.S. Pattichis, "Despeckle filtering for ultrasound imaging and video, Volume I: Algorithms and software", 2nd Ed., Synthesis lectures on algorithms and software in engineering, Ed. Morgran & Claypool Publishers, 1537 Fourth street, Suite 228, San Rafael, CA 94901 USA, vol. 7, no. 1, pp. 1–180, April 2015. ISBN: 9781627056687.

[2] C.P. Loizou, C.S. Pattichis, "Despeckle filtering for ultrasound imaging and video," Vol. II: Selected applications, Synthesis lectures on algorithms and software in engineering, Ed. Morgan & Claypool Publishers, 1537 Fourth Street, Suite 228, San Rafael, CA 94901 USA, vol. 7, no. 2, pp. 1–180, August 2015, ISBN-9781627058148.

[3] C.P. Loizou, C. Theofanous, M. Pantziaris, T. Kasparis, "Despeckle filtering software toolbox for ultrasound imaging of the common carotid artery," *Comput. Meth. Progr. Biomed.*, vol. 114, no. 1, pp. 109–124, 2014.

[4] C.P. Loizou, C. Theofanous, M. Pantziaris, *et al.*, "Despeckle filtering toolbox for medical ultrasound video," *Int. J. Monit. Surveill. Technol. Res.*

(IJMSTR): Special issue Biomed. Monitor. Technol., vol. 4, no. 1, pp. 61–79, 2013.

[5] Z. Wang, A. Bovik, H. Sheikh, E. Simoncelli, "Image quality assessment: from error measurement to structural similarity," *IEEE Trans. Image Process.*, vol. 13, no. 4, pp. 600–612, 2004.

[6] T. Elatrozy, A. Nicolaides, T. Tegos, *et al.*, "The effect of B-mode ultrasonic image standardization of the echodensity of symptomatic and asymptomatic carotid bifurcation plaque," *Int. Angiol.*, vol. 17, no. 3, 179–186, 1998.

[7] J.S. Lee, "Speckle analysis and smoothing of synthetic aperture radar images," *Comput. Graph. Image Proces.*, vol. 17, pp. 24–32, 1981.

[8] C.P. Loizou, C.S. Pattichis, C.I. Christodoulou, *et al.*, "Comparative evaluation of despeckle filtering in ultrasound imaging of the carotid artery," *IEEE Trans. Ultrason. Ferroelectr. Freq. Control*, vol. 52, no. 10, pp. 1653–1669, 2005.

[9] C.P. Loizou, C.S. Pattichis, M. Pantziaris, T. Tyllis, A.N. Nicolaides, "Quantitative quality evaluation of ultrasound imaging in the carotid artery," *Med. Biol. Eng. Comput.*, vol. 44, no. 5, pp. 414–426, 2006.

[10] C.P. Loizou, C.S. Pattichis, M. Pantziaris, A.N. Nicolaides, "An integrated system for the segmentation of atherosclerotic carotid plaque," *IEEE Trans. Inform. Techn. Biomed.*, vol. 11, no. 5, pp. 661–667, 2007.

[11] T. Greiner, C.P. Loizou, M. Pandit, J. Mauruschat, F.W. Albert, "Speckle reduction in ultrasonic imaging for medical applications," *Proc. ICASSP91, Int. Conf. Acoustic Sign. Speech & Proc.*, Toronto Canada, May 14–17, pp. 2993–2996, 1991.

[12] C.P. Loizou, C.S. Pattichis, "Despeckle filtering algorithms and Software for Ultrasound Imaging", Synthesis Lectures on Algorithms and Software for Engineering, Ed. Morgan & Claypool Publishers, San Rafael, CA, USA, 2008.

[13] C.P. Loizou, V. Murray, M.S. Pattichis, M. Pantziaris, A.N. Nicolaides, C.S. Pattichis, "Despeckle filtering for multiscale amplitude-modulation frequency-modulation (AM-FM) texture analysis of ultrasound images of the intima-media complex," *Int. J. Biomed. Imag.*, vol. 2014, Art. ID. 518414, 13 pages, 2014.

[14] C.P. Loizou, S. Petroudi, C.S. Pattichis, M. Pantziaris, A. N. Nicolaides, "An integrated system for the segmentation of atherosclerotic carotid plaque in ultrasound video," *IEEE Trans. Ultrason. Ferroelectr. Freq. Control*, vol. 61, no. 1, pp. 86–101, 2014.

[15] C.P. Loizou, T. Kasparis, P. Christodoulides, *et al.*, "Despeckle filtering in ultrasound video of the common carotid artery," *12th Int. Conf. Bioinf. & Bioeng. Proc. (BIBE)*, Larnaca, Cyprus, Nov. 11–13, pages 4, 2012.

[16] L. Busse, T.R. Crimmins, J.R. Fienup, "A model based approach to improve the performance of the geometric filtering speckle reduction algorithm," *IEEE Ultrasonic Symposium*, pp. 1353–1356, 1995.

[17] D.T. Kuan, A.A. Sawchuk, T.C. Strand, P. Chavel, "Adaptive restoration of images with speckle," *IEEE Trans. Acoust. Speech Signal Proc.*, vol. ASSP-35, pp. 373–383, 1987.

[18] M.F. Insana, T.J. Hall, G.G. Cox, S.J. Rosenthal, "Progress in quantitative ultrasonic imaging," *SPIE Vol. 1090 Medical Imaging III, Image Formation*, pp. 2–9, 1989.

[19] V.S. Frost, J.A. Stiles, K.S. Shanmungan, J.C. Holtzman, "A model for radar images and its application for adaptive digital filtering of multiplicative noise," *IEEE Trans. Pattern Anal. Mach. Intell.*, vol. 4, no. 2, pp. 157–165, 1982.

[20] J.S. Lee, "Digital image enhancement and noise filtering by using local statistics," *IEEE Trans. Pattern Anal. Mach. Intell.*, vol. PAMI-2, no. 2, pp. 165–168, 1980.

[21] D. Lamont, L. Parker, M. White, *et al.*, "Risk of cardiovascular disease measured by carotid intima-media thickness at age 49–51: life course study," *BMJ*, vol. 320, pp. 273–278, 29 January 2000.

[22] C.B. Burckhardt, "Speckle in ultrasound B-mode scans," *IEEE Trans. Sonics Ultrason.*, vol. SU-25, no. 1, pp. 1–6, 1978.

[23] R.F. Wagner, S.W. Smith, J.M. Sandrik, H. Lopez, "Statistics of speckle in ultrasound B-scans," *IEEE Trans. Sonics Ultrason.*, vol. 30, pp. 156–163, 1983.

[24] J.W. Goodman, "Some fundamental properties of speckle," *J. Opt. Soc. Am.*, vol. 66, no. 11, pp. 1145–1149, 1976.

[25] Y. Yongjian, S.T. Acton, "Speckle reducing anisotropic diffusion," *IEEE Trans. Image Process.*, vol. 11, no. 11, pp. 1260–1270, 2002.

[26] R.W. Prager, A.H. Gee, G.M. Treece, L. Berman, "Speckle detection in ultrasound images using first order statistics," University of Cambridge, Dept. of Engineering, GUED/F-INFENG/TR 415, pp. 1–17, 2002.

[27] C.I. Christodoulou, C.P. Loizou, C.S. Pattichis, *et al.*, "Despeckle filtering in ultrasound imaging of the carotid artery," *2nd Joint EMBS/BMES Conference*, Houston, TX, USA, pp. 1027–1028, Oct. 23–26, 2002.

[28] J.S. Lee, "Refined filtering of image noise using local statistics," *Comp. Graph. Imag. Proces.*, vol. 15, pp. 380–389, 1981.

[29] V. Dutt, "Statistical analysis of ultrasound echo envelope," Ph.D. dissertation, Mayo Graduate School, Rochester, MN, 1995.

[30] M. Amadasun and R. King, "Textural features corresponding to textural properties," *IEEE Trans. Syst. Man Cybern.*, vol. 19, no. 5, pp. 1264–1274, 1989.

[31] C.M. Wu, Y.C. Chen, K.-S. Hsieh, "Texture features for classification of ultrasonic images," *IEEE Trans. Med. Imaging*, vol. 11, pp. 141–152, 1992.

[32] T.J. Chen, K.S. Chuang, J. Wu, *et al.*, "A novel image quality index using Moran I statistics," *Phys. Med. Biol.*, vol. 48, pp. 131–137, 2003.

[33] S. Winkler, "Vision models and quality metrics for image processing applications," PhD, University of Lausanne-Switzerland, 2000.

[34] C. Christodoulou, C.S. Pattichis, M. Pantziaris, A. Nicolaides, "Texture-based classification of atherosclerotic carotid plaques," *IEEE Trans. Med. Imaging*, vol. 22, no. 7, pp. 902–912, 2003.

[35] E. Kyriakou, M.S. Pattichis, C.I. Christodoulou, *et al.*, "Ultrasound imaging in the analysis of carotid plaque morphology for the assessment of stroke," *In Plaque Imaging: Pixel to molecular level*, ed. Suri JS, Yuan C, Wilson DL, Laxminarayan S, IOS Press, pp. 241–275, 2005.

[36] J. Grosby, B.H. Amundsen, T. Hergum, *et al.*, "3D Speckle tracking for assessment of regional left ventricular function," *Ultrasound Med. Biol.*, vol. 35, pp. 458–471, 2009.

[37] J.A. Noble, N. Navab, H. Becher, "Ultrasonic image analysis and image guided interventions," *Interface Focus*, vol. 1, pp. 673–685, 2011.

[38] D.T. Kuan, A.A. Sawchuk, "Adaptive noise smoothing filter for images with signal dependent noise," *IEEE Trans. Pattern Anal. Mach. Intell.*, vol. PAMI-7, no. 2, pp. 165–177, 1985.

[39] M. Nagao, T. Matsuyama, "Edge preserving smoothing," *Comput. Graph. Image Proces.*, vol. 9, pp. 394–407, 1979.

[40] T. Huang, G. Yang, G. Tang, "A fast two-dimensional median filtering algorithm," *IEEE Trans. Acoustics Speech Signal Proces.*, vol. 27, no. 1, pp. 13–18, 1979.

[41] R. Gonzalez, R. Woods, Digital image processing, Second Edition, Upper Saddle River, NJ: Prentice-Hall Inc., 2002.

[42] S. Solbo, T. Eltoft, "Homomorphic wavelet based-statistical despeckling of SAR images," *IEEE Trans. Geosci. Remote Sensing*, vol. 42, no. 4, pp. 711–721, 2004.

[43] J. Saniie, T. Wang, N. Bilgutay, "Analysis of homomorphic processing for ultrasonic grain signal characterization," *IEEE Trans. Ultrason. Ferroelectr. Freq. Control*, vol. 3, pp. 365–375, 1989.

[44] A. Nieminen, P. Heinonen, Y. Neuvo, "A new class of detail-preserving filters for image processing," *IEEE Trans. Pattern Anal. Mach. Intell.*, vol.9, pp. 74–90, 1987.

[45] M. Kuwahara, K. Hachimura, S. Eiho, M. Kinoshita, "Digital processing of biomedical images," K. Preston Jr. and M. Onoe, eds. Boston, MA: Springer Verlag US, pp. 187–203, 1976.

[46] A. Buades, B. Coll, J.-M. Morel, "Nonlocal image and movie denoising," *Int. J. Comput. Vis.*, vol. 76, pp. 123–139, 2008.

[47] S. Jin, Y. Wang, J. Hiller, "An adaptive non-linear diffusion algorithm for filtering medical images," *IEEE Trans. Inform. Technol. Biomed.*, vol. 4, no. 4, pp. 298–305, December 2000.

[48] J. Weickert, B. Romery, M. Viergever, "Efficient and reliable schemes for nonlinear diffusion filtering," *IEEE Trans. Image Process.*, vol. 7, pp. 398–410, 1998.

[49] N. Rougon, F. Preteux, "Controlled anisotropic diffusion," *Conference on Nonlinear Image Processing VI*, IS&T/SPIE Symposium on Electronic

Imaging, Science and Technology, San Jose, California, pp. 1–12, 5–10 February 1995.

[50] M. Black, G. Sapiro, D. Marimont, D. Heeger, "Robust anisotropic diffusion," *IEEE Trans. Image Process.*, vol. 7, no. 3, pp. 421–432, March 1998.

[51] P. Rerona, J. Malik, "Scale-space and edge detection using anisotropic diffusion," *IEEE Trans. Pattern Anal. Mach. Intell.*, vol. 12, no. 7, pp. 629–639, July 1990.

[52] K. Abd-Elmoniem, A.-B. Youssef, Y. Kadah, "Real-time speckle reduction and coherence enhancement in ultrasound imaging via nonlinear anisotropic diffusion," *IEEE Trans. Biomed. Eng.*, vol. 49, no. 9, pp. 997–1014, September 2002.

[53] R. Bernardes, C. Mduro, P. Serranho, *et al.*, "Improved adaptive complex diffusion despeckling filter," *Opt. Exp.*, vol. 18, pp. 24048–24059, 2010.

[54] S. Zhong, V. Cherkassky, "Image denoising using wavelet thresholding and model selection," *Proc. IEEE Int. Conf. Image Process.*, Vancouver, Canada, pp.1–4, November 2000.

[55] A. Achim, A. Bezerianos, P. Tsakalides, "Novel Bayesian multiscale method for speckle removal in medical ultrasound images," *IEEE Trans. Med. Imag.*, vol. 20, no. 8, pp. 772–783, 2001.

[56] X. Zong, A. Laine, E. Geiser, "Speckle reduction and contrast enhancement of echocardiograms via multiscale nonlinear processing," *IEEE Trans. Med. Imaging*, vol. 17, no. 4, pp. 532–540, 1998.

[57] X. Hao, S. Gao, X. Gao, "A novel multiscale nonlinear thresholding method for ultrasonic speckle suppressing," *IEEE Trans. Med. Imaging*, vol. 18, no. 9, pp. 787–794, 1999.

[58] D. L. Donoho, "Denoising by soft thresholding," *IEEE Trans. Inform. Theory*, vol. 41, pp. 613–627, 1995.

[59] F.N.S Medeiros, N.D.A. Mascarenhas, R.C.P Marques, C.M. Laprano, "Edge preserving wavelet speckle filtering," *5th IEEE Southwest Symp. Image Anal. & Interpret.*, Santa Fe, New Mexico, pp. 281–285, 7–9 April 2002.

[60] S. Finn, M. Glavin, E. Jones, "Echocardiographic speckle reduction comparison," *IEEE Trans. Ultrason. Ferroelectr. Freq. Control*, vol. 58, no. 1, pp. 82–101, 2011.

[61] M. Zain, M. Luqman, I. Elamvazuthi, K. M. Begam, "Enhancement of bone fracture image using filtering techniques," *Int. J. Video Image Process. Netw. Secur. (IJVIPNS)*, vol. 9, no. 10, pp. 49–54, 2009.

[62] H.G. Senel, R.A. Peters, B. Dawant, "Topological median filter," *IEEE Trans. Image Process.*, vol. 11, no. 2, pp. 89–104, 2002.

[63] Q. Sun, J. A. Hossack, J. S. Tang, S. T. Acton, "Speckle reducing anisotropic diffusion for 3D ultrasound images" *Comput. Med. Imaging Graph.*, vol. 28, pp. 461–470, 2004.

[64] Y.S. Kim, J.B. Jong Beom Ra, "Improvement of ultrasound image based on wavelet transform: speckle reduction and edge enhancement," *Proc. SPIE, Image Processing Medical Imaging*, 5747, 2005.

[65] E. Nadernejad, "Despeckle filtering in medical ultrasound imaging," *Contemp. Eng. Sci.*, vol. 2, no. 1, pp. 17–36, 2009.

[66] G. Amara, "An introduction to wavelets," *IEEE Comput. Sci. Eng.*, vol. 2, no. 2, pp. 50–61, 1995.

[67] A. Pižurica, W. Philips, I. Lemahieu, M. Acheroy, "A versatile wavelet domain noise filtration technique for medical imaging," *IEEE Trans. Med. Imaging*, vol. 22, no. 3, pp. 323–331, 2003.

[68] Y. Zhan, M. Ding, L. Wu, X. Zhang, "Nonlocal means method using weight refining for despeckling of ultrasound images," *Sign. Proces.*, vol. 103, pp. 201–213, 2014.

[69] M. Maggioni, G. Boracchi, A. Foi, K. Engiazarian, "Video denoising, deblocking and enhancement through separable 4-D nonlocal spatiotemporal transforms," *IEEE Trans. Imaging Proc.*, vol. 21, no. 9, pp. 3952–3966, 2012.

[70] C. Lui, W.T. Freeman, "A high-quality video denoising algorithm based on reliable motion estimation," *Proc. ECCV 10 11th Eur. Conf. Comput. Vis.*, Part III, pp. 706–719, 2010.

[71] T.W. Chan, O.C. Au, T.S. Chong, W.S. Chau, "A novel content-adaptive video denoising filter, *IEEE Proc. Vis. Image Signal Process.*, vol. 2, no. 2, pp. 649–652, 2005.

[72] G. Varghese, Z. Wang, "Video denoising using a spatiotemporal statistical model of wavelet coefficients," *IEEE Int. Conf. Acoust. Speech Sign. Proc.*, Las Vegas, NV, USA, pp. 1257–1260, 2008.

[73] N. Biradar, M.L. Dewal, M.K. Rohit, "Edge preserved speckle noise reduction using integrated fuzzy filters," *Int. Scholarly. Res. Not.*, vol. 2014, pp. 1–14, 2014.

[74] P. Coupé, P. Hellier, C. Kervrann, C. Barillot, "Nonlocal means-based speckle filtering for ultrasound images," *IEEE Trans. Image Proces.*, vol. 18, no. 10, pp. 2221–2229, 2009.

[75] V. Zlokolica, W. Philips, D. van de Ville, "Robust non-linear filtering for video processing," *IEEE 14th Int. Conf. on Digit. Sign. Process.*, Santorini, Greece, pp. 1–4, 1–3 July 2002.

[76] V. Zlokolica, A. Pizurica, W. Philips, "Recursive temporal denoising and motion estimation of video," *Int. Conf. Image Proc.*, vol. 3 no. 3, pp. 1465–1468, 2008.

[77] T. Loupas, W.N. McDicken, P.L. Allan, P.L., "An adaptive weighted median filter for speckle suppression in medical ultrasonic images," *IEEE Trans. Circuits Syst.*, vol. 36, pp. 129–135, 1989.

[78] F.M. Cardoso, M.M. Matsumoto, S.S. Furuie, "Edge-preserving speckle texture removal by interference-based speckle filtering followed by anisotropic diffusion," *Ultrasound Med. Biol.*, vol. 38, no 8, pp. 1414–1428, 2012.

[79] S.K. Narayanan, R.S.D. Wahidabanu, "Despeckling of ultrasound images, using median regularized coupled Pde," *ACEEE Int. J. Contr. Syst. Instrum.*, vol. 2, no. 2, pp. 40–44, 2011.

[80] J.S. Ullom, M.L. Oelze, J.R. Sanchez, "Speckle reduction for ultrasonic imaging using frequency compounding and despeckling filters along with coded excitation and pulse compression," *Adv. Acoust. Vibr.*, vol. 2012, pp. 1–16, 2012.

[81] P.C. Tay, C.D. Garson, S.T. Acton, J.A. Hossack, "Ultrasound despeckling for contrast enhancement," *IEEE Trans. Image Process.*, vol. 19, no. 7, pp. 1847–1860, 2010.

[82] G. Ramos-Llorden, G. Vegas-Sanchez-Ferrero, M. Martin-Fernandez, C. Alberola-Lopez, S. Aia-Fernandez, "Anisotropic diffusion filter with memory based on speckle statistics for ultrasound images," *IEEE Trans. Image Process.*, vol. 24, no. 1, pp. 345–358, 2015.

[83] B.A. Abrahim, Z.A. Mustafa, I.A. Yassine, N. Zayed, Y.M. Kadah, "Hybrid total variation and wavelet thresholding speckle reduction for medical ultrasound imaging," *J. Med. Image Health Inform.*, vol. 2, pp. 114–124, 2012.

[84] J.M. Bioucas-Dias, M.A.T. Figueiredo, "Multiplicative noise removal using variable splitting and constrained optimization," *IEEE Trans. Image Process.*, vol. 9, no. 10, pp. 1720–1730, 2010.

[85] K. Dabov, A. Foi, K. Egiazarian, "Video denoising by sparse 3D transform-domain collaborative filtering," *Proc. of the 15th Eur. Sign. Proc. Conf.*, pp. 1–5, 2007.

[86] D. Rusanovskyy, K. Dabov, K. Egiazarian, "Moving-window varying size 3D transform-based video denoising," *Proc. Int. Workshop Video Proc. Quality Metrics*, pp. 1–4, 2006.

[87] S. Gupta, R.C. Chauhan, S.C. Sexana, "Wavelet-based statistical approach for speckle reduction in medical ultrasound images," *Med. Biol. Eng. Comput.*, vol. 42, pp. 189–192, 2004.

[88] Y. Yue, M.M. Croitoru, A. Bidani, J.B. Zwischenberger, J.W. Clark, Jr., "Nonlinear multiscale wavelet diffusion for speckle suppression and edge enhancement in ultrasound images," *IEEE Trans. Med. Imaging*, vol. 25, no. 3, pp. 297–311, March 2006.

[89] R. Sivakumar, M.K. Gayathri, D. Nedumaran, "Speckle filtering of ultrasound B-scan images-A comparative study of single scale spatial adaptive filters, multiscale filter and diffusion filters," *IACSIT Int. J. Eng. Technol.*, vol. 2, no. 6, pp. 514–523, 2010.

[90] J. Zhang, C. Wang, Y. Cheng, "Comparison of despeckle filters for breast ultrasound images," *Circuits Syst. Process.*, vol. 34, pp. 185–208, 2015.

[91] S.H. Contrera Ortiz, T. Chiu, M.D. Fox, "Ultrasound image enhancement: A review," *Biomed. Sign. Process. Contr.*, vol. 7, no. 5, 419–428, 2012.

[92] N. Biradar, M.L. Dewal, M.K. Rohit, "Comparative analysis of despeckle filters for continuous wave Doppler images," *Biomed. Eng. Lett.*, vol. 5, no. 1, pp. 33–44, 2015.

Chapter 7

Linear despeckle filtering

Christos P. Loizou[1] and Constantinos S. Pattichis[2]

This chapter provides the basic theoretical background of linear despeckle filtering techniques together with their algorithmic implementation, MATLAB® code for selected filters and practical examples on phantom and real ultrasound images. There are three groups of filters presented in this chapter, first-order statistics filtering, local statistics filtering and homogeneous mask area filtering (see also Table 6.1 in Chapter 6). Despeckle filtering was evaluated for all filters presented in this chapter on phantom ultrasound carotid artery images (see Figure 7.2) and real ultrasound images and videos (see Figure 7.5) of the common carotid artery (CCA). Furthermore, we present an evaluation and comparison of five linear despeckle filtering algorithms presented in this chapter. The evaluation is carried out on a phantom image, an artificial image and on real carotid and cardiac ultrasound images. Furthermore, findings on video despeckling are presented.

7.1 First-order statistics filtering (*DsFlsmv*, *DsFwiener*)

Most of the techniques for speckle reduction filtering in the literature use linear filtering based on local statistics. Their working principle may be described by a weighted average calculation using subregion statistics to estimate statistical measures over different pixel windows varying from 3×3 up to 15×15. All these techniques assume that the speckle noise model has a multiplicative form as given in [1–108]:

$$g_{i,j} \approx f_{i,j} n_{i,j} \tag{7.1}$$

with $g_{i,j}$ the observed noisy pixel on the ultrasound image display and $f_{i,j}$, and $n_{i,j}$ the noise-free pixel and noise component of the image, respectively.

The filters utilizing the first-order statistics such as the variance and the mean of the neighborhood may be described with the model as in (7.1). Hence, the

[1]Department of Electrical Engineering, Computer Engineering and Informatics, Cyprus University of Technology, Cyprus
[2]Department of Computer Science, University of Cyprus, Cyprus

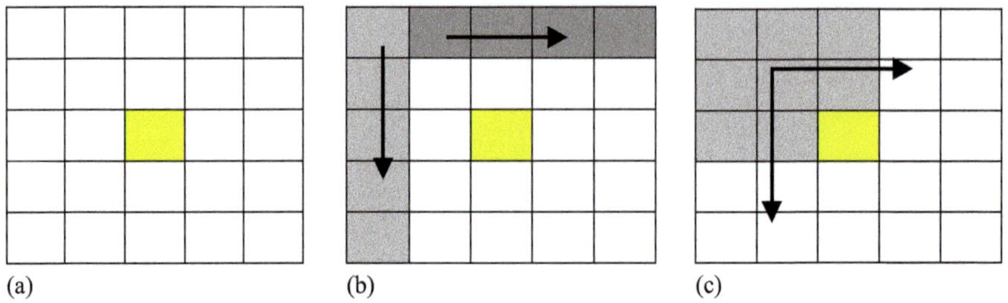

Figure 7.1 (a) Pixel moving window of 5×5 pixels, (b) schematical operation of the filters DsFlsminv1d with a 1D sliding moving window and (c) DsFlsmv with a 2D sliding moving window. © 2015, Reprinted from [77]

algorithms in this class may be traced back to the following equation [7,13,29,49,77,78] (see also Figure 7.1):

$$f_{i,j} = \overline{g} + k_{i,j}\left(g_{i,j} - \overline{g}\right) \tag{7.2}$$

where $\overline{g}$ is the local mean value of an $N_1 \times N_2$, region surrounding and including pixel $g_{i,j}$, $k_{i,j}$ is a weighting factor, with $k \in [0\ldots 1]$, and i,j are the pixel coordinates. The factor $k_{i,j}$ is a function of the local statistics in a moving window. It can be found in the literature [7,13,36,38,45,77,78] and may be derived in different forms that

$$k_{i,j} = \left(1 - \overline{g}^2\sigma^2\right)/\left(\sigma^2\left(1 + \sigma_n^2\right)\right) \tag{7.3}$$

$$k_{i,j} = \sigma^2/\left(\overline{g}^2\sigma_n^2 + \sigma^2\right) \tag{7.4}$$

$$k_{i,j} = \left(\sigma^2 - \sigma_n^2\right)/\sigma^2. \tag{7.5}$$

The values σ^2 and σ_n^2 represent the variance in the moving window and the variance of noise in the whole image, respectively. The noise variance may be calculated for the logarithmically compressed image or video, by computing the average noise variance over a number of windows with dimensions considerable larger than the filtering window. In each window, the noise variance is computed as

$$\sigma_n^2 = \sum_{i=1}^{p} \sigma_p^2/\overline{g}_p \tag{7.6}$$

where σ_p^2 and $\overline{g}_p$ are the variance and mean of the noise in the selected windows, respectively, and p is the index covering all windows in the whole image or video [3,37,40,69,77,78]. If the value of $k_{i,j}$ is 1 (in edge areas), this will result to an unchanged pixel, whereas a value of 0 (in uniform areas) replaces the actual pixel by the local average, $\overline{g}$, over a small region of interest (see (7.2)). In this work, the filter *DsFlsmv* uses (7.3).

The filter *DsFwiener* uses a pixel-wise adaptive wiener method [13,32–35,46,77,78] implemented as given in (7.2), with the weighting factor $k_{i,j}$, as given in (7.5).

For both despeckle filters *DsFlsmv* and *DsFwiener*, the moving window size was 5×5 (see also Figure 7.1(a)).

Algorithm 7.1 Linear filtering: linear scaling filter (*DsFlsmv*)

1. *Load the image (first frame) for filtering*
2. *Specify the region of interest to be filtered, the moving window size (n hood) and the number of iterations (n)*
3. *Compute the noise variance* σ_n^2 *with* (7.6) *for the whole image (frame)*
4. *Starting from the left upper corner of the image (frame), compute for each moving window the coefficient* $k_{i,j}$ *in* (7.3)
5. *Compute* $f_{i,j}$ *in* (7.2) *and replace the noisy middle point in each moving window* $g_{i,j}$, *with the new computed value* $f_{i,j}$
6. *Repeat steps* 4 *and* 5 *for the whole image (frame) by sliding the moving window from left to right. For video despeckling repeat steps* 1 *to* 6 *for all consecutive video frames*
7. *Repeat steps* 3 *to* 6 *for* n *iterations*
8. *Compute the image quality evaluation metrics and the texture features for the original and the despeckled images (videos)*
9. *Display the original and despeckled images (or videos), the image (video) quality and evaluation metrics, and the texture features*

Algorithm 7.1 presents the algorithmic steps for the implementation of the *DsFlsmv* despeckle filter for image despeckling. For video despeckling, the procedure described above is repeated for each consecutive video frame or selected video frames depending on the application.

Figure 7.2 illustrates the application of the despeckle filter *DsFlsmv* on the phantom image. Table 7.1 illustrates selected statistical and image quality metrics for the phantom image of Figure 7.2 for the original and the despeckled images.

(a) (b)

Figure 7.2 Example of DsFlsmv despeckle filtering on a phantom ultrasound image. (a) Original phantom image, (b) DsFlsmv ([7×7] window, 5 iterations). © 2015, Reprinted from [77]

Table 7.1 Selected statistical and image quality features for Figure 7.2 before and after despeckle filtering for the DsFlsmv *filter. © 2015, Reprinted from [77]*

Features	μ	**Median**	σ^2	σ^3	σ^4	**Contrast**	**C**	**CSR**	**MSE**	**SNR**	**Q**	**SSIN**	**AD**	**SC**	**MD**	**NAE**
Original	36	37	21	0.2	2.8	76	58	–	–	–	–	–	–	–	–	–
DsFlsmv	35	40	**17**	0.3	2.0	74	**48**	0.5	1,757	28	0.5	0.54	0.7	1.1	74	0.22

Bold values show improvement after despeckle filtering. C, speckle index, $C = (\sigma^2/\mu)100$; CSR, contrast-speckle ratio; MSE, mean square error; SNR, peak signal-to-noise ratio; Q, universal quality index; SSIN, structural similarity index; AD, average difference; SC, structural content; MD, maximum difference; NAE, normalized absolute error.

The despeckle filter *DsFlsmv* was applied on the phantom image varying the number of iterations (from 1 to 15) where the size of the sliding moving window was [5×5] as illustrated in Figure 7.3. Table 7.2 tabulates the statistical and image quality features for the phantom image of Figure 7.3, after the application of the *DsFlsmv* despeckle filter for increasing number of iterations. It is shown in Table 7.2, that increasing the number of iterations, the mean, median, skewness,

Figure 7.3 Original phantom ultrasound image given in (a) and the despeckled phantom images after the application of the DsFlsmv filter for increasing number of iterations from 1 to 15 given in (b)–(l), respectively. The window size was [5×5]. © 2015, Reprinted from [77]

Table 7.2 Selected statistical and image quality evaluation features for Figure 7.3 before and after despeckle filtering with the DsFlsmv filter for increasing the number of iterations and constant window size ([5×5]). © 2015, Reprinted from [77]

Features	Number of iterations												
	Original	**1**	**2**	**3**	**4**	**5**	**6**	**7**	**8**	**9**	**10**	**15**	**20**
μ	36	36	36	36	36	36	36	35	35	35	35	35	35
Median	37	38	39	39	40	40	40	40	40	40	40	40	39
σ^2	21	19	18	18	17	17	17	17	17	17	16	16	16
σ^3	0.2	0.01	0.2	0.2	0.3	0.3	0.3	0.3	0.3	0.4	0.4	0.4	0.4
σ^4	2.8	2.6	2.4	2.3	2.1	2.1	2	2	2	1.9	1.9	1.8	1.8
Contrast	76	35	17	9	6	3.8	2.9	2	1.7	1.4	1.3	0.8	0.6
C	58	53	50	50	47	47	47	49	49	49	46	46	46
CSR	–	0.43	0.43	0.44	0.44	0.44	0.44	0.45	0.45	0.45	0.46	0.46	0.46
MSE	–	1,757	1,758	1,759	1,760	1,760	1,762	1,763	1,764	1,766	1,778	1,770	1,771
SNR	–	21	17	18	16	15	14	13.7	13.3	12	12.5	12.9	12.5
Q	–	0.86	0.58	0.36	0.36	0.24	0.21	0.13	0.10	0.09	0.07	0.05	0.03
SSIN	–	0.88	0.71	0.55	0.55	0.51	0.49	0.47	0.45	0.43	0.42	0.41	0.39
MD	–	30	39	54	65	74	82	88	93	96	100	114	117
LMSE	–	0.58	0.88	0.91	0.95	1.02	0.99	0.99	0.99	1.01	1.01	1.01	1.02

σ^3, and kurtosis, σ^4, are preserved, whereas the standard deviation, σ^2, is slightly reduced. Furthermore, it is shown that increasing the numbers of iterations for the *DsFlsmv* filter, reduced contrast dramatically as demonstrated also in Figure 7.3. Moreover, *C* is reduced with the number of iterations, whereas an increase of *C* for iterations 7, 8 and 9 was observed. The CSR (contrast-speckle ratio) increases slightly with the number of iterations. It is furthermore shown that the SNR (signal-to-noise ratio) is reduced significantly with increasing number of iterations. The Q (universal quality index) and SSIN (structural similarity index) are reduced significantly with the number of iterations. The despeckled phantom images of Figure 7.3 were also visually assessed by the experts, where the best visual results were given for iterations 4, 5 and 6. For these iterations, the filtered image statistics remain the same, but contrast is further reduced.

The despeckle filter *DsFlsmv* was applied on the phantom image for different sliding moving window sizes (from [3×3] to [23×23]) where the number of iterations was kept constant to five as demonstrated in Figure 7.4. Table 7.3 tabulates the statistical and image quality evaluation features for the phantom image after the application of the *DsFlsmv* filter illustrated in Figure 7.4. It is shown that increasing the sliding moving window size, the mean and median are preserved and the variance is decreased for the window sizes [3×3] and [5×5].

Contrast is significantly reduced for window sizes [3×3] and [5×5] and then exhibits very small variations. Furthermore, it is shown that for increasing the number of iterations the filter *DsFlsmv* reduced the speckle index, C, especially for the first three window sizes, and then it exhibits smaller variations, whereas the CSR remains constant. Table 7.3 also shows that the MSE remains relatively unchanged while the SNR is reduced significantly with increasing window size. The Q and SSIN are reduced significantly with the number of iterations. The despeckled phantom images of Figure 7.4 were also visually assessed by the two experts, where the best visual results were given for the sliding window sizes of [3×3] and [5×5].

Figure 7.5 illustrates the application of the despeckle filter *DsFlsmv* on a video acquired from a symptomatic male subject at the age of 62 with 40% stenosis and a plaque at the far wall of the CCA. Despeckle filtering was applied on frames 1, 50, 100, 150, 200 and 250 for a moving window size of 5×5 pixels and two iterations.

The despeckle filter *DsFlsmv* was applied on the CCA ultrasound image of Figure 7.5 for different number of iterations (from 1 to 20) where the sliding moving window was kept constant to [5×5] and the results are demonstrated in Table 7.4, where the statistical and image quality evaluation features for the application of the *DsFlsmv* filter are tabulated. It is shown that increasing the number of iterations, the mean, median and variance are preserved up to the third iteration and then are reduced.

Contrast and SNR are reduced with increasing the number of iterations. Furthermore, it is shown that for increasing the number of iterations the filter *DsFlsmv* increases the speckle index, C, and decreases the CSR. The Q and SSIN

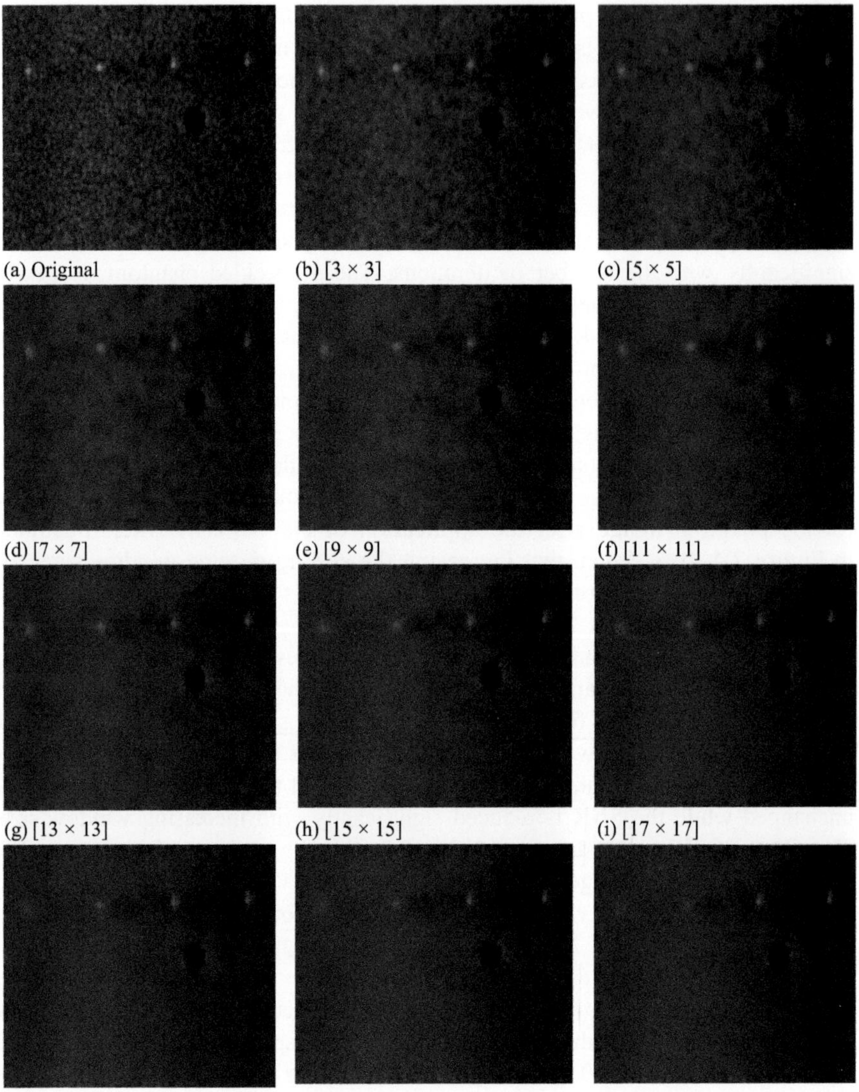

(a) Original (b) [3 × 3] (c) [5 × 5]
(d) [7 × 7] (e) [9 × 9] (f) [11 × 11]
(g) [13 × 13] (h) [15 × 15] (i) [17 × 17]
(j) [19 × 19] (k) [21 × 21] (l) [25 × 25]

Figure 7.4 Original phantom ultrasound image given in (a) and the despeckled phantom images after the application of the DsFlsmv filter for increasing pixel moving window size from [3×3] to [25×25] windows given in (b)–(l). The number of iterations was five for all cases. © 2015, Reprinted from [77]

are reduced with the number of iterations. The despeckled phantom images of Figure 7.4 were also visually assessed by the expert, where the best visual results were given for iterations 2 and 3.

Table 7.3 Selected statistical and image quality evaluation features for Figure 7.4 before and after despeckle filtering with the DsFlsmv filter for increasing window size (from [3×3] to [25×25] window) and for five iterations. © 2015, Reprinted from [77]

Feature	**Window size**												
	Original	**×3**	**×5**	**×7**	**×9**	**×11**	**×13**	**×15**	**×17**	**×19**	**×21**	**×23**	**×25**
μ	36	35	36	36	36	36	36	36	36	36	36	36	35
Median	37	38	39	40	40	41	41	41	41	41	41	41	41
σ^2	21	18	18	17	17	17	17	17	17	16	16	16	16
σ^3	0.2	0.06	0.2	0.3	0.3	0.4	0.4	0.4	0.4	0.4	0.4	0.4	0.5
σ^4	2.8	2.4	2.1	2	2	2	2	2	2	1.9	1.9	1.9	1.9
Contrast	76	14	6	4	3	3	3	4	4	4	5	5	6
C	58	51	50	47	47	47	47	47	47	44	44	44	46
CSR	–	0.44	0.44	0.44	0.44	0.44	0.44	0.44	0.44	0.44	0.44	0.44	0.46
MSE	–	1,754	1,757	1,758	1,760	1,762	1,764	1,765	1,766	1,767	1,768	1,768	1,770
SNR	–	19	16	15	14	14	13	12	12	11	11	10	9
Q	–	0.82	0.67	0.47	0.39	0.35	0.29	0.24	0.20	0.18	0.16	0.13	0.11
SSIN	–	0.80	0.61	0.59	0.57	0.56	0.54	0.52	0.50	0.49	0.48	0.46	0.45
MD	–	38	62	67	80	95	124	157	189	214	223	254	267
LMSE	–	0.78	0.93	0.94	0.99	2.5	3.4	4.5	5.6	6.2	7.1	8.02	8.3

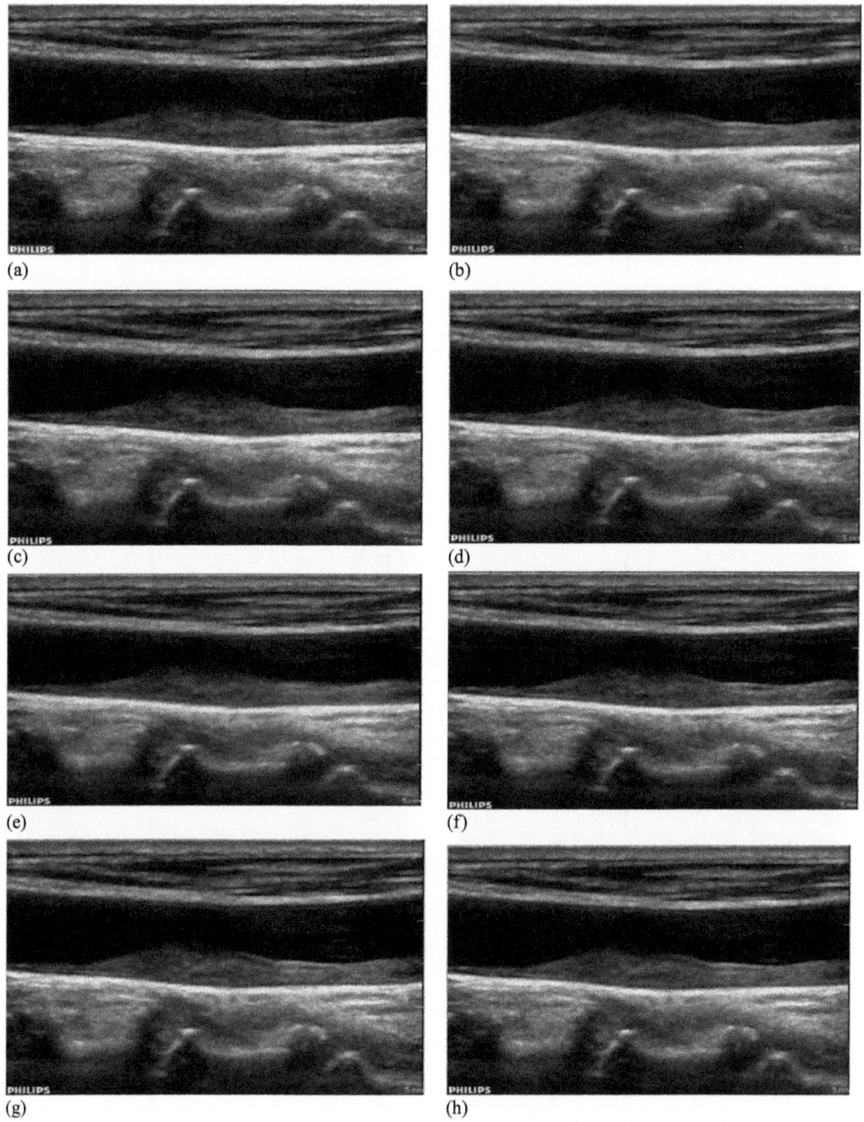

Figure 7.5 Examples of despeckle filtering with the filter DsFlsmv *on a symptomatic video of the CCA with plaque at the far wall on frames 1, 50, 100, 150, 200, 250 and 250 illustrated in (b)–(h), respectively. (a) illustrates the original image of frame 1 of the video, before despeckle filtering. © 2015, Reprinted from [77]*

Algorithm 7.2 presents the algorithmic steps for the implementation of the *DsFwiener* despeckle filter for image despeckling. For video despeckling, the procedure described above is repeated for each consecutive video frame or selected video frames depending on the application.

Table 7.4 Selected statistical and image quality evaluation features for Figure 7.5 before and after despeckle filtering with the DsFlsmv filter for increasing the number of iterations and constant window size of [5×5]. © 2015, Reprinted from [77]

Features	**Number of iterations**												
	Original	**1**	**2**	**3**	**4**	**5**	**6**	**7**	**8**	**9**	**10**	**15**	**20**
μ	77	76	76	75	75	73	72	71	70	69	68	65	45
Median	68	68	68	67	65	64	63	62	62	60	59	57	49
σ^2	67	64	63	62	61	60	58	57	55	54	53	46	39
σ^3	0.63	0.58	0.56	0.53	0.49	0.47	0.44	0.41	0.39	0.37	0.36	0.31	0.26
σ^4	2.4	2.4	2.4	2.4	2.5	2.5	2.6	2.6	2.7	2.7	3.0	3.2	3.6
Contrast	334	313	310	308	307	305	303	300	296	292	286	272	243
C	87	89	89	90	91	93	35	97	98	100	102	115	126
CSR	–	0.09	0.09	0.08	0.08	0.07	0.07	0.07	0.06	0.06	0.05	0.03	0.03
MSE	–	10,480	10,482	10,485	10,490	10,493	10,496	10,499	10,501	10,555	10,555	10,560	10,656
SNR	–	25	25	24	22	21	20	19	18	17	15	12	10
Q	–	0.87	0.85	0.81	0.78	0.75	0.72	0.68	0.63	0.54	0.46	0.39	0.27
SSIN	–	0.89	0.86	0.83	0.79	0.77	0.73	0.70	0.62	0.52	0.47	0.38	0.26
MD	–	167	171	182	189	192	198	203	212	225	230	245	267
LMSE	–	0.18	0.32	0.35	0.41	0.47	0.54	0.67	0.74	0.88	0.92	1.92	2.01

Figure 7.6 illustrates the application of the despeckle filter *DsFwiener* on the phantom image of the CCA with the original and the despeckled images shown on the left and right column, respectively. Table 7.5 illustrates selected statistical and image quality features for the phantom image of Figure 7.6 for the original and the despeckled images.

Algorithm 7.2 Linear filtering: linear scaling filter (*DsFwiener*)

1. *Load the image for filtering*
2. *Specify the region of interest to be filtered, the moving sliding window size and the number of iterations*
3. *Compute the noise variance* σ_n^2 *with* (7.6) *for the whole image (frame)*
4. *Starting from the left upper corner of the image (frame), compute for each sliding moving window the coefficient* $k_{i,j}$ *in* (7.5)
5. *Compute* $f_{i,j}$ *in* (7.2) *and replace the noisy middle point in each moving window* $g_{i,j}$, *with the new computed value* $f_{i,j}$
6. *Repeat steps* 4 *and* 5 *for all the pixels in the image (frame) by sliding the moving window from left to right*
   For video despeckling, repeat steps 1 *to* 6 *for all consecutive video frames*
7. *Repeat steps* 3 *to* 6 *for a second iteration of despeckle filtering*
8. *Compute the image quality evaluation metrics and the texture features for the original and the despeckled images (video frames)*
9. *Display the original and despeckled images (videos), the image quality and evaluation metrics, and the texture features*

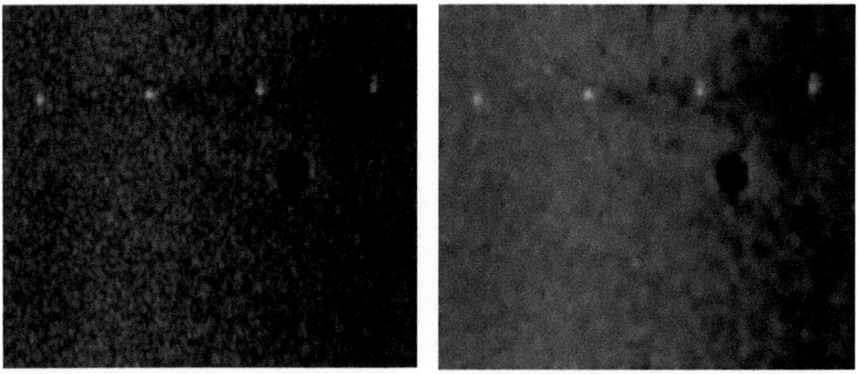

(a) (b)

Figure 7.6 Example of DsFwiener despeckle filtering on a phantom ultrasound image. (a) Original phantom image, (b) DsFwiener ([5×5] window, four iterations)

Table 7.5 Selected statistical and image quality features for Figure 7.6 before and after despeckle filtering for the DsFwiener despeckle filter. © 2015, Reprinted from [77]

Features	μ	Median	σ^2	σ^3	σ^4	Contrast	C	CSR	MSE	PSNR	Q	SSIN	AD	SC	MD	NAE
Original	36	37	21	0.2	2.8	76	58	–	–	–	–	–	–	–	–	–
DsFwiener	**36**	39	**18**	0.06	3.0	65	50	10	1,730	29	0.4	0.58	0.1	1.1	34	0.21

Bold values show improvement after despeckle filtering.

7.2 Local statistics filtering with higher moments (*DsFlsminv1d, DsFlsmvsk2d*)

As discussed earlier, many of the despeckle filters proposed in the literature suffer from smoothing effects in edge areas. Because of their statistical working principle, the edges may be better detected by incorporating higher statistical variance moments (variance, skewness, kurtosis) [60], calculated from the local moving window. The variance in every window, σ_w^2, may thus be described as a function of the variance, σ^2, skewness, σ^3, and kurtosis, σ^4, in the sliding moving local window and is calculated for the filter *DsFlsminv1d* as (see also Figure 7.1(b)):

$$\sigma_w^2 = \left(c_2\sigma^2 + c_3\sigma^3 + c_4\sigma^4\right)/(c_2 + c_3 + c_4) \tag{7.7}$$

The constants c_2, c_3, c_4, in (7.7), may be calculated using [7]:

$$R = 1 - \frac{1}{1+\sigma^2}, \tag{7.8}$$

which represents the smoothness of the image. Specifically, the constants c_2, c_3, c_4 are calculated, by replacing, the variance σ^2, in (7.8), the skewness, σ^3, and the kurtosis, σ^4, in the moving pixel window, respectively. The higher moments are each, weighted with a factor, c_2, c_3, c_4, which receives values, $0 < c < 1$. Equations (7.7) and (7.8) will be applied in windows where

$$c_3\sigma^3 \leq c_2\sigma^2 \leq c_4\sigma^4. \tag{7.9}$$

In regions where (7.9) is not valid, the window variance can be calculated as

$$\sigma_w^2 = \left(c_2\sigma^2 + c_4\sigma^4\right)/(c_2 + c_4). \tag{7.10}$$

The final value for the σ_w^2 will be used to replace the variance, σ^2, and will be further used for calculating the coefficient of variation in (7.5). The *DsFlsminv1d* despeckle filter operates in the 1D direction, by calculating the σ_w^2 for each row and each column in the sliding moving window (see Figure 7.1(b)), where the introduction of the higher moments in the filtering process should preserve the edges and should not smooth the image in areas with strong pixel variations. The middle pixel in the window is then replaced with (7.8), by replacing the $k_{i,j}$ weighting factor with the σ_w^2. The σ_w^2 in (7.10) can be interpreted as a generalized moment weighting factor with the weighting coefficients c_2, c_3, c_4. The moving window size for the *DsFlsminv1d* filter was 5×5 and its operation is shown in Figure 7.1(b).

The despeckle filter *DsFlsmvsk2d* [7] is the 2D realization of the *DsFlsminv1d* utilizing the higher statistical moments, σ^3 and σ^4, of the image in a 5×5 pixel moving window.

Algorithm 7.3 presents the algorithmic steps for the implementation of the *DsFlsmvsk2d* despeckle filter.

Algorithm 7.3 Linear filtering: linear scaling filter (*DsFlsmvsk2d*)

1. *Load the image for filtering*
2. *Specify the region of interest to be filtered, the moving window size and the number of iterations (n)*
3. *Compute the noise variance* σ_n^2 *with* (7.6) *for the whole image*
4. *Starting from the left upper corner of the image, compute for each moving window the coefficient* win_var *as follows:*
5. *If* (7.9) *is true, use* (7.7) *otherwise use* (7.10)
6. *Compute* $f_{i,j}$ *in* (7.2) *and replace the noisy middle point in each moving window* $g_{i,j}$, *with the new computed value* $f_{i,j}$, *by using the* win_var *for the coefficient of variation* $k_{i,j}$
7. *Repeat steps* 4 *to* 6 *for all the pixels in the image by sliding the moving window from left to right*
8. *Repeat steps* 3 *to* 7 *for* n *iterations*
9. *Compute the image quality evaluation metrics and the texture features for the original and the despeckled images*
10. *Display the original and despeckled images, the image quality and evaluation metrics, and the texture features*

Figure 7.7 illustrates the application of the despeckle filters *DsFlsminv1d* and *DsFlsmvsk2d* on the phantom ultrasound image of the CCA with the original shown in Figure 7.7(a) and the despeckled images shown in Figure 7.7(b), (c) and (d), respectively. Table 7.6 illustrates selected statistical and image quality features for the phantom image of Figure 7.7 for the original and the despeckled images. Bold values show improvement after despeckle filtering. It is shown that both filters preserve the mean, while the *DsFlsmvsk2d* increases enormously the CSR.

7.3 Homogeneous mask area filtering (*DsFlsminsc*)

The *DsFlsminsc* is a 2D filter operating in a 5×5 pixel neighborhood by searching for the most homogenous neighborhood area around each pixel, using a 3×3 subset window [78], as shown in Figure 7.1(c). The middle pixel of the 5×5 neighborhood is substituted with the average gray level of the 3×3 mask with the smallest speckle index, C, where C for log-compressed images is given in [77]. The window with the smallest C is the most homogenous semi-window, which presumably, does not contain any edge. The filter is applied iteratively until the gray levels of almost all pixels in the image do not change.

The operation of the *DsFlsminsc* filter may be described as follows (see also Figure 7.1(c)):

1. Slide the 3×3 mask with the (5×5 pixel) selected window.
2. Detect the position of the mask for which the C is minimum.

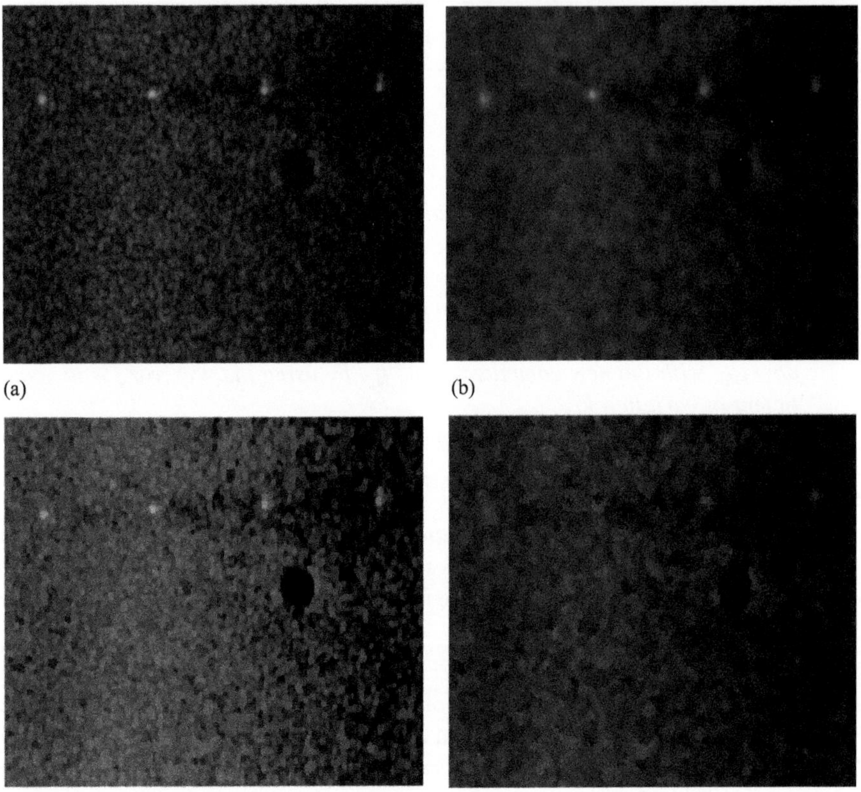

(a) (b) (c) (d)

Figure 7.7 Example of DsFlsminv1d in (b) and DsFlsmvsk2d despeckle filtering on a phantom ultrasound image of the CCA in (c) and (d), respectively. (a) Original phantom image, (b) DsFlsminv1d ([1×5] window, 2 iterations), (c) DsFlsmvsk2d ([5×5] window, 1 iteration), (d) DsFlsmvsk2d ([5×5] window, 2 iterations)

3. Assign the average gray level of the mask to the middle pixel of the 5×5 window.
4. Apply steps 1 to 3 for all pixels in the image.
5. Iterate the above process until the gray levels of almost all pixels in the image do not change.

Algorithm 7.4 presents the algorithmic steps for the implementation of the DsFlsminsc despeckle filter. Figure 7.8 shows the application of the despeckle filter DsFlsminsc on a phantom ultrasound image for a moving window size 5×5 pixels and three iterations.

Table 7.6 Selected statistical features for Figure 7.7 before and after despeckle filtering for the DsFlsminv1d *and* DsFlsmvsk2d *(for 1 iteration) despeckle filters*

Features	μ	**Median**	σ^2	σ^3	σ^4	**Contrast**	**C**	**CSR**	**MSE**	**PSNR**	**Q**	**SSIN**	**AD**	**SC**	**MD**	**NAE**
Original	36	37	21	0.2	2.8	76	58	–	–	–	–	–	–	–	–	–
DsFlsminvld	**34**	36	**19**	0.12	2.0	54	**56**	3	1746	16	0.5	0.65	0.09	1.2	44	0.21
DsFlsmvsk2d	**36**	43	**18**	0.19	2.1	49	**52**	10	1735	14	0.5	0.79	1.2	1.1	1,112	0.20

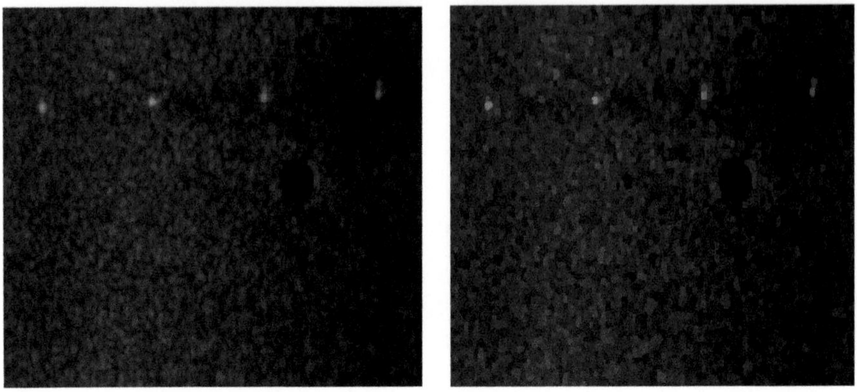

(a) (b)

Figure 7.8 Example of the DsFlsminsc despeckle filtering on a phantom ultrasound image. (a) Original phantom image, (b) DsFlsminsc *([5×5] window, 2 iterations)*

Table 7.7 illustrates selected statistical and image quality features for the phantom image of Figure 7.8, the original and the despeckled images. Bold values show improvement after despeckle filtering. It is shown that filter DsFlsminsc preserves almost all features very well and decreases C.

Algorithm 7.4 Linear filtering: homogeneous mask area filtering (*DsFlsminsc*)

---

1. *Load the image for filtering*
2. *Specify the region of interest to be filtered, the moving window size, the number of iterations (n) and the edge detector to be used*
3. *Starting from the left upper corner of the image, rotate a mask around the middle pixel of the window for each moving window*
4. *Detect the position of the mask for which the speckle index, C is minimum*
5. *Assign the average gray level of the mask at the selected position to the middle pixel in the* 5×5 *window*
6. *Repeat steps* 4 *and* 5 *for all the pixels in the image by sliding the moving window from left to right*
7. *Repeat steps* 3 *to* 6 *for a second iteration of despeckle filtering*
8. *Compute the image quality evaluation metrics and the texture features for the original and the despeckled images*
9. *Display the original and despeckled images, the image quality and evaluation metrics, and the texture features*

Table 7.7 Selected statistical and image quality features for Figure 7.8 before and after despeckle filtering for the DsFlsminsc *despeckle filter*

Features	μ	Median	σ^2	σ^3	σ^4	Contrast	C	CSR	MSE	SNR	Q	SSIN	AD	SC	MD	NAE
Original	36	37	21	0.2	2.8	76	58	–		–	–	–	–	–	–	–
DsFlsminsc	36	36	22	0.2	2.8	75	**48**	21	1,757	20	0.84	0.86	0.22	0.98	54	0.13

Bold values show improvement after despeckle filtering.

7.4 Despeckle filtering evaluation on an artificial carotid artery image

Despeckle filtering was evaluated on an artificial carotid artery image corrupted by speckle noise (see Figure 7.9(a)). Figure 7.9 shows the original noisy image of the artificial carotid artery, degraded by speckle noise, together with the despeckled images. Figure 7.10 shows line profiles (intensity), for the line marked in Figure 7.9(a) for all despeckle filters. The profile results show that most of the filters (DsFlsmv, DsFwiener and DsFlsminsc) preserved the edge boundaries. Best results were obtained for the filters *DsFwiener*, *DsFlsmv* and *DsFlsminsc* that preserved the edge boundaries preserving the locality and minimally affecting the reference values in each region. The despeckled images of Figure 7.9 were also assessed by two experts. Filters that showed an improved smoothing after filtering, as assessed by visual perception criteria, were in the following order: *DsFlsmv*, *DsFlsminsc* and *DsFwiener*.

The upper part of Table 7.8 tabulates the statistical features μ, median, σ^2, σ^3, σ^4, the contrast, the speckle index, C [77,78] and the contrast-speckle ratio, CSR [77,78], for the artificial image and the 16 filters illustrated in Figure 7.9. Also, the number of iterations (no. of iterations), for each despeckle filter is given, which was

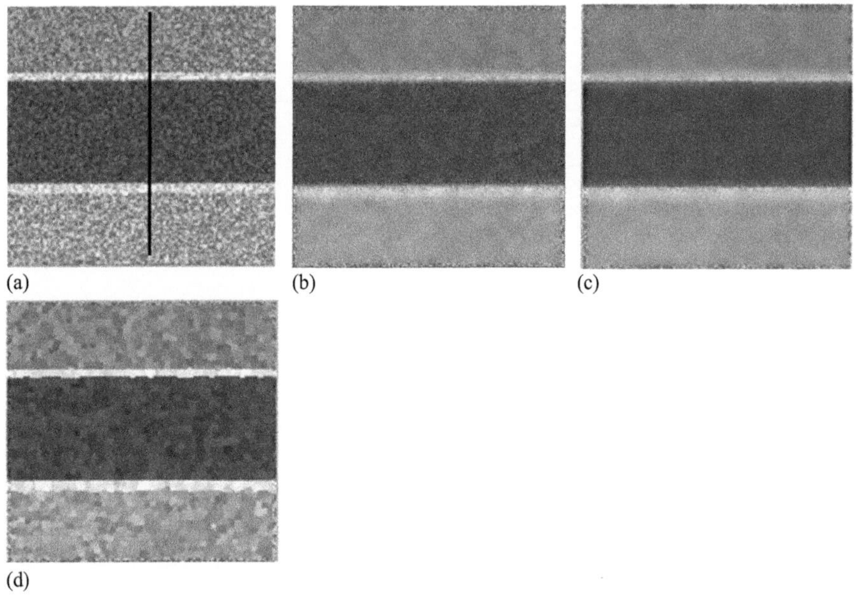

Figure 7.9 Original noisy image of an artificial carotid artery given in (a) and the application of the three despeckle filters given in (b)–(d). (Vertical line given in (a) defines the position of the line intensity profiles plotted in Figure 7.10). (a) Original phantom image, (b) DsFlsmv ([5×5], 3 iterations, (c) DsFwiener ([5×5], 3 iterations), (d) DsFlsminsc ([5×5], 4 iterations)

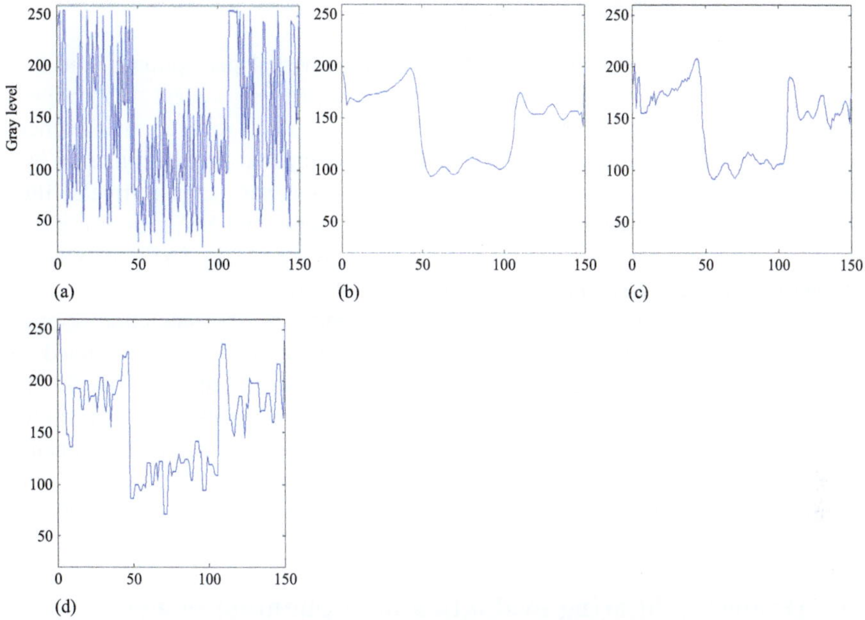

Figure 7.10 Line profiles of the line illustrated in Figure 7.9(a) for the original noisy image (a), and the three despeckled images given in (b)–(d). (a) Original phantom carotid image, (b) DsFlsmv, (c) DsFwiener and (d) DsFlsminsc

Table 7.8 Selected statistical features and image quality evaluation metrics for images of Figure 7.9 before and after despeckle filtering

Feature No. of iterations Window size	**Original image**	**Linear filtering**		
		DsFlsmv 2 5×5	**DsFLsminsc 1 5×5**	**DsFwiener 2 5×5**
μ	138	145	157	145
Median	132	151	162	157
σ^2	53	41	46	37
σ^3	0.85	−0.1	0.09	−0.2
σ^4	2.0	2.0	1.8	1.6
Contrast	124	68	239	27
C	38	28	29	26
CSR		99	263	101
MSE		24,510	24,516	24,520
RMSE		31	33	47
Err3		32	37	58
SNR		18	17	14
Q		0.79	0.59	0.46
SSIN		0.81	0.51	0.33
SC		1.31	1.06	0.98
MD		125	127	188
NAE		0.22	0.18	0.23

selected based on the speckle index, C, and on the visual perception of the two experts. When C was minimally changing then the filtering process was stopped. As shown in Table 7.8, all filters reduced the C. Filters that reduced the variance, σ^2, while preserving the mean, μ, and the median compared to the original image were *DsFlsmv* and *DsFwiener*. The contrast of the image was increased by the filter *DsFlsminsc*, and it was decreased by the filter *DsFwiener* and *DsFlsmv*. It is noted that filters *DsFlsmv* and *DsFlsminsc* reduced C, increased CSR; *DsFlsmv* reduced the contrast, whereas *DsFlsminsc* increased the contrast.

The lower part of Table 7.8 tabulates the image quality evaluation metrics presented [77,78] for the artificial carotid artery ultrasound image illustrated in Figure 7.9. The quality metrics were calculated between the original (see Figure 7.9(a)) and the despeckled images (see Figure 7.1(b) and (d)). Best values were obtained for the *DsFlsmv and DsFlsminsc* with higher SNR. Best values for the universal quality index, Q, and the SSIN, were obtained for the filter *DsFlsmv*. The SC was best for the filters *DsFlsmv* and *DsFlsminsc*. The smallest MD values were given for the *DsFlsmv* and *DsFlsminsc* filters.

7.5 Despeckle filtering evaluation on a phantom image

Despeckle filtering was evaluated on a phantom carotid (see Figure 7.9(a) and used in introducing the filters in this chapter). Figure 7.9(a) shows the original phantom ultrasound images and the despeckled phantom images (see Figure 7.9(b) and (d)) after the application of the linear despeckle filters DsFlsmv, DsFwiener and DsFlsminsc, for different window sizes (given in brackets) and number of iterations (shown in parentheses). Best results were obtained for the filters DsFlsmv, DsFlsminsc and DsFwiener which preserves edges.

Furthermore, diameter and area measurements were carried out for the anechoic cylinder of Figure 7.11(a) and tabulated in Table 7.9. The following measurements were carried out: (i) two measurements of the diameter (where each measurement was perpendicular to the other), (ii) area of the anechoic cylinder using the average of the two diameter measurements and (iii) the percentage area error difference between the original area and the area estimated in (ii).

The upper part of Table 7.9 tabulates the statistical features, μ, median, σ^2, σ^3, σ^4, the contrast, the speckle index, C, and the contrast-speckle-radio, CSR, for the phantom image and the three despeckle filters illustrated in Figures 7.9 and 7.10. As shown in Table 7.9, all filters reduced C. The CSR is better for the *DsFlsmv*. Filters that reduced the variance, σ^2, while preserving the mean, μ, and the median compared to the original image were *DsFwiener* and *DsFlsmv*. The contrast of the image is increased by the filter *DsFlsminsc* (enormously). It is decreased by the filters *DsFlsmv* and *DsFwiener*. It is noted that filters *DsFlsmv* and *DsFlsminsc* reduced C; *DsFlsmv* reduced the contrast, whereas *DsFlsminsc* increased the contrast. The despeckled images of Figure 7.11 were also assessed by the two experts. Filter that showed an improved smoothing after filtering, as assessed visually by the two experts, using visual perception criteria was the *DsFlsmv*. Filters that showed a blurring effect especially on the edges were the *DsFlsminsc* and *DsFwiener*.

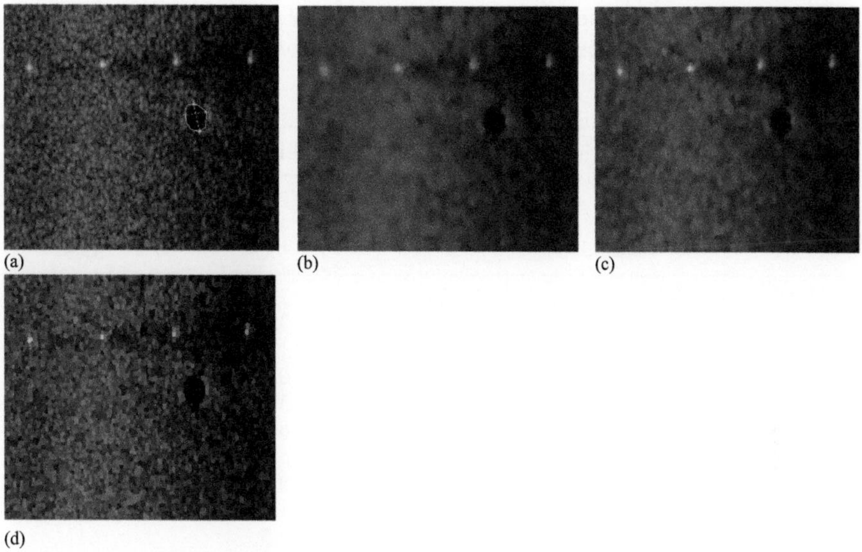

Figure 7.11 Original phantom image given in (a) and the application of three despeckle filters for different number of iterations and different pixel moving window sizes, shown in brackets, given in (b)–(d). See Table 7.10 for number of iterations and window size. (a) Original phantom image, (b) DsFlsmv([5×5], 5 iterations), (c) DsFwiener ([5×5], 4 iterations), (d) DsFlsminsc([5×5], 4 iterations)

The lower part of Table 7.9 tabulates the image quality evaluation metrics for the phantom carotid artery ultrasound image illustrated in Figure 7.11. The image quality metrics were calculated between the original (see Figure 7.11(a)) and the despeckled images (see Figure 7.11(b) and (d)). Best values were obtained for the *DsFlsmv* and *DsFlsminsc* with lower RMSE and Err3, and higher SNR. Best values for the universal quality index, Q, and the SSIN, were obtained for the filter *DsFlsmv*. The SC was best for the filters *DsFlsmv* and *DsFlsminsc*. The smallest MD was given by *DsFwiener* filter, while for the NAE best values were obtained for the filter *DsFlsminsc*. Finally, the lowest part of Table 7.9 illustrates the manual measurements of diameter 1 and diameter 2 and the area of the anechoic cylinder in Figure 7.11. The percentage area error for most of the filters was small of the order of a few percent.

7.6 Despeckle filtering evaluation on real ultrasound images and video

Figure 7.12 shows an ultrasound image of the carotid artery together with the despeckled images. Table 7.10 tabulates the statistical features and image quality

Table 7.9 Selected statistical features, image quality evaluation metrics and shape[a] measurements for Figure 7.11 before and after despeckle filtering

Feature No. of iterations Window	Original	Linear filtering		
		DsFlsmv **2** **5×5**	**DsFwiener** **4** **5×5**	**DsFlsminsc** **4** **5×5**
μ	36	35	36	36
Median	37	40	39	37
σ^2	21	17	18	22
σ^3	0.2	0.3	0.06	0.2
σ^4	2.8	2	3	3
Contrast	76	4	6	114
C	58	48	50	51
CSR*100		0.5	0.02	0.09
MSE		1,741	1,754	1,734
RMSE		8.4	9.5	9.1
Err3		10.4	10.9	14.2
SNR		14.8	15.8	13.7
Q		0.73	0.36	0.22
SSIN		0.74	0.58	0.43
SC		1.31	1.11	1.22
MD		74	34	81
NAE		0.92	0.94	0.87
Diameter 1	5.77	5.78	5.74	5.86
Diameter 2	5.61	5.64	5.73	5.77
Area[a]	17.87	17.93	18.01	18.26
%Area		0.35	0.79	2.19

[a]Shape measurements refer to the anechoic cylinder of Figure 7.11 (marked in Figure 7.11(a)).

evaluation metrics of the despeckled images. The best visual results as assessed by the two experts were obtained for the filters *DsFlsmv* and *DsFlsminsc* Those filters performed filtering without destroying subtle details and preserving the edges. The filter that showed a blurring effect was the *DsFwiener*, which also showed poorer visual results, when compared with the rest of the filters. The corresponding number of iterations and window size for each filter is given in Table 7.10. The intima-media complex (IMC) was automatically segmented [25], and the intima-media thickness (IMT) measurements for each despeckled image are shown in millimeters in the last two rows of Table 7.10. Additionally, the percentage difference (%) between the original and despeckled IMT measurements is shown. The smallest percentage difference was obtained by the filter *DsFlsminsc*.

Figure 7.13 shows two original ultrasound cardiac images in (a) and (b) and the despeckled images in (c) and (d) with the filter *DsFlsmv*. The corresponding

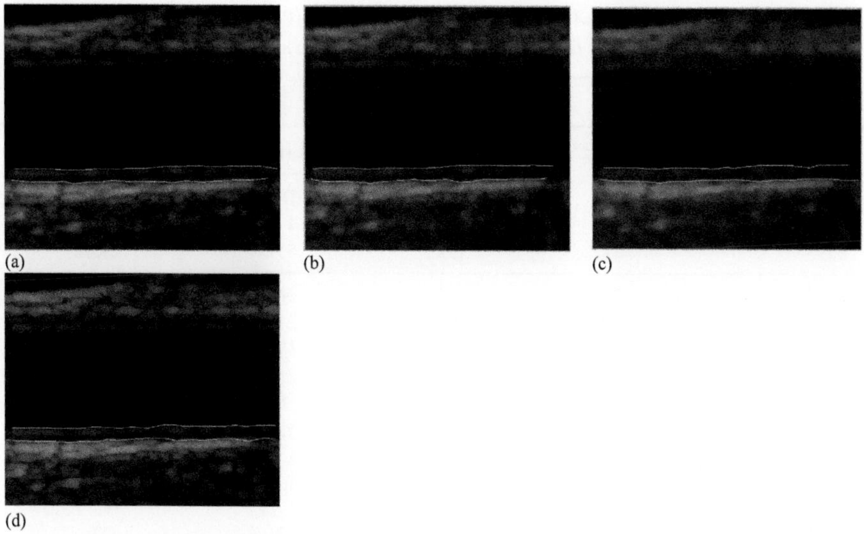

Figure 7.12 Original ultrasound image of the carotid artery (2–3 cm proximal to bifurcation) given in (a) and the despeckled filtered images given in (b)–(d). (a) Original image, (b) DsFlsmv *([5×5], 5 iterations), (c)* DsFwiener *([5×5], 4 iterations), (d)* DsFlsminsc*([5×5], 4 iterations). The corresponding number of iterations and window size for each filter is given in Table 7.10. Also, the IMC segmentation derived using snakes as documented in [25] is demonstrated in the far wall of the image. In addition, the corresponding measurements of IMT are tabulated in the last row of Table 7.10*

number of iterations and the moving sliding windows applied were the same as in Figure 7.12. The filter *DsFlsmv* preserved the mean (see also Table 7.11).

Figure 7.14 shows the original (see Figure 7.14(a), (c) and (e)) and despeckled (see Figure 7.14(b), (d) and (f)) frames numbered 1, 100 and 200 from an ultrasound CCA video consisting of 300 frames, with a width of 211 and a height of 256 pixels, captured at 30 frames/second. The *DsFlsmv* despeckle filter was iteratively applied for two iterations at consecutive video frames with a moving sliding window size of 5×5 pixels. The filtering was only applied to the luminance channel of the video (Y-channel). The speckle index (C), for the original and despeckled frames, was also calculated and it is given in parentheses. It is clear that C is reduced after despeckle filtering for all frames. Table 7.12 tabulates selected statistical features and image quality metrics for the original and the despeckled video frames for the despeckle filter *DsFlsmv*. It is observed that the effect of despeckle filtering is similar with that on images and also that there is variability in the tabulated statistical and quality metrics among the video frames investigated.

Table 7.10 Selected statistical features, image quality evaluation metrics and intima-media thickness (IMT) (mean±std) [mm] measurements for images of Figure 7.12 before and after despeckle filtering

Feature	**Original**	**Linear filtering**		
No. of iterations				
Window size		**DsFlsmv**	**DsFwiener**	**DsFIsminsc**
		2	**4**	**4**
		5×5	**5×5**	**5×5**
μ	24	27	26	26
Median	21	19	21	9
σ^2	34	40	37	32
σ^3	1.99	2.42	2.41	1.79
σ^4	7.55	9.75	10.12	5.81
Contrast	143	392	321	49
C	1.45	1.44	1.42	1.23
CSR*100	–	1.47	1.36	0.87
MSE	–	1,718	1,717	1,717
RMSE	–	27	22	23
Err3	–	48	43	43
SNR	–	8	9	9
Q	–	0.83	0.67	0.69
SSIN	–	0.91	0.85	0.82
SC	–	0.75	0.86	0.85
MD	–	199	204	203
NAE	–	0.36	0.32	0.32
IMT_{mean} [mm]	0.72	0.69	0.71	0.72
IMT_{std} [mm]	0.90	0.11	0.9	0.12
Difference [%]		4.17	1.37	0.001

Difference [%]: Percentage difference
[(Original_IMT_{mean}–Despeckled_IMT_{mean})/Original_IMT_{mean}]*100%.

7.7 Summary findings on despeckle filtering evaluation

Despeckle filtering is an important operation in the enhancement of ultrasound images of the carotid artery. In this chapter, a total of five despeckle filters were presented and three were evaluated on artificial, phantom and real ultrasound images and videos.

As given in Table 7.13, filter DsFlsmv improved the statistical and texture features analysis, the measurements and shape features, the image quality evaluation and the optical perception evaluation. This was observed for both filters on the artificial image phantom and the real ultrasound images. The filter DsFlsminsc improved the statistical and texture image analysis and the image quality evaluation in real carotid ultrasound images. The DsFlsmv filter, which is a simple filter, is based on local image statistics gave very good performance. It was first introduced in [36,38,47] by Jong-Sen Lee *et al.*, and it was tested on a few SAR images with very satisfactory results. It was also used for SAR imaging in [46] and image restoration in [49], again with very satisfactory results.

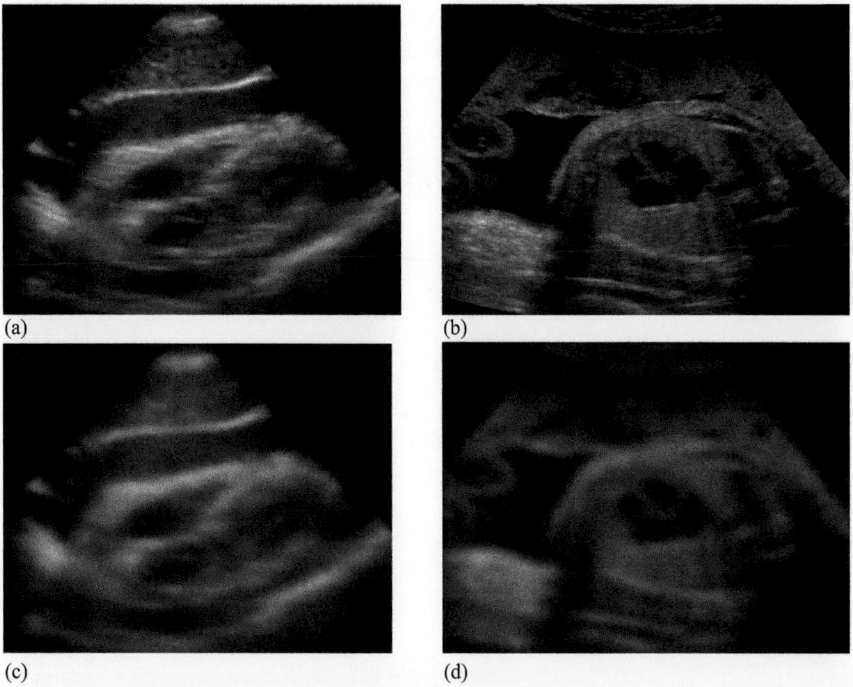

Figure 7.13 *(a) and (b) Original cardiac ultrasound images and the despeckled images with the filters DsFlsmv ([5×5], 5 iterations) in (c) and (d), respectively. The corresponding number of iterations and the window size used were the same used in Figure 7.12*

Despeckle filtering was investigated by other researchers and also in our study, on an artificial carotid image (Figure 7.9), [7,29] on line profiles (Figure 7.10) of different ultrasound images, [2,3,7,28,59], on phantom ultrasound images [3,5,40], SAR images [50,53–55], real longitudinal ultrasound images of the carotid artery (Figure 7.12) [3,7,29] and cardiac ultrasound images (see Figure 7.13). There are only two studies [29,7] where despeckle filtering was investigated on real and artificial longitudinal ultrasound image of the carotid artery. Four different despeckle filters were applied in [29], namely the DsFlsmv [38], Frost [46], anisotropic diffusion (DsFad) [27] and a despeckle reducing anisotropic diffusion (DsFsrad) filter [29]. The despeckle window used for the DsFlsmv, and Frost filters was 5×5 pixels. To evaluate the performance of these filters, the mean and the standard deviation were used, which were calculated in different regions of the carotid artery image, namely in lumen, tissue and at the vascular wall. The mean gray level values of the original image for the lumen, tissue and wall regions were 1.03, 5.31 and 22.8, whereas the variances were 0.56, 2.69 and 10.61. The mean after despeckle filtering with the DsFsrad gave brighter values for the lumen and tissue. Specifically, the mean for the lumen, tissue and wall for the DsFsrad was (1.19, 6.17,

Table 7.11 Selected statistical features and image quality evaluation metrics for Figure 7.13(a) (-/) and Figure 7.13(g) (/-) (original images) and Figure 7.13 (c) (-/) and Fig. 7.13 (d) (/-) (despeckled images with filter DsFlsmv)

Feature	**Original**	**DsFIsmv**
No. of iterations		**2**
Window size		**5×5**
μ	42/37	43/33
Median	27/18	29/22
σ^2	48/33	41/33
σ^3	1.18/1.14	1.03/1.04
σ^4	3.87/3.73	3.34/3.58
Contrast	91/82	87/56
C	114/112	95/99
CSR*100	–	0.51/0.01
MSE	–	3612/2438
RMSE	–	6.2/12.2
Err3	–	54/17
SNR	–	11/15
Q	–	0.78/0.67
SSIN	–	0.89/0.71
SC	–	0.93/1.12
MD	–	225/217
NAE	–	0.19/0.25

Table 7.12 Selected statistical features and image quality evaluation metrics for Figure 7.14 for the despeckle filter DsFlsmv *on selected video frames before and after despeckle filtering*

Feature	**Original**	**DsFlsmv**	**Original**	**DsFlsmv**	**Original**	**DsFlsmv**
No. of iterations	**Frame 1**		**Frame 100**		**Frame 200**	
μ	40.14	44.88	44.64	44.79	44.86	45.06
Median	38.23	45.35	42.05	45.05	42.34	45.81
σ^2	34.42	37.43	38.99	37.34	38.86	37.22
σ^3	0.65	0.72	0.61	0.72	0.62	0.73
σ^4	2.99	4.01	2.69	4.03	2.72	4.09
Contrast	215	307	231	305	234	309
C	85	82	87	84	87	83
CSR*100	–	1.1	–	0.36	–	0.65
MSE	–	3281	–	3780	–	3787
RMSE	–	4.76	–	22.4	–	11.4
Err3	–	9.58	–	41.77	–	13.51
SNR	–	25	–	12	–	18
Q	–	0.99	–	0.65	–	0.71
SSIN	–	0.99	–	0.77	–	0.84
SC	–	1.05	–	1.11	–	1.18
MD	–	51	–	254	–	82
NAE	–	0.002	–	0.22	–	0.15

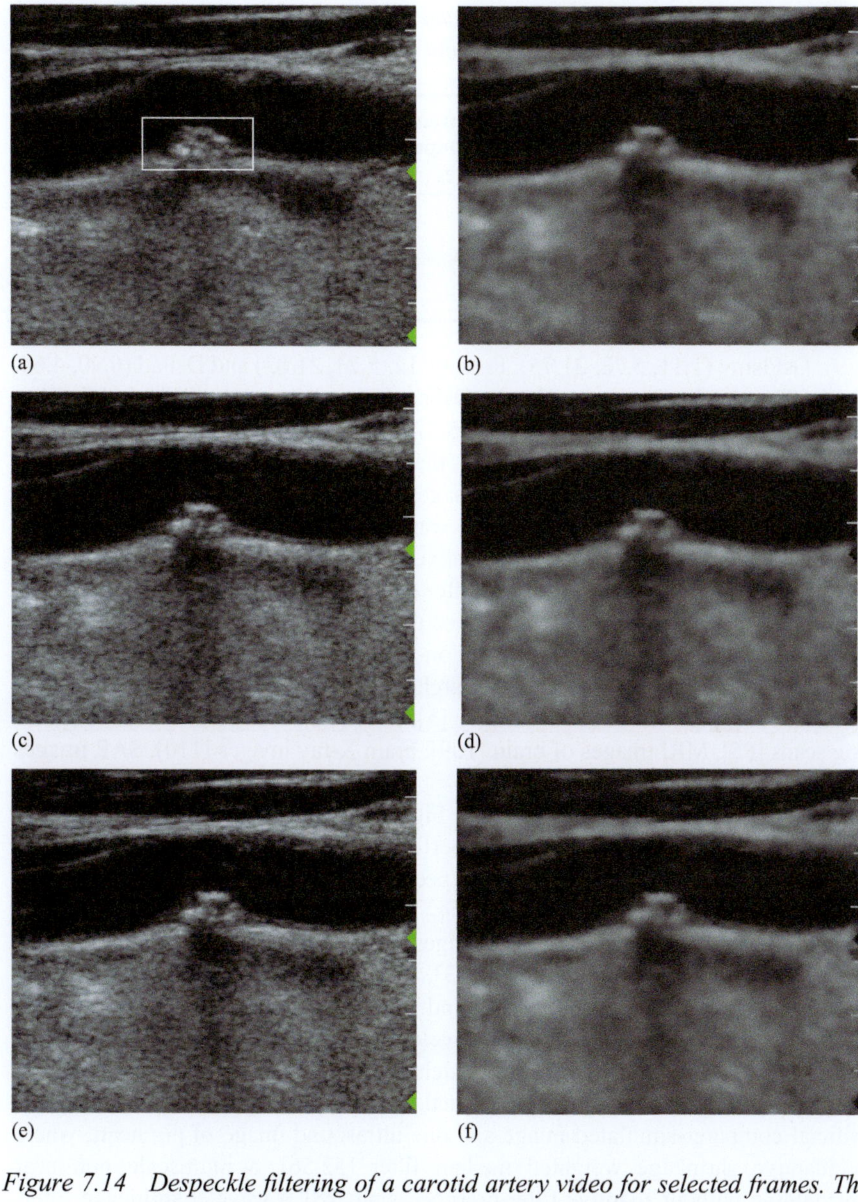

Figure 7.14 *Despeckle filtering of a carotid artery video for selected frames. The despeckle filter DsFlsmv was iteratively applied for two iterations at each video frame, using a sliding moving window of size [5×5]. The carotid plaque is indicated with an ROI in the first frame at the far wall of the artery. The despeckle index (C) is also given for the corresponding despeckled frames. (a) Original frame 1 (C = 0.863), (b) despeckled frame 1 (C = 0.844), (c) original frame 100 (C = 0.861), (d) despeckled frame 100 (C = 0.831), (e) original frame 200 (C = 0.0855), (f) despeckled frame 200 (C = 0.825)*

Table 7.13 Summary findings of despeckle filtering in an artificial carotid image (A), a phantom image (P) and real ultrasound image (C)

Despeckle filter	Statistical and texture features	Measurements and shape features	Image quality evaluation	Optical perception evaluation
	A/P/C	*A/P/C*	*A/P/C*	*A/P/C*
Linear filtering				
DsFlsmv	✓/✓/✓	–/✓/✓	✓/✓/✓	–/✓/✓
DsFlsminsc	–/–/✓	–/–/–	–/–/✓	–/–/–

18.9), DsFlsmv (1.11, 5.72, 21.75), Frost (1.12, 5.74, 21.83) and DsFad (0.90, 4.64, 14.64). The standard deviation for the DsFsrad gave lower values (0.15, 0.7, 2.86) when compared with Lee (0.33, 1.42, 5.37), Frost (0.32, 1.40, 5.30) and DsFad (0.20, 1.09, 3.52). It was thus shown that the DsFsrad filter preserves the mean and reduces the variance. The number of images investigated in [29], was very small, visual perception evaluation by experts was not carried out, as well as only two statistical measures were used to quantitatively evaluate despeckle filtering, namely the mean, and the variance before and after despeckle filtering as explained above. We believe that the mean and the variance used in [29] are not indicative and may not give a complete and accurate evaluation result as in [7]. Furthermore, despeckle filtering was investigated by other researchers on ultrasound images of heart [3], pig heart [28], pig muscle [108], kidney [5], liver [52], echocardiograms [51], CT lung scans [85], MRI images of brain [109], brain X-ray images [110], SAR images [50] and real world images [56].

Line plots, as used in our study (see Figure 7.10), were also used in few other studies to quantify despeckle filtering performance. Specifically, in [110], a line profile through the original and the despeckled ultrasound image of kidney was plotted, using adaptive Gaussian filtering. In [1], line profiles were plotted on 4 simulated and 15 ultrasound cardiac images of the left ventricle, in order to evaluate the median filter. In another study [3], line profiles through one phantom, one heart, one kidney and one liver ultrasound image were plotted where an adaptive shrinkage weighted median [52,56], wavelet shrinkage method [70] and wavelet shrinkage coherence enhancing [51] models were used and compared with a nonlinear coherent diffusion model [70]. Finally, in [28], line plots were used in one artificial computer-simulated image and one ultrasound image of pig heart, where an adaptive shrinkage weighted median filter [52,56], a multiscale nonlinear thresholding without adaptive filter preprocessing [28], a wavelet shrinkage filtering method [70] and a proposed adaptive nonlinear thresholding with adaptive preprocessing method [28] were evaluated. In all of the above studies, visual perception evaluation by experts, statistical and texture analysis, on multiple images, as performed in our study, was not performed.

Different aspects of despeckle filtering were surveyed in [111,112] where various speckle characterization methods were introduced. In [113], a comprehensive review on despeckle filtering techniques was presented. It was also shown in [111] that the speckle pattern from one specific area will ideally be unique and, therefore, it is identifiable. This makes speckle regarded as a fundamental source of information which is to be exploited for driving different applications. These applications include adaptive speckle suppression or filtering as shown in this book, speckle decorrelation [114], classification [115], freehand 3D reconstruction of ultrasound images [116], elastography [117], speckle-tracking echocardiography [118], tissue characterization [112], ultrasound image deconvolution and segmentation [119,120], and other methods where data-driven terms are crucial, e.g., level-sets [121], graph-cuts [122] or power watershed [36]. Once the speckle regions of interest are identified, it is also possible to track their patterns in the case of a continuously moving organ, such as the heart. This procedure is habitually referred to as "speckle tracking" whose essence is to compare two consecutive image frames and to follow the speckle regions of interest.

Most of the papers published in the literature for video filtering are limited to the reduction of additive noise, mainly by frame averaging. More specifically, in [123], the Wiener filtering method was applied to 3D image sequences for filtering additive noise, but results have not been thoroughly discussed and compared with other methods. The method was superior when compared to the purely temporal operations implemented earlier [124]. The pyramid thresholding method was used in [124], and wavelet-based additive denoising was used in [125] for additive noise reduction in image sequences. In another study [126], the image quality and evaluation metrics were used for evaluating the additive noise filtering and the transmission of image sequences through telemedicine channels. An improvement of almost all the quality metrics extracted from the original and processed images was demonstrated. An additive noise reduction algorithm, for image sequences, using variance characteristics of the noise was presented in [127]. Estimated noise power and sum of absolute difference employed in motion estimation were used to determine the temporal filter coefficients. A noise measurement scheme using the correlation between the noisy input and the noise-free image was applied for accurate estimation of the noise power. The experimental results showed that the proposed noise reduction method efficiently removes noise. An efficient method for movie denoising that does not require any motion estimation was presented in [128]. The method was based on the fact that averaging several realizations of a random variable reduces the variance. The method was unsupervised and was adapted to denoise image sequences with an additive white noise while preserving the visual details on the movie frames. Very little attention has been paid to the problem of missing data (impulsive distortion) removal in image sequences. In [129], a 3D median filter for removing impulsive noise from image sequences was developed. This filter was implemented without motion compensation and so the results did not capture the full potential of these structures. Further, the median operation, although quite successful in the additive noise filtering in images, invariably introduces distortion when filtering of image sequences [129]. This distortion primarily takes the form of blurring fine image details. Further, the median operation, although quite successful in the additive noise filtering in images, invariably introduces distortion when filtering of image sequences [130].

This distortion primarily takes the form of blurring fine image details. Finally, despeckle filtering may also be applied in video encoding and wireless video transmission as it was shown in [131]. More specifically, it was shown in [131] that despeckle filtering reduces the cost of video transmission, increases the transportation speed while preserving video quality.

The application of despeckle filters, the extraction of texture features, the calculation of image quality metrics and the visual perception evaluation by experts may also be applied to video. The video is broken into frames, which can then be processed one by one and then grouped together to form the processed video. Preliminary results for the application of despeckle filtering in an ultrasound carotid and an ultrasound cardiac video. However, significant work still remains to be carried out.

Despeckle filtering has been a rapidly emerging research area in recent years. The basic principles, the theoretical background and the algorithmic steps of a representative set of despeckle filters were covered in this book. Moreover, selected representative applications of image despeckling covering a variety of ultrasound image processing tasks will be presented in two monographs [77,78]. Most importantly, a despeckle filtering and evaluation protocol for imaging and video is documented in Table 7.14. The source code of the algorithms discussed in this book has been made available on the web, thus enabling researchers to more easily exploit the application of despeckle filtering in their problems under investigation.

For those readers, whose principal need is to use existing image despeckle filtering technologies and apply them on different type of images, there is no simple answer regarding which specific filtering algorithm should be selected without a significant understanding of both the filtering fundamentals and the application environment under investigation. A number of issues would need to be addressed. These include availability of the images to be processed/analyzed, the required

Table 7.14 Despeckle filtering and evaluation protocol

1. *Recording of ultrasound images:* Ultrasound images are acquired by ultrasound equipment and stored for further image processing. Regions of interest (ROI) could be selected for further processing
2. *Normalize the image:* The stored images may be retrieved and a normalized procedure may be applied
3. *Apply despeckle filtering:* Select the set of filters to apply despeckling together with their corresponding parameters (like moving window size, iterations and other)
4. *Texture features analysis:* After despeckle filtering the user may select ROI's (i.e., the plaque or the area around the intima-media thickness) and extract texture features. Distance metrics between the original and the despeckled images may be computed (as well as between different classes of if applicable)
5. *Compute image quality evaluation metrics:* On the elected ROI's compute image quality evaluation metrics between the original noisy and the despeckled images
6. *Visual quality evaluation by experts:* The original and/or despeckled images may be visually evaluated by experts
7. *Select the most appropriate despeckle filter/filters:* Based on steps 3 to 6 and construct a performance evaluation table and select the most appropriate filter(s) for the problem under investigation

level of filtering, the application scope (general purpose or application specific), the application goal (for extracting features from the image or for visual enhancement), the allowable computational complexity, the allowable implementation complexity and the computational requirements (e.g., real time or offline). We believe that a good understanding of the contents of this book can help the readers make the right choice of selecting the most appropriate filter for the application under development. Furthermore, the despeckle filtering evaluation protocol documented in Table 7.14 could also be exploited.

References

[1] B. Fetics, E. Wong, T. Murabayashi, *et al.*, "Enhancement of contrast echocardiography by image variability analysis," *IEEE Trans. Med. Imaging*, vol. 20, no. 11, pp. 1123–1130, Nov. 2001.

[2] C.I. Christodoulou, C. Loizou, C.S. Pattichis, *et al.*, "Despeckle filtering in ultrasound imaging of the carotid artery," *Second Joint EMBS/BMES Conference*, Houston, TX, USA, pp. 1027–1028, Oct. 23–26, 2002.

[3] K. Abd-Elmoniem, A.-B. Youssef, and Y. Kadah, "Real-time speckle reduction and coherence enhancement in ultrasound imaging via nonlinear anisotropic diffusion," *IEEE Trans. Biomed. Eng.*, vol. 49, no. 9, pp. 997–1014, Sep. 2002.

[4] J.E. Wilhjelm, M.S. Jensen, S.K. Jespersen, B. Sahl, and E. Falk, "Visual and quantitative evaluation of selected image combination schemes in ultrasound spatial compound scanning," *IEEE Trans. Med. Imaging*, vol. 23, no. 2, pp. 181–190, 2004.

[5] A. Achim, A. Bezerianos, and P. Tsakalides, "Novel Bayesian multiscale method for speckle removal in medical ultrasound images," *IEEE Trans. Med. Imaging*, vol. 20, no. 8, pp. 772–783, 2001.

[6] C. Christodoulou, C. Pattichis, M. Pantziaris, and A. Nicolaides, "Texture-based classification of atherosclerotic carotid plaques," *IEEE Trans. Med. Imaging*, vol. 22, no. 7, pp. 902–912, 2003.

[7] T. Elatrozy, A. Nicolaides, T. Tegos, A. Zarka, M. Griffin, and M. Sabetai, "The effect of B-mode ultrasonic image standardization of the echodensity of symptomatic and asymptomatic carotid bifurcation plaque," *Int. Angiol.*, vol. 17, no. 3, pp. 179–186, Sep. 1998.

[8] C.P. Loizou, C.S. Pattichis, M. Pantziaris, T. Tyllis, and A. Nicolaides, "Quantitative quality evaluation of ultrasound imaging in the carotid artery," *Med. Biol. Eng. Comput.*, vol. 44, no. 5, pp. 414–426, 2006.

[9] C.P. Loizou, C.S. Pattichis, M. Pantziaris, and A. Nicolaides, "An integrated system for the segmentation of atherosclerotic carotid plaque," *IEEE Trans. Inf. Technol. Biomed.*, vol. 11, no. 5, pp. 661–667, Nov. 2007.

[10] C.I. Christodoulou, S.C. Michaelides, and C.S. Pattichis, "Multi-feature texture analysis for the classification of clouds in satellite imagery," *IEEE Trans. Geosci. Remote Sens.*, vol. 41, no. 11, pp. 2662–2668, Nov. 2003.

[11] C.P. Loizou, C.S. Pattichis, C.I. Christodoulou, R.S.H. Istepanian, M. Pantziaris, and A. Nicolaides "Comparative evaluation of despeckle filtering in ultrasound imaging of the carotid artery," *IEEE Trans. Ultrason. Ferroelectr. Freq. Control*, vol. 52, no. 10, pp. 1653–1669, 2005.

[12] C.P. Loizou, V. Murray, M.S. Pattichis, M. Pantziaris, A.N. Nicolaides, and C.S. Pattichis, "Despeckle filtering for multiscale amplitude-modulation frequency-modulation (AM-FM) texture analysis of ultrasound images of the intima-media complex," *Int. J. Biomed. Imaging*, vol. 2014, Art. ID. 518414, 13 pages, 2014.

[13] C.P. Loizou, C. Theofanous, M. Pantziaris, and T. Kasparis, "Despeckle filtering software toolbox for ultrasound imaging of the common carotid artery," *Comput. Methods Programs Biomed.*, vol. 114, no. 1, pp. 109–124, 2014.

[14] C.P. Loizou, S. Petroudi, C.S. Pattichis, M. Pantziaris, and A.N. Nicolaides, "An integrated system for the segmentation of atherosclerotic carotid plaque in ultrasound video," *IEEE Trans. Ultrason. Ferroelectr. Freq. Control*, vol. 61, no. 1, pp. 86–101, 2014.

[15] C.P. Loizou, C. Theofanous, M. Pantziaris, *et al.*, "Despeckle filtering toolbox for medical ultrasound video," *Int. J. Monit. Surveill. Technol. Res. (IJMSTR): Special Issue Biomed. Monit. Technol.*, vol. 4, no. 1, pp. 61–79, 2013.

[16] K.T. Dussik, "On the possibility of using ultrasound waves as a diagnostic aid," *Neurol. Psychiatry*, vol. 174, pp. 153–168, 1942.

[17] A. Kurjak, "Ultrasound scanning – Prof. Ian Donald (1910–1987)," *Eur. J. Obstet. Gynecol. Reprod. Biol.*, vol. 90, no. 2, pp. 187–189, Jun. 2000.

[18] S.-M. Wu, Y.-W. Shau, F.-C. Chong, and F.-J. Hsieh, "Non-invasive assessment of arterial dimension waveforms using gradient-based Hough transform and power Doppler ultrasound imaging," *J. Med. Biol. Eng. Comput.*, vol. 39, pp. 627–632, 2001.

[19] R. Gonzalez and R. Woods, Digital image processing, Second Edition, Upper Saddle River, NJ: Prentice-Hall Inc., 2002.

[20] W.R. Hedrick and D.L. Hykes, "Image and signal processing in diagnostic ultrasound imaging," *J. Diagn. Med. Sonogr.*, vol. 5, no. 5, pp. 231–239, 1989.

[21] F.J. Polak, "Doppler sonography: an overview," in *Peripheral vascular sonography: a practical guide*, Baltimore, USA: Williams and Wilkins, 1992.

[22] A Philips Medical System Company, "Comparison of image clarity, SonoCT real-time compound imaging versus conventional 2D ultrasound imaging," in *ATL ultrasound, report*, Phillips Ltd, 2001.

[23] J.-C. Tradif and H Lee, "Applications of intravascular ultrasound in cardiology," in *What's new in cardiovascular ultrasound imaging*, J. Reiber and E. van der Wall, eds., pp. 133–148, Dordrecht: Kluwer Academic Publisher, 1998.

[24] M. Cilingiroglu, A. Hakeem, M. Feldman, and M. Wholey, "Optical coherence tomography imaging in asymptomatic patients with carotid artery stenosis," *Cardiovasc. Revasc. Med.*, vol. 14, no. 1, pp. 53–56, 2012.

[25] C.P. Loizou, C.S. Pattichis, M. Pantziaris, T. Tyllis, and A. Nicolaides, "Snakes based segmentation of the common carotid artery intima media," *Med. Biol. Eng. Comput.*, vol. 45, no. 1, pp. 35–49, Jan. 2007.

[26] C.S. Pattichis, C. Christodoulou, E. Kyriakou, *et al.*, "Ultrasound imaging of carotid atherosclerosis," in *Wiley encyclopaedia of biomedical engineering*, M. Akay, ed., Hoboken, USA: Wiley, John Wiley & Sons, Inc., 2006.

[27] P. Rerona and J. Malik, "Scale-space and edge detection using anisotropic diffusion," *IEEE Trans. Pattern Anal. Mach. Intell.*, vol. 12, no. 7, pp. 629–639, Jul. 1990.

[28] X. Hao, S. Gao, and X. Gao, "A novel multiscale nonlinear thresholding method for ultrasonic speckle suppressing," *IEEE Trans. Med. Imaging*, vol. 18, no. 9, pp. 787–794, 1999.

[29] Y. Yongjian and S.T. Acton, "Speckle reducing anisotropic diffusion," *IEEE Trans. Image Process.*, vol. 11, no. 11, pp. 1260–1270, Nov. 2002.

[30] D. Lamont, L. Parker, M. White, *et al.*, "Risk of cardiovascular disease measured by carotid intima-media thickness at age 49–51: life course study," *BMJ*, vol. 320, pp. 273–278, Jan. 29, 2000.

[31] C.P. Loizou, T. Kasparis, P. Papakyriakou, L. Christodoulou, M. Pantziaris, and C.S. Pattichis, "Video segmentation of the common carotid artery intima-media complex," *12th Int. Conf. Bioinf. & Bioeng. Proc. (BIBE)*, Larnaca, Cyprus, pages 4, Nov. 11–13, 2012.

[32] C.B. Burckhardt, "Speckle in ultrasound B-mode scans," *IEEE Trans. Son. Ultrason.*, vol. SU-25, no. 1, pp. 1–6, 1978.

[33] R.F. Wagner, S.W. Smith, J.M. Sandrik, and H. Lopez, "Statistics of speckle in ultrasound B-scans," *IEEE Trans. Son. Ultrason.*, vol. 30, pp. 156–163, 1983.

[34] J.W. Goodman, "Some fundamental properties of speckle," *J. Opt. Soc. Am.*, vol. 66, no. 11, pp. 1145–1149, 1976.

[35] R.W. Prager, A.H. Gee, G.M. Treece, and L. Berman, "Speckle detection in ultrasound images using first order statistics," London, UK: University of Cambridge, Dept. of Engineering, GUED/F-INFENG/TR 415, pp. 1–17, Jul. 2002.

[36] J.S. Lee, "Speckle analysis and smoothing of synthetic aperture radar images," *Comput. Graphics Image Process.*, vol. 17, pp. 24–32, 1981.

[37] C.P. Loizou, T. Kasparis, P. Christodoulides, *et al.*, "Despeckle filtering in ultrasound video of the common carotid artery," *12th Int. Conf. Bioinf. & Bioeng. Proc. (BIBE)*, Larnaca, Cyprus, pages 4, Nov. 11–13, 2012.

[38] J.S. Lee, "Digital image enhancement and noise filtering by using local statistics," *IEEE Trans. Pattern Anal. Mach. Intell.*, vol. PAMI-2, no. 2, pp. 165–168, 1980.

[39] M. Black, G. Sapiro, D. Marimont, and D. Heeger, "Robust anisotropic diffusion," *IEEE Trans. Image Process.*, vol. 7, no. 3, pp. 421–432, Mar. 1998.

[40] V. Dutt, "Statistical analysis of ultrasound echo envelope," Ph.D. dissertation, Mayo Graduate School, Rochester, MN, 1995.

[41] J.C. Dainty, Laser speckle and related phenomena, New York: Springer-Verlag Berlin Heidelberg, 1974.

[42] J.M. Thijssen, B.J. Oosterveld, P.C. Hartman, *et al.*, "Correlations between acoustic and texture parameters from RF and B-mode liver echograms," *Ultrasound Med. Biol.*, vol. 19, pp. 13–20, 1993.

[43] L. Busse, T.R. Crimmins, and J.R. Fienup, "A model based approach to improve the performance of the geometric filtering speckle reduction algorithm," *IEEE Ultrason. Symp.*, pp. 1353–1356, 1995.

[44] J.U. Quistgaard, "Signal acquisition and processing in medical diagnostic ultrasound," *IEEE Signal Process. Mag.*, vol. 14, no. 1, pp. 67–74, Jan. 1997.

[45] H. Paul and H.P. Schwann, "Mechanism of absorption of ultrasound in liver tissue," *J. Acoust. Soc. Am.*, vol. 50, pp. 692, 1971.

[46] V.S. Frost, J.A. Stiles, K.S. Shanmungan, and J.C. Holtzman, "A model for radar images and its application for adaptive digital filtering of multiplicative noise," *IEEE Trans. Pattern Anal. Mach. Intell.*, vol. 4, no. 2, pp. 157–165, 1982.

[47] J.S. Lee, "Refined filtering of image noise using local statistics," *Comput. Graphics Image Process.*, vol. 15, pp. 380–389, 1981.

[48] D.T. Kuan, A.A. Sawchuk, T.C. Strand, and P. Chavel, "Adaptive restoration of images with speckle," *IEEE Trans. Acoust. Speech Signal Process.*, vol. ASSP-35, pp. 373–383, 1987.

[49] D.T. Kuan and A.A. Sawchuk, "Adaptive noise smoothing filter for images with signal dependent noise," *IEEE Trans. Pattern Anal. Mach. Intell.*, vol. PAMI-7, no. 2, pp. 165–177, 1985.

[50] C.P. Loizou, C. Christodoulou, C.S. Pattichis, R. Istepanian, M. Pantziaris, and A. Nicolaides, "Speckle reduction in ultrasound images of atherosclerotic carotid plaque," *DSP 2002, Proc., IEEE 14th Int. Conf. Digital Signal Process.*, Santorini, Greece, pp. 525–528, Jul. 1–3, 2002.

[51] X. Zong, A. Laine, and E. Geiser, "Speckle reduction and contrast enhancement of echocardiograms via multiscale nonlinear processing," *IEEE Trans. Med. Imaging*, vol. 17, no. 4, pp. 532–540, 1998.

[52] M. Karaman, M.A. Kutay, and G. Bozdagi, "An adaptive speckle suppression filter for medical ultrasonic imaging," *IEEE Trans. Med. Imaging*, vol. 14, no. 2, pp. 283–292, 1995.

[53] S.M. Ali and R.E. Burge, "New automatic techniques for smoothing and segmenting SAR images," *Signal Process.*, North-Holland, vol. 14, pp. 335–346, 1988.

[54] A. Baraldi and F. Pannigianni, "A refined gamma MAP SAR speckle filter with improved geometrical adaptivity," *IEEE Trans. Geosci. Remote Sens.*, vol. 33, no. 5, pp. 1245–1257, Sep. 1995.

[55] E. Trouve, Y. Chambenoit, N. Classeau, and P. Bolon, "Statistical and operational performance assessment of multi-temporal SAR image filtering," *IEEE Trans. Geosci. Remote Sens.*, vol. 41, no. 11, pp. 2519–2539, 2003.

[56] H.-L. Eng and K.-K. Ma, "Noise adaptive soft-switching median filter," *IEEE Trans. Image Process.*, vol. 10, no. 2, pp. 242–251, 2001.

[57] S. Solbo and T. Eltoft, "Homomorphic wavelet based-statistical despeckling of SAR images," *IEEE Trans. Geosci. Remote Sens.*, vol. 42, no. 4, pp. 711–721, 2004.

[58] J. Saniie, T. Wang, and N. Bilgutay, "Analysis of homomorphic processing for ultrasonic grain signal characterization," *IEEE Trans. Ultrason. Ferroelectr. Freq. Control*, vol. 3, pp. 365–375, 1989.

[59] T. Huang, G. Yang, and G. Tang, "A fast two-dimensional median filtering algorithm," *IEEE Trans. Acoust. Speech Signal Process.*, vol. 27, no. 1, pp. 13–18, 1979.

[60] J. Weickert, B. Romery, and M. Viergever, "Efficient and reliable schemes for nonlinear diffusion filtering," *IEEE Trans. Image Process.*, vol. 7, pp. 398–410, 1998.

[61] S. Jin, Y. Wang, and J. Hiller, "An adaptive non-linear diffusion algorithm for filtering medical images," *IEEE Trans. Inf. Technol. Biomed.*, vol. 4, no. 4, pp. 298–305, Dec. 2000.

[62] M. Larsson, B. Heyde, F. Kremer, L.-A. Brodin, and J. D'hooge, "Ultrasound speckle tracking for radial, longitudinal and circumferential strain estimation of the carotid artery – An in vitro validation via sonomicrometry using clinical and high-frequency ultrasound," *Ultrasonics*, vol. 56, pp. 399–408, 2015.

[63] J. D'hooge, E. Konofagou, F. Jamal, *et al.*, "Two-dimensional ultrasonic strain rate measurement of the human heart in vivo," *IEEE Trans. Ultrason. Ferroelectr. Freq. Control*, vol. 49, pp. 281–286, 2002.

[64] C.L. de Korte, H.H. Hansen, and A.F. van der Steen, "Vascular ultrasound for atherosclerosis imaging," *Interface Focus*, vol. 1, pp. 565–575, 2001.

[65] M. Catalano, A. Lamberti-Castronuovo, A. Catalano, D. Filocamo, and C. Zimbalatti, "Two-dimensional speckle-tracking strain imaging in the assessment of mechanical properties of carotid arteries: feasibility and comparison with conventional markers of subclinical atherosclerosis," *Eur. J. Echocardiogr.*, vol. 12, pp. 528–535, 2001.

[66] M. Cinthio, Å. Rydén Ahlgren, T. Jansson, A. Eriksson, H.W. Persson, and L. Kjell, "Evaluation of an ultrasonic echo-tracking method for measurements of arterial wall movements in two dimensions," *IEEE Trans. Ultrason. Ferroelectr. Freq. Control*, vol. 52, pp. 1300–1311, 2005.

[67] M. Larsson, F. Kremer, P. Claus, T. Kuznetsova, L.-Å. Brodin, and J. D'hooge, "Ultrasound-based radial and longitudinal strain estimation of the carotid artery: a feasibility study," *IEEE Trans. Ultrason. Ferroelectr. Freq. Control*, vol. 58, pp. 2244–2251, 2011.

[68] R. Bernardes, C. Mduro, P. Serranho, A. Araujo, S. Barbeiro, and J. Cunha-Vaz, "Improved adaptive complex diffusion despeckling filter," *Opt. Express*, vol. 18, pp. 24048–24059, 2010.

[69] S. Zhong and V. Cherkassky, "Image denoising using wavelet thresholding and model selection," *Proc. of IEEE Int. Conf. Image Proces.*, Vancouver, Canada, pp. 1–4, Nov. 2000.

[70] D.L. Donoho, "Denoising by soft thresholding," *IEEE Trans. Inf. Theory*, vol. 41, pp. 613–627, 1995.

[71] T.W. Chan, O.C. Au, T.S. Chong, and W.S. Chau, "A novel content-adaptive video denoising filter," *Proc. IEEE Vision, Image Signal. Process.*, vol. 2, no. 2, pp. 649–652, 2005.

[72] K. Dabov, A. Foi, and K. Egiazarian, "Video denoising by sparse 3D transform-domain collaborative filtering," *Proc. 15th Eur. Sign. Proc. Conf.*, pp. 1–5, 2007.

[73] M. Maggioni, G. Boracchi, A. Foi, and K. Engiazarian, "Video denoising, deblocking and enhancement through separable 4-D nonlocal spatiotemporal transforms," *IEEE Trans. Image Process.*, vol. 21, no. 9, pp. 3952–3966, 2012.

[74] D. Rusanovskyy, K. Dabov, and K. Egiazarian, "Moving-window varying size 3D transform-based video denoising," *Proc. Int. Workshop on Video Proc. & Quality Metrics*, 1–4, 2006.

[75] V. Zlokolica, W. Philips, and van de Ville, "Robust non-linear filtering for video processing,", *IEEE 14th Int. Conf. on Digit. Sign. Process.*, Santorini, Greece, pp. 1–4, 1–3 July 2002.

[76] V. Zlokolica, A. Pizurica, and W. Philips, "Recursive temporal denoising and motion estimation of video," *Int. Conf. Image Process.*, vol. 3, no. 3, pp. 1465–1468, 2008.

[77] C.P. Loizou and C.S. Pattichis, "Despeckle filtering for ultrasound imaging and video, Vol. II: selected applications," in *Synthesis lectures on algorithms and software in engineering*, Ed. Morgan & Claypool Publishers, 1537 Fourth Street, Suite 228, San Rafael, CA, vol. 7, no. 2, pp. 1–180, Aug. 2015, ISBN-9781627058148.

[78] C.P. Loizou and C.S. Pattichis, "Despeckle filtering for ultrasound imaging and video, Vol. I: algorithms and software," in *Synthesis lectures on algorithms and software in engineering*, Ed. Morgan & Claypool Publishers, 1537 Fourth street, Suite 228, San Rafael, CA, vol. 7, no. 1, pp. 1–180, Apr. 2015. ISBN: 9781627056687.

[79] M. Nagao and T. Matsuyama, "Edge preserving smoothing," *Comput. Graphics. Image Process.*, vol. 9, pp. 394–407, 1979.

[80] T. Greiner, C.P. Loizou, M. Pandit, J. Mauruschat, and F.W. Albert, "Speckle reduction in ultrasonic imaging for medical applications," *Proc. of the ICASSP91, 1991 Int. Conf. Acoustic Signal Speech Processing*, Toronto Canada, pp. 2993–2996, May 14–17,1991.

[81] A. Nieminen, P. Heinonen, and Y. Neuvo, "A new class of detail-preserving filters for image processing," *IEEE Trans. Pattern Anal. Mach. Intell.*, vol. 9, pp. 74–90, 1987.

[82] M. Kuwahara, K. Hachimura, S. Eiho, and M. Kinoshita, "Digital processing of biomedical images," K. Preston and M. Onoe, eds., pp. 187–203, Plenum. Pub. Corp., 1976.

[83] A. Buades, B. Coll, and J.-M. Morel, "Nonlocal image and movie denoising," *Int. J. Comput. Vision*, vol. 76, pp. 123–139, 2008.

[84] A.M. Wink and J.B.T.M. Roerdink, "Denoising functional MR images: a comparison of wavelet denoising and Gaussian smoothing," *IEEE Trans. Med. Imaging*, vol. 23, no. 3, pp. 374–387, 2004.

[85] N. Rougon and F. Preteux, "Controlled anisotropic diffusion," *Conf. on Nonlinear Image Processing VI, IS&T/SPIE Symposium on Electronic Imaging, Science and Technology*, San Jose, California, pp. 1–12, 5–10 Feb. 1995.

[86] F.N.S Medeiros, N.D.A. Mascarenhas, R.C.P Marques, and C.M. Laprano, "Edge preserving wavelet speckle filtering," *5th IEEE Southwest Symp. Image Anal. & Interpr.*, Santa Fe, New Mexico, pp. 281–285, 7–9 Apr. 2002.

[87] P. Moulin, "Multiscale image decomposition and wavelets," in *Handbook of image & video processing*, A. Bovik, ed., pp. 289–300, New York: Academic Press, 2000.

[88] P. Scheunders, "Wavelet thresholding of multivalued images," *IEEE Trans. Image Process.*, vol. 13, no. 4, pp. 475–483, 2004.

[89] C.P Loizou, "Ultrasound image processing for the evaluation of the risk of stroke," PhD thesis, Kingston University, UK, 2005.

[90] J.T. Bushberg, J.A. Seibert, E.M. Leidholdt, Jr., and J.M. Boone, The essential physics of medical imaging, Philadelphia, USA: Lippincott Williams & Wilkins, 2002.

[91] J. Stoitsis, S. Golemati, V. Koropouli, and K.S. Nikita, "Simulating dynamic B-mode ultrasound image data of the common carotid artery," *IEEE Int. Work. Imag. Synth. & Techn.*, p. 4, 2008.

[92] E. Krupinski, H. Kundel, P. Judy, and C. Nodine, "The medical image perception society, key issues for image perception research," *Radiology*, vol. 209, pp. 611–612, 1998.

[93] Z. Wang, A. Bovik, H. Sheikh, and E. Simoncelli, "Image quality assessment: from error measurement to structural similarity," *IEEE Trans. Image Process.*, vol. 13, no. 4, pp. 600–612, Apr. 2004.

[94] A. Ahumada and C. Null, "Image quality: a multidimensional problem," in *Digital images and human vision*, AB Watson, ed., Cambridge, MA: Bradford Press, pp. 141–148, 1993.

[95] E.A. Fedorovskaya, H. De Ridder, and F.J. Blomaert, "Chroma variations and perceived quality of colour images and natural scenes," *Color Res. Appl.*, vol. 22, no. 2, pp. 96–110, 1997.

[96] G. Deffner, "Evaluation of display image quality: experts vs. non-experts," *Symp. Soc. Inf. Disp. Dig.*, vol. 25, pp. 475–478, 1994.

[97] T.J. Chen, K.S. Chuang, J. Wu, S.C. Chen, I.M. Hwang, and M.L. Jan, "A novel image quality index using Moran I statistics," *Phys. Med. Biol.*, vol. 48, pp. 131–137, 2003.

[98] S. Winkler, "Vision models and quality metrics for image processing applications," PhD, University of Lausanne, Switzerland, Dec. 21, 2000.

[99] D. Sakrison, "On the role of observer and a distortion measure in image transmission," *IEEE Trans. Commun.*, vol. 25, pp. 1251–1267, Nov. 1977.

[100] Z. Wang and A. Bovik, "A Universal quality index," *IEEE Signal Process. Lett.*, vol. 9, no. 3, pp. 81–84, Mar. 2002.

[101] V.S. Vora, A.C. Suthar, Y.N. Makwana, and S.J. Davda, "Analysis of compressed image quality assessments," *Int. J. Adv. Eng. Appl.*, vol. 1, pp. 225–229, 2010.

[102] A. Pommert and K. Hoehne, "Evaluation of image quality in medical volume visualization: the state of the art," T. Dohi and R. Kikinis, eds., Medical image computing and computer-assisted intervention, *Proc., MICCAI, 2002, Part II, Lecture Notes in Computer Science*, 2489, pp. 598–605, Springer Verlag, Berlin, 2002.

[103] M. Eckert, "Perceptual quality metrics applied to still image compression," in *Canon information systems research*, Sydney, Australia: Faculty of Engineering, University of Technology, pp. 1–26, 2002.

[104] A. Efros and T. Leung, "Texture synthesis by non-parametric sampling," *Proc. Int. Conf. Comput. Vision*, vol. 2, pp. 1033–1038, 1999.

[105] Y. Zhan, M. Ding, L. Wu, and X. Zhang, "Nonlocal means method using weight refining for despeckling for ultrasound images," *Sign. Proc.*, vol. 103, pp. 201–213, 2014.

[106] A. Buades, B. Coll, and J. Morel, "On image denoising methods," in *Technical report*, CMLA, 2004–2015.

[107] G. Gilboa, N. Sochen, and Y.Y. Zeevi, "Image enhancement and denoising by complex diffusion processes," *IEEE Trans. Pattern Anal. Mach. Intell.*, vol. 26, no 8, pp. 1020–1036, 2004.

[108] R.N. Czerwinski, D.L. Jones, and W.D. O'Brien, "Detection and boundaries in speckle images-Application to medical ultrasound," *IEEE Trans. Med. Imaging*, vol. 18, no. 2, pp. 126–136, Feb. 1999.

[109] A.M. Wink and J.B.T.M. Roerdink, "Denoising functional MR images: a comparison of wavelet denoising and Gaussian smoothing," *IEEE Trans. Med. Imaging*, vol. 23, no. 3, pp. 374–387, 2004.

[110] S. Jin, Y. Wang, and J. Hiller, "An adaptive non-linear diffusion algorithm for filtering medical images," *IEEE Trans. Inf. Technol. Biomed.*, vol. 4, no. 4, pp. 298–305, Dec. 2000.

[111] V. Damerjian, O. Tankyevych, N. Souag, and E. Petit, "Speckle characterisation methods in ultrasound images-A review," *Innov. Res. Biomed. Eng. (IRBM)*, vol. 35, pp. 202–213, 2014.

[112] J.A. Noble, "Ultrasound image segmentation and tissue characterization," *Proc. Inst. Mech. Eng.*, vol. 224, no. 2, pp. 307–316, 2010.

[113] C.P. Loizou, "A review on ultrasound common carotid artery image and video segmentation techniques," *Med. Biol. Eng. Comput.*, vol. 52, no. 12, pp. 1073–1093, 2014.

[114] R.J. Housden, A.H. Gee, G.M. Treece, and R.W. Prager, "Sensorless reconstruction of unconstrained freehand 3D ultrasound data," *Ultrasound Med. Biol.*, vol. 33, no. 3, pp. 408–419, 2007.

[115] J.C. Seabra, F. Ciompi, O. Pujol, J. Mauri, P. Radeva, and J. Sanches, "Rayleigh mixture model for plaque characterization in intravascular ultrasound," *IEEE Biomed. Eng.*, vol. 58, no. 5, pp. 1314–1324, 2001.

[116] M.A.H Khan, "3D reconstruction of ultrasound images," MSc in vision and robotics, University of Burgundy, University of Girona and University of Heriot Watt., 2008.

[117] J. Revell, M. Mirmehdi, and D. McNally, "Computer vision elastography: speckle adaptive motion estimation for elastography using ultrasound sequences," *IEEE Med. Imaging*, vol. 24, no. 6, pp. 755–766, 2005.

[118] H. Geyer, G. Caracciolo, H. Abe, *et al.*, "Assessment of myocardial mechanics using speckle tracking echocardiography: fundamentals and clinical applications," *J. Am. Soc. Echocardiogr.*, vol. 23, no. 4, pp. 351–369, 2010.

[119] M. Alessandrini, "Statistical methods for analysis and processing of medical ultrasound: applications to segmentation and restoration," PhD thesis, Universita di Bologna, 2011.

[120] F. Destrempes, G. Soulez, M.-F. Giroux, J. Meunier, and G. Cloutier, "Segmentation of plaques in sequences of ultrasonic B-mode images of carotid arteries based on motion estimation and Nakagami distributions," *IEEE Int. Ultrason. Symp. (IUS)*, pp. 2480–24833, 20–23 Sept. 2009.

[121] N. Paragios and R. Deriche, "Geodesic active contours and level sets for the detection and tracking of moving objects," *IEEE Trans. Pattern. Anal. Mach. Intell.*, vol. 22, no. 3, pp. 266–280, 2000.

[122] Y.Y. Boykov and M.-P. Jolly, "Interactive graph cuts for optimal boundary & region segmentation of objects in ND images," *Computer Vision, ICCV 2001. Proc. 8th IEEE Int. Conf.*, pp. 105–112, 2001.

[123] M. Oezkan, A. Erdem, M. Sezan, and A. Tekalp, "Efficient multi-frame Wiener restoration of blurred and noisy image sequences," *IEEE Trans. Image Process.*, vol. 1, pp. 453–476, Oct. 1992.

[124] P.M.B. Van Roosmalen, S.J.P Westen, R.L. Lagendijk, and J. Biemond, "Noise reduction for image sequences using an oriented pyramid threshold technique," *IEEE Int. Conf. Image Process.*, vol. 1, pp. 375–378, 1996.

[125] M. Vetterli and J. Kovacevic, Wavelets and subband coding, Englewood Cliffs, NJ: Prentice Hall, 1995.

[126] S. Winkler, "Digital video quality," in *Vision models and metrics*, Chichester, West Sussex, England: John Wiley & Sons Ltd., 2005.

[127] J.-H. Jung, K. Hong, and S. Yang, "Noise reduction using variance characteristics in noisy image sequence," *Int. Conf. Consumer Electronics*, pp. 213–214, Jan. 8–12, 2005.

[128] M. Bertalmio, V. Caselles, and A. Pardo, "Movie denoising by average of warped lines," *IEEE Trans. Image Process.*, vol. 16, no. 9, pp. 233–2347, 2007.

[129] B. Alp, P. Haavisto, T. Jarske, K. Oestaemoe, and Y. Neuro, "Median based algorithms for image sequence processing," *Proc. SPIE Vis. Commun. Image Process.*, Lausanne, Switzerland, vol. 1360, pp. 122–133, 1990.

[130] A. Panayides, M.S. Pattichis, C.S. Pattichis, C.P. Loizou, M. Pantziaris, and A. Pitsillides, "Atherosclerotic plaque ultrasound video encoding, wireless transmission, and quality assessment using H.264," *IEEE Trans. Inf. Tech. Biomed.*, vol. 15, no. 3, pp. 387–397, 2011.

Chapter 8

Nonlinear despeckle filtering

Santiago Aja-Fernández[1], *Gabriel Ramos-Llordén*[2], *and Gonzalo Vegas-Sánchez-Ferrero*[3,4]

In this chapter, we will review some of the methods proposed in literature to remove the speckle pattern from ultrasound data based on nonlinear processing. Note that some filters that can also be considered as *nonlinear* are left aside since they will be deeply treated in other chapters. That is the case of the wavelet-based methods and Bayesian methods. Other methods also treated in other chapters, like diffusion-based schemes are only briefly reviewed in order to place them inside the global partial differential equation (PDE) classification. On the other hand, note that some of the filters here reviewed are not initially proposed for ultrasound imaging but derived for Synthetic Aperture Radar (SAR) images, where noise can be modeled similarly. In those images, the multiplicative model for speckle holds and therefore, many of the methods defined in literature for SAR can be easily extrapolated to ultrasound denoising. This is the case of some of the most popular speckle filters. In addition, we would like to remark that the effectiveness of many of these schemes lays on a proper modeling of the speckle statistics. For some purposes, a simple multiplicative model will suffice, while for some specific applications, more accurate models must be used. Finally, as we stated in the previous chapter, the filtering method must be selected following the specific needs of the problem. There is no all-purpose filter that, with the same configuration parameters, could perform excellent in all situations.

8.1 Filtering based on local windows

The most direct approaches to speckle filtering are based on the kernel-based convolutions commonly used in classical image processing. These convolutions

[1]ETSI Telecomunicación, Universidad de Valladolid, Spain
[2]Imec-Vision Lab, Department of Physics, University of Antwerp, Belgium
[3]Applied Chest Imaging Laboratory (ACIL), Brigham and Women's Hospital, Harvard Medical School, USA
[4]Biomedical Image Technologies Laboratory (BIT), ETSI Telecomunicación, Universidad Politécnica de Madrid, and CIBER-BBN, Spain

implied linear operations that use a predefined kernel to smooth the image and statistical approaches like those derived by Lee or Kuan.

The applications reviewed here take advantage of the local filtering philosophy by replacing the convolution by nonlinear operations. The implementation of such methods is usually slower than the linear ones, but they may present important advantages, mainly on the preservation of structures. We will focus on two of the most popular methodologies in ultrasound imaging, the median and the Gamma filters and some of their extensions.

8.1.1 Median filter

The median filter [1–4] is a well-known methodology that, in its basic form, calculates the median value of the pixels of a neighborhood centered around a particular pixel. Let $I(\mathbf{x})$ be a certain noisy image. We define the median filtering as

$$I_{\text{MED}}(\mathbf{x}) = \underset{\eta(\mathbf{x})}{\text{median}}\, I(\mathbf{x}) \tag{8.1}$$

where $\eta(\mathbf{x})$ is a centered neighborhood. Assuming a $P \times P$ window, the median filter works as follows:

1. The P^2 values of the pixels in the neighborhood are extracted.
2. Those values are ordered.
3. The output of the filter corresponds to the value placed in the $\frac{P^2+1}{2}$ position.

An example of the filtering of one particular neighborhood is depicted in Figure 8.1 and compared to the result of a linear *mean* filter. This particular example illustrates one of the distinct features of the median filter: the output value is one of the values already present in the image. This effect has two advantages: first, no new values are introduced into the image; second, there is no smoothness or blurring of edges.

One of the main drawbacks of the median filter is its computational cost, with the number of operations growing exponentially with the size of the window. An alternative would be the so-called *pseudomedian* filter [5]. If $\{M_N\}$ is a sequence of elements $m_1, m_2, \ldots, m_N$, the pseudomedian of the sequence is defined as

$$\text{pmed}\{M_N\} = \frac{\text{maximim}\{M_N\} + \text{minimax}\{M_N\}}{2} \tag{8.2}$$

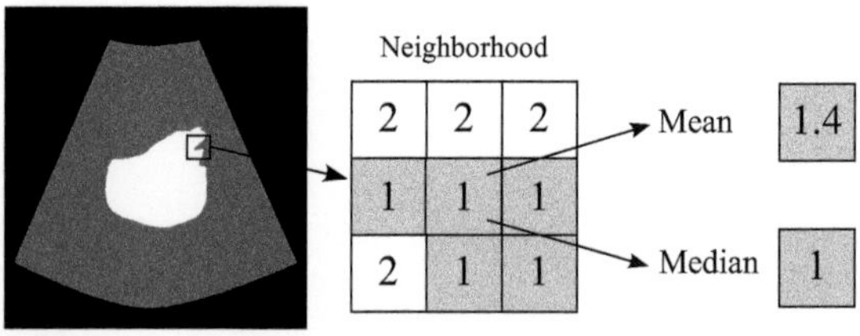

Figure 8.1 Example of median filtering in a 3 × 3 neighborhood compared to a mean filter of the same area

where

$$\text{maximin}\{M_N\} = \max\{\min(m_1, \dots, m_L), \min(m_2, \dots, m_{L+1}), \dots, \min(m_{N-L+1}, \dots, m_N)\}$$

and

$$\text{maximin}\{M_N\} = \min\{\max(m_1, \dots, m_L), \max(m_2, \dots, m_{L+1}), \dots, \max(m_{N-L+1}, \dots, m_N)\},$$

with $L = (N + 1)/2$.

Although median filtering has been used in all kind of image modalities, there are some implementations specifically adapted to cope with the specificity of speckle. Some examples are the adaptive weighted median filter [6], the detail-preserving median filter [7], the directional median filter [8] and the modified hybrid median proposed in [9].

8.1.2 Gamma filter

Some of the filters used in ultrasound imaging were initially derived for SAR images, where noise can be modeled similarly. In those images, the multiplicative model for Speckle holds and therefore, many of the methods defined in literature for SAR can be easily extrapolated to ultrasound. This is the case of the Gamma filter proposed in [10,11].

The Gamma filter assumes that the speckle present in the image follows a Gamma distribution. This model has also been used lately in real ultrasound data, showing a great capability to model the acquired signal after processes like interpolation, filtering and compression [12]. The Gamma filter is a Maximum a Posteriori (MAP) approach in which the original signal is estimated. In its original formulation in [10], it was designed under a Gaussian assumption and extended to a Gamma in [11]. The estimated signal is defined as

$$\widehat{I(\mathbf{x})} = \begin{cases} \overline{I(\mathbf{x})} & C_I(\mathbf{x}) < C_N \\ \dfrac{(\alpha - L - 1)\overline{I(\mathbf{x})} + \sqrt{\overline{I(\mathbf{x})}^2(\alpha - L - 1) + 4\alpha L I(\mathbf{x})\overline{I(\mathbf{x})}}}{2\alpha} & C_N \le C_I(\mathbf{x}) \le C_{\max} \\ I(\mathbf{x}) & C_I(\mathbf{x}) > C_{\max} \end{cases} \tag{8.3}$$

with

$$\alpha = \frac{C_N^2 + 1}{C_I^2(\mathbf{x}) - C_N^2}. \tag{8.4}$$

$C_I(\mathbf{x})$ is the (sample) coefficient of variation of the noisy image, C_N is the coefficient of variation of noise, $\overline{I(\mathbf{x})}$ is a sample estimate of the local mean of the image, $C_{\max}$ is an upper bound usually set to $C_{\max} = 2C_B$ and L is the *number of looks* in the RADAR image. Note that some of the noise parameters must be properly estimated from data [13,14].

Some extensions of the original formulation can be found in [15], where authors included geometrical adaptivity and in the multiscale formulation proposed in [16].

8.1.3 Region-oriented schemes

Similar to the philosophy of the Gamma filter, there exist other nonlinear modifications of known linear filters by adding information about the different regions present in ultrasound B-scan images. Implicitly, these methods assume a Rayleigh distribution of the data. The purpose of the filters is to differentiate between homogenous areas, areas with structures and isolated points. To that end, in [11] for instance, authors modified the well-known speckle filters of Frost and Lee. For the sake of illustration, the enhanced Lee filter is defined as

$$\widehat{I(\mathbf{x})} = \begin{cases} \overline{I(\mathbf{x})} & C_I(\mathbf{x}) < C_N \\ I(\mathbf{x})W(\mathbf{x}) + (1 - W(\mathbf{x}))\overline{I(\mathbf{x})} & C_N \leq C_I(\mathbf{x}) \leq C_{\max} \\ I(\mathbf{x}) & C_I(\mathbf{x}) > C_{\max} \end{cases} \tag{8.5}$$

with $W(\mathbf{x})$ a weighting function defined as

$$W(\mathbf{x}) = \exp\left(\frac{-k(C_I(\mathbf{x}) - C_N)}{C_{\max} - C_I(\mathbf{x})}\right), \tag{8.6}$$

and k is a constant.

8.2 Nonlocal means schemes

The nonlocal means (NLM) was first described in [17] to denoise 2D natural images corrupted by an additive white Gaussian noise. This methodology has lately gained an increasing popularity due to its excellent performance and has been successfully extended to more complex noise models. NLM is a nonlinear filter based on a weighted average of pixels inside a search window that is relatively large compared to traditional neighborhood techniques, hence the term nonlocal. The structure of the image is preserved by applying an adaptive weight according to a similarity measure (usually the mean squared difference for natural images). NLM has proven to be optimal for Gaussian additive and multiplicative noise.

In its original formulation, the output of a NLM filter is computed as follows [17]:

$$I_{\mathrm{NLM}}(\mathbf{x}) = \sum_{\mathbf{y}\in\Omega} w(\mathbf{x},\mathbf{y})I(\mathbf{y}) \tag{8.7}$$

where w is a set of weights computed as

$$w(\mathbf{x},\mathbf{y}) = \frac{1}{Z(\mathbf{x})}\exp\left(-\frac{d(\mathbf{x},\mathbf{y})}{h^2}\right), Z(\mathbf{x}) = \sum_{\mathbf{y}\in\Omega}\exp\left(-\frac{d(\mathbf{x},\mathbf{y})}{h^2}\right) \tag{8.8}$$

where h is a parameter related to the noise power in the image and $d(\mathbf{x},\mathbf{y})$ is a distance between the voxels at positions p and q. Instead of using a geometrical distance, NLM uses a distance in the domain of the gray levels of the image, defined as

$$d(\mathbf{x},\mathbf{y}) = \left(\mathbf{I}(\mathcal{N}_{\mathbf{x}}) - \mathbf{I}(\mathcal{N}_{\mathbf{y}})\right)^T G_\rho\left(\mathbf{I}(\mathcal{N}_{\mathbf{x}}) - \mathbf{I}_i(\mathcal{N}_{\mathbf{y}})\right) \tag{8.9}$$

where $\mathbf{I}(\mathcal{N}_{\mathrm{x}})$ and $\mathbf{I}(\mathcal{N}_{\mathrm{y}})$ are column vectors containing the gray values of the voxels in the neighborhoods $\mathcal{N}_{\mathrm{x}}$ and $\mathcal{N}_{\mathrm{y}}$ of voxels $\mathbf{x}$ and $\mathbf{y}$, respectively. G_ρ is a matrix that accounts for a Gaussian weighting that gives a higher weight to the voxels of the neighborhood closer to the central voxel.

The computational cost associated to (8.7) is prohibitive, so the domain Ω is usually substituted by a neighborhood $\mathcal{N}'_{\mathbf{x}}$ of voxel $\mathbf{x}$. Besides, it is proposed in [18] to change the weight $w(\mathbf{x}, \mathbf{x})$ in (8.8) by the maximum of $w(\mathbf{x}, \mathbf{y})$ with $\mathbf{x} \neq \mathbf{y}$ to avoid over-weighting the central voxel of $\mathcal{N}'_{\mathbf{x}}$. A similar procedure is applied to the central coefficient of G_ρ.

An alternative approach to decrease the computational burden is the so-called *blockwise approach*, which performs the NLM on overlapping supports. Finally, the resulting image is calculated as the mean of all overlapped results [19].

The NLM was adapted to ultrasound images in [19,20], where the following speckle model is assumed

$$I(\mathbf{x}) = A(\mathbf{x}) + A^\gamma(\mathbf{x})n(\mathbf{x}) \tag{8.10}$$

where $A(\mathbf{x})$ is the noiseless image, $I(\mathbf{x})$ is the observed image and $n(\mathbf{x})$ is a zero-mean Gaussian noise. Thus, $I(\mathbf{x})$ is a Gaussian distributed variable with mean $A(\mathbf{x})$ and variance $A^{2\gamma}(\mathbf{x})\sigma^2$. This model was proposed to describe the image-dependent nature of noise, where the factor γ depends on the image formation and is assumed to be 1/2. According to the noise model of (8.10), the authors proposed a different distance function based on the conditional probability

$$p(I|A) \propto \exp - \frac{(I(\mathbf{x}) - A(\mathbf{x}))^2}{2A^{2\gamma}(\mathbf{x})\sigma^2}. \tag{8.11}$$

This analysis can be applied for each block B_i where the likelihood is factorized assuming conditional independence as

$$p(B_i, B_j) = \prod_{\mathbf{x},\mathbf{y}} p(I(\mathbf{x})|I(\mathbf{y})) \propto \exp - \sum_{\mathbf{x},\mathbf{y}} \frac{(I(\mathbf{x}) - I(\mathbf{y}))^2}{2I^{2\gamma}(\mathbf{y})\sigma^2} \tag{8.12}$$

where $\mathbf{x}$ and $\mathbf{y}$ are the corresponding locations within each block B_i and B_j. Note that this formulation assumes that the compared block B_j is the noiseless signal. So, the distance applied for comparing blocks is defined as

$$d_P(B_i, B_j) = \sum_{\mathbf{x},\mathbf{y}} \frac{(I(\mathbf{x}) - I(\mathbf{y}))^2}{I^{2\gamma}(\mathbf{y})} \tag{8.13}$$

with $\mathbf{x} \in B_i$ and $\mathbf{y} \in B_j$. Finally, the filtered image is obtained as the conditional mean calculated as

$$I_{\mathrm{NLM}}(\mathbf{x}) = \frac{\sum_j I(B_j)p(B_i, B_j)}{\sum_j p(B_i, B_j)} \tag{8.14}$$

where the index j refers to all the overlapping blocks, B_j, containing location $\mathbf{x}$.

An alternative formulation of a nonlocal-based filter was proposed in [21] to deal with Rayleigh distributed noise. This approach is performed in two steps. First, the maximum likelihood is employed to calculate an initial noise-free intensity. Then, the nonlocal (NL)-means method is used to restore the details missing from the ML step.

During the estimation step, the maximum-likelihood (ML) estimator used assumes independent and identically distributed Rayleigh samples in a local neighborhood and the following noise model:

$$I(\mathbf{x}) = A(\mathbf{x})R(\mathbf{x}|\sigma) \tag{8.15}$$

where σ is the noise parameter, $A(\mathbf{x})$ is the noise-free intensity and $R(\mathbf{x})$ is a Rayleigh distributed random variable of parameter and mean value equals 1.

The authors assume local stationarity of noise within a neighborhood of each location $\mathcal{N}_{\mathbf{x}}$. In those conditions, the resulting ML estimator for a Rayleigh distribution becomes

$$I_{\mathrm{NLM}}(\mathbf{x}) = \hat{A}(\mathbf{x}) = \left(\frac{1}{2|\mathcal{N}_{\mathbf{x}}|\sigma^2} \sum_{\mathbf{y} \in \mathcal{N}_{\mathbf{x}}} I(\mathbf{y})^2 \right)^{1/2} \tag{8.16}$$

This coarse estimation is prone to errors due to the inclusion of different tissues within the local neighborhood $\mathcal{N}_{\mathbf{x}}$. To compensate this effect, the authors propose to calculate the distance between patches from the ML estimate and provide the filtered value with the NLM philosophy.

8.3 Speckle filtering based on partial differential equations

An important type of speckle filters are those that are rooted in concepts of calculus of variations and PDEs. Within these approaches, the filtered image is either the solution of a given continuous optimization problem (variational framework) or the steady-state solution of a given temporal PDE. In this section, we just focus on two paradigmatic cases, diffusion filtering and total-variation (TV) techniques.

8.3.1 Diffusion filters

Probably the most well-known PDE-based filtering technique is the so-called diffusion filtering. In this section, we begin by providing a very general description of the genuine diffusion filter approach, after which we describe adaptations of such formulation so as to consider the speckle nature properly. The reader should be aware that our aim is to provide a general survey of this kind of speckle filtering and not to dig into the details of every specific diffusion technique. The interested reader is referred to the chapter that is fully devoted to diffusion filtering.

8.3.1.1 Original formulation

The cornerstone in diffusion filtering is well-known diffusion equation [22]:

$$\frac{\partial I(\mathbf{x},t)}{\partial t} = \mathrm{div}(\mathbf{D}\cdot\nabla I(\mathbf{x},t)) \tag{8.17}$$

where a noisy image $I(\mathbf{x})$ feeds the PDE with initial condition $I(\mathbf{x}, t=0) = I(\mathbf{x})$ and the temporal evolution is represented by variable t. Such a temporal evolution is governed by the divergence and gradient operator, denoted by div and ∇, respectively, and importantly, by $\mathbf{D}$, a symmetric positive definite tensor that depends on the local structure of the filtered image at time t, that is, $I(\mathbf{x}, t)$. When $\mathbf{D}$ becomes a tensor of order zero, i.e., a scalar function, the filter is usually termed as *isotropic nonhomogeneous* diffusion filter. On the other hand, regarding the two-order tensor case, that is, when $\mathbf{D}$ is represented by a matrix, the term anisotropic diffusion filter is usually adopted [22]. Note that, to be strictly considered as *anisotropic*, the diffusion must be controlled by a tensor of order two. However, in most of the seminal papers, it was called *anisotropic diffusion* even in the case of non-homogeneous diffusion (scalar function).

Most of diffusion filters are modifications of the work of Perona and Malik [23] and its practical implementation by Gerig [24]. Both works focused on the zero-order tensor case, where $\mathbf{D} = c(\mathbf{x}, t)$ is called the *diffusion coefficient*, which attempts to avoid diffusion closing to the boundaries (edges should be preserved) while filtering (diffusion) should be encouraged in homogeneous areas. To that end, since a natural approach to detect edges is looking at the gradient, the diffusion coefficient $c(\mathbf{x}, t)$ is defined as a decreasing function, $g(\cdot)$, of $\nabla I(\mathbf{x}, t)$

$$c(\mathbf{x},t) = g(\|\nabla I(\mathbf{x},t)\|). \tag{8.18}$$

where $\|\cdot\|$ is a prescribed norm, commonly the l_2 norm. When $\nabla I(\mathbf{x}, t) \to \infty$, $c(\mathbf{x}, t) \to 0$, since $c(\mathbf{x}, t)$ is, by construction, nonnegative. Thus, $\frac{\partial I(\mathbf{x},t)}{\partial t} \to 0$ and smoothing is not applied. For practical implementation, $g(.)$ is usually defined as a decreasing function of $\|\nabla I(\mathbf{x}, t\|$, as for instance,

$$g_1(\|\nabla I(\mathbf{x},t)\|) = \exp\left(-\left(\frac{\|\nabla I(\mathbf{x},t)\|}{K}\right)^2\right)$$

$$g_2(\|\nabla I(\mathbf{x},t)\|) = \left(1+\left(\frac{\|\nabla I(\mathbf{x},t)\|}{K}\right)^2\right)^{-1}$$

where K is the *diffusivity parameter*, which plays the role of thresholding mechanism in order to control the sensitivity of edge detection. Under this formulation, the parameter K must be manually selected. However, it could be also automatically tuned using some estimation of the level of noise present in the image [14,25]. Some further proposals improve the robustness of the original implementation in the presence of noise, like the ones in [26,27].

One of the most important issues to take into account when designing a PDE-based method is the selection of a proper numerical approach. Traditional methodologies, such as [23,24], use an explicit discretization scheme that yields the final solution via an iterative process, which is usually slow. In [22], Weickert proposed a semi-implicit discretization that allows a boost in convergence acceleration to get the final steady-state image. For other interesting modifications of the original formulation, the reader is referred to [28,29].

8.3.1.2 Speckle-adapted diffusion filtering

Original diffusion filtering formulation may provide excellent visual results, and it can be a useful tool for edge enhancement while making any further segmentation easier and more accurate. However, the technique was not initially conceived for speckle data but for general images. Thus, results are far from optimal when dealing with ultrasound imaging, due to the nature of the speckle. Accordingly, substantial improvements can be made if the filters are properly adapted to the features of the ultrasound data. Note that speckle images often look drastically different from images in photography or in other medical imaging modalities.

In 2002, Yu and Acton [25] proposed one of the first approaches to include speckle information into a PDE scheme, the so-called speckle-reducing anisotropic diffusion (SRAD). In order to add noise statistics into the diffusion process, the authors take the well-known Lee's filter as a starting point. Lee's filter can be seen as the linear minimum mean square error estimator of a signal corrupted with Gaussian multiplicative noise. It depends on the local coefficient of variation of signal and noise. Yu and Acton found an equivalence between this filter and the discrete formulation of the diffusion equation in (8.17). Instead of a tensor, they use the scalar diffusion coefficient that was defined as

$$c(C_s(\mathbf{x},t),t) = \left[1 + \frac{C_s(\mathbf{x},t)^2 - C_u^2(t)}{C_u^4(t) + C_u^2(t)}\right]^{-1} \tag{8.19}$$

where $C_s(\mathbf{x}, t)$ is *instantaneous coefficient of variation* of the image, given by

$$C_s(\mathbf{x},t) = \sqrt{\frac{(1/2)(|\nabla I(\mathbf{x},t)|/I(\mathbf{x},t))^2 - (1/16)(\nabla^2 I(\mathbf{x},t)/I(\mathbf{x},t))^2}{(1 + (1/4)(\nabla^2 I(\mathbf{x},t)/I(\mathbf{x},t)))^2}} \tag{8.20}$$

and $C_u(t)$ is the *coefficient of variation of noise* at time instant t. Note that, under this approach, the diffusion process is not governed solely the gradient, as in the original formulation, but by a more sophisticated mechanism, the *instantaneous coefficient of variation*, which can be seen as a continuous generalization of the so-called local coefficient of variation. It is precisely the *instantaneous coefficient of variation* that makes SRAD a speckle-adapted diffusion filter. Such a coefficient exhibits high values at edges and high contrast features and produces low values in homogeneous region.

The key of the success of the method lies on the correct estimation of $C_u(t)$. The estimation proposed in [25] was based on a homogeneous region and a time-decay model of the coefficient of variation. This was improved by the authors in a following paper [30].

The proper estimation of the noise features of the image motivated the derivation of the detailed-preserving anisotropic diffusion (DPAD) filter by Aja-Fernández and Alberola-López [14]. The DPAD filter relies on Kuan's filter (instead of Lee's) and mostly decouples the problem of noise estimation and image filtering, by using different window sizes for each task. The authors showed that, by using improved noise estimators, DPAD and SRAD may provide similar results, thus highlighting the importance of a proper noise estimation. The same authors proposed a more accurate estimation for $C_u(t)$ in [13].

Interestingly, neither SRAD nor DPAD can be strictly considered anisotropic, if we adhere to the strict terminology, since they both use a scalar value (and not a tensor) as a diffusion function.

The oriented speckle reducing anisotropic (OSRAD) filter, proposed by Krissian *et al.* in [31], is properly an anisotropic approach. The method uses a tensor **D** that is diagonalized with eigenvalues λ_1, λ_2 and λ_3 and eigenvectors $\mathbf{v}_1$, $\mathbf{v}_2$ and $\mathbf{v}_3$, respectively. The authors select $\mathbf{v}_1$ as the direction of the gradient and $\mathbf{v}_2$ and $\mathbf{v}_3$ being the maximal and minimal curvature directions computed on the Gaussian smoothed image. These directions are acquired as the eigenvectors of the projection of the Hessian matrix **H** in the plane orthogonal to the gradient. Krissian *et al.* define λ_1 as $1 - k_{\mathrm{Kuan}}(\mathbf{x})$ and fixed λ_2 and λ_3 to constants $c_{\max}$ and $c_{\min}$ with $c_{\max} >> c_{\min} > 0$. Hence, along the direction of $\mathbf{v}_1$, the filter is effectively detecting the presence of an edge in order to preserve the boundaries or smooth the region in case of negative detection.

The filtered image with OSRAD filter is the solution $I(\mathbf{x}, t)$ of (8.17) with

$$\mathbf{D} = [\mathbf{v}_1, \mathbf{v}_2, \mathbf{v}_3] \begin{bmatrix} 1 - k_{\mathrm{Kuan}}(\mathbf{x}) & 0 & 0 \\ 0 & c_{\max} & 0 \\ 0 & 0 & c_{\min} \end{bmatrix} \begin{bmatrix} \mathbf{v}_1^T \\ \mathbf{v}_2^T \\ \mathbf{v}_3^T \end{bmatrix} \tag{8.21}$$

The key of a proper filtering in the OSRAD is the definition of the diffusion tensor **D**. To improve the accuracy of the method, Vegas-Sánchez-Ferrero *et al.* proposed in [32] the probabilistic-driven oriented speckle reducing anisotropic diffusion (POSRAD) filter and extension of the OSRAD filter. The new method employs a probabilistic framework to better define the diffusion tensor **D** and accounts for speckle distribution models. The intensity of the image X is modeled as a random variable that follows a J-component mixture of density probability functions,

$$f_X(x;\pi_1,\ldots,\pi_J,\theta_1,\ldots,\theta_J)=\sum_{j=1}^{J}\pi_j f_{X_j}(x;\theta_j), \tag{8.22}$$

where $\pi_j > 0$, $\sum_{j=1}^{J}\pi_j = 1$ and f_{X_j} are probability density functions with parameters vector θ_j. Speckle modeling is inherently accounted for due to the J-component mixture model.

With the a posteriori probabilities, $P(x \in C_j \mid X = x;\theta_j)$, the authors define a structure tensor for each class C_j as the Weickert's local structure tensor [22],

$$\mathbf{T}_j = G_\sigma * \nabla_\sigma\big(P(x \in C_j \,|\, X = x;\theta_j)\nabla_\sigma P(x \in C_j \,|\, X = x;\theta_j)\big)^T \tag{8.23}$$

The diffusion tensor **D** is diagonalized with eigenbase $\{\mathbf{e}_1, \mathbf{e}_2, \mathbf{e}_3\}$. Such an eigenbase is extracted from the $\hat{j}$-th structure tensor, $\mathbf{T}_{\hat{j}}$, whose maximum eigenvalue, μ_1^j, is maximal for all j, i.e., $\hat{j} = \mathrm{argmax}_j\,\mu_1^j$. Thereby, the most probable boundary is preserved during the filtering process. The eigenvalues λ_1, λ_2 and λ_3 are defined as

$$\begin{aligned}\lambda_1 &= 1 - |\nabla_\sigma P\big(x \in C_{\hat{j}} \,|\, X = x;\theta_{\hat{j}}\big)\cdot \mathbf{e}_1|,\\ \lambda_2 &= 1 - |\nabla_\sigma P\big(x \in C_{\hat{j}} \,|\, X = x;\theta_{\hat{j}}\big)\cdot \mathbf{e}_2|,\\ \lambda_3 &= 1.\end{aligned} \tag{8.24}$$

In homogeneous areas, **D** becomes isotropic and in the presence of boundaries, it turns out to be anisotropic, with the main orientation aligned along the most probable boundaries. The least eigenvalue, λ_3, is defined in this way to perform filtering just in the direction of the least probable boundary.

Recently, an extension of the POSRAD filter was proposed by Ramos-Llordén *et al.* [33]. Perhaps, the most striking feature of the new diffusion filter is that it includes a tissue-selective memory mechanism to overcome the over-filtering problem that typically occurred in diffusion filtering. Such a memory mechanism is implemented in terms of a delay differential equation for the diffusion tensor, whose behavior depends on the statistics of tissues, by accelerating the diffusion in meaningless region but preserving as well speckled in regions where details should be kept intact.

The novel diffusion filter is formulated as follows:

$$\frac{\partial I(\mathbf{x},t)}{\partial t} = \mathrm{div}(\mathbf{L}(\mathbf{x},t)\nabla I(\mathbf{x},t)), \tag{8.25}$$

$$\frac{\partial \mathbf{L}(\mathbf{x},t)}{\partial t} = \frac{1}{\tau(\mathbf{x})}(\mathbf{L}(\mathbf{x},t) - S\{\mathbf{D}(\mathbf{x},t)\}), \tag{8.26}$$

The evolution of the novel diffusion tensor **L(x**, *t*) is dictated by **D(x**, *t*), defined as in POSRAD, and importantly, by the spatially variant terms $\tau(\mathbf{x})$ and operator

$S\{\cdot\}$. Such terms introduces memory in a tissue-distinctive manner, since they depend on tissue characterization via the probability of detecting the specific type of speckle to be removed.

8.3.2 Total-variation methods

Another popular PDE-based filtering methods in image are the so-called TV techniques. TV denoising is a concept pioneered by Rudin *et al.* in the early 1990s [34]. It relies on the minimization of the TV of a given image, let say $I(\mathbf{x})$, which is defined as,

$$\int_{\Omega} |\nabla I(\mathbf{x})| d\mathbf{x}. \tag{8.27}$$

The rationale behind TV denoising is that, by seeking for restored images whose TV is minimum, impulsive noise, e.g., speckle noise, is effectively suppressed and sharp discontinuities (edges) are well preserved. Indeed, TV denoising techniques promotes piece-wise or cartoon-like reconstructed images, which can be quite handful for segmentation purposes, though the appearance may look quite unrealistic. Most of the TV approaches are formulated under the following variational framework,

$$\inf_{I_{\mathrm{TV}}(\mathbf{x})} \int_{\Omega} |\nabla I_{\mathrm{TV}}(\mathbf{x})| d\mathbf{x} + \lambda \int_{\Omega} (I_{\mathrm{TV}}(\mathbf{x}) - I(\mathbf{x}))^2 d\mathbf{x} \tag{8.28}$$

The second term in (8.28) is called the data-fidelity term and promotes that the optimal $I_{\mathrm{TV}}(\mathbf{x})$ is in agreement with the given noisy image $I(\mathbf{x})$. The influence in the final result of the data-fidelity term compared to the TV term is controlled by the user-parameter λ. Very low values of λ effectively suppress speckle but produces heavy cartoon-like images, while high values of λ can be seen as conservative choices and may even preserve speckle. Tractable algorithms to solve (8.28) involve the derivation of the Euler–Lagrange equation, yielding a nonlinear equation of the form $F(I(\mathbf{x})) = 0$, with $F(\cdot)$ depending on (8.28). A popular approach then consists of formulating the following (temporal) PDE,

$$\frac{\partial I(\mathbf{x}, t)}{\partial t} + F(I(\mathbf{x}, t)) = 0 \tag{8.29}$$

and solving it iteratively. The steady-state solution, $\frac{\partial I(\mathbf{x},t)}{\partial t} \approx 0$, is considered the solution of the Euler–Lagrange equations and hence the solution of problem (8.28).

Some specific implementation of TV schemes for ultrasound despeckling are [35,36]. In both cases, authors assume a multiplicative Rayleigh model for Speckle. In the latter, the logarithm compression is also taken into account.

8.4 Homomorphic filtering

The homomorphic technique is based on the assumption that the speckle is multiplicative in nature and therefore signal dependent. In order to achieve a noise component additive and signal independent, the logarithm is taken and filtering methods are carried out over the logarithm-transformed signal. In its simplest form, if $I(\mathbf{x})$ is the observed signal, then

$$I(\mathbf{x}) = A(\mathbf{x})\eta_N(\mathbf{x}).$$

where $A(\mathbf{x})$ is the underlying signal and $\eta_N(\mathbf{x})$ is a multiplicative noise, then

$$\log I(\mathbf{x}) = \log A(\mathbf{x}) + \log \eta_N(\mathbf{x}),$$

and the filtering is done over log $I(\mathbf{x})$. Different techniques have been proposed as suitable filters over the separated components. In [37], authors introduce a homomorphic gamma wavelet MAP, which is equivalent to the gamma-MAP previously reviewed, properly adapted to work over the wavelet domain.

In [38], a simpler method was proposed by using a filter on the Fourier domain of log $I(\mathbf{x})$. The filter is defined to be a band-pass or a high-boost Butterworth filter with impulse response:

$$H(u,v) = \gamma_L + \frac{\gamma_H}{1 + (D_0/D(u,v))^2} \tag{8.30}$$

with

$$D(u,v) = \sqrt{(u - N/2)^2 + (v - N/2)^2}. \tag{8.31}$$

$D_0 = 1.8$ is the cut of frequency of the filter and $\gamma_L = 0.4$ and $\gamma_H = 0.6$ are the gains for the low and high frequencies, respectively. u and v are the spatial coordinates of the Fourier domain and N is the dimension of the image in that domain.

Other approaches based on homomorphic decomposition of the signal are those in [39,40], where deconvolution schemes were used to restore the underlying signal is used, and [41], also using a wavelet thresholding to remove the noise component.

8.5 Bilateral filters

A bilateral filter is a well-known nonlinear and noniterative technique that has proved its suitability in edge-preserving and noise reduction across different image modalities. In the original formulation of Tomasi and Manduchi [42], the concept of bilateral filtering was introduced by using the following integral expression,

$$I_F(\mathbf{x}) = k^{-1}(\mathbf{x}) \int c(\mathbf{x},\mathbf{y}) s(I(\mathbf{x}), I(\mathbf{y})) I(\mathbf{y}) d\mathbf{y}, \tag{8.32}$$

where $I_F(\mathbf{x})$ is the filtered image. $c(\cdot, \cdot)$ is a spatial kernel called the *closeness function*, which merely depends on a given distance between variables $\mathbf{y}$ and $\mathbf{x}$. Its purpose is to smooth the differences in coordinates and it is usually built using a Gaussian kernel. Function $s(\cdot, \cdot)$, dubbed the *similarity function*, depends on the image intensity via a nonlinear operation. Finally, function $k(\cdot)$ is used to provide a proper normalization.

In the bilateral filtering framework, in order to average similar pixels, not only the geometrical similarity (closeness) is considered but also the similarity based on the intensity. In this way, the methodology incorporates (quoting the authors): domain filtering, that is, a conventional convolution and range filtering, i.e., filtering based on intensity similarity. This motivates the terminology bilateral. Bilateral filtering prevents smoothing near the boundaries. This is because, even though nearby pixels of different regions are considered similar according to $c(\cdot, \cdot)$, they will be substantially dissimilar in terms of $s(\cdot, \cdot)$. For practical purposes, a discretization of (8.32) is used:

$$I_F(\mathbf{x}) = \frac{1}{W_p} \sum_{\mathbf{y} \in \eta(\mathbf{x})} c(\|\mathbf{y} - \mathbf{x}\|) s(I(\mathbf{y}), I(\mathbf{x})) I(\mathbf{y}), \tag{8.33}$$

with W_p the normalization term calculated as

$$W_p = \sum_{\mathbf{y} \in \eta(\mathbf{x})} c(\|\mathbf{y} - \mathbf{x}\|) s(I(\mathbf{y}), I(\mathbf{x})). \tag{8.34}$$

To the best of our knowledge, the first application of bilateral filtering to ultrasound despeckling was done by Balocco *et al.* [43]. Their starting point is the fact that a proper design of the similarity function is key for the good behavior of a bilateral filtering. Thus, authors define function $s(\cdot, \cdot)$ using the specific statistics of speckle. First, they assume image $I(\mathbf{x})$ to be a random variable that follows a Rayleigh distribution, with shape parameter α, that is,

$$f_{I(\mathbf{x})}\left(I(bx), \alpha^2\right) = \frac{I(\mathbf{x})}{\alpha^2} e^{-\frac{I^2(\mathbf{x})}{2\alpha^2}} \quad I(\mathbf{x}) \geq 0. \tag{8.35}$$

The value of the shape parameter α is then estimated using a maximum likelihood estimator for Rayleigh:

$$\hat{\alpha}(\mathbf{x}) = \sqrt{\frac{1}{2|\eta(\mathbf{x})|} \sum_{\mathbf{q} \in \eta(\mathbf{x})} I(\mathbf{q})^2}. \tag{8.36}$$

For the practical implementation, authors assume that if two points $\mathbf{x}$ and $\mathbf{y}$ are similar in intensity, it is because $I(\mathbf{y})$ also belongs to a Rayleigh distribution with same $\hat{\alpha}(\mathbf{x})$. Consequently, in that case, $tf_{I(\mathbf{x})}\left(I(\mathbf{y}), \hat{\alpha}^2(\mathbf{x})\right)$ must take high values. To simplify the expression, they just reduce the sum over $\eta(\mathbf{x})$ in (8.36) to just one single value $I(\mathbf{x})$. Under this simplification, $f_{I(\mathbf{x})}\left(I(\mathbf{y}), \hat{\alpha}^2(\mathbf{x})\right)$ only depends on $I(\mathbf{x})$ and $I(\mathbf{x})$ and

$$s(I(\mathbf{x}), I(\mathbf{y})) = f_{I(\mathbf{x})}\left(I(\mathbf{y}), \hat{\alpha}^2(\mathbf{x})\right). \tag{8.37}$$

Finally, a Gaussian kernel is adopted for $c(\cdot, \cdot)$ and its standard deviation is determined from the estimated speckle size. The adaptive support in combination with the incorporation of speckle statistics into the similarity function yields a more homogeneous smoothing and a better edge preservation.

There are other adaptations of the bilateral filtering philosophy to cope with speckle, like the ones in [44–46]. In general, bilateral filters provide an attractive trade-off between speckle suppression and boundaries preservation. Its main drawback is the sensitivity of the similarity function definition. The reader should be aware that common similarity functions used for bilateral filters are adequate for photographs, where regions present clear well-defined structures or quasi-constant areas. However, as we have mentioned throughout this chapter, ultrasound speckle images do not share the same lenient characteristics as images in photography. Consequently, a proper definition of similarity metrics may be a seriously complicated task, yielding a specific research line on its own.

8.6 Geometric filtering

In 1986, Crimmins proposed an ingenious way to reduce speckle in SAR images [47]. The filtering technique was termed geometric speckle filter. The algorithm relies on morphological operations applied to binary images. In particular, the iterative binary algorithm, named the eight convex hull algorithm, reduces the curvature of the boundaries appearing in binary images. In other words, suppose that a given binary image contains some geometric objects with sharp edges. The eight convex hull algorithm effectively reduces the curvature of boundaries or equivalently, sharp discontinuities are greatly diminished.

To convert the speckle noisy image $I(\mathbf{x})$ into a binary image, and hence, be in condition to apply the algorithm, Crimmins came up with the following idea. Let us think on $I(x, y)$ as a 2D surface in a 3D domain (note that we have made explicit the dependence on x and y in contrast to previous despeckle filtering cases), that is,

$$(x, y, I(x, y)) \in \mathbb{R}^3, \tag{8.38}$$

where, by convenience, variable x represents the *width*, y represents the *depth* and $I(x, y)$ represents the *height*. Let us think on a vertical plane $y = y_0$. If that plane intersects the surface of (8.38), the result is a 1D curve. The height of that curve for each x is, precisely, given by $I(x, y_0)$. Due to the spurious nature of speckle, $I(x, y_0)$ looks quite sharp/abrupt except in the presence of edges between regions, where a soft plateau is expected.

Crimmins suggested to create a binary image $B(x, z)$ based on such a curve. In particular, he defined

$$B(x, z) = \begin{cases} 1 & \text{if} \quad z > I(x, y_0) \\ 0 & \qquad \text{otherwise} \end{cases}$$

Note that the boundary of the binary image, $B(x, z)$ is exactly $(x, I(x, y_0))$. Therefore, reduction in its curvature is equivalent to despeckling $I(x, y_0)$.

In order to filter the whole image, $I(x, y)$, the process is repeated for all vertical planes y, after which is also applied for horizontal planes x. The new speckle-filtered image is used as input in the second iteration of the whole algorithm. Geometric speckle filter is notably effective for speckle reduction since speckle normally appears as narrow winding walls and valleys when we look at its 2D surface visualization.

Although the geometric filter originated for speckle reduction in SAR, it was later successfully extended to Ultrasound speckle denoising in [38,48].

8.7 Other filtering methodologies

Finally, let us focus on those other nonlinear filtering methodologies that do not strictly adhere to previous philosophies and cannot be classified accordingly. We have intentionally left aside speckle filtering based on MAP and maximum likelihood reconstruction since they will be addressed in a specific section.

A stochastic nonlinear approach named the *squeeze box filter* was introduced by Tay *et al.* in [49] intended to despeckle B-mode ultrasound images. The key idea of the squeeze box filter is that the local extrema of $I(\mathbf{x})$ are treated as outliers and just those values are smoothed with a locally averaging filter. Next, local extrema of the thus smoothed image are again extracted and the same procedure repeated.

Some authors introduce controllers based on fuzzy logic in order to fine tune different parameters of speckle filters. In [50], Aja-Fernández *et al.* used fuzzy logic over a speckle anisotropic diffusion framework. Specifically, the diffusion coefficient definition was reconsidered and guided by fuzzy reasoning. Since then, other several nonlinear filters based on fuzzy logic have been applied to speckle denoising. Guo *et al.* in [51] proposed a fuzzy-logic-based filter was presented and applied to breast ultrasound image enhancement. The whole approach consists of image normalization, fuzzy logic application, edge and textural information extraction and contrast enhancement. According to the authors, details of breast lesions may be enhanced without over-filtering. Fuzzy filtering was also used in combination of geometric filters so as to enhance edge details in echocardiographic images while reducing speckle noise [52].

Recently, Gupta *et al.* presented an interesting technique [53] that deals with speckle removal by using the Ripplet transform, a generalization of the Curvelet transformation [54]. The complete despeckling method comprises of a logarithmic transformation and a filtering process of the Ripplet transform coefficients with a bilateral filter. The final image is recovered by computing the inverse Ripple transform after which the logarithmic transformation is reversed.

8.8 Some final remarks

Different filtering nonlinear methods for speckle have been reviewed in this chapter. Many more can be found in the literature, together with all those reviewed in other chapters. For sure that many more will arise along the following years.

The reader must see all these methods not as a complete closed survey of the only possible filtering schemes for speckle, but as an outlook to the possibilities and opportunities that noise filtering methods offer to ultrasound processing. As stated at the chapter of this part, the selection of the specific filter must be totally aligned with the final purpose of the filtered image. When dealing with ultrasound data, denoising must not be a cosmetic operation, but a way to enhance the features already present in the data. Accordingly, we should not search for the *best* speckle filter, but, instead, for the most suitable filter for any specific application. If you are measuring some distance in the heart that may be indicative of mitral failure, you need precision and you cannot erode or blur any edge. In addition, image does not need to look nice, since you are using it to extract a measure. On the other hand, if the purpose of your filtering is to enhance fetal ultrasound 3D data to achieve a nice 3D+t rendering, you are precisely looking for *nicer looking* effects.

Accordingly, since the final purpose of speckle filters may differ, so must the way of validating and comparing filters. Performance assessment of filtering methods has been traditionally done using visual comparison and some measures like the Figure of Merit, mean square errors or structural measures. However, we really think that the evaluation of a specific technique should be done attending to the specific use of the technique inside the whole processing pipeline.

Acknowledgments

This work was supported by Ministerio de Ciencia e Innovación (Spain) with research grant TEC2013-44194-P. Gonzalo Vegas-Sánchez-Ferrero acknowledges Consejería de Educación, Juventud y Deporte of Comunidad de Madrid and the People Programme (Marie Curie Actions) of the European Union's Seventh Framework Programme (FP7/2007–2013) for REA grant agreement no. 291820.

References

[1] Tyan S. Median filtering: deterministic properties. In: Two-Dimensional Digital Signal Processing II. Berlin, Heidelberg, New York: Springer Verlag; 1981. p. 197–217.

[2] Yang GJ. Median filters and their applications to image processing. Dissertation Abstr Int Part B: Sci Eng. 1980;41(6): 1980.

[3] Narendra PM. A separable median filter for image noise smoothing. IEEE Trans Pattern Anal Mach Intell. 1981;(1):20–29.

[4] Ko SJ, Lee YH. Center weighted median filters and their applications to image enhancement. IEEE Trans Circuits Syst. 1991;38(9): 984–993.

[5] Pratt WK. Digital Image Processing. 4th ed. New Jersey: John Wiley and Sons; 2007.

[6] Loupas T, McDicken W, Allan P. An adaptive weighted median filter for speckle suppression in medical ultrasonic images. IEEE Trans Circuits Syst. 1989;36(1): 129–135.

[7] Sun T, Neuvo Y. Detail-preserving median based filters in image processing. Pattern Recognit Lett. 1994;15(4): 341–347.

[8] Czerwinski RN, Jones DL, O'Brien WD. Ultrasound speckle reduction by directional median filtering. In: Image Processing, 1995. Proceedings, International Conference on. vol. 1. IEEE; 1995. p. 358–361.

[9] Vanithamani R, Umamaheswari G, Ezhilarasi M. Modified hybrid median filter for effective speckle reduction in ultrasound images. In: Proceedings of the 12th International Conference on Networking, VLSI and Signal Processing; 2010. p. 166–171.

[10] Kuan D, Sawchuk A, Strand T, Chavel P. Adaptive restoration of images with speckle. IEEE Trans Acoust Speech Signal Process. 1987;35(3): 373–383.

[11] Lopes A, Nezry E, Touzi R, Laur H. Structure detection and statistical adaptive speckle filtering in SAR images. Int J Remote Sens. 1993;14(9): 1735–1758.

[12] Vegas-Sanchez-Ferrero G, Seabra J, Rodriguez-Leor O, *et al.* Gamma mixture classifier for plaque detection in intravascular ultrasonic images. IEEE Trans Ultrason Ferroelectr Freq Control. 2014;61(1): 44–61.

[13] Aja-Fernández S, Vegas-Sánchez-Ferrero G, Martín-Fernández M, Alberola-López C. Automatic noise estimation in images using local statistics. Additive and Multiplicative Cases. Image Vision Comput. 2009 May;27(6): 756–770.

[14] Aja-Fernández S, Alberola-López C. On the estimation of the coefficient of variation for anisotropic diffusion speckle filtering. IEEE Trans Image Process. 2006;15(9): 2694–2701.

[15] Baraldi A, Parmiggiani F. A refined Gamma MAP SAR speckle filter with improved geometrical adaptivity. IEEE Trans Geosci Remote Sens. 1995;33(5): 1245–1257.

[16] Foucher S, Bénié GB, Boucher JM. Multiscale MAP filtering of SAR images. IEEE Trans Image Process. 2001;10(1): 49–60.

[17] Buades A, Coll B, Morel JM. A review of image denoising algorithms, with a new one. Multiscale Model Simul. 2005;4(2): 490–530.

[18] Manjón J, Carbonell-Caballero J, Lull J, García-Martí G, Martí-Bonmatí L, Robles M. MRI denoising using non-local means. Med Image Anal. 2008;12:514–523.

[19] Coupé P, Hellier P, Kervrann C, Barillot C. Nonlocal means-based speckle filtering for ultrasound images. IEEE Trans Image Process. 2009;18(10): 2221–2229.

[20] Coupé P, Hellier P, Kervrann C, Barillot C. Bayesian non local means-based speckle filtering. In: 2008 5th IEEE Int. Symp. on Biomedical Imaging: from Nano to Macro. IEEE; 2008. p. 1291–1294.

[21] Guo Y, Wang Y, Hou T. Speckle filtering of ultrasonic images using a modified non local-based algorithm. Biomed Signal Process Control. 2011;6(2): 129–138.

[22] Weickert J. Anisotropic Diffusion in image processing. Stuttgart, Germany: Teubner-Verlag; 1998.

[23] Perona P, Malik J. Scale-space and edge detection using anisotropic diffusion. IEEE Trans Pattern Anal Mach Intell. 1990 Jul;12(7): 629–639.
[24] Gerig G, Kübler O, Kikinis R, Jolesz FA. Nonlinear anisotropic filtering of MRI data. IEEE Trans Med Image. 1992 Jun;11(2): 221–232.
[25] Yu Y, Acton ST. Speckle reducing anisotropic diffusion. IEEE Trans Image Process. 2002;11(11): 1260–1270.
[26] Alvarez L. Images and PDE's. In: Lecture Notes in Control and Information Sciences. Heidelberg, Germany: Springer, vol. 219, pp. 3–14, 1996.
[27] Catté F, Lions PL, Morel JM, Coll T. Image selective smoothing and edge detection by nonlinear diffusion. SIAM J Numer Anal. 1992;29:182–193.
[28] Black MJ, Sapiro G, Marimont DH, Heeger D. Robust anisotropic diffusion. IEEE Trans Image Process. 1998 Mar;7(3): 421–432.
[29] Sapiro G, Ringach DL. Anisotropic diffusion of multivalued images with applications to color filtering. IEEE Trans Image Process. 1996;5: 1582–1586.
[30] Yu Y, Acton ST. Edge detection in ultrasound imagery using the instantaneous coefficient of variation. IEEE Trans Image Process. 2004;13 (12): 1640–1655.
[31] Krissian K, Westin CF, Kikinis R, Vosburgh KG. Oriented speckle reducing anisotropic diffusion. IEEE Trans Image Process. 2007;16(5): 1412–1424.
[32] Vegas-Sánchez-Ferrero G, Aja-Fernandez S, Martín-Fernández M, Frangi AF, Palencia C. Probabilistic-driven oriented speckle reducing anisotropic diffusion with application to cardiac ultrasonic images. In: International Conference on Medical Image Computing and Computer-Assisted Intervention. Springer; 2010. p. 518–525.
[33] Ramos-Llordén G, Vegas-Sánchez-Ferrero G, Martin-Fernandez M, Alberola-López C, Aja-Fernández S. Anisotropic diffusion filter with memory based on speckle statistics for ultrasound Images. IEEE Trans Image Process. 2015;24(1): 345–358.
[34] Rudin LI, Osher S, Fatemi E. Nonlinear total variation based noise removal algorithms. Physica D. 1992;60(1): 259–268.
[35] Sanches J, Bioucas-Dias JM, Marques JS. Minimum total variation in 3D ultrasound reconstruction. In: IEEE International Conference on Image Processing 2005. vol. 3. IEEE; 2005. p. III–597.
[36] Afonso M, Sanches JM. Image reconstruction under multiplicative speckle noise using total variation. Neurocomputing. 2015;150:200–213.
[37] Solbo S, Eltoft T. Homomorphic wavelet-based statistical despeckling of SAR images. IEEE Trans Geosci Remote Sens. 2004;42(4): 711–721.
[38] Loizou CP, Pattichis CS, Christodoulou CI, Istepanian RSH, Pantziaris M, Nicolaides A. Comparative evaluation of despeckle filtering in ultrasound imaging of the carotid artery. IEEE Trans Ultrason Ferroelectr Freq Control. 2005 Oct;52(10): 1653–1669.
[39] Taxt T. Restoration of medical ultrasound images using two-dimensional homomorphic deconvolution. IEEE Trans Ultrason Ferroelectr Freq Control. 1995;42(4): 543–554.

[40] Taxt T, Strand J. Two-dimensional noise-robust blind deconvolution of ultrasound images. IEEE Trans Ultrason Ferroelectr Freq Control. 2001; 48(4): 861–866.

[41] Gupta S, Chauhan R, Saxena S. Homomorphic wavelet thresholding technique for denoising medical ultrasound images. J Med Eng Technol. 2005;29(5): 208–214.

[42] Tomasi C, Manduchi R. Bilateral filtering for gray and color images. In: Computer Vision, 1998. Sixth International Conference on. IEEE; 1998. p. 839–846.

[43] Balocco S, Gatta C, Pujol O, Mauri J, Radeva P. SRBF: speckle reducing bilateral filtering. Ultrasound Med Biol. 2010;36(8): 1353–1363.

[44] Tang J, Guo S, Sun Q, Deng Y, Zhou D. Speckle reducing bilateral filter for cattle follicle segmentation. BMC Genomics. 2010;11(2): 1.

[45] Loganayagi T, Kashwan K. An analysis of speckle reduction in ultrasound kidney images by adaptive bilateral filter. Int J Digital Content Technol Appl. 2015;9(5): 1.

[46] Konyar MZ, Ertürk S. Enhancement of ultrasound images with bilateral filter and Rayleigh CLAHE. In: 2015 23nd Signal Processing and Communications Applications Conference (SIU). IEEE; 2015. p. 1861–1864.

[47] Crimmins TR. Geometric filter for reducing speckle. Opt Eng. 1986;25(5): 255651.

[48] Busse L, Crimmins T, Fienup J. A model based approach to improve the performance of the geometric filtering speckle reduction algorithm. In: Ultrasonics Symposium, 1995. Proceedings, 1995 IEEE. vol. 2. IEEE; 1995. p. 1353–1356.

[49] Tay PC, Acton ST, Hossack JA. Ultrasound despeckling using an adaptive window stochastic approach. In: 2006 International Conference on Image Processing. IEEE; 2006. p. 2549–2552.

[50] Aja S, Alberola C, Ruiz A. Fuzzy anisotropic diffusion for speckle filtering. In: Acoustics, Speech, and Signal Processing, 2001. Proceedings (ICASSP'01). 2001 IEEE International Conference on. vol. 2. IEEE; 2001. p. 1261–1264.

[51] Guo Y, Cheng H, Huang J, *et al.* Breast ultrasound image enhancement using fuzzy logic. Ultrasound Med Biol. 2006;32(2): 237–247.

[52] Biradar N, Dewal M, Rohit MK. Edge preserved speckle noise reduction using integrated fuzzy filters. Int Sch Res Not. pp. 1–11, vol. 2014;2014.

[53] Gupta D, Anand R, Tyagi B. Ripplet domain non-linear filtering for speckle reduction in ultrasound medical images. Biomed Signal Process Control. 2014;10:79–91.

[54] Xu J, Yang L, Wu D. Ripplet: a new transform for image processing. J Visual Commun Image Represent. 2010;21(7): 627–639.

Chapter 9

Wavelet despeckle filtering

Savita Gupta[1] *and Lakhwinder Kaur*[2]

9.1 Introduction

In signal and image processing, locating the transients, i.e. image discontinuities, help to select the most important information from a vast amount of data. To aid the analysis of transient signals, that is to localize both the frequency and the time information in a signal, various transforms and bases are proposed [1,2]. Among them, the wavelet transform (WT) and the short time Fourier transform (STFT) are quite standard in signal processing applications. In STFT transform, also called windowed Fourier transform (FT) or Gabor transform, the signal is multiplied by a smooth window function, typically Gaussian and the Fourier integral is applied to the windowed signal. The main drawback of STFT is its fixed time-frequency resolution, which means that once a window is chosen for STFT, the time-frequency resolution becomes fixed over the entire time-frequency plane because the same window is used at all frequencies. This limitation of STFT can be resolved using WT, which acts as a microscope, focusing on smaller time phenomena [2].

A 'wavelet' is a function that oscillates, in a manner similar to a wave, for a limited portion of space or time and vanishes outside. The important characteristic of wavelet is that it allows simultaneous time and frequency analysis that makes it a convenient and suitable tool for analysis and processing of transient, non-stationary or time-varying signals. In wavelet analysis, the scale can be interpreted as the inverse of frequency permitting a local characterization of signals, which is not feasible with the conventional FT and the windowed FT (STFT). Other advantageous properties of the WT are multi-resolution, edge detection, sparsity and fast implementation. Further, the importance of wavelet analysis in image processing applications is increased from the psychophysical aspects of human vision as it corresponds well to the way the human beings perceive the images [3].

[1]Department of CSE, UIET, Panjab University, India
[2]Department of CSE, UCoE, Punjabi University, India

9.2 Discrete wavelet transform

The discrete WT (DWT) is a linear transform for which wavelets are discretely sampled. The practical applicability of DWT comes from its multi-resolution analysis ability [3] and efficient perfect reconstruction (PR) filter bank structures. The implementation of an analysis filter bank for a single-level two-dimensional (2-D) DWT is shown in Figure 9.1. This structure produces three detailed sub-images (HL, HL and HH) corresponding to three different directional-orientations, namely, horizontal, vertical and diagonal as well as a lower resolution sub-image (LL).

The filter bank structure can be iterated in a similar manner on the LL channel to provide multi-level decomposition. The multi-level decomposition hierarchy of an image is illustrated in Figure 9.2.

Each decomposition breaks the parent image into four child images. Each of such sub-images is one-fourth of the size of a parent image. The sub-images are placed according to the position of each sub-band in the 2-D partition of frequency plane.

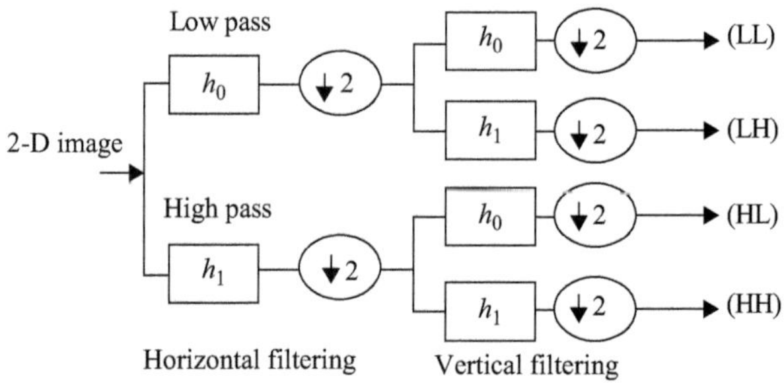

Figure 9.1 Single-level analysis filter bank for 2-D DWT (Section 9.2)

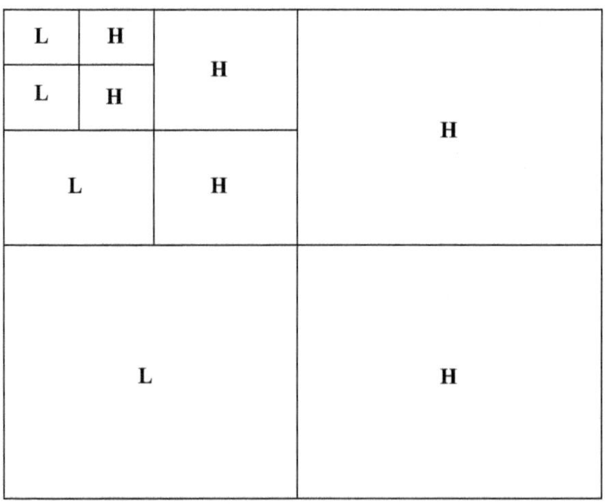

Figure 9.2 Multi-level decomposition with 2-D DWT (Section 9.2)

The DWT of an image yields adequately de-correlated wavelet coefficients. However, these coefficients are not independent. The large-magnitude coefficients tend to occur near each other within sub-bands and also at the same relative spatial locations in sub-bands at adjacent scales and orientations [4]. The positions of the large wavelet coefficients indicate image edges, i.e. the DWT can act as local edge detectors in the horizontal (0° sub-band), vertical (90°) and diagonal (±45°) directions.

9.3 Limitations of DWT and its improvements in de-noising

The standard DWT is a compact and non-redundant representation of signal in transform domain. However, the decimation step after filtering makes the standard DWT time shift-variant, which means that a small shift in an image can cause a major variation in the distribution of energy of the wavelet coefficients at different levels and mild ringing artefacts around the edges. The solution to this problem is to use the redundant representation of the orthogonal WT, which omits the down-sampling operation. The redundant WT (RDWT) has a similar tree-structured implementation without any decimation (sub-sampling) step. The balance for PR is preserved through level dependent zero-padding interpolation of respective low pass and high pass filters in the filter bank structures.

The DWT in its redundant and non-decimated form (RDWT) has established an impressive reputation as a tool for image de-noising due to its shift-invariance property. However, it too suffers from two main disadvantages. First, the high redundancy introduced in the output information increases the storage and computation requirements of the applications, and second, the poor directional selectivity for diagonal features does not allow discrimination between features at positive and negative frequencies as the wavelet filters are separable and real. As an alternative to the un-decimated DWT, many authors have used best-basis methods or optimal wavelet designs to reduce DWT shift sensitivity without any increase in transform redundancy [5–7]. More recently, Selenick and Sendur [8] formulated double density WT (DDWT), a low redundancy DWT extension with reduced sensitivity. However, the DDWT has poor directionality and offers no phase information.

A radiçally different approach to shift-invariance and directional selectivity was pioneered by Simoncelli *et al.* [9]. They designed the steerable pyramid, a highly redundant, non-separable, directional and multi-scale transform that attains approximate shiftability. The main drawback of this method is that it does not allow principally PR and has high transform redundancy. In 1997, Magarey and Kingsbury [10,11] demonstrated that these two key problems of shift sensitivity and poor directional selectivity could be overcome by using complex WT (CWT) at the cost of limited redundancy. However, a further problem arises here because PR becomes difficult to achieve for complex wavelet decompositions beyond level 1, when the input to each level becomes complex. To overcome this, more recently, Kingsbury developed the dual tree-CWT (DT-CWT), which added PR to the other attractive properties of complex wavelets [12–14].

DT-CWT gives much better directional selectivity when filtering multi-dimensional signals while maintaining the low redundancy (independent of the number of scales; 2:1 for 1-D; 2^m:1 for m-dimensional signal), as compared to that of RDWT (($J(2^m - 1) + 1$):1 for J-scale transform). Moreover, it allows efficient computation of the order-N, less than 2^m times than that of the RDWT for m-D signal. Motivated by these key features of DT-CWT, Choi *et al.* [15] incorporated the DT-CWT with a Hidden Markov Tree (HMT) model and achieved a significant improvement in the de-noising of natural images. However, the HMT-based methods are computationally very expensive [16].

Recently, the wavelet domain Bayesian approaches have become quite popular due to the good performance and low complexity. Bayesian algorithms that exploit the wavelet coefficient dependencies give better results compared to the ones derived using an independent assumption [17–19]. In this respect, the locally adaptive despeckling algorithms designed using *maximum a posteriori* estimates are the powerful and low-complexity tools for exploiting the intra-scale dependencies of the wavelet coefficients [20–22]. In the present work, all these algorithms have been extended in the complex wavelet domain to mitigate the shortcomings of RDWT and to find the optimal wavelet basis for image de-noising applications.

9.4 Dual tree-complex wavelet transform

Like DWT, the 1-D DT-CWT decomposes a signal $f(t)$, in terms of a complex shifted and dilated mother wavelet [12]:

$$f(t) = \sum_{j \geq j_0}^{J} \sum_{k=-\infty}^{\infty} D_f(j,k)\psi_{j,k}(t) + \sum_{k=-\infty}^{\infty} C_f(J,k)\phi_{J,k}(t) \tag{9.1}$$

where $\phi_{J,k}$ and $\psi_{j,k}$ are complex; $\phi_{J,k} = \phi^r_{J,k} + \sqrt{-1}\phi^i_{J,k}, \psi_{j,k} = \psi^r_{j,k} + \sqrt{-1}\psi^i_{j,k}$. The $\psi^r_{j,k}$ and $\psi^i_{j,k}$ are themselves real wavelets. The real and imaginary parts of the DT-CWT are computed using separate filter bank structures (hence the name 'dual tree') with wavelet h_{0a}, h_{1a} for the real part and h_{0b}, h_{1b} for the imaginary part.

In 2-D, the CWT decomposes an image $f(t)$, $t = (t_1, t_2) \in R^2$ using a complex scaling function and six complex wavelet functions as

$$f(t) = \sum_{b \in B} \sum_{j \geq j_0}^{J} \sum_{k=-\infty}^{\infty} D_f(j,k)\psi_{j,k}(t) + \sum_{k=-\infty}^{\infty} C_f(J,k)\phi_{J,k}(t) \tag{9.2}$$

The six sub-bands of the 2D-CWT are labelled as $B = \{+15°, +45°, +75°, -15°, -45°, -75°\}$ for the six-oriented direction of the wavelet function. For a separable 2-D CWT, based on 1-D complex scaling function (ϕ) and wavelet function (ψ), the relations are

$$\psi^{+15°}(t) = \phi(t_1)\psi(t_2), \quad \psi^{+45°}(t) = \psi(t_1)\psi(t_2), \quad \psi^{+75°}(t) = \psi(t_1)\phi(t_2),$$
$$\psi^{-15°}(t) = \phi(t_1)\psi^*(t_2), \quad \psi^{+45°}(t) = \psi(t_1)\psi^*(t_2) \text{ and } \psi^{-75°}(t) = \psi^*(t_1)\phi(t_2)$$

where ψ^* is the complex conjugate of ψ. The 2D-CWT expansion represents $f(t)$ using a tight frame with four times redundancy. The real parts of complex

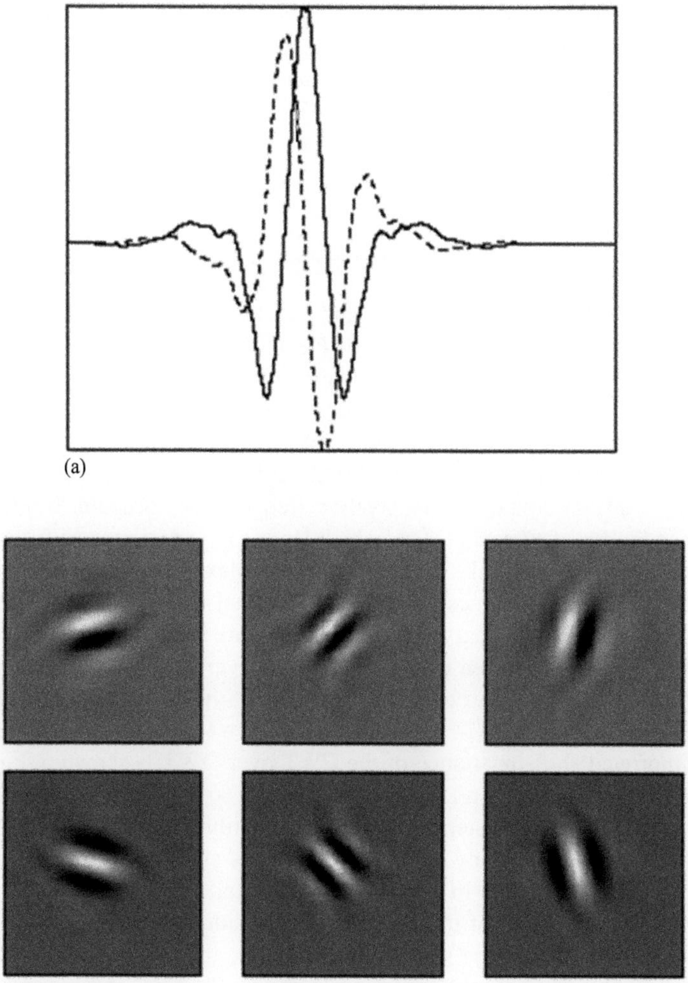

Figure 9.3 (a) Real (solid) and imaginary (dashed) parts of a 1-D complex wavelet-basis function. (b) Real parts of the six 2-D wavelet-basis functions (Sections 9.4 and 9.5)

wavelet-basis functions are shown in Figure 9.3(b). As in the DWT case, the complex wavelet coefficients are indexed using one number, writing $D_f(j,k)$ in place of $D_f^b(j,k)$.

9.5 DT-CWT and shift-invariance

It is a known fact that the wavelet coefficients of a signal $f(t)$ enjoy shift-invariance if either the scaling coefficients $C_f(j,k)$ at every scale (j) or the wavelet filters

(h_0 and h_1) are appropriately band-limited. The approximate shift-invariance can also be achieved using complex filters that suppress negative frequencies. One approach is to analyse only the positive frequencies in the input signal ($f(t)$) using a DWT with real mother wavelet (ψ^r) [23,24]. Let $f^+(t)$ be the projection of f onto the positive frequencies; if $F(\omega)$ and $F^+(\omega)$ are the FTs of f and f^+, then

$$F^+(\omega) = \begin{cases} F(\omega) & \omega \geq 0 \\ 0 & \omega < 0 \end{cases} \tag{9.3}$$

For real $f(t)$, the FT ($F(\omega)$) is symmetric and $f(t)$ can be recovered from $f^+(t)$. Since $F^+(\omega)\Psi^r(2^{-j}\omega)$ has half the bandwidth of $F(\omega)\Psi^r(2^{-j}\omega)$, the aliasing in each sub-band is greatly reduced and the wavelet coefficients are approximately shift-invariant. This approach analyses a complex signal $f^+(t)$ with real wavelets $\psi^r_{j,k}(t)$.

Equivalently, $f(t)$ can be analysed with two wavelets ψ^r and ψ^i, which represent a Hilbert transform pair [14,25,26]. Now, the relation $\psi^+_{j,k}(t) = \psi^r_{j,k}(t) + \sqrt{-1}\psi^i_{j,k}(t)$ contains only positive frequencies, so again $F(\omega)\Psi^+(2^{-j}\omega)$ has half bandwidth of $F(\omega)\Psi^r(2^{-j}\omega)$, which leads to approximate shift-invariance. This approach analyses a real signal $f(t)$ with complex wavelets $\psi^+_{j,k}(t)$.

Figure 9.3(a) shows an example of a 1-D dual-tree complex wavelet-basis function. The real and imaginary-basis functions share the same locale, but are '90° out of phase'; ψ^r is large when ψ^i is small and vice versa. The same is also true for symmetry properties, i.e. if we design ψ^r to be even symmetric, then ψ^i will be odd symmetric.

The improved shift-invariance of the CWT over DWT is shown in Figure 9.4. As the basis functions ($\psi_{j,k}$) in DWT are oscillatory, so their step responses are also oscillatory. When the 1-D step edge is shifted within the locale of some basis wavelet function, the resulting wavelet coefficients swing wildly and come very close to zero for some shifts. In contrast, the magnitudes of CWT coefficients vary smoothly with the location of the 1-D step edge inside the basis function's locale. The closer the edge is to the centre of the locale, the larger the corresponding magnitude. As the edge moves from one locale to the next, the energy transfers smoothly between the corresponding CWT coefficients.

Due to good shift-invariance of CWT, the image de-noising techniques developed in CWT domain yield better performance than the DWT-based methods. Figure 9.5 shows a simple 2-D contour reconstructed from one scale of its real and CWTs. As the contour moves through space, the reconstruction using the DWT coefficients changes erratically, while the CWT reconstructs all local shifts and orientations in the same manner.

9.6 CWT and directional selectivity

In 1-D, the CWT can be viewed as performing a sub-band analysis on only the positive signal frequencies. In 2-D, this allows to distinguish between a feature oriented at an angle α and one oriented at angle $-\alpha$. Figure 9.6 shows that the CWT

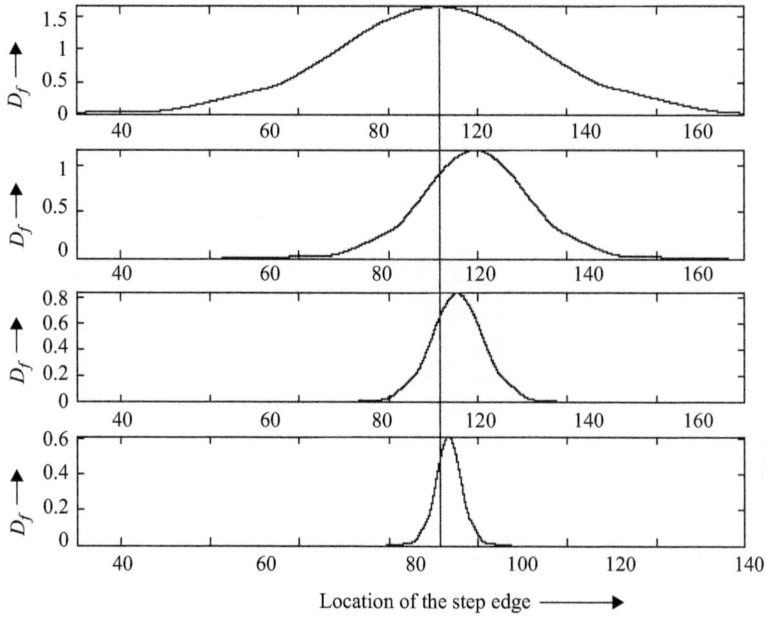

Figure 9.4 Magnitude of the 1-D step response of complex wavelet coefficients at four consecutive scales (Section 9.5)

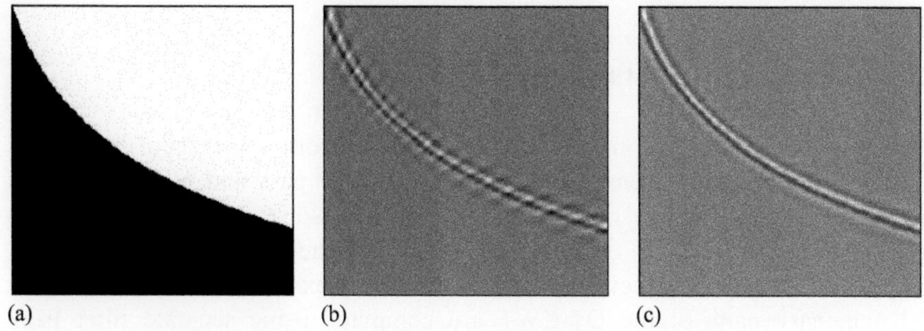

Figure 9.5 Visual appearance of (a) an edge contour in the plane (b) reconstructed using wavelet coefficients of real DWT and (c) reconstructed using wavelet coefficients of CWT (Section 9.5)

has separate sub-bands for features at $\pm 15^\circ$, whereas the DWT lumps these into one 'horizontal' sub-band.

An edge in an image at 15° angle causes the CWT coefficients in the '$+15^\circ$' sub-band to be large, while an edge at -15° causes the CWT coefficients in the '-15°' sub-band to be large. In contrast, both edges would cause the real coefficients in the '0' (horizontal) sub-band of the DWT to be large. Hence, the 2-D CWT provides greater directional selectivity than the DWT.

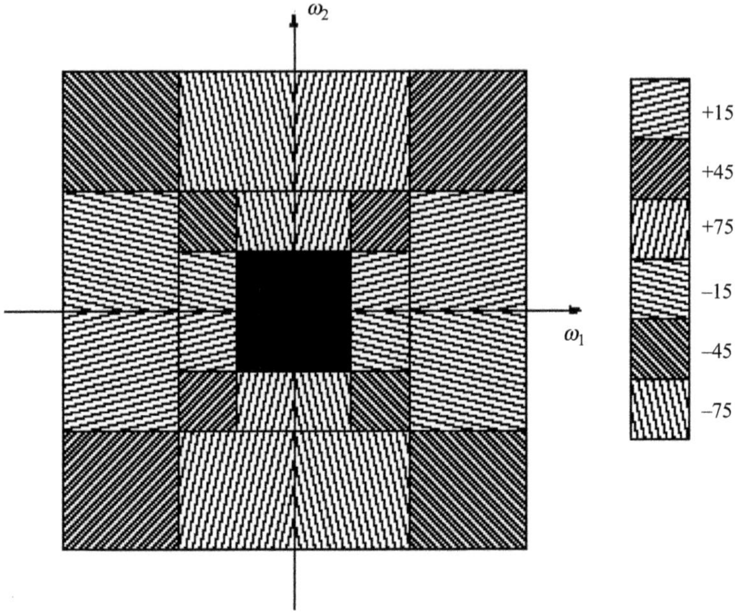

Figure 9.6 Frequency plane tilings for the CWT. The six sub-bands of the complex wavelet transform can capture features along lines at six different angles (Section 9.6)

9.7 Filter implementation of DT-CWT

The DT-CWT is an over-complete PR separable transform with Gabor-like filters. It uses two trees per dimension each with short low pass and high pass filters to synthesize a single linear-phase complex low pass/high pass filter pair. The implementation of CWT is the same as DWT, with the difference that the CWT filters have complex coefficients and generate complex output samples. The real and imaginary parts of the DT-CWT are computed using separate filter bank structures with wavelet filters (h_{0a} and h_{1a}) for the real part and (h_{0b} and h_{1b}) for the imaginary part. The filters in the two trees are just time reverse of each other as are the analysis and reconstruction filters. Since the output sampling rates are unchanged from the DWT, but each sample contains a real and imaginary part, a redundancy of 2:1 is introduced that becomes 4:1 in two dimensions.

DT-CWT was developed by observing that the approximate shift-invariance can be achieved with a real DWT by doubling the sampling rate at each level of the tree. For this, the samples must be evenly spaced. In the present work, a more recent form of dual tree known as Q-shift DT-CWT has been used. This tree is shown in Figure 9.7 [14]. There are two sets of filters, the filters at level 1 and the filters at all higher levels. The filters beyond level 1 have even length but are no longer strictly linear phase. Instead, they are designed to have a group delay of

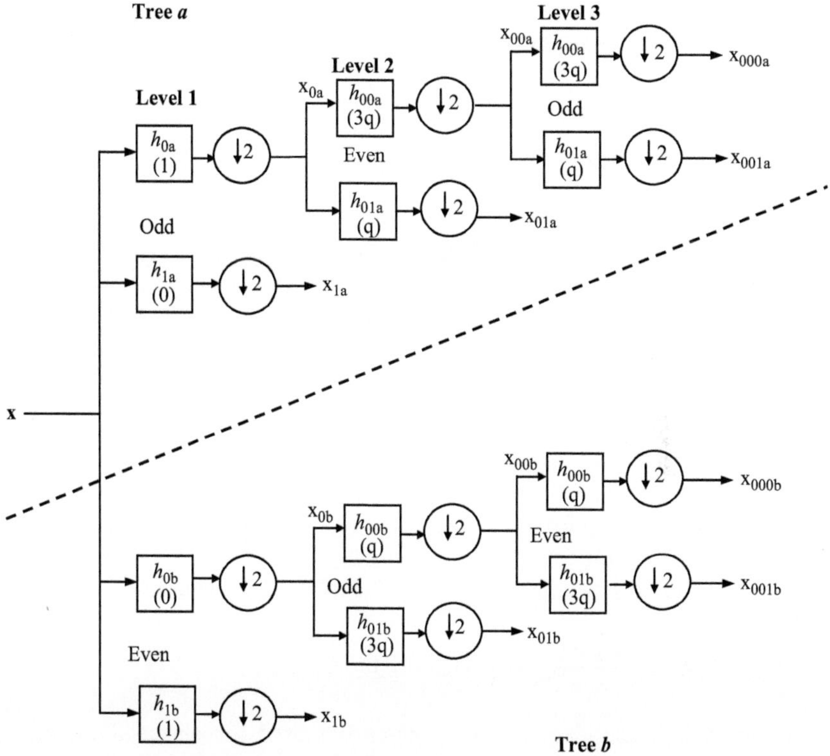

Figure 9.7 The Q-shift version of DT-CWT giving real and imaginary parts of complex coefficients from trees a and b, respectively (Section 9.7)

approximately 1/4. In Figure 9.7, the values in brackets indicate the delay for each filter with $q = 1/4$ sample.

The required delay difference of 1/2 sample is achieved using the time reverse of 'tree *a*' filters in 'tree *b*'. The PR filters used are chosen to be orthonormal so that the reconstruction filters are just the time reverse of the equivalent analysis filters. There are a number of choices for possible filter combinations. In the present research work, the near-Symmetric 5,7 tap filters at level 1 together with the 18-tap Q-shift filters beyond level 1 are chosen [14]. The Q-shift transform retains the good shift-invariance and directionality properties of the original DT-CWT along with improvement in sampling structure.

In Q-shift implementation, the two trees are very closely matched and have a more symmetric sub-sampling structure. For Q-shift CWT, each complex wavelet basis is centred on the equivalent complex scaling function basis, and each of these is centred between a pair of adjacent complex bases from the previous (finer) level. In this way, each complex wavelet coefficient at level j has two complex *children* located symmetrically above it, i.e. at level $(j - 1)$. For the odd/even DT-CWT, such symmetries do not occur. Moreover, the Q-shift CWT leads to a transform, which can use shorter filters and is orthonormal beyond level 1. Due to these features, the Q-shift filters have been used for implementing the CWT domain speckle suppressors.

9.8 Practical algorithm

The implementation of a despeckling algorithm in DT-CWT domain is very similar to the RDWT case. The principle difference is that the shrinkage rule is applied to the magnitudes of the complex coefficients so as to achieve nearly shift-invariance. The magnitude information is more reliable than either real or imaginary parts because the small signal shifts do not affect the magnitudes, however, they may affect the real and imaginary parts. The implementation of the DT-CWT domain-de-noising algorithm is summarized as follows:

1. *Apply the log-transform operation to the speckled image (f)
2. Compute the DT-CWT
3. Specify the value of tuning parameter (K), which controls the degree of speckle suppression
4. Estimate the noise variance (σ^2) using the following equation:

$$\hat{\sigma}^2 = \left[K\frac{\text{median}\,(|Y_l|)}{0.6745}\right]^2 \quad Y_l \in \{\text{HH}_1, \text{HH}_2\} \tag{9.4}$$

   where K is a user-defined tuning parameter used to balance the degree of speckle suppression against the level of feature preservation. As the value of K goes on increasing, the degree of smoothing increases. To preserve more details, it should be kept low
5. For each resolution scale, j, $1 \leq j \leq J$, and
   (i) For each direction (negative and positive), D, $1 \leq D \leq 2$,
      (a) For each orientation, $i \in \{\text{HH}_j^D, \text{LH}_j^D, \text{HL}_j^D\}$
      (b) For all the spatial locations, $l = 1,2,\ldots,M$
         (I) Compute the standard deviation, σ_X
         (II) If $\sigma_X > 0$, estimate the coefficient, $\hat{x}_l$, using following equations, otherwise set $\hat{x}_l = 0$

$$\hat{x} = \text{sign}(y)\left(\max\left(0, |y| - \frac{\Omega + \sqrt{\Omega^2 + 4m\sigma_x^2\Omega(2m-1)}}{2\sqrt{2}m\sigma_x}\right)\right) \tag{9.5}$$

$$\hat{x} = \text{sign}(y)\left(\max\left(0, \frac{|y|(\Omega + 4m\sigma_x^2) - \sqrt{\Omega^2 y^2 + 4\Omega\sigma_x^2(2m-1)(\Omega + 2m\sigma_x^2)}}{2(\Omega + 2m\sigma_x^2)}\right)\right) \tag{9.6}$$

The symbol Ω corresponds to noise variance and m is the Nakagami shape parameter computed from the speckled wavelet coefficients using the following relation:

$$m = \frac{\mu_2^2}{\mu_4 - \mu_2^2} \tag{9.7}$$

where μ_2 and μ_4 are the second and fourth moments of data belonging to the diagonal detail sub-bands (HH_1 and HH_2), respectively

$$\hat{x} = \mathrm{sign}(y)\left(\max\left(0, \frac{(4As+\Omega)|y| - \sqrt{\Omega^2 y^2 - 8Ay^2(s-1)(2As-\Omega) + 4C(AB+\Omega)}}{2(AB+\Omega)}\right)\right) \tag{9.8}$$

$$\hat{x} = \mathrm{sign}(y)\left(\max\left(0, \frac{2s|y|}{B} - \frac{\Omega + \sqrt{\Omega^2 - 8As(s-1)\left(Ay^2 - \sqrt{2}\Omega y\right) + 2ABC}}{\sqrt{2}AB}\right)\right) \tag{9.9}$$

where $A = ms\sigma_x\ y^{2s-2}$ $B = 2s(2s-1)$ and $C = (2ms-1)\Omega\sigma_x$. The estimators derived in (9.5), (9.6), (9.8) and (9.9) are the expressions for the shrinkage functions of *HomoGenThresh*, *HomoGenShrink*, *GNDShrink* and *GNDThresh*, respectively

6. Apply the inverse DT-CWT to get the de-noised image
7. *Perform the exponential operation on the image obtained from previous step to convert the image back to the non-logarithmic format
8. *Apply mean-bias correction using (9.10) to restore the mean of the original image

$$\widehat{g} = \hat{g} + \mu_f - \mu_{\hat{g}} \tag{9.10}$$

where μ_f and $\mu_{\hat{g}}$ are the mean of the original speckled image (*f*) before log transform and of the filtered image ($\hat{g}$), respectively.

*For non-homomorphic techniques, the steps 1, 7 and 8 are not required.

9.9 Results and discussions

In judging the performance of a noise suppression technique, the major aspects to evaluate are: the ability to retain small details, retaining edges and gradual changes in grey level. In this work, these aspects have been evaluated both quantitatively and qualitatively on two sets of US images that are collected from the website http://telin.rug.ac.be/~sanja.

1. Realistic US image (US1) in which natural speckle noise was previously suppressed (shown in Figure 9.8(a)). US1 test image is highly textured.

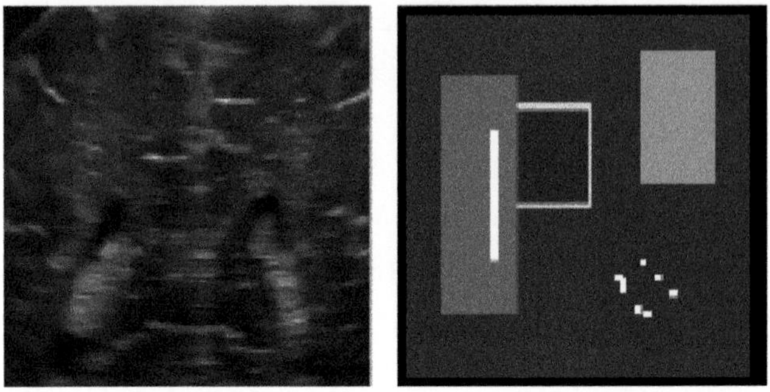

(a) US1 test image (b) US2 test image

Figure 9.8 (a) Speckle-free US test image and (b) a purely synthetic US test image (Section 9.9)

2. A purely synthetic image, which consists of regions with uniform intensity, sharp edges and strong scatterers (US2 test image shown in Figure 9.8(b)).

To evaluate the performance gain of DT-CWT, a number of experiments have been performed on these US images with four different Bayesian processors (*HomoGenThresh*, *HomoGenShrink*, *GNDShrink* and *GNDThresh*) in three alternative wavelet domains (the standard DWT, RDWT and DT-CWT). Each WT is designed to produce a four-level wavelet decomposition of an image. The DT-CWT is implemented using 5,7 tap near-symmetric linear-phase filters at level 1 and the 18-tap orthogonal Q-shift filters at levels beyond 1 for non-homomorphic processors. For homomorphic processors, standard Antonini 9,7 tap near-orthogonal linear-phase filter is used at level 1 [13]. For DWT and RDWT, the experiments are conducted using the Haar wavelet (*db*1), which has been reported to be optimum for US images [20–22].

To quantify the performance gain, three measures of quality evaluation, namely, signal-to-noise ratio (SNR), coefficient of correlation (CoC) and edge-preservation index (EPI) have been used. In the case of multiplicative noise, SNR is usually defined as [27]

$$\mathrm{SNR} = 10 \log 10\left(\frac{\sigma_g^2}{\sigma_e^2}\right) \tag{9.11}$$

where σ_g^2 is the variance of the noise-free reference image and σ_e^2 is the variance of error (between the original and de-noised image). The larger SNR values correspond to good image quality. This objective performance measure treats an image simply as a matrix of numbers. As such, it does not reflect exactly the human perception about the image. However, the other two objective criteria, namely, CoC and EPI evaluate the noise suppression and edge preservation capability.

These two quality metrics are computed as given below [28–30]:

$$\mathrm{CoC} = \frac{\sum (g - \bar{g}) \cdot (\hat{g} - \bar{\hat{g}})}{\sqrt{\sum (g - \bar{g})^2 \cdot \sum (\hat{g} - \bar{\hat{g}})^2}} \tag{9.12}$$

$$\mathrm{EPI} = \frac{\sum \left(\Delta g - \overline{\Delta g}\right) \cdot \left(\Delta \hat{g} - \overline{\Delta \hat{g}}\right)}{\sqrt{\sum \left(\Delta g - \overline{\Delta g}\right)^2 \cdot \sum \left(\Delta \hat{g} - \overline{\Delta \hat{g}}\right)^2}} \tag{9.13}$$

where $\bar{g}$ and $\bar{\hat{g}}$ are the mean of original and de-noised image, respectively. Δg is the high pass filtered version of g obtained with a 3×3 pixel standard approximation of the Laplacian operator. The value of CoC and EPI should be close to unity for good diagnostic quality in medical domain [18,29,30].

Table 9.1 tabulates these measures of quality evaluation on two different US test (realistic and pure synthetic) images. The highest values in each set are shaded and highest values among all the sets are shown boldface. The results are very interesting, which show that on certain types of images, the RDWT performs better, while on others, DT-CWT-based methods are the best. Specifically, on the realistic US images (textured), the DT-CWT performs better than the RDWT at low-to-moderate noise level. However, at high noise levels, the performance of RDWT starts approaching the DT-CWT. For example, at an input SNR of 17.09 dB, the SNR of DT-CWT-based methods is better than that of RDWT-based methods by more than 0.43 dB and at low input SNR the difference is negligible. The values of other metrics like EPI and CoC also show the same behaviour.

To verify this observation, the SNR results at various noise levels on two different realistic US test images are plotted in Figures 9.9–9.12. Each figure contains two SNR plots comparing the different WTs. Each plot is dedicated

Table 9.1 Quantitative comparison of the various de-noising methods in three different wavelet domains on US1 test image

Method	SNR (dB)	CoC	EPI	SNR(dB)	CoC	EPI
Speckled image (input)	17.09	0.9904	0.9499	09.03	0.9426	0.7711
BiShrink-DT-CWT	18.67	0.9932	0.9745	11.42	0.9643	0.8935
GenLik-RDWT	16.57	0.9891	0.9637	11.33	0.9625	0.8796
GNDThresh-DT-CWT	**18.82**	**0.9934**	**0.9752**	11.86	0.9669	0.8952
GNDThresh-RDWT	18.39	0.9929	0.9721	11.79	0.9663	0.8882
GNDThresh-DWT	16.97	0.9899	0.9317	10.45	0.9551	0.8042
HomoGenThresh-DT-CWT	18.78	0.9934	0.9744	11.76	0.9663	0.8916
HomoGenThresh-RDWT	17.84	0.9923	0.9697	11.82	0.9675	0.8917
HomoGenThresh-DWT	16.46	0.9887	0.9162	10.56	0.9552	0.7835
GNDShrink-DT-CWT	18.60	0.9931	0.9732	**11.88**	**0.9670**	**0.8956**
GNDShrink-RDWT	18.18	0.9927	0.9715	11.78	0.9663	0.8901
GNDShrink-DWT	16.99	0.9900	0.9331	10.61	0.9562	0.8081
HomoGenShrink-DT-CWT	18.51	0.9930	0.9724	11.75	0.9668	0.8949
HomoGenShrink-RDWT	17.42	0.9918	0.9686	11.64	0.9667	0.8943
HomoGenShrink-DWT	16.36	0.9885	0.9164	10.62	0.9557	0.7867

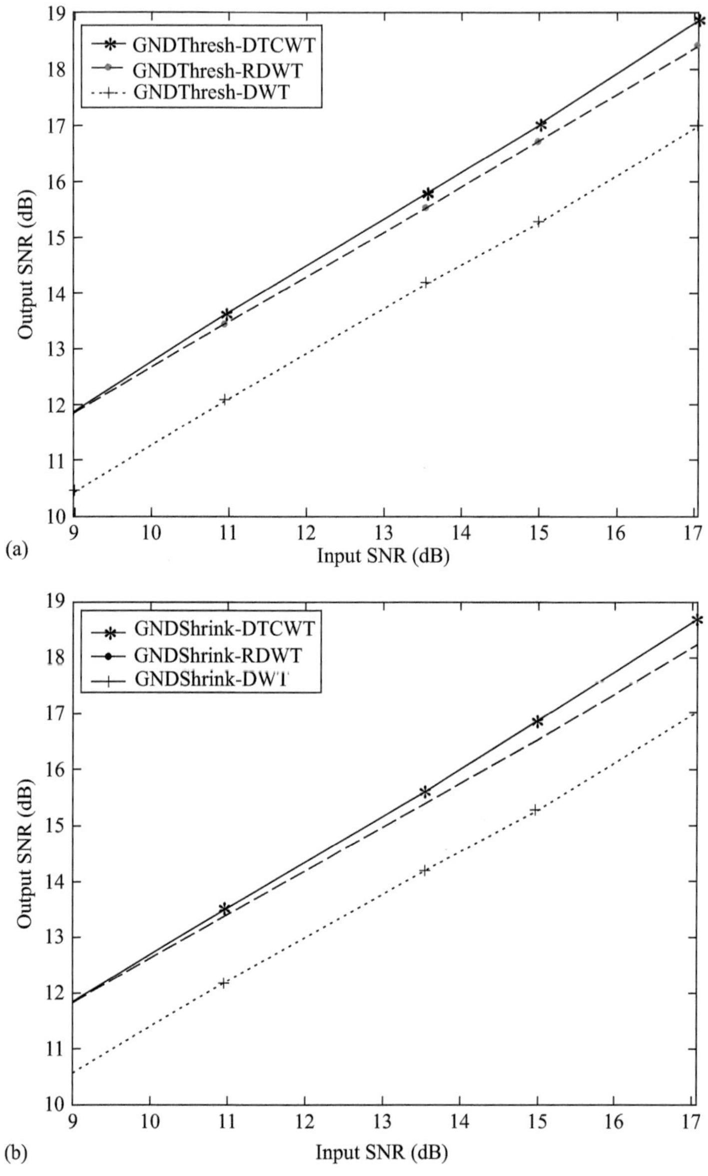

Figure 9.9 SNR comparison of various non-homomorphic speckle suppression techniques in three different transform domains (DT-CWT, RDWT and DWT) on US1 test image (Section 9.9). (a) using eq. (9.9) and (b) using eq. (9.8)

to a particular despeckling method. Within each figure, it can be observed that DT-CWT does better than the RDWT and the RDWT does better than the DWT. The results for other images also follow the same tendency. At very high

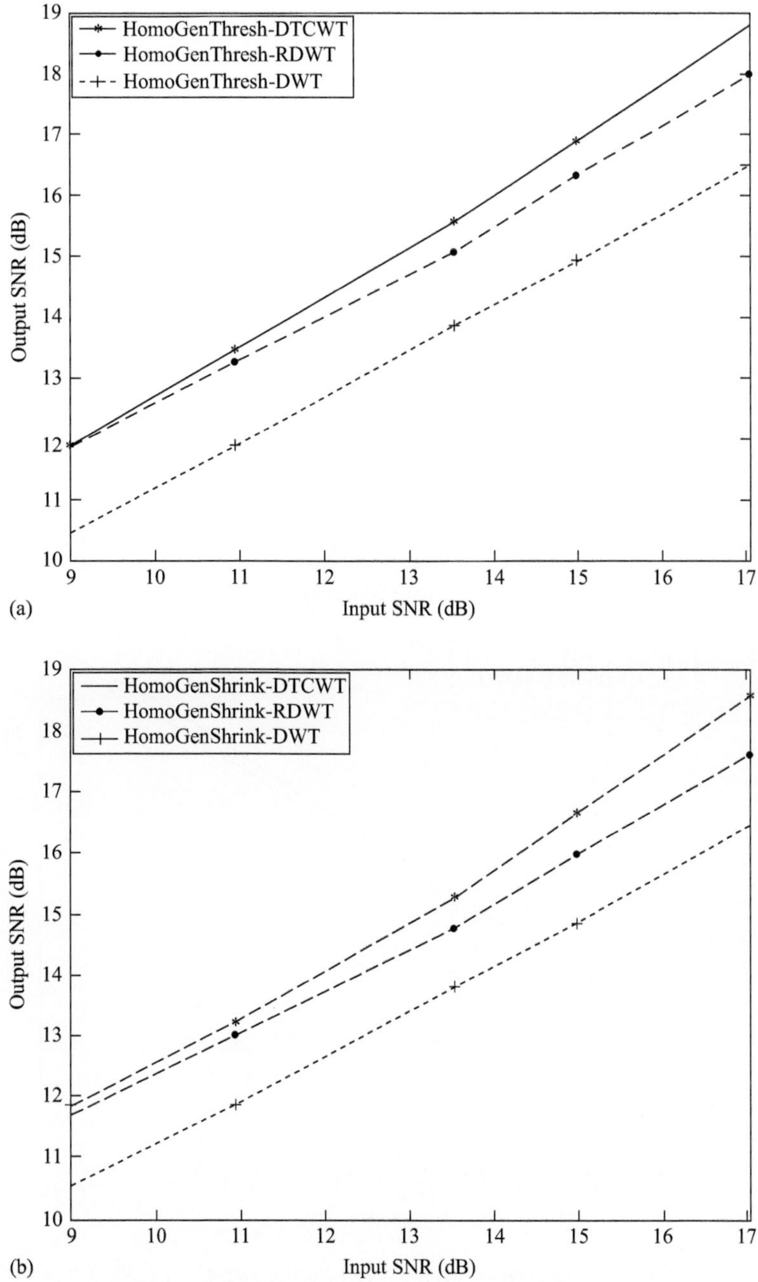

Figure 9.10 SNR comparison of various homomorphic speckle suppression techniques in three different transform domains (DT-CWT, RDWT and DWT) on realistic US1 test image (Section 9.9). (a) using eq. (9.9) and (b) using eq. (9.8)

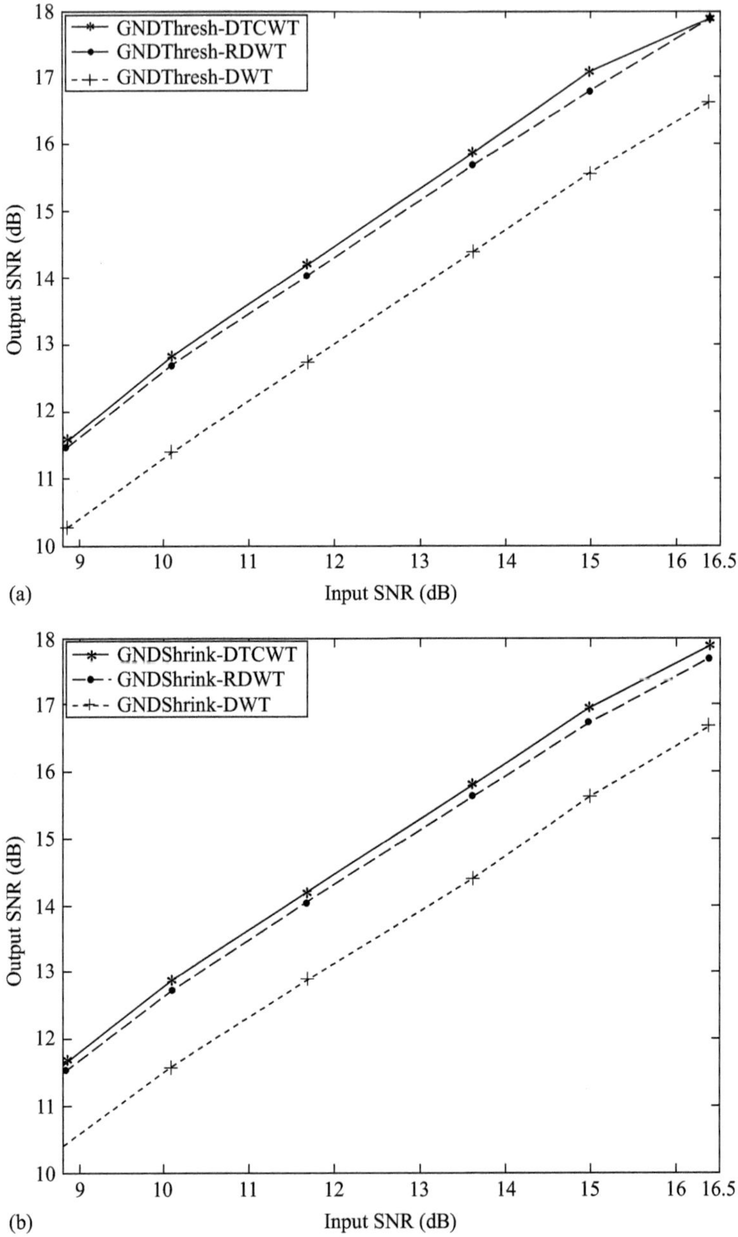

Figure 9.11 SNR comparison of various non-homomorphic speckle suppression techniques in three different transform domains (DT-CWT, RDWT and DWT) on realistic US2 test image (Section 9.9). (a) using eq. (9.9) and (b) using eq. (9.8)

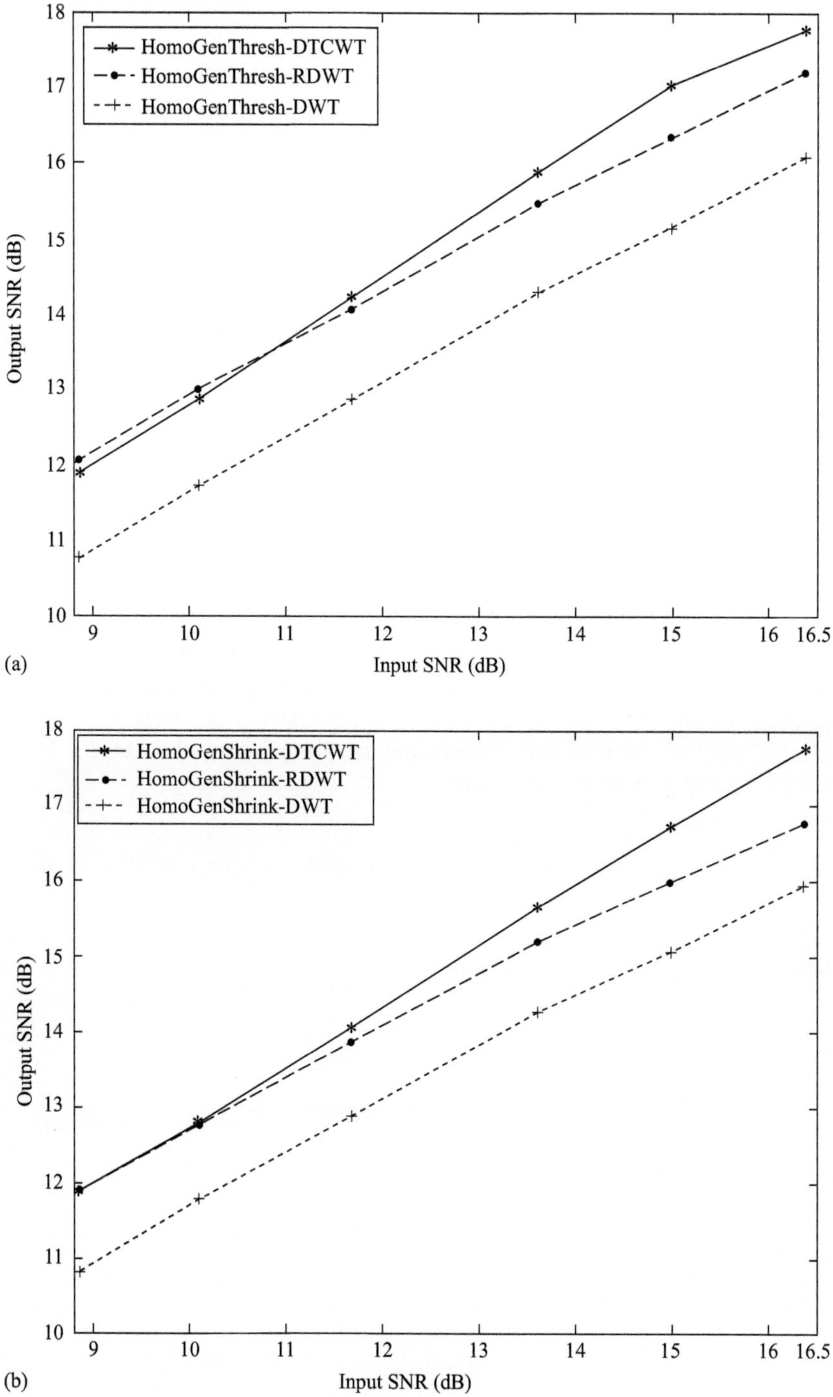

Figure 9.12 SNR comparison of various homomorphic speckle suppression techniques in three different transform domains (DT-CWT, RDWT and DWT) on realistic US2 test image (Section 9.9). (a) using eq. (9.9) and (b) using eq. (9.8)

noise levels, when noise dominates the texture, the performance difference is small and hardly visible. The performance behaviour reveals that on the texture-rich images, the DT-CWT-based methods usually outperform the RDWT-based methods.

Table 9.2 shows the quantitative results on the synthetic US2 test image. On the basis of results presented in Table 9.2, it is observed that on images that are dominated by large areas of uniform or slightly varying intensity intercepted by sharp edges and/or thin lines, the RDWT methods yield superior performance over the DT-CWT methods. Similar observations can be made from the SNR plots given in Figure 9.13. From these results, it can be concluded that on uniform images, the performance of RDWT is significantly better than the DT-CWT.

The reason for this performance behaviour may be that in the complex domain, the short-support filters matching the US speckle statistics (analogous to *db*1) are not available. To justify the effect of filter length (support size) on the noise suppression performance, the results of RDWT with long filter (*Sym*4) are also included for comparison in Table 9.2 and Figure 9.13. From the results, it can be observed that as the filter length increases, the despeckling performance decreases. The visual comparison (from the processed images shown in Figure 9.14) also depicts the same thing. Hence, it is expected that by designing short-support complex domain filters (well matched to the US image characteristics) analogous to '*db*1' mother wavelet, the despeckling performance of the DT-CWT-based methods can be enhanced significantly.

Table 9.2 Quantitative comparison of the various de-noising methods in three different wavelet domains on US2 test image

Method	SNR (dB)	S/MSE (dB)	CoC	EPI
Speckled image (input)	18.09	**23.74**	0.9923	0.9302
BiShrink-DT-CWT	21.50	27.15	0.9965	0.9805
GenLik-RDWT	17.16	22.61	0.9906	0.9798
GNDShrink-RDWT (*Sym*4)	21.95	27.60	0.9968	0.9796
GNDThresh-RDWT (*Sym*4)	22.06	27.71	0.9969	0.9795
GNDShrink-RDWT (*db*1)	23.99	29.64	0.9981	0.9888
***GNDThresh-RDWT* (*db*1)**	**25.12**	**30.77**	**0.9985**	**0.9906**
GNDShrink-DT-CWT	21.97	27.63	0.9968	0.9806
GNDThresh-DT-CWT	22.17	27.83	0.9970	0.9824
Speckled image (input)	**12.03**	**17.68**	**0.9699**	**0.7891**
BiShrink-DT-CWT	15.70	21.34	0.9865	0.9339
GenLik-RDWT	14.93	20.44	0.9839	0.9442
GNDShrink-RDWT (*Sym*4)	15.66	21.31	0.9865	0.9234
GNDThresh-RDWT (*Sym*4)	16.10	21.75	0.9877	0.9257
***GNDShrink-RDWT* (*db*1)**	17.92	23.57	0.9924	0.9552
GNDThresh-RDWT (*db*1)	**18.98**	**24.63**	**0.9938**	**0.9649**
GNDShrink-DT-CWT	15.91	21.56	0.9871	0.9240
***GNDThresh*-DT-CWT**	16.15	21.80	0.9878	0.9317

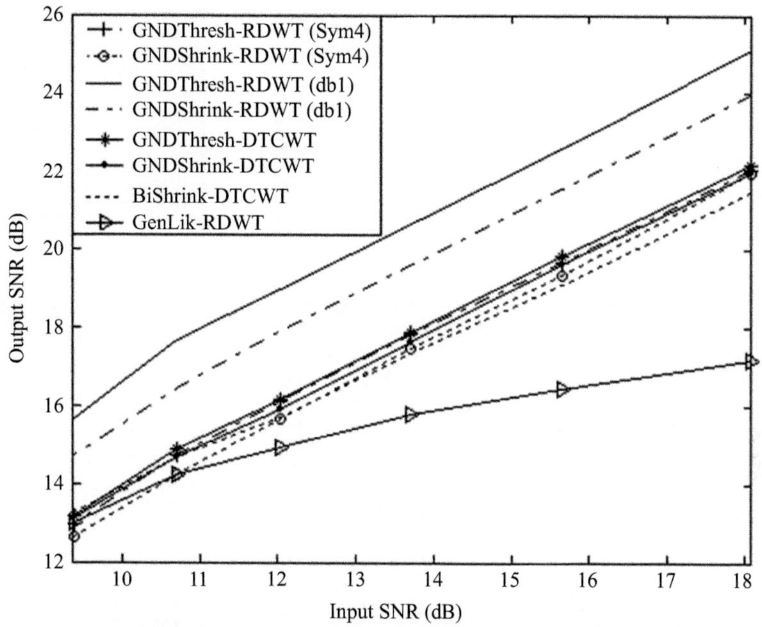

Figure 9.13 SNR comparison of RDWT-based despeckling methods with that of DTCWT on US2 test image using different wavelet filters (Section 9.9)

Further, to benchmark our algorithms against the recently published DT-CWT and RDWT domain methods, the results are also compared with two state-of-the-art methods.

BiShrink [19] designed in the DT-CWT domain and the *GenLik* [27] implemented in the RDWT domain. For comparison, SNR plots are shown in Figure 9.15. The results clearly indicate that the methods based on the DT-CWT perform better than the RDWT-based methods, *GenLik* at all noise levels and among the DT-CWT-based methods, the non-homomorphic methods (*GNDThresh* and *GNDShrink*) yield the best performance at all noise levels and for both the test images.

Next, Figures 9.16 and 9.17 show the speckled and despeckled US images processed by various methods for visual quality evaluation. Visually, the differences are hardly noticeable between the images processed by RDWT and DT-CWT methods (see Figures 9.16 and 9.17). The latter conclusion is valid for many images, i.e. the two methods generally yield a similar visual appearance.

However, in certain cases, if the image contains strong diagonal features, the differences can be visualized clearly. In this respect, a good example is the hat of standard Lena image (shown in Figure 9.18). In this case, the result of DT-CWT-based methods is better than that of the RDWT by 0.22 dB. The improvement of the DT-CWT relative to the RDWT is seen more in terms of feature preservation

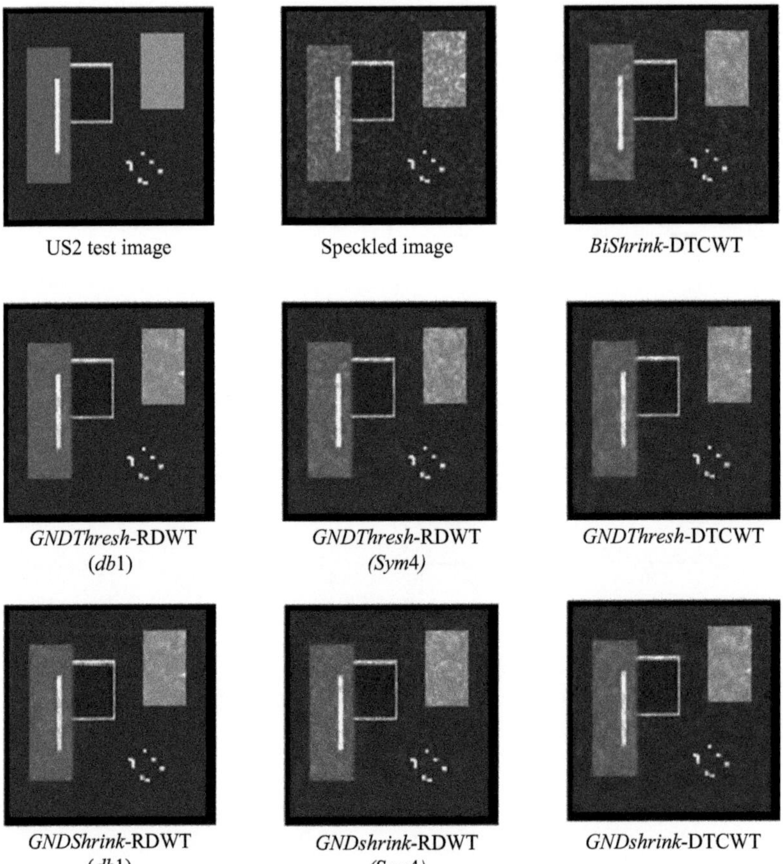

Figure 9.14 Visual comparison of the output of various RDWT-based methods (using shorter support, db1, and longer filter, Sym4) and DT-CWT-based techniques on a synthetic US2 test image (Section 9.9)

(see the difference in the geometrical pattern of the hat Figure 9.18). The reason being that the DT-CWT can separate features near 45° from those near −45° while the RDWT combines such features.

All these experimental investigations reveal that that the despeckling performance of DWT is worst as it fails to represent the images optimally whereas the performance of RDWT and DTCWT is comparable. Hence, it can be concluded that the shift-invariance of a transform has a very significant effect on the despeckling performance of a de-noising algorithm (as reflected in the performance gain of RDWT and DT-CWT over DWT) whereas high transform directionality is very essential for representing the image features optimally.

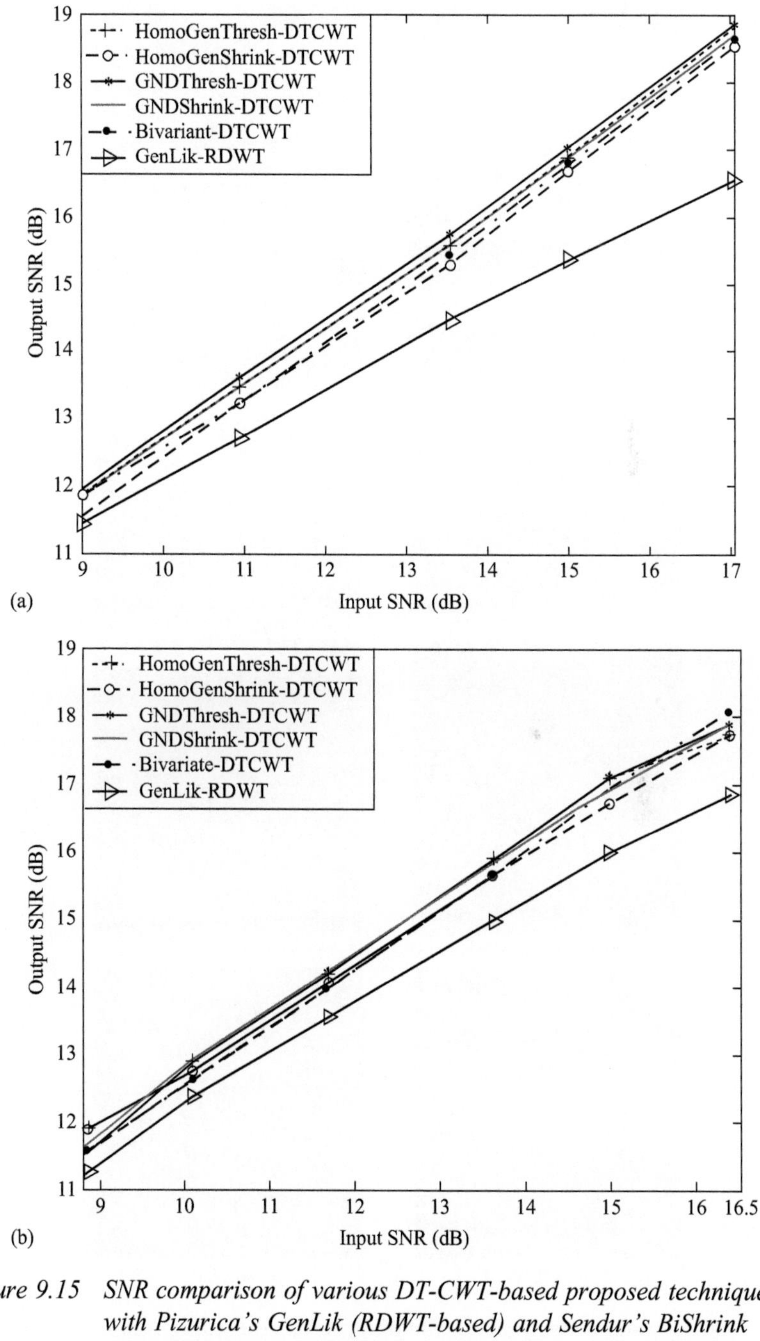

Figure 9.15 SNR comparison of various DT-CWT-based proposed techniques with Pizurica's GenLik (RDWT-based) and Sendur's BiShrink (DT-CWT-based) method on (a) US1 test image and (b) US2 test image 2 (Section 9.9)

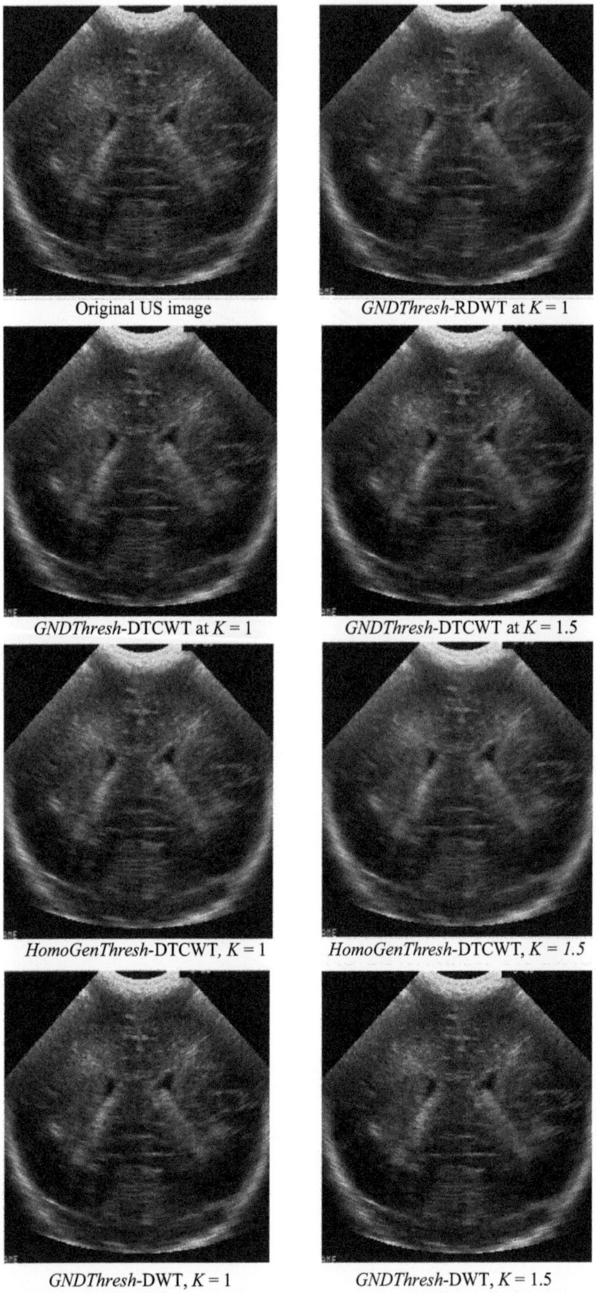

Figure 9.16 Visual comparison of the proposed thresholding techniques on real US image (Section 9.9)

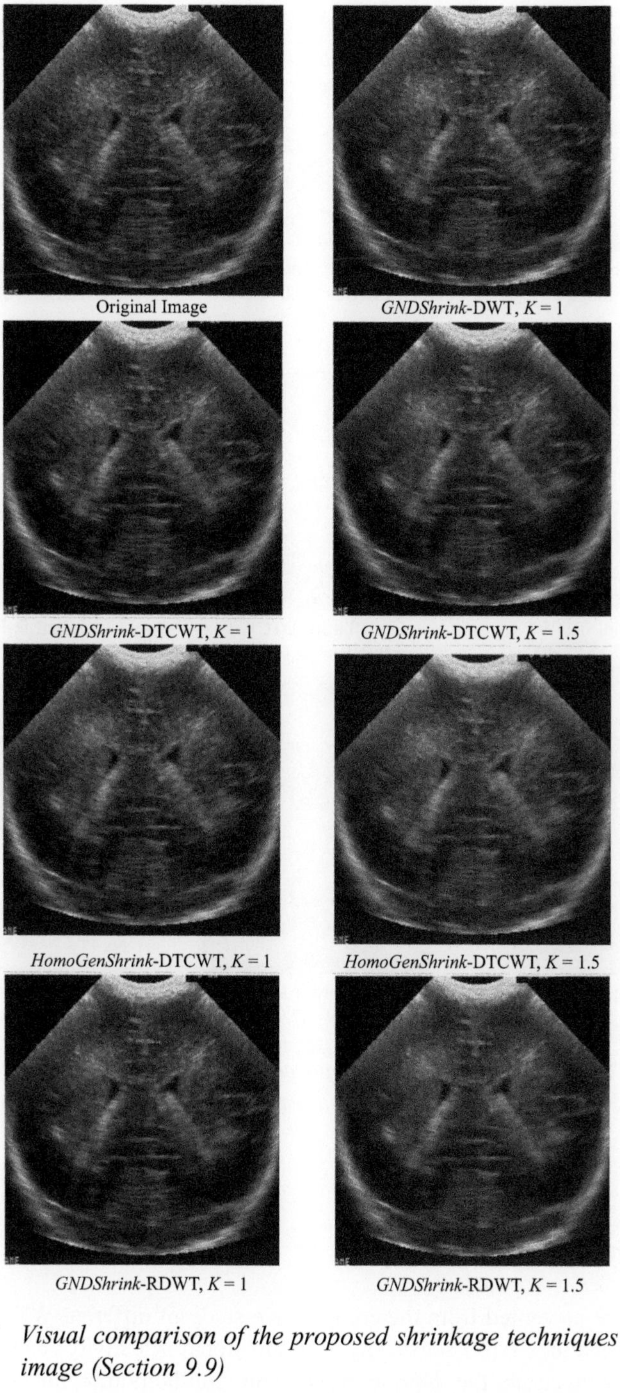

Figure 9.17 Visual comparison of the proposed shrinkage techniques on real US image (Section 9.9)

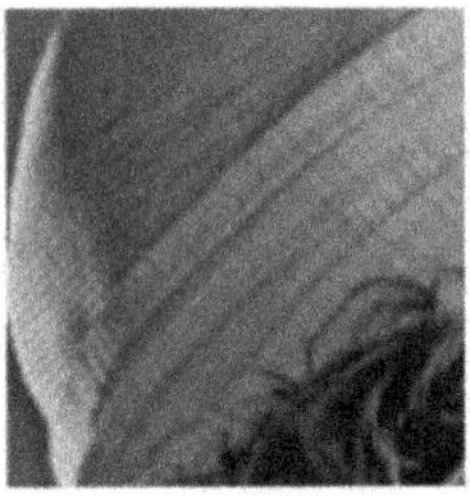

Hat of original
Lena image

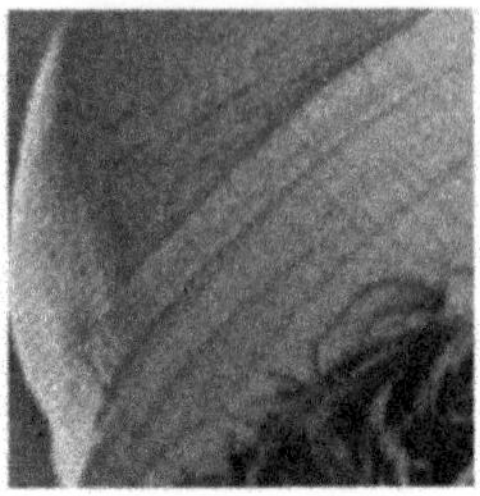

Noisy image
PSNR = 28.08 dB

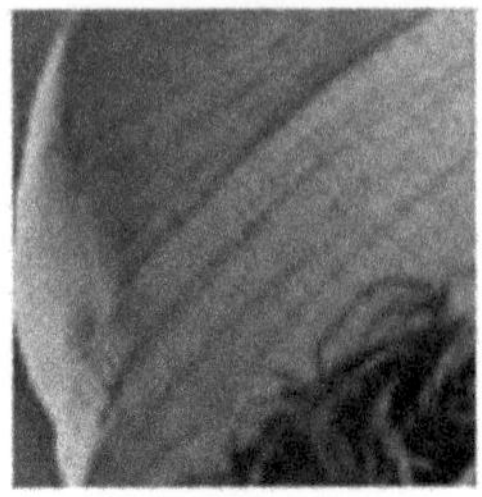

GNDThresh-DWT,
PSNR = 32.68 dB

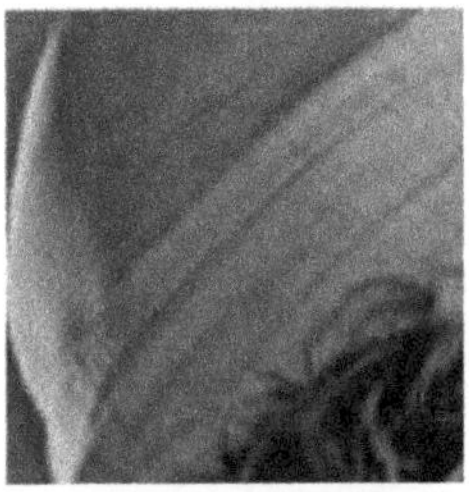

GNDShrink-RDWT
PSNR = 32.73 dB

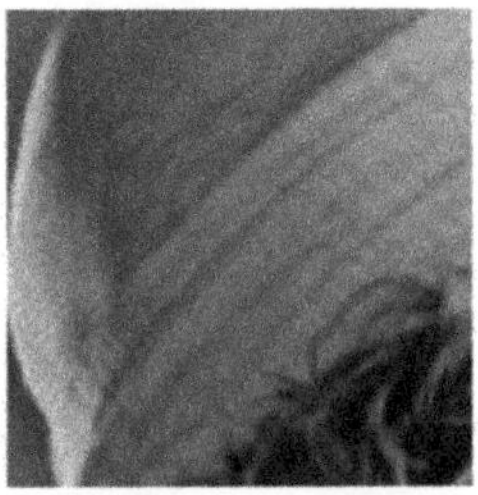

GNDShrink-DTCWT
PSNR = 32.97 dB

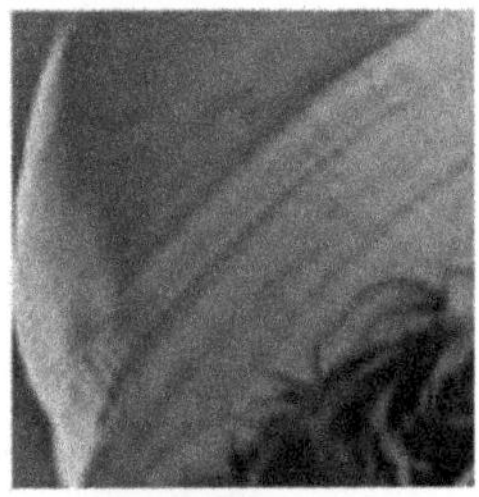

GenLik-RDWT
PSNR=32.33 dB

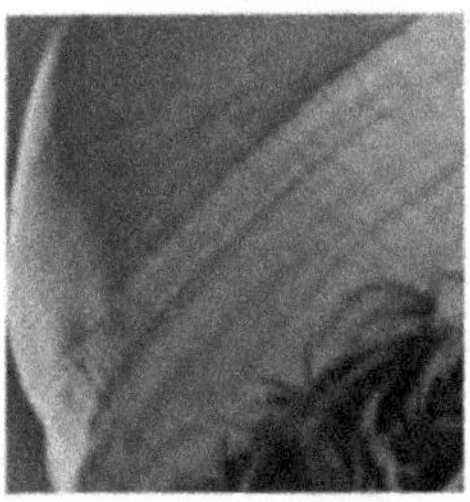

GNDThresh-RDWT
PSNR=32.68 dB

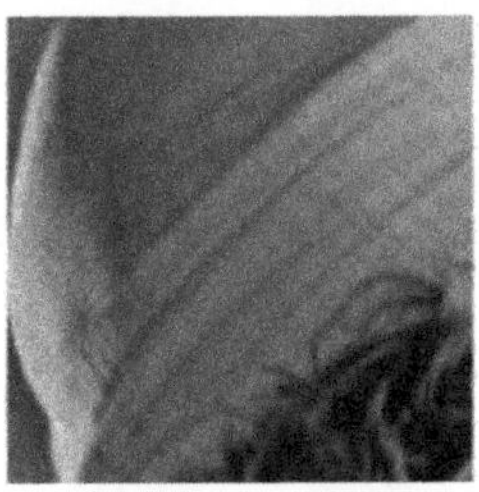

GNDThresh-DTCWT
PSNR=32.95 dB

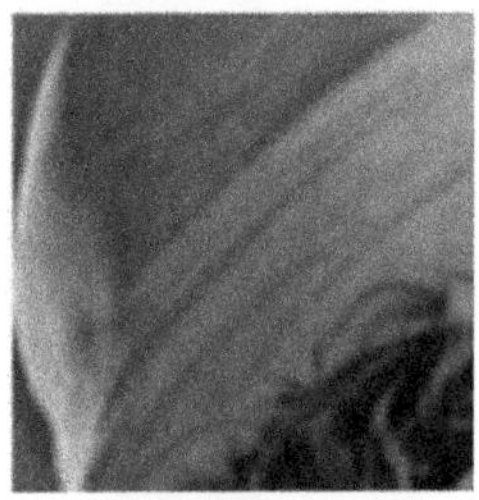

Bishrink-DTCWT
PSNR=31.03 dB

Figure 9.18 Visual comparison of proposed techniques in three different transforms domains (on natural image, 'Lena' at optimum tuning) (Section 9.9)

9.10 Conclusions

The results are presented from the comparative study of different WTs. The effect of transform features (shift sensitivity and directional selectivity) has been examined by implementing the homomorphic and non-homomorphic speckle suppressors in three alternative wavelet domains—DWT, RDWT and CWT.

The experimental results demonstrate that performance of DWT is worst on all type of images whereas the performance of RDWT and DT-CWT is comparable. On certain types of images (images dominated by uniform areas), RDWT performs better while on others (textured images), DT-CWT-based methods are the best. This shows that the shift-dependence of a transform causes a significant degradation in performance of a despeckling technique and good directional selectivity is essential for representing the textured images optimally.

From these investigations, it is concluded that both DT-CWT and RDWT are equally good for designing wavelet-based de-noising applications. However, the low computational complexity of DT-CWT and the textured nature of medical US images, favours the use of DT-CWT in comparison to RDWT for despeckling applications. More work is required to develop shorter length filters for the DT-CWT (e.g. analogous to *Haar* wavelet) in order to further improve the despeckling performance of the US images.

References

[1] Mallat S. *A wavelet tour of signal processing*. New York: Academic Press; 1998.

[2] Vetterli M., Kovacevic. *Wavelets and Subband Coding* (No. LCAV-BOOK-1995–001, Prentice-Hall).

[3] Mallat S. 'A theory for multi-resolution signal decomposition: The wavelet representation'. *IEEE Transactions on Patterns Analysis and Machine Intelligence*. 1989; **11**: 674–692.

[4] Simoncelli E. P. 'Modeling the joint statistics of image in the wavelet domain'. *Proceedings of SPIE's International Symposium on Optical Science, Engineering, and Instrumentation*; Denver, Colorado, 1999. **3813**, pp. 188–195.

[5] Liang J., Parks T. W. 'A translation invariant wavelet representation algorithm with applications'. *IEEE Transactions on Signal Processing*. 1996; **44**(2): 225–232.

[6] Benno S. A., Moura J. M. F. 'Scaling functions robust to translation'. *IEEE Transactions on Signal Processing*. 1998; **46**(12): 3269–3281.

[7] Bao F., Erdol N. 'The optimal wavelet transform and translation invariance'. *Proceedings of IEEE Conference on Acoustics, Speech, Signal Processing*; 1994. **3**, pp. III-13.

[8] Selenick I. W., Sendur L. 'Iterated over-sampled filter banks and wavelet frames'. *Proceedings of SPIE, In Wavelet Applications VII*; 2000.

[9] Simoncelli E. P., Freeman W. T., Adelson E. H., Heeger D. J. 'Shiftable multi-scale transforms'. *IEEE Transactions Information Theory*. 1992; **38**(2): 587–607.

[10] Magarey J. F., Kingsbury N. G. 'Motion estimation using complex wavelets'. *SPIE's International Symposium on Optical Science, Engineering and Instrumentation;* 1996. pp. 674–685.

[11] Kingsbury N. G., Magarey J. 'Wavelet transforms in image processing'. *Proceedings of First European Conference on Signal Analysis and Prediction*; Prague; June 1997. pp. 23–34.

[12] Kingsbury N. 'Image processing with complex wavelets'. *Philosophical Transactions of the Royal Society of London*. 1999; **357**: 2543–2560.

[13] Kingsbury N. 'A dual-tree complex wavelet transform with improved orthogonality and symmetry properties'. *Proceedings of International Conference on Image Processing*; Vancouver; 2000.

[14] Kingsbury N. 'Complex wavelets for shift-invariant analysis and filtering of signals'. *Journal of Applied and Computational Harmonic Analysis*. 2001; **10**(3): 234–253.

[15] Choi H., Romberg J. K., Baraniuk R. G., Kingsbury N. 'A Hidden Markov Tree model for the complex wavelet transform'. *Proceedings of ICASSP 2000*; Istanbul; June 2000.

[16] Pizurica A. '*Image denoising using wavelets and spatial context modeling*' (Doctoral dissertation, Ghent University, 2002).

[17] Chang G., Yu B., Vetterli M. 'Adaptive wavelet thresholding for image denoising and compression'. *IEEE Transactions on Image Processing*. 2000; **9**(9): 1532–1546.

[18] Achim A., Bezeriano A., Tsakalides P. 'Novel Bayesian multiscale method for speckle removal in medical ultrasound images'. *IEEE Transactions of Imaging*. 2001; **20**(8): 772–783.

[19] Sendur L., Selenick I. W. 'Bivariate Shrinkage functions for wavelet based denoising exploiting inter-scale dependencies'. *IEEE Transactions on Signal Processing*. 2002; **50**(11): 2744–2756.

[20] Gupta S., Chauhan R. C., Saxena S. C. 'Wavelet-based statistical approach for speckle reduction in medical ultrasound images'. *Medical and Biological Engineering and Computing*. 2004; **42**(2): 189–192.

[21] Gupta S., Chauhan R. C., Saxena S. C. 'Homomorphic wavelet thresholding technique for denoising medical ultrasound images'. *Journal of Medical Engineering & Technology*. 2005; **29**(5): 208–214.

[22] Gupta S., Chauhan R. C., Saxena S. C. 'Robust non-homomorphic approach for speckle reduction in medical ultrasound images'. *Medical and Biological Engineering and Computing*. 2005; **43**(2): 189–195.

[23] Fernandes F., Spaendonck V. R., Coates M., Burrus C. S. 'Directional complex wavelet processing in wavelet applications'. *VII Proceedings of SPIE*; 2000.

[24] Romberg J. K., Choi H., Baraniuk R. G. 'Bayesian tree structured image modeling using wavelet-domain hidden Markov models'. *IEEE Transactions on Image Processing*. 2001; **10**(7): 1056–1068.

[25] Selenick I. W. 'Hilbert transform pairs of wavelet bases'. *IEEE Signal Processing Letters*. 2001; **8**: 170–173.

[26] Spaendonck R., Blue T., Baraniuk R., Vetterli M. 'Orthogonal Hilbert transform filter banks and wavelets'. *Proceedings of IEEE Conference on Acoustics, Speech, Signal Processing 2003*; April 2003.

[27] Pižurica A., Philips W., Lemahieu I., Acheroy M. 'A versatile wavelet domain noise filtration technique for medical imaging'. *IEEE Transactions on Medical Imaging*. 2003; **22**(3): 323–331.

[28] Singh S., Kumar V., Verma H. K., 'Reduction of blocking artifacts in JPEG compressed images'. *Digital Signal Processing*, vol. **17**, no. 1, pp. 225–243, 2007.

[29] Sattar F., Floreby L., Salomonsson G., Lovstrom B. 'Image enhancement based on a nonlinear multi scale method'. *IEEE Transactions of Image Processing*. 1997; **6**(9): 888–895.

[30] Ives R. W., Eichel P., Magotra, N. 'A new SAR image quality metric'. *Proceedings of 42nd IEEE Midwest Symposium on Circuits and Systems*; 1999. **2**, pp. 1143–1145.

Chapter 10

A comparative evaluation on linear and nonlinear despeckle filtering techniques

Christos P. Loizou[1]

In this chapter, the methods of texture analysis, image quality evaluation, distance measures, univariate statistical analysis and the k-nearest-neighbor (kNN) classifier, which are used to evaluate despeckle filtering [1,2] on ultrasound imaging and video, are presented. For speckle reduction, 16 different despeckle filtering methods, already described in [1,2] (as well as in Chapters 2–9), were applied to each image or video prior to intima-media complex (IMC) or atherosclerotic plaque segmentation. Despeckle filtering was applied after image or video normalization (see [1]), either to the entire image or to an ROI, selected by the user (see also Figure 10.1). The selected area of interest (ROI) can be of any shape but the image despeckle filtering (IDF) software [3] doesn't support multiple ROIs selection. In the latter case, where the user of the system is interested only in the selected ROI, the area outside the ROI can be blurred using the DsFlsmv filter (see Chapter 6) operating with a sliding moving window of $[15 \times 15]$ pixels and a number iterations 5 (see also Figure 10.1). It should be noted that the blurring is applied outside of the ROI if the user of the system is not interested to subjectively evaluate this area. The input parameters of the 16 different despeckle filters for the IDF and video despeckle filtering (VDF) software toolboxes can be selected by the user as it was documented in [1–4]. The 16 despeckle filters evaluated in this chapter were applied on a large number of asymptomatic (AS) and of symptomatic (SY) ultrasound images (220 vs 220) of the common carotid artery (CCA). Four despeckle filters (DsFlsmv, DsFhmedian, DsFkuwahara, DsFsrad) were further applied to ten videos of the carotid artery bifurcation [4]. A large number of texture features (61 different texture features) [1] were extracted from the original and despeckle images and videos, and the most discriminant ones are presented. The performance of these filters is investigated for discriminating between AS and SY images using the statistical kNN classifier. Moreover, 16 different image quality evaluation metrics [1,5] were computed, as well as visual evaluation scores carried out by two experts [5].

[1]Cyprus University of Technology, Department of Electrical Engineering, Computer Engineering and Informatics, Cyprus

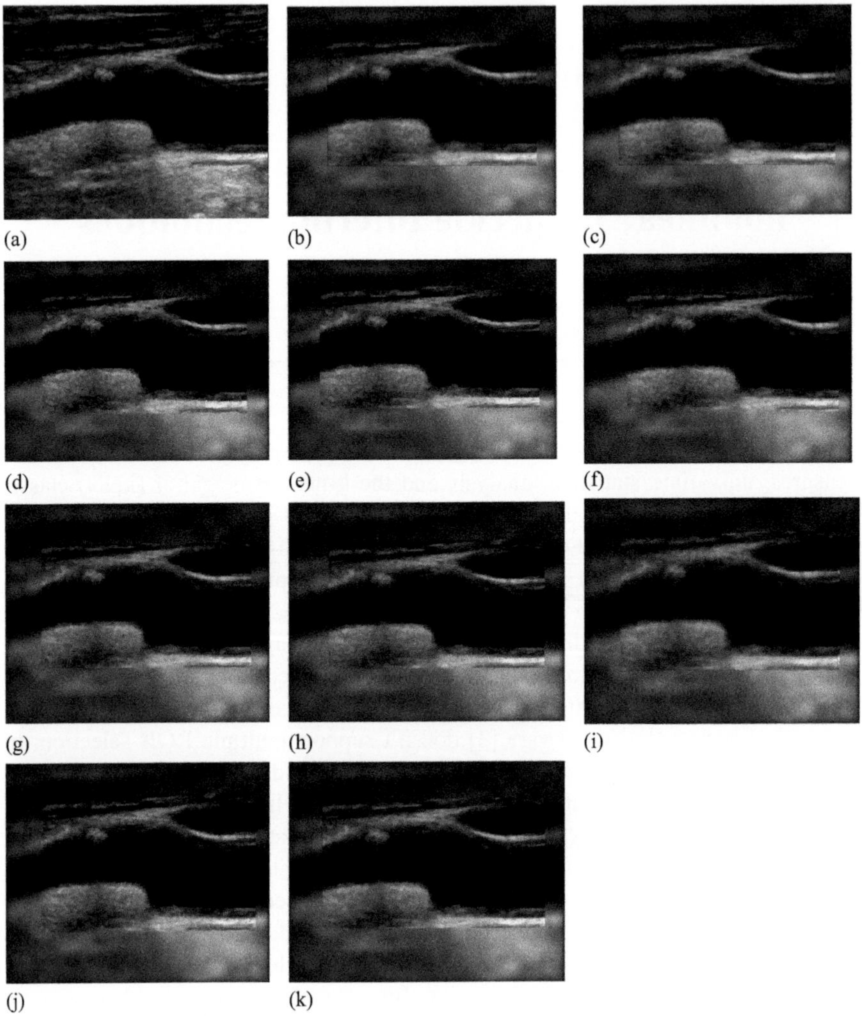

Figure 10.1 Examples of despeckle filtering in an ROI selected by the user of the system, of an ultrasound image of the CCA acquired from a symptomatic subject at risk of atherosclerosis (67-year-old male with a stenosis of 65% and a plaque at the far wall of the CCA) for (a) original, (b) DsFlsmv, (c) DsFwiener, (d) DsFlsminsc, (e) DsFkuwahara, (f) DsFgf, (g) DsFmedian, (h) DsFhmedian, (i) DsFad, (j) DsFnldif, and (k) DsFsrad. © 2014 Reprinted with the permission from [3]

We will further consider, in this chapter, the problem of filtering multiplicative noise in ultrasound videos of the CCA in order to increase the visual interpretation by experts and facilitate the automated analysis of the videos. We will apply and demonstrate the video despeckling techniques by investigating their performance on ten ultrasound videos of the CCA. The despeckling filtering techniques were evaluated through visual perception evaluation, performed by two medical experts as well as through a number of texture characteristics and video quality metrics [5]. These were extracted from the original and the despeckled videos. Figure 10.1 presents an ultrasound image of the CCA acquired from a SY subject at risk of atherosclerosis with a stenosis of 65% and a plaque at the far wall of the CCA, where ten different despeckle filters are applied in an ROI, selected by the user. The area outside of the ROI is blurred with the DsFlsmv filter. It is observed that filters DsFlsmv and DsFhmedian smoothed the image without destroying subtle details.

10.1 Despeckle filtering evaluation of carotid plaque imaging based on texture analysis

After the application of the despeckling, texture features [5] may be extracted from the original and the despeckled images and videos using the IDF [2] and VDF [3] toolboxes respectively. Texture image and video analysis is one of the most important features used in image processing and pattern recognition [5]. It can provide information about the arrangement and spatial properties of fundamental image elements. Furthermore, image or video texture characteristics extracted may provide additional useful information for the characterization of atherosclerotic plaque as documented in [6]. In this chapter, a total of 65 different texture features were used and extracted both from the original and the despeckled ultrasound images and videos as follows [6,7]:

Statistical features (SF): (1) Mean, (2) median, (3) variance (σ^2), (4) skewness (σ^3), (5) kurtosis (σ^4), and (6) speckle index (σ^2/m).

Spatial gray level dependence matrices (SGLDM) [7]: (1) Angular second moment, (2) contrast, (3) correlation, (4) sum of squares: variance (SOV), (5) inverse difference moment (IDM), (6) sum average (SA), (7) sum variance (SV), (8) sum entropy, (9) entropy, (10) difference variance (DV), (11) difference entropy, and (12) and (13) information measures of correlation. Each feature was computed using a distance of one pixel. Also, for each feature, the mean values and the range of values were computed and were used as two different feature sets.

Gray level difference statistics (GLDS) [8]: (1) Contrast, (2) angular second moment, (3) entropy, and (4) mean.

Neighborhood gray tone difference matrix (NGTDM) [9]: (1) Coarseness, (2) contrast, (3) business, (4) complexity, and (5) strength.

Statistical feature matrix (SFM) [10]: (1) Coarseness, (2) contrast, (3) periodicity, and (4) roughness.

Laws texture energy measures (TEM) [10]: For the laws TEM extraction, vectors of length $l=7$, $L=(1,6,15,20,15,6,1)$, $E=(-1,-4,-5,0,5,4,1)$, and $S=(-1,-2,1,4,1,-2,-1)$ were used, where L performs local averaging, E acts as an edge detector and S acts as a spot detector. The following TEM features were extracted: (1) LL—texture energy (TE) from LL kernel, (2) EE—TE from EE kernel, (3) SS—TE from SS kernel, (4) LE—average TE from LE and EL kernels, (5) ES—average TE from ES and SE kernels, and (6) LS—average TE from LS and SL kernels.

Fractal dimension texture analysis (FDTA) [10]: Hurst coefficient, $H^{(k)}$, for resolutions $k = 1, 2, 3, 4$.

Fourier power spectrum (FPS) [10]: (1) Radial sum and (2) angular sum.

Shape parameters: (1) X-coordinate maximum length, (2) Y-coordinate maximum length, (3) area, (4) perimeter, (5) perimeter2/area, (6) eccentricity, (7) equivalence diameter, (8) major axis length, (9) minor axis length, (10) centroid, (11) convex area, and (12) orientation.

Above presented texture features may be computed on an ROI, for example, the region prescribed by the atherosclerotic carotid plaque contour that may be automatically or manually computed [1–5].

10.1.1 Distance measures

Despeckle filtering and texture analysis were carried out on ultrasound images of the CCA. For identifying the most discriminant features separating the two classes under investigation i.e., AS and SY ultrasound images (i.e., identify features that have the highest discriminatory power), before and after despeckle filtering, the distance as shown in (10.1) between AS and SY images was calculated for the set of all ultrasound images, before and after despeckle filtering for each feature [6]:

$$dis_{zc} = |m_{za} - m_{zs}| / \sqrt{\sigma_{za}^2 + \sigma_{zs}^2} \tag{10.1}$$

where z is the feature index, c if o indicates the original image set and if f indicates the despeckled image set, m_{za} and m_{zs} are the mean values and σ_{za} and σ_{zs} are the standard deviations of the AS and SY classes, respectively. The features which are most discriminant are the ones with the highest distance values [6]. If the distance, as shown in (10.2), after despeckle filtering is increased, i.e.,

$$dis_{zf} > dis_{zo} \tag{10.2}$$

then it can be concluded that the two different classes investigated (AS, SY) may be better separated.

For each feature, a percentage distance was computed with

$$feat\_dis_z = (dis_{zf} - dis_{zo})100. \tag{10.3}$$

For each feature set, a score distance was computed with

$$Score\_Dis = (1/N)\sum_{z=1}^{N}(dis_{zf} - dis_{zo})100 \tag{10.4}$$

with N representing the number of features in the feature set. It is expected that a larger distance will show an improvement, for all features investigated.

Table 10.1 illustrates the results of $feat\_dis_z$ (10.3), and *Score_Dis* (10.4), for SF, SGLDM range of values and NGTDM feature sets for the 16 despeckle filters investigated. The filters are categorized in linear filtering, nonlinear filtering,

Table 10.1 *Feature distance (see (10.3)) and Score_Dis (see (10.4)) for statistical features (SF), spatial gray level dependence matrices (SGLDM) range of values, and neighborhood gray tone difference matrix (NGTDM) texture feature sets between AS and SY carotid plaque ultrasound images. © 2015. Reprinted with the permission from [2]*

Feature	Linear filtering			Nonlinear filtering								Diffusion				Wavelet
	DsF lsmv	**DsF wiener**	**DsF lsminsc**	**DsF ls**	**DsF homog**	**DsF gf4d**	**DsF homo**	**DsF median**	**DsF hmedian**	**DsF Kuwahara**	**DsF nlocal**	**DsF ad**	**DsF srad**	**DsF nldif**	**DsF ncdif**	**DsF waveltc**
No. of iterations	2	4	4	3	5	4	4	4	4	2	2	30	50	20	20	10
Window size	5×5	5×5	5×5	5×5	5×5	5×5	5×5	5×5	5×5	5×5	5×5	–	–	–	–	5×5
SF																
μ	**14**	**19**	**22**	**20**	**11**	**3**	**164**	**4**	**9**	**12**	**13**	**18**	**5**	**5**	**4**	**15**
Median	−5	−26	−17	−21	−5	−15	110	−5	**2**	−22	−19	−29	−31	−6	−3	−15
σ^2	**18**	**18**	38	34	13	−2	140	**7**	**9**	**11**	**17**	**9**	**10**	**7**	**6**	**18**
σ^3	**12**	**5**	**16**	15	**7**	−0.1	149	**9**	**11**	**8**	**6**	**17**	1	**7**	**2**	**8**
σ^4	−12	−7	−14	−11	−4	−3	117	−6	−13	−8	−6	−21	2	6	−3	−9
C	0.4	0.3	0.3	0.3	0.3	0.4	0.08	0.4	0.4	0.3	0.4	0.3	0.3	0.4	0.3	0.3
Score_Dis	27	9	45	37	22	−17	680	9	21	1	11	−6	−13	19	6	17
SGLDM range of values																
ASM	−21	−29	−0.5	−6	−4	−8	−47	2	−4	−8	−6	−25	−11	−17	−19	−20
Contrast	**47**	**14**	**107**	**33**	**32**	−3	**165**	**64**	**55**	**55**	**59**	**104**	**29**	**13**	**47**	**22**
Correlation	**12**	**15**	**59**	**23**	−5	**2**	**10**	**24**	**22**	**19**	**17**	**54**	**17**	−4	**11**	−4
SOSV	**9**	**18**	**40**	11	**16**	−2	**101**	**10**	**15**	7	**11**	**9**	3	**8**	**9**	**20**
IDM	−50	−48	−11	−34	−29	−8	**94**	2	**4**	−12	−14	−54	−22	−34	−41	−43
SAV	**17**	**23**	**24**	**21**	**15**	**3**	**169**	7	**9**	**27**	**22**	**22**	**14**	**6**	**14**	**18**
$\sum Var$	**19**	**18**	**38**	15	**15**	−2	**90**	**9**	**15**	**19**	**21**	**9**	**4**	**8**	7	**20**
$\sum Entr$	−34	−49	−14	−19	−19	−4	−11	**3**	**12**	−21	−17	−47	−59	−30	−22	−36

(Continues)

Table 10.1 (Continued)

Feature	Linear filtering			Nonlinear filtering								Diffusion				Wavelet
	DsF lsmv	DsF wiener	DsF lsminsc	DsF ls	DsF homog	DsF gf4d	DsF homo	DsF median	DsF hmedian	DsF Kuwahara	DsF nlocal	DsF ad	DsF srad	DsF nldif	DsF ncdif	DsF waveltc
Score_Dis	−1	−38	243	44	21	−22	571	121	128	86	93	72	−35	−50	6	−23
NGTDM–neighborhood gray tone difference matrix																
Coarseness	**30**	**4**	**87**	**6**	−16	−7	72	**9**	11	**5**	**4**	−36	5	−37	−11	−33
Contrast	7	−9	−0.3	−0.1	0.4	−4	**105**	8	12	−3	−4	**5**	4	−27	−19	−15
Busyness	**17**	−30	26	−10	**1**	−4	48	**8**	**7**	2	**6**	−14	9	−39	5	8
Completion	**64**	**21**	**151**	**45**	**80**	**2**	**150**	**53**	55	**26**	**21**	**63**	21	**18**	14	**27**
Score_Dis	118	−14	264	41	66	−13	375	78	85	30	27	18	39	−85	−11	−13
Score_Dis_T	144	−43	551	122	108	−52	1626	208	267	117	131	84	8	−116	1	−19

Bold values show improvement after despeckle filtering. ASM, angular second moment; SOSV, sum of squares variance; IDM, inverse difference moment; SAV, sum average; $\sum_{var}$, sum variance.

diffusion filtering, and wavelet filtering, as introduced in the earlier chapters as well as in [1]. We also provide the number of iterations (No. of It.) for each filter. This was selected based on the speckle index (*C*) and on the visual evaluation of the two experts. When *C* was minimally changing then the filtering process was stopped. Values that showed an improvement after despeckle filtering compared to the original are shown with bold text in Table 10.1. We also present an additional score measure, *Score_Dis*, in the last row in each sub-table, where the highest value indicates the best filter.

Furthermore, we compute the total score distance *Score_Dis_T* for all feature sets, which is shown in the last row of Table 10.1. A number of texture features are changing after despeckle filtering, by some of the despeckle filters, as shown in Table 10.1, and thus increasing the distance between the two classes (AS vs SY) (see the positive values in Table 10.1). This feature distance increases between the features of the two classes, enables the better identification and separation between AS and SY plaques. A positive feature distance shows improvement after despeckle filtering, whereas a negative shows deterioration.

The first part of Table 10.1 presents the results of the SF features, where the best *Score_Dis* is given for the filter *DsFhomo*, followed by the *DsFlsminsc, DsFlsmv, DsFhomog, DsFnldif, DsFwaveltc, DsFmedian,* and *DsFwiener*, with the worst *Score_Dis* given by *DsFgf4d*. The speckle index, C, is reduced by all filters investigated. Furthermore, it is shown that the variance, σ^2, and the kurtosis, σ^3, of the histogram are also reduced (see bold values in the first part of Table 10.1).

The results of the SGLDM range of values features set are tabulated in the second part of Table 10.1.

It is shown for the SGLDM range of values features set, that the filters with the highest *Score_Dis*, are *DsFhomo,DsFlsminsc, DsFhmedian, DsFmedian, DsFnlocal, DsFKuwahara, DsFad,* and *DsFhomog,* whereas all the other filters (*DsFlsmv, DsFwiener, DsFwaveltc, DsFgf4d, DsFlsrad,* and *DsFnldif*) are presenting a negative *Score_Dis*. Texture features which were most benefited from despeckle filtering were the contrast, correlation, sum of squares variance, SA, and SV. The third part of Table 10.1 illustrates the NGTDM feature set, where it is shown, that almost all filters improved the *Score_Dis*. In the NGTDM feature set, the best filters were the *DsFhomo, DsFlsminsc, DsFhomog*, and *DsFlsmv*. The texture features completion, coarseness, and contrast were improved at most. All filters increase the completion of the image.

Finally, the total score distance, *Score_Dis_T,* in the last row of Table 10.1 for all measures is shown. The best values for *Score_Dis_T* were obtained by the filters *DsFhomo*, *DsFlsminsc*, *DsFhmedian*, *DsFmedian*, *DsFlsmv*, *DsFls*, and *DsFKuwahara.*

10.1.2 Univariate statistical analysis

Since texture features and image/video quality metrics are not normally distributed, the Wilcoxon rank sum test for paired samples was used. This is a nonparametric alternative for the paired samples *t*-test, when the distribution of the samples is not normal. The Wilcoxon test for paired samples ranks the absolute values of the differences between the paired observations in samples 1 and 2 and calculates a statistic on the number of negative and positive differences. If the resulting p-value is small ($p < 0.05$), it can be accepted that the median of the differences between the paired observations is statistically significant different from 0. We want to investigate if for each texture feature extracted, a significant (S) difference or not significant (NS) exists between the original and the despeckled images and videos at $p < 0.05$. We use therefore the Wilcoxon matched pairs signed rank sum test. We apply the test on all the original and despeckled images and videos of the CCA.

Table 10.2 illustrates results of the rank sum test. This was performed on the features set presented in Table 10.1 for the SGLDM range of values, for all the 16 despeckle filters. We want to check if significant differences exist between the features computed on the 440 original and the 440 despeckled CCA ultrasound images. The filters resulted with the most significant number of features after despeckle filtering are illustrated in the score row of Table 10.2 (last row in table) as follows: DsFlsmv (7), DsFgf4d (6), DsFlsminsc (5), and DsFnldif (4). All other despeckle filters investigated, filters gave a lower number of significantly different features. The features angular second moment (ASM), IDM, sum entropy, correlation SOV, contrast, $\sum Var$ and SAV showed a significant difference after filtering (number of significant features after filtering for each filter: 10, 8, 8, 4, 4, 3, 3, 1, see also Table 10.2).

10.1.3 The kNN classifier

The statistical pattern recognition kNN classifier using the Euclidean distance with $k = 7$ was used to classify a plaque as AS or SY [6]. The kNN classifier was chosen because it is simple to implement and computationally very efficient. This is highly desired due to the many feature sets and filters tested [10]. In the kNN algorithm, in order to classify a new pattern, its kNNs from the training set are identified. The new pattern is classified to the most frequent class among its neighbors based on a similarity measure that is usually the Euclidean distance. In this work, the kNN carotid plaque classification system was implemented for values of $k = 1, 3, 5, 7$, and 9 using for input the eight texture feature sets and morphology features described above.

The leave-one-out method was used for evaluating the performance of the classifier, where each case is evaluated in relation to the rest of the cases. This procedure is characterized by no bias concerning the possible training and evaluation bootstrap sets. This method calculates the error or the classifications score by using $n - 1$ samples in the training set and testing or evaluating the performance of the classifier on the remaining sample. It is known that for large n, this method is computationally expensive. However, it is approximately unbiased, at the expense of an increase in the variance of the estimator [11]. The kNN classifier was chosen because it is simple to implement and computationally very efficient. This is highly desired due to the many feature sets and filters tested [10].

Table 10.2 Wilcoxon rank-sum test for the SGLDM range of values texture features applied on 440 ultrasound images of carotid plaque before and after despeckle filtering. © 2015. Reprinted with the permission from [2]

Feature	**Linear filtering**			**Nonlinear filtering**								**Diffusion**				**Wavelet**	
	DsF lsmv	**DsF wiener**	**DsF lsminsc**	**DsF ls**	**DsF homog**	**DsF gf4d**	**DsF homo**	**DsF median**	**DsF hmedian**	**DsF Kuwahara**	**DsF nlocal**	**DsF ad**	**DsF srad**	**DsF nldif**	**DsF ncdif**	**DsF waveltc**	**Score**
ASM	S	NS	S	NS	S	S	NS	NS	NS	S	NS	S	S	S	S	S	10
Contrast	S	NS	NS	NS	NS	S	NS	NS	NS	NS	NS	NS	NS	S	NS	NS	3
Correlation	S	NS	S	NS	NS	S	NS	NS	NS	NS	NS	NS	NS	NS	S	NS	4
SOSV	S	NS	NS	S	NS	S	NS	NS	S	NS	NS	NS	NS	NS	NS	NS	4
IDM	S	NS	S	NS	S	S	S	S	NS	NS	NS	NS	NS	S	NS	S	8
SAV	NS	NS	NS	NS	NS	NS	NS	NS	NS	NS	S	NS	NS	NS	NS	NS	1
$\sum Var$	S	NS	S	NS	NS	NS	NS	NS	NS	S	NS	NS	NS	NS	NS	NS	3
$\sum Entr$	S	NS	S	S	NS	S	NS	NS	NS	S	NS	NS	S	S	NS	S	8
Score	7	0	5	2	2	6	1	1	1	3	1	1	2	4	2	3	

Score: illustrates the number of *S*. The test shows with *S* significant difference after filtering at $p < 0.05$ and *NS* no significant difference after filtering at $p \geq 0.05$. ASM, angular second moment; SOSV, sum of squares variance; IDM, inverse difference moment; SAV, sum average; $\sum Var$, sum variance.

The percentage of correct classifications score for the kNN classifier with $k = 7$ for classifying a subject as AS or SY is shown in Table 10.3. We use the leave-one-out method [10] to evaluate the classifier, on the original and despeckled images (220 AS vs 220 SY images of the CCA). We provide the percentage of correct classifications score for the following feature sets: SF, spatial gray level dependence matrix mean values (SGLDMm), spatial gray level dependence matrix range of values (SGLDMr), GLDS, NGTDM, SFM, TEM, FDTA, and FPS. Following despeckle filters showed an improvement in classifications success score compared to that of the original image set (see also last row of Table 10.4): DsFhomo (3%), DsFgf4d (1%), and DsFlsminsc (1%).

In the last column of Table 10.3, we illustrate the feature sets which were benefited mostly by the despeckle filtering [SF (11), TEM (10), SFM (5), SGLDM (4), GLDS (4), and NGTDM (4)], when counting the number of cases that the correct classifications score was improved. For the feature sets FDTA, FPS, and SGLDMr, less improvement was obtained. The only filter that showed an improvement for the SGLDMr feature class was the DsFlsminsc filter (2% improvement). The DsFlsmv filter showed the best improvement for the TEM feature set (9% improvement), whereas the DsFlsminsc filter gave the best improvement for the FPS feature set (5% improvement). In the GLDS and NGTDM feature sets, the filter DsFlsminsc gave best performance, the filter DsFlsmv showed improvement for the feature sets SF and TEM whereas the filter DsFhmedian in SFM, SF, and GLDS.

10.1.4 Image and video quality and visual evaluation

The image quality evaluation metrics (also presented in [1]) for the 220 AS and 220 SY ultrasound images between the original and the despeckled images are presented in Table 10.4. Filters DsFnldif, DsFlsmv, and DsFwaveltc demonstrated the best values with lower mean square error (MSE), randomized mean square error (RMSE), Err3, and Err4 and higher signal-to-noise ratio (SNR) and peak signal-to-noise ratio (PSNR). For all case investigated, the geometric average error was 0.00. This can be attributed to the fact that the information between the original and the despeckled images remains unchanged. For the universal quality index, Q, and the structural similarity index, SSIN, best values were obtained for the despeckle filters DsFlsmv, DsFnldif, and DsFhmedian.

As also presented in [1,2] (see Figs. 7.4 and 7.6 and Tables 7.3 and 7.5), best visual evaluation results, which were assessed by two different experts (a cardiovascular surgeon and a neurovascular specialist), were obtained for the filters DsFlsmv, DsFlsminsc, and DsFkuwahara, whereas the filters DsFgf4d, DsFad, DsFncdif, and DsFnldif also showed good visual results but smoothed the image, loosing subtle details and affecting the edges. Filters that showed a blurring effect were the DsFmedian, DsFwiener, DsFhomog, and DsFwaveltc. Filters DsFwiener, DsFls, DsFhomog, and DsFwaveltc showed poorer visual results. The experts evaluated an artificial carotid artery image, a phantom ultrasound image, and a real ultrasound image of the CCA.

Table 10.3 Percentage of correct classifications score for the kNN classifier with k=7 for the original and the filtered image set. © 2015. Reprinted with the permission from [2]

Feature set	No. of feat	Original	Linear filtering			Nonlinear filtering							Diffusion				Wavelet	
			DsF lsmv	**DsF wiener**	**DsF lsminsc**	**DsF ls**	**DsF homog**	**DsF gf4d**	**DsF homo**	**DsF median**	**DsF hmedian**	**DsF Kuwahara**	**DsF nlocal**	**DsF ad**	**DsF srad**	**DsF nldif**	**DsF ncdif**	**DsF waveltc**	**Score**
SF	5	59	**62**	**61**	**61**	57	**63**	59	**65**	**60**	**61**	59	**60**	**60**	58	52	**60**	**61**	11
SGLDMm	13	65	63	62	64	65	**69**	**67**	**68**	62	64	64	62	61	64	**66**	63	63	4
SGLDMr	13	70	66	64	**72**	68	65	70	69	70	69	**71**	69	64	69	65	69	65	2
GLDS	4	64	63	61	**66**	64	64	**66**	**72**	63	**66**	62	52	59	61	58	61	62	4
NGTDM	5	64	63	60	**68**	**65**	63	**65**	57	59	63	64	61	60	63	61	**65**	62	4
SFM	4	62	62	62	60	62	55	**65**	**68**	58	**64**	**63**	61	59	**63**	56	57	55	5
TEM	6	59	**68**	**60**	52	54	**66**	**60**	**65**	**61**	**61**	58	**60**	53	60	**60**	59	**60**	10
FDTA	4	64	63	53	**66**	63	53	62	**73**	63	63	62	61	55	62	54	61	62	3
FPS	2	59	54	59	**64**	57	59	59	59	52	59	**60**	59	52	56	48	**60**	55	3
Average		63	63	60	**64**	62	62	**64**	**66**	61	63	63	61	58	62	58	62	61	

Score: illustrates the number of *S*. Bold values indicate improvement after despeckling. SGLDMm, spatial gray level dependence matrix mean values; SGLDMr, spatial gray level dependence matrix range of values; ASM, angular second moment; SOSV, sum of squares variance; IDM, inverse difference moment; SAV, sum average; $\sum Var$, sum variance.

Table 10.4 Image quality evaluation metrics extracted for the 220 AS and 220 SY images. © 2015. Reprinted with the permission from [2]

Feature set	Linear filtering			Nonlinear filtering								Diffusion				Wavelet
	DsF lsmv	DsF wiener	DsF lsminsc	DsF ls	DsF homog	DsF gf4d	DsF homo	DsF median	DsF hmedian	DsF Kuwahara	DsF nlocal	DsF ad	DsF srad	DsF nldif	DsF ncdif	DsF waveltc
Asymptomatic images																
MSE	13	19	86	22	42	182	758	131	112	21	15	132	111	8	9	11
RMSE	3	4	9	5	6	13	27	10	27	4	2	11	19	2	7	3
Err3	7	5	17	9	14	25	38	25	22	5	9	21	21	5	6	4
Err4	11	7	26	11	24	40	49	41	23	9	24	32	29	10	11	5
GAE	0	0	0	0	0	0	0	0	0	0	0	0	0	0	0	0
SNR	25	23	17	7	21	14	5	16	9	22	7	14	12	28	16	25
PSNR	39	36	29	29	34	27	20	29	30	30	19	28	27	41	22	39
Q	0.83	0.74	0.78	0.71	0.72	0.77	0.28	0.80	0.81	0.74	0.74	0.68	0.69	0.83	0.79	0.65
SSIN	0.97	0.92	0.88	0.93	0.97	0.88	0.43	0.94	0.96	0.89	0.81	0.87	0.89	0.97	0.81	0.9
AD	0.9	0.2	0.3	0.86	0.2	−0.67	−0.99	0.44	0.51	0.4	0.6	0.3	−11	−0.1	0.3	−0.1
SC	1.3	1.1	1.0	1.2	0.9	0.75	0.04	1.8	1.2	1.1	1.1	1.2	0.9	1.1	1.1	1.2
MD	55	35	55	59	32	98	122	54	130	54	67	55	74	129	125	55
Symptomatic images																
MSE	33	44	374	45	110	557	1452	169	131	26	19	374	134	8	11	23
RMSE	5	6	19	16	10	23	37	13	22	6	14	19	22	3	8	5
Err3	10	9	33	22	20	43	51	25	29	8	21	31	33	5	12	6
Err4	16	11	47	41	30	63	64	38	36	5	16	43	41	7	11	8
GAE	0	0	0	0	0	0	0	0	0	0	0	0	0	0	0	0
SNR	24	22	13	22	17	12	5	16	14	28	19	12	15	29	19	25
PSNR	34	33	23	17	28	21	17	26	26	24	21	23	19	39	20	36
Q	0.82	0.71	0.77	0.74	0.77	0.75	0.24	0.79	0.80	0.78	0.78	0.63	0.71	0.81	0.77	0.49
SSIN	0.97	0.86	0.85	0.82	0.84	0.85	0.28	0.81	0.88	0.82	0.84	0.81	0.77	0.97	0.81	0.87
AD	2.1	0.9	0.5	1.9	0.5	−0.61	−0.96	0.67	0.62	0.6	0.9	0.4	−17	−0.3	0.3	−0.3
SC	1.5	1.3	1.4	1.7	1.0	0.98	0.05	1.4	1.4	1.3	1.6	1.4	0.7	0.9	1.4	1.4
MD	88	39	59	78	31	76	139	52	121	67	53	59	67	111	110	63

MSE, mean square error; RMSE, randomized mean square error; Err3, Err4, Minkowski metrics; GAE, geometric average error; SNR, signal-to-noise ratio; PSNR, peak signal-to-noise ratio; Q, universal quality index; SSIN, structural similarity index; AD, average difference; SC, structural content, maximum difference.

Table 10.5A illustrates the results of the visual evaluation of the original and despeckled images made by the two experts [2]. They evaluated before and after despeckle filtering 100 ultrasound images (50 AS and 50 SY). For each case, the experts evaluated one original and nine filtered (a total of ten images were evaluated). The experts assigned a score in the one-to-five scale based on subjective criteria, for each case, for each image. If the score of five for all the 100 images is assigned by the expert, the maximum score for a filter is 500. Furthermore, in order to express the result in percentage format, for each filter, the score was divided by five. The overall average percentage (%) score assigned by both experts for each filter is also presented in the last row of Table 10.5B.

The average score for the cardiovascular surgeon showed that the best score was obtained by the DsFlsmv filter with 62%. The filters DsFgf4d, DsFhmedian, DsFhomog, and original followed with scores of 52%, 50%, 45%, and 41%, respectively.

The average score for the neurovascular specialist showed that the best filter is the DsFgf4d (score: 72%), followed by DsFlsmv (score: 71%), original (score: 68%), DsFlsminsc (score: 68%), and DsFhmedian (score: 66%). The highest score, which is shown by the overall average percentage score, was given to the filter DsFlsmv (score: 67%), followed by DsFgf4d (score: 62%), DsFhmedian (score: 58%), and the original (score: 54%). We may observe that the despeckle filter DsFlsmv is the only filter that was graded with a higher score than the original by both experts for the AS and SY image sets.

A difference in the scorings between the two vascular specialists is observed when inspecting Tables 10.5A and 10.5B. This may be attributed to the fact that the cardiovascular surgeon is primarily interested in the plaque composition and texture evaluation, whereas the neurovascular specialist is interested to evaluate the degree of stenosis and the lumen diameter in order to identify the plaque contour. The best despeckle filters as identified, by both specialists, wee the DsFlsmv and DsFgf4d. Both filters improved visual perception with overall average scores of 67% and 62%, respectively. The lowest overall average scores were given to the filters DsFwaveltc and DsFhomo, by both specialists (28% vs 29%).

Results of the visual perception evaluation made by same experts, one year after the first visual evaluation, are also tabulated in Table 10.5B. Both experts repeated the visual perception evaluation in order to assess the intraobserver variability between the same experts. The procedure was performed under the same conditions as the first visual evaluation.

The average score for the cardiovascular surgeon indicated that the best despeckle filter is the DsFlsmv (score: 61%), followed by DsFhmedian (score: 60%), DsFgf4d (score: 52%), DsFls (score: 49%), DsFhomog (score: 40%), and the original (score: 36%), respectively. The average score for the neurovascular expert showed that the best filter is the DsFlsminsc (score: 68%), followed by DsFgf4d (score: 67%), DsFlsmv (score: 64%), original (score: 63%), and DsFhmedian (score: 61%), respectively. The highest score given, which is shown by the overall average percentage score, was to the filter DsFlsmv (score: 63%), followed by DsFhmedian (score: 61%), DsFgf4d (score: 60%), DsFls (score: 54%), and the

Table 10.5A *Visual evaluation percentage scoring of the original and despeckled images (50 AS and 50 SY) performed by the experts [1]. Reprinted with the permission from [1] © 2014, [2] © 2015*

Experts	**A/S**	**Original**	**Linear filtering**		**Nonlinear filtering**				**Diffusion**	**Wavelet**
			DsF lsmv	**DsF lsminsc**	**DsF hmedian**	**DsF homog**	**DsF gf4d**	**DsF homo**	**DsF nldif**	**DsF waveltc**
Cardiovascular	AS	33	75	33	43	47	61	19	43	32
surgeon	SY	48	49	18	57	43	42	20	33	22
Average %		41	62	26	50	45	52	19	38	27
Neurovascular	AS	70	76	73	74	63	79	23	52	29
specialist	SY	66	67	63	58	45	65	55	41	28
Average %		68	71	68	66	54	72	39	47	28
Overall average %		54	67	47	58	50	62	29	43	28

Table 10.5B *Visual evaluation percentage scoring of the original and despeckled images (50 AS and 50 SY) performed by the experts one year after the first visual evaluation [1]. Reprinted with the permission from [1] © 2014, [2] © 2015*

Experts	**A/S**	**Original**	**Linear filtering**		**Nonlinear filtering**					**Diffusion**	**Wavelet**
			DsF lsmv	**DsF lsminsc**	**DsF hmedian**	**DsF ls**	**DsF homog**	**DsF gf4d**	**DsF homo**	**DsF nldif**	**DsF waveltc**
Cardiovascular	AS	28	57	43	62	49	41	53	16	39	31
surgeon	SY	44	65	24	57	49	39	51	23	37	21
Average %		36	61	34	60	49	40	52	20	38	26
Neurovascular	AS	62	65	64	69	67	51	65	19	49	24
expert	SY	64	62	71	53	51	49	69	49	44	26
Average %		63	64	68	61	59	50	67	34	47	25
Overall average %		50	63	51	61	54	45	60	27	43	26

original (score: 50%). Table 10.5B shows a consistency in almost all results for the intraobserver variability between the experts, with only small differences between filters. The DsFlsmv despeckle filter is the only filter that was graded with a higher score than the original by both vascular experts for the AS and SY images.

Both experts came into a final agreement for the best despeckle filters for visual perception. They agreed that the DsFlsmv, DsFlsminsc, DsFgf4d, and DsFhmedian were the best, whereas the worst filters were the DsFwaveltc followed by the DsFhomo and DsFnldif (see also Tables 10.5A and 10.5B). Both experts also agreed that almost all despeckle filters reduced the noise substantially and thus ultrasound images may be better visualized after the application of despeckle filtering. When studying the results of Tables 10.1–10.4 and the visual evaluation of Tables 10.5A and 10.5B, we may conclude that the best despeckle filters are the DsFlsmv and the DsFgf4d. The two filters may be used for both plaque composition enhancement and plaque texture analysis, whereas the filters DsFlsmv, DsFgf4d, and DsFlsminsc are more appropriate to identify the degree of stenosis and therefore may be used when the primary interest is to outline the plaque borders.

10.2 Despeckle filtering based on texture analysis (discussion)

As shown from the results on texture analysis (see Tables 10.2–10.4), the filters DsFlsmv, DsFgf4d, and DsFlsminsc improved the class separation between the AS and the SY classes by increasing the distance between them. These filters (DsFlsmv, DsFgf4d, and DsFlsminsc) gave the highest number of significantly different features (see also Table 10.2, with 7, 6, and 5, respectively) but gave only a marginal improvement in the percentage of correct classification success rate (see Table 10.3).

The high number of significantly different features for these filters showed that the two classes (AS, SY) may be better separated after despeckle filtering using the filters DsFlsmv, DsFgf4d, and DsFlsminsc. The distance between the AS and the SY images, as shown in Table 10.1, was increased for almost all despeckle filters thus making the identification of a class more easily to identify. It is also shown from Table 10.1 that most of the filters reduced the asymmetry, σ^3, and the skewness, σ^4, of the histogram. Despeckle filtering influenced more some SF, such as the IDM, the ASM, and the $\sum Entr$, while other SF were less influenced by despeckle filtering as shown in Table 10.2. These features, which were more influenced by despeckle filtering, may thus be used to evaluate despeckle filtering. The *Score_Dis_T*, which is shown in the last row of Table 10.2, showed that best feature distance was given by the filters DsFhomo, DsFlsminsc, DsFmedian, and DsFlsmv. Table 10.3 also showed that not all feature sets equally benefited from despeckle filtering. Specifically, the SF and TEM feature sets benefited from almost all despeckle filters (7), whereas the feature sets SGLDMm, GLDS, and NGTDM benefited from four despeckle filters, FDTA three, and SFM two. The features sets SGLDMr, and FPS, benefited from only one despeckle filter.

Results on texture analysis of ultrasound images were also given in the literature for the classification of atherosclerotic carotid plaque [5,12], liver ultrasound images [10], electron microscopic muscle images [13], detection of breast masses [14], cloud images [15], and SAR images [16,17]. Some results were also given on artificial images from the pioneer researchers in texture analysis [7,8]. To the best of our knowledge, there is no other study reported in the literature, where texture analysis (as the one presented here in Tables 10.1–10.3) was used to the extent, that is used in our study, to evaluate despeckle filtering in ultrasound imaging. In [15,18], some of the texture measures, also used in our study (see Table 10.3), were used on a total of 230 ultrasound images of the carotid plaque (115 AS, 115 SY). These were used to characterize carotid plaques as safe or unsafe and identify patients at risk of stroke. More specifically, in [10,15], all nine different features, also used in our study (see Table 10.3), were used to classify a plaque as AS or SY, where comparable values as in our study were obtained for all feature sets. Further examples on the use of texture features analysis are provided in [14], for classifying malignant and benign tumors of breast, for classifying clouds and predicting weather [15], and to automatically classify terrain texture [8].

Despeckle filtering was in this chapter as well as by other researchers on an artificial carotid image [1–5,19–21], on line profiles of different ultrasound images [1–5,19–21], on phantom ultrasound images [1–5,19–21], SAR images [1,16,17], real longitudinal ultrasound images of the CCA [1,19,21], and cardiac ultrasound images. There are only few studies [1–5,19] where despeckle filtering was investigated on real, and artificial longitudinal ultrasound image of the CCA. Four different despeckle filters were applied in [19], namely the DsFlsmv, Frost, DsFad, and a DsFsrad filter [19]. For the DsFlsmv and Frost filters, the despeckle sliding pixel window used was 7×7 pixels. The performance of these filters was evaluated using the mean and the standard deviation extracted from the original and the despeckled images, in different regions of the carotid artery image, namely in lumen, tissue, and at the vascular wall. For the original image, the mean gray level values for the lumen/tissue/wall regions were 1.1/5.3/23, whereas the variances were 0.57/2.7/10.6, respectively. The mean after despeckle filtering with the DsFsrad gave brighter values for the lumen and tissue. Specifically, the mean of the lumen/tissue/wall for the DsFsrad was 1.2/6.2/19, DsFlsmv (1.1/5.7/22), Frost (1.1/5.8/22), and DsFad (0.9/4.6/15). The standard deviation for the DsFsrad gave lower values (0.2, 0.7, 3) when compared with the Lee (0.3, 1.4, 5.4), Frost (0.3, 1.4, 5.3), and DsFad (0.2, 1.1, 3.5). It was thus shown that the DsFsrad filter preserves the mean and reduces the variance. The number of images investigated in [19], was relatively small, where visual perception evaluation was not carried out by experts. Additionally, only two statistical measures were used to quantitatively evaluate despeckle filtering (the mean and the variance). We are confident that the mean and the variance used in [19] are not indicative and may not give a complete and accurate evaluation result as in [5]. Furthermore, despeckle filtering was investigated by other researchers on ultrasound images of heart [1,21], pig heart [22], pig muscle [23], liver [24], kidney [25], echocardiograms [26], computed tomography

(CT) lung scans [27], brain X-ray images [20], magnetic resonance image (MRI) images of brain [28], SAR images [16], and real-world images [29].

Line plots, as used in our study (see also Fig. 7.2 in [20]), were used in few other studies to quantify despeckle filtering performance. In [1], a line profile through the original and the despeckled ultrasound image of kidney was plotted, using adaptive Gaussian filtering. In [30], line profiles were plotted on four simulated and 15 ultrasound cardiac images of the left ventricle, in order to evaluate the DsFmedian despeckle filter. In another study [21], line profiles through one phantom, one heart, one kidney, and one liver ultrasound image were plotted where an adaptive shrinkage weighted median [24,29], DsFwaveltc (wavelet shrinkage) [31], and wavelet shrinkage coherence enhancing [26] models were used and compared with a nonlinear coherent diffusion model [31]. Finally, in [22], line plots were used in one artificial computer-simulated image, and one ultrasound image of pig heart, where an adaptive shrinkage weighted median filter [24,29], a multi-scale nonlinear thresholding without adaptive filter preprocessing [22], a wavelet shrinkage filtering method [31], and a proposed adaptive nonlinear thresholding with adaptive preprocessing method [22] were evaluated. In all of the above studies, visual perception evaluation by experts, statistical and texture analysis, on multiple images, as performed in our study, was not performed.

Phantom images were used in [1–3] and by other researchers in order to evaluate despeckle filtering in carotid ultrasound imaging. Specifically, in [21], a synthetic carotid ultrasound image of the CCA was used to evaluate the DsFsard filtering (speckle reducing anisotropic filtering) which was compared with the DsFlsmv (Lee filter) [32] and the DsFad filter (conventional anisotropic diffusion) [33]. The edges of the phantom image used in [21] were studied, and it was shown that the DsFsrad does not blur edges as with the other two despeckle filtering techniques evaluated (DsFlsmv and DsFad).

While there are a number of despeckle filtering techniques and commercial software packages proposed in the literature for despeckling of ultrasound images, which are presented in [1–5], we found no other studies in the literature for despeckle filtering in ultrasound videos of the CCA with the exception of [3]. More specifically, we proposed in [3] a freeware despeckle filtering toolbox which was based on four despeckle filtering methods (DsFlsmv, DsFhmedian, DsFkuwahara, and DsFsrad) for video despeckling.

10.3 Image despeckle filtering based on visual quality evaluation (discussion)

The visual perception evaluation performed in Tables 10.5A and 10.5B showed that the filters DsFlsmv, DsFgf4d, and DsFlsminsc improved the visual assessment which is performed by experts. The intraobserver variability test (Table 10.5A which was repeated one year after the first visual evaluation Table 10.5B) showed that the differences between the visual evaluations made by the two experts were very small. The results of the two tables were thus in agreement.

By inspecting the two tables (Tables 10.5A and 10.5B), it was shown that the highest scores were obtained, for the filter DsFlsmv for both tables. There are differences observed in the ratings between the two experts, and these were due to the fact that each expert was interested in a different tissue area in the ultrasound image of the CCA. Specifically, the cardiovascular surgeon was interested in the plaque composition and texture, whereas the neurovascular expert was interested in the degree of stenosis and the lumen diameter of the CCA. The neurovascular expert rated the DsFlsminsc despeckle filter with the highest score in Table 10.5B. He found that the filter was helpful in identifying and inspecting the degree of stenosis, the lumen diameter, and the surrounding tissue.

The images were furthermore evaluated by the two experts before and after despeckle filtering and gave additional comments which are briefly outlined below. The primary interest of the two experts were the borders between intima media thickness (IMT), plaque, artery wall, and blood as they were interested to be able to exactly make a separation between them. There were also some important points which were taken into consideration from both experts during this examination. These were the texture of the atherosclerotic carotid plaque, as the texture may give additional indication about the risk of stroke [1–6]. Both experts commented the fact that the DsFlsmv despeckle filter was adequate for visualizing the borders between blood, plaque, and wall but not between wall and surrounding tissue. The despeckle filter DsFlsminsc helped specifically for the visualization of plaque borders which were displayed after filtering. Finally, the DsFgf4d despeckle filter sharpened the edges; thus, it may be used for plaque visualization and to separate the borders between blood and plaque.

We found no other studies in the current literature (with the exception of [1–5]) performed for the visual evaluation of ultrasound images by using despeckle filtering and image normalization with two experts [20]. More specifically, in [5], 56 different textures features and ten different image quality evaluation metrics were used to compare the effect of despeckle filtering in 440 ultrasound images of the CCA, where two different experts optically evaluated the images. It was found that a linear order statistics filter, based on first order statistics, may be successfully used for despeckling CCA ultrasound images. Furthermore, in [1,2], two ultrasound imaging scanners from different manufacturers, namely the ATL HDI-3000 and the ATL HDI-5000, were compared based on texture features and image quality metrics. The features were extracted from 80 ultrasound images of the carotid bifurcation, before and after despeckle filtering. It was shown that normalization and despeckle filtering favors image quality. In a large number of despeckle filtering studies [19,32,16,21,26,22], the procedure of visual evaluation was carried out by nonexperts. There are very few results reported in the literature, where visual perception evaluation was carried out in ultrasound images. Two experts manually delineated 60 echocardiographic images and visually evaluated them before and after despeckle filtering in [26]. The mean of absolute border difference and the mean of border area differences were estimated for quantitative evaluating the delineations. It was shown by the visual evaluation performed in [26] that the borders manually defined by the experts were improved after despeckle filtering.

Ten photo interpreters were evaluated in [11], the performance assessment of multi-temporal SAR image despeckling between the original and three filtered results. The images were presented in a random order, and they evaluated the accuracy of manual detection of geographical features (lines, points, and surfaces). It was concluded that despeckle filtering improves the identification of the above criteria and that specific filters may be used to enhance points, lines, or surfaces as required. In [34], image quality was evaluated for compressed still images. The images were presented to an unknown number of not expert observers over 18 years old (from a university population), in a random order.

The results of Table 10.4 showed that the best values for the quality evaluation were obtained by the despeckle filters DsFnldif, DsFlsmv, and DsFwaveltc. Table 10.4 also showed that the effect of despeckle filtering was more obvious on the AS images, where generally better image quality evaluation results were obtained. Moreover, it is obvious that all quality evaluation metrics presented here were equally important for image quality evaluation. It is also important to indicate that a higher PSNR (or equivalently, a lower RMSE) does not necessarily imply a higher subjective image quality, although they do provide some measure of relative quality. There are some quality metrics studied for different images as proposed in the literature, such as for MRI [35], natural and artificial images [36], but to the best of our knowledge, no other comparative study exists except [5], which have investigated the application of the above metrics together with visual perception evaluation, on ultrasound images of the carotid artery. In previous studies [16,19,25,32], researchers evaluated image quality on real-world images using either only the visual perception by experts or some of the evaluation metrics presented in Table 10.4. In all abovementioned studies, the researchers compared the proposed method with another one, based on image quality evaluation metrics such as the MSE [1–5,20–22,29], the PSNR [29], the SNR [1–5,20], the C [1–5], the mean, and the variance [19,16,24] and line plots [21,22,32]. The comparison was made between the original and some preprocessed images, thus the usefulness of these measures was not investigated for the despeckling of ultrasound images. Furthermore, normalization and despeckling also proposed in this chapter was not taken into consideration. In [37], image quality on ultrasound images of the CCA was investigated, and it was shown that despeckle filtering increases the quality of images as well as increases the accuracy of the IMT [38] and plaque [39] segmentation.

In [40], ultrasound spatial compound scanning was evaluated based on PSNR and SSIN [36], for comparing the quality of joint photographic experts group (JPEG) images before and after compression. Image quality metrics were also investigated for the evaluation of ultrasound spatial compound scanning [40], to compare the quality of JPEG images before and after compression using the PSNR, and SSIN [36] (PSNR: 8.45, SSIN: 0.96 vs this study PSNR: 39, and SSIN: 0.97 with the DsFlsmv filter). In [41], real-world images were evaluated before and after a preprocessing procedure based on their compression ratios using the MSE and Q (–/–) (histogram equalization (1,144/0.74), median filtering (15/0.78), wavelet compression (16/0.68), and spatial displacement (141/0.5)).

In [29], various median filtering techniques were investigated on real-world images, where the MSE and PSNR were used to compare the original and the filtered images. In [42], MSE, SNR, PSNR, M3, and M4 were used to evaluate JPEG compression on still real-world images. In [21], despeckle filtering was investigated on artificial and ultrasound images of heart, kidney, and abdomen by measuring the MSE before and after despeckle filtering using four different despeckle filtering methods, namely the adaptive weighted median filtering [29], wavelet shrinkage enhanced [26], wavelet shrinkage [26], and nonlinear coherence diffusion method [31] (MSE: 289, 271, 132, and 121). In the majority of studies investigated, the researchers used image quality measures such as the MSE [21,22,29], SNR [1–5,16,19,22], and PSNR [1–5,16,29], in order to compare the original with the processed images. Original and four despeckled SAR images were compared in [25] before and after despeckle filtering (MSE: 133, 43, 49, 26, 22), using the despeckle filters Lee [32], gamma MAP filter [23], soft thresholding, and the WIN-SAR filter [25], which used a 7×7 pixel filtering window.

In [25], MSE values between original and despeckle kidney ultrasound images were for the filters median (13.7), DsFwiener [16] (13.8), after soft thresholding [31] (13.6), 13.5 after hard thresholding [31] (13.5), and 12.74 after Bayesian denoising (12.74) [25]. In the present work, the MSE values for the filter DsFlsmv, DsFwiener, DsFnldif, and DsFwaveltc (see also Table 10.5) were 13, 19, 8, 11, for the ASY, and 33, 44, 8, 23, for the SY images, respectively, which are better or comparable with other studies reported above.

It was shown that normalization and speckle reduction produces better images [1–5,37]. The procedure of image normalization was also proposed in other studies using blood echogenicity as a reference and applied in CCA images [40]. In [1–5,37,39], it was shown that image normalization improves the comparability of the image by reducing the variability, which is introduced by different gain settings, operators, and equipment. It should be noted that the order of applying these processes (normalization and speckle reduction filtering) affects the final result. Based on unpublished results, we have observed that by applying first speckle reduction filtering and then normalization produces distorted edges. The preferred method is to apply first normalization and then speckle reduction filtering for better results.

In two recent studies [38,39], it was shown that the preprocessing of ultrasound images of the CCA with normalization followed by speckle reduction filtering improves the performance of the automated segmentation of the intima-media thickness [38] and plaque [39]. More specifically, it was shown in [27] that a smaller variability in segmentation results was observed when performed on images after normalization and speckle reduction filtering, compared with the manual delineation results made by two medical experts. In study [5], it was furthermore shown that speckle reduction filtering improves the percentage of correct classifications score of AS and SY images of the CCA. Speckle reduction filtering was also investigated by other researchers on ultrasound images of liver and kidney [43], and on natural scenery [32], using an adaptive two-dimensional filter similar to the DsFlsmv speckle reduction filter used in this study. In these studies [32,43], speckle reduction filtering was evaluated based only on visual perception evaluation made by the researches.

Verhoeven *et al.* [44] applied mean and median filtering in simulated ultrasound images and in ultrasound images with blood vessels. The lesion-SNR was used in order to quantify the detectability of lesions after filtering. Filtering was applied on images with fixed and adaptive size windows in order to investigate the influence of the filter window size. It was shown that the difference in performance between the filters was small but the choice of the correct window size was important. Kotropoulos *et al.* [45] applied adaptive speckle reduction filtering in simulated tissue mimicking phantom and liver ultrasound B-mode images, where it was shown that the proposed maximum likelihood estimator filter was superior to the mean filter.

Although in this book, speckle has been considered as noise, there are other studies where speckle, approximated by the Rayleigh distribution, was used to support automated segmentation. Specifically, in [46], an automated luminal contour segmentation method based on a statistical approach was introduced, whereas in [47] ultrasound intravascular images were segmented using knowledge-based methods. Furthermore, in [48], a semiautomatic segmentation method for intravascular ultrasound images, based on gray-scale statistics of the image, was proposed, where the lumen, IMT, and the plaque were segmented in parallel by utilizing a fast-marching model.

10.4 Despeckle filtering evaluation on carotid plaque video based on texture analysis

Figure 10.2 presents the application of the DsFlsmv (see Figure 10.2(a)–(f)) and the DsFhmedian (see Figure 10.2(g)–(l)) despeckle filters, which showed best performance (see Tables 10.6–10.8) on consecutive video frames (1, 50, and 100) of an SY subject, for the cases where the filtering was applied on the whole video frame (see left column of Figure 10.2) and on an ROI selected by the user (see right column of Figure 10.2). Despeckle filtering was evaluated on ten videos of the CCA where texture features were extracted from the original and the despeckled videos from the whole video and the ROI (see also Figure 10.2). Table 10.6 presents the results of selected SF (from the SF and SGLDM feature sets, see Section 10.1) that showed significant difference after despeckle filtering ($p \leq 0.05$). The features were extracted from the original video frame and the despeckled video frames for the whole video frame and the ROI, for all ten videos investigated. These features were the median, variance, SOV, IDM, entropy, difference entropy, and coarseness. It is shown that the filters DsFlsmv and DsFhmedian comparatively preserved the features median, variance, and entropy but increased coarseness. It should be noted that these findings cannot be compared with the results presented in [5,37] as the texture features in these two studies were computed for the whole despeckled plaque images (and not the ROIs as defined in this example).

Table 10.7 tabulates selected video quality metrics between the original and the despeckled videos for whole frame filtering and when the filtering was applied on an ROI. It is clearly shown that the despeckle filter DsFlsmv performs better in

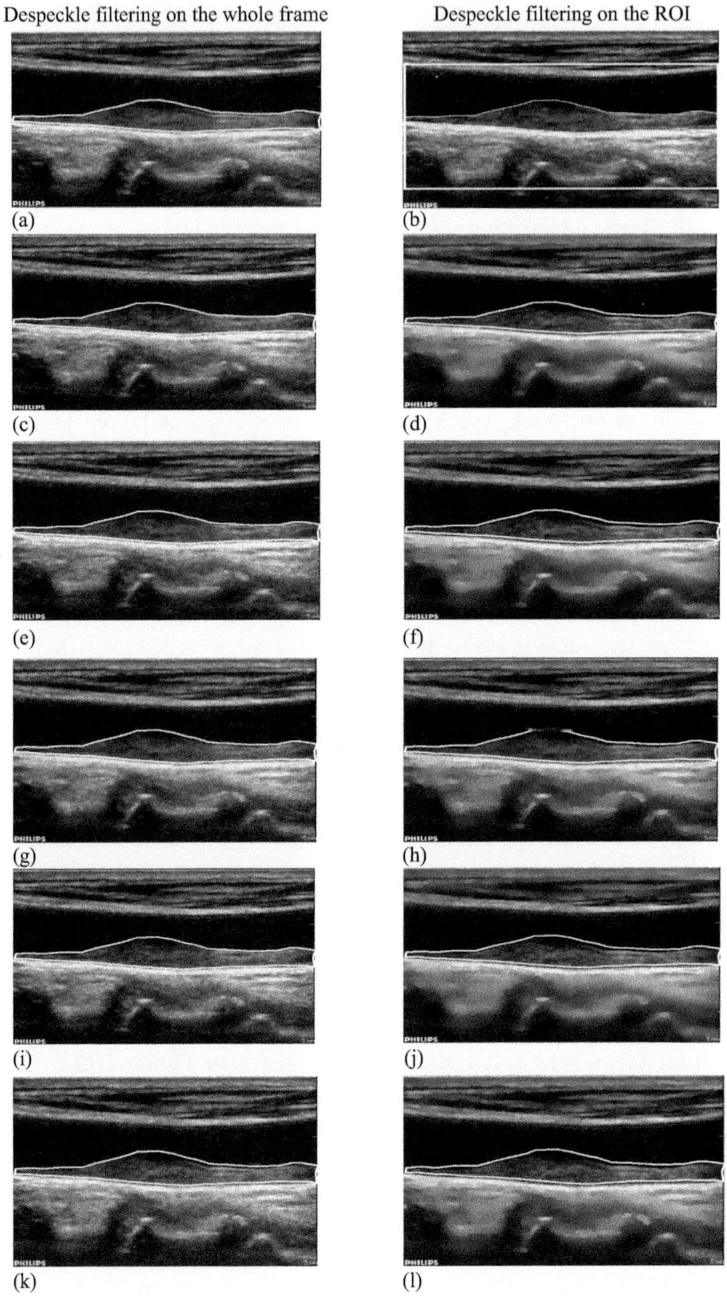

Figure 10.2 *Examples of despeckle filtering with the filter DsFlsmv (a)–(f) and DsFhmedian (g)–(l) on a video of the CCA (male SY subject at the age of 62, with 40% stenosis and a plaque at the far wall of the CCA), on frames 1, 50, and 100 for the whole image frame in the left column, and on an ROI (shown in (b)), in the right column. The automated plaque segmentations are shown in all examples*

Table 10.6 Texture features (mean±SD) that showed significant difference (based on the statistical Wilcoxon rank-sum test at $p \leq 0.05$) after despeckle filtering, for all ten videos of the CCA extracted from the original and the despeckled videos from the whole video and the ROI (–/–). © 2013. Reprinted with the permission from [4]

Features	Original	DsFlsmv	DsFhmedian	DsFkuwahara	DsFsrad
Median	43±14/23±17	43±14/28±18	43±14/26±12	42±14/26±17	43±14/26±14
Variance	54±7/58±8	53±6/58±9	54±6/58±8	55±8/59±9	54±6/62±8
SOV	8±6/7±4	12±11/9±3	8±7/14±22	11±7/7±5	10±9/12±13
IDM	0.27±0.07/0.29±0.14	0.29±0.07/0.43±0.09	0.39±0.05/0.48±0.09	0.41±0.07/0.51±0.089	0.38±0.06/0.38±0.094
Entropy	7.8±0.5/7±0.96	7.7±0.4/6.7±0.9	7.5±0.4/.6±0.9	7.5±0.6/6.6±1.1	7.4±0.5/7.01±0.8
DE	0.74±0.15/0.9±0.2	0.74±0.12/0.77±0.15	0.69±0.12/0.74±0.13	0.7±0.11/0.72±0.1	0.61±0.09/0.56±0.16
Coarseness	38±7/61±11	93±13/110±22	52±10/84±21	37±4/55±12	54±22/33±18

IQR, interquartile range; SOV, sum of squares variance; IDM, inverse difference moment; DE, difference entropy.

Table 10.7 Video quality metrics (mean±SD) for all ten videos of the CCA extracted between the original and the despeckled videos from the whole video and the ROI (–/–). © 2013. Reprinted with the permission from [4]

Features	DsFlsmv	DsFhmedian	DsFkuwahara	DsFsrad
SSI	0.98±0.01/0.98±0.05	0.97±0.001/0.96±0.06	0.77±0.025/0.84±0.03	0.96±0.025/0.88±0.08
VSNR	36±3.77/41±3.0	30±1.86/38±5.3	15±1.1/24.7±2.3	37±5.7/32±10
IFC	7.2±0.93/6.2±0.98	6.1±0.6/4.6±1.3	1.9±0.08/1.4±0.21	6.6±2.3/3.7±2.1
NQM	35.3±1.9/29±1.9	34±1.4/26.7±5.1	17.7±1.1/14.2±1.3	34.8±4.9/24.1±6.7
WSNR	34.8±1.8/38±0.91	33.1±1.1/35±5.4	18.8±0.9/20.6±1.3	39.1±5.2/25±8
PSNR	39.6±2.1/42.9±1.6	38.9±1.1/40.1±4.5	29.1±1.1/29.9±1.2	43.9±4.3/34.9±6.9

SSI, structural similarity index; VSNR, visual signal-to-noise ratio; IFC, information fidelity criterion; NQM, noise quality measure; WSNR, weighted signal-to-noise ratio; PSNR, peak signal-to-noise ratio.

Table 10.8 Percentage scoring of the original and despeckle videos by the experts. © 2013. Reprinted with the permission from [4]

Experts	Original	DsFlsmv	DsFhmedian	DsFkuwahara	DsFsrad
Expert 1	33	75	71	65	61
Expert 2	40	72	75	77	51
Average %	37	74	73	71	56
Ranking	–	1	2	3	4

terms of quality evaluation for the metrics structural SSI (similarity index), VSNR (visual signal-to-noise ratio), IFC (information fidelity criterion), NQM (noise quality measure), and WSNR (weighted signal-to-noise ratio) when applied on the whole frame. Moreover, all the investigated evaluation metrics gave better results when the DsFlsmv was applied only on the ROI, followed by the DsFhmedian.

Table 10.8 presents results of the visual perception evaluation of the original and despeckled videos made by the two experts (expert 1: a cardiovascular surgeon, expert 2: neurovascular specialist). The evaluation was performed on the whole despeckle video frame as well as to the ROI, where both methods gave similar visual evaluation scorings. The last two rows of Table 9.8 present the overall average percentage (%) score assigned by both experts for each filter and the filter ranking. It is shown in Table 9.8 that marginally the best video despeckle filter is the DsFlsmv with a score of 74%, followed by the filter DsFhmedian and DsFkuwahara with scores of 73% and 71%, respectively. It is interesting to note that the three filters, DsFlsmv, DsFhmedian, and DsFkuwahara, were scored with high evaluation markings by both experts. The filter DsFsrad gave poorer performance with an average score of 56%.

10.5 Video despeckle filtering based on texture analysis and visual quality evaluation (discussion)

Most of the papers published in the literature for video filtering are limited to the reduction of additive noise, mainly by frame averaging. More specifically, in [49], the Wiener filtering method was applied to 3D image sequences for filtering additive noise, but results have not been thoroughly discussed and compared with other methods. The method was superior when compared to the purely temporal operations implemented earlier [50]. The pyramid thresholding method was used in [50], and wavelet-based additive denoising was used in [51] for additive noise reduction in image sequences. In another study [52], the image quality and evaluation metrics were used for evaluating the additive noise filtering and the transmission of image sequences through telemedicine channels. An improvement of almost all the quality metrics extracted from the original and processed images was demonstrated. An additive noise reduction algorithm, for image sequences, using variance characteristics of the noise was presented in [53]. Estimated noise power and sum of absolute difference employed in motion estimation were used to determine the temporal filter coefficients. A noise measurement scheme using the correlation between the noisy input and the noise-free image was applied for accurate estimation of the noise power. The experimental results showed that the proposed noise reduction method efficiently removes noise. An efficient method for movie denoising that does not require any motion estimation was presented in [54]. The method was based on the fact that averaging several realizations of a random variable reduces the variance. The method was unsupervised and was adapted to denoise image sequences with an additive white noise while preserving the visual details on the movie frames. Very little attention has been paid to the problem of missing data (impulsive distortion) removal in image sequences. In [55], a 3D median filter for removing impulsive noise from image sequences was developed. This filter was implemented without motion compensation and so the results did not capture the full potential of these structures. Further, the median operation, although quite successful in the additive noise filtering in images, invariably introduces distortion while filtering of image sequences [55]. This distortion primarily takes the form of blurring fine image details.

The basic principles of despeckle filtering for still images presented in [1], i.e., the proposed despeckle filtering algorithms as well as the extraction of texture features, quality evaluation metrics and the optical perception evaluation procedure by experts, can also be applied to video. The application of despeckle filters, the extraction of texture features, the calculation of image quality metrics, and the visual perception evaluation by experts may also be applied to video. The video can be broken into frames, which can then be processed one by one and then grouped together to form the processed video. Preliminary results for the application of despeckle filtering in ultrasound carotid and cardiac video were presented in this chapter. However, significant work still remains to be carried out.

In a work made by our group [4], we evaluated four different video despeckling filtering techniques (DsFlsmv, DsFhmedian, DsFkuwahara, and DsFsrad) and applied them on ten ultrasound videos of the CCA. Our effort was to achieve multiplicative noise reduction in order to increase visual perception by the experts but also to make the videos suitable for further analysis such as video segmentation and coding. The video despeckle results were evaluated based on visual perception evaluation by two experts, different texture descriptors, and video quality metrics. The results showed that the best filtering method for ultrasound videos of the CCA is the DsFlsmv, followed by the despeckle filter DsFhmedian. Both filters performed best with respect to the visual evaluation by the experts as well as by the video quality metrics. It is noted that the evaluation performance for the DsFlsmv was slightly better. Our results in [4] are also consistent with our previous despeckle filtering results found in other studies performed by our group [5,37] on ultrasound images of the CCA, where the DsFlsmv filter was also found to be the preferred filter in terms of optical perception evaluation and classification accuracy between AS and SY plaques.

While there are a number of despeckle filtering techniques proposed in the literature for despeckle filtering on ultrasound images of the CCA, we have found no other studies in the literate for despeckle filtering in ultrasound videos of the CCA (with the exception of [4]). As it has been mentioned in the introduction, a number of studies investigated additive noise filtering in natural video sequences [56,57]. The usefulness of these methods in ultrasound video denoising of multiplicative noise still remains to be investigated.

It was shown in this chapter that despeckle filtering is an important operation in the enhancement of ultrasonic video of the carotid artery. Initial findings show some promises of the proposed techniques; however, more work is needed to further evaluate the performance of the despeckle filters presented. Future work will investigate the application of the proposed VDF methods in a larger video dataset as well as between AS and SY patients in order to select the most appropriate filleting method for the two different classes. Furthermore, the proposed despeckle filtering techniques will be investigated and evaluated as a preprocessing step in CCA automated ultrasound video segmentation and in a mobile health telemedicine system.

There are several studies reported in the literature for filtering additive noise from natural video sequences [56–60], but we have found no other studies (with the exception of [4]), where despeckle filtering on ultrasound medical videos (of the CCA) was investigated. Previous researches on the use of despeckle filtering of the CCA images [1–3,15,37], and videos [4], were also reported by our group where improved results were presented in terms of visual quality and classification accuracy between AS and SY plaques. Moreover, it should be mentioned that a significant number of studies investigated different despeckle filters in various medical ultrasound video modalities with very promising results [1,2].

The performance of the proposed VDF methods was evaluated in [4] after video normalization and despeckle filtering using visual perception evaluation, texture features, and image quality evaluation metrics.

The need for image standardization or postprocessing has been suggested in the past, and normalization using only blood echogenicity as a reference point has been applied in ultrasound images of carotid artery [61]. Brightness adjustments of the ultrasound images and videos have been used in this book as this has been shown to improve image compatibility by reducing the variability introduced by different gain settings and facilitate ultrasound tissue comparability [5,37,61].

The images and videos used for the image texture analysis and quality evaluation were normalized manually by linearly adjusting the image so that the median gray level value of the blood was 0–5, and the median gray level of the adventitia (artery wall) was 180–190. The scale of the gray level of the images ranged from 0 to 255 [61]. The normalization can be made using the IDF [3] and VDF [4] toolboxes for image and videos, respectively. This normalization using blood and adventitia as reference points was necessary in order to extract comparable measurements in case of processing images obtained by different operators or different equipment [61]. The image normalization procedure was implemented in MATLAB® software (version 6.1.0.450, release 12.1, May 2010, by The Mathworks, Inc.) and tested on a Pentium III desktop computer, running at 1.9 GHz, with 512 MB of RAM memory. The same software and computer station were also used for all other methods employed in this book.

10.6 Concluding remarks and future directions

Despeckle filtering is an important operation in the enhancement of ultrasound images and videos of the carotid artery, in the case of segmentation, texture analysis, quality evaluation, and visual evaluation by the experts. In this chapter, a total of 16 despeckle filters were comparatively evaluated on three sets of ultrasound images videos of the CCA, and the validation results are summarized below.

The filter DsFlsmv improved the feature distance (see Table 10.1), the image quality evaluation (see Table 10.4), and the optical perception (see Tables 10.5A and 10.5B) for both images and videos of the CCA (see Tables 10.2–10.5). The DsFlsmv filter also improved the accuracy of the IMC and plaque segmentation in ultrasound video. The filters DsFlsminsc, DsFhomo, and DsFhmedian improved the feature distance. Filters DsFlsmv, DsFlsminsc, DsFgf4d, DsFnldif, and DsFwaveltc improved the class separation between the AS and the SY classes (see also Table 10.2) for image despeckling. The filters DsFgf4d, DsFlsminsc, and DsFhomo improved the correct classification rate (see also Table 10.3) for image despeckling. Filters DsFlsmv, and DsFgf4d, and DsFhmedian improved the visual assessment carried out by the experts for images and videos of the CCA (see Tables 10.5A and 10.5B). Moreover, the filter DsFlsmv improved the accuracy of the IMC and plaque segmentation in ultrasound images and videos.

It is clearly shown that filter DsFlsmv gave the best performance for both images and videos of the CCA. It is followed by filters DsFgf4d, DsFlsminsc, and DsFhmedian. Filter DsFlsmv or DsFgf4d can be used for despeckling AS images, where the expert is interested mainly in the plaque composition and texture analysis. Filters DsFlsmv or DsFgf4d or DsFlsminsc of DsFhmedian can be used for despeckling of SY images, where the expert is interested in identifying the degree of stenosis and the plaque borders. Filters DsFhomo, DsFnldif, and DsFwaveltc gave poorer performance.

The results of our study showed that observer variability and sensitivity are important in image quality evaluation and can only be compensated when assessments are made against a standard scale of quality, such as the image quality evaluation metrics proposed in this study. Observer variability may also be compensated by additional tests employing image quality and texture measures, as proposed in this study, for quantifying image quality.

Despeckle filtering may also be applied in the preprocessing of ultrasound images for other organs, including the detection of hyperechoic or hypoechoic lesions in the kidney, liver, spleen, thyroid, kidney, echocardiographic images, mammography, and others. It may be particularly effective when combined with harmonic imaging since both can increase tissue contrast. Speckle reduction can also be extremely valuable when attempting to fuse ultrasound with CT, MRI, positron emission tomography, or optical coherence tomography images. For example, when a lesion is suspected on a CT scan but it is not clearly visible, ultrasound despeckle filtering can be applied in order to accentuate subtle borders that may be masked by speckle.

Great efforts are also currently made in optimizing the despeckle filtering algorithms in order to achieve better performance [1–5]. It is foreseen that optimization of a despeckling algorithm would be dependent on transducer geometry, operating frequency, focal point(s), distribution of pixel values due to speckle, subject being scanned, etc. Automatic selection of optimal despeckling algorithm's parameters would provide a useful tool for research and clinical applications.

Ultrasound imaging instrumentation, linked with imaging hardware and software technology, has been rapidly advancing in the last two decades. Although these advanced imaging devices produce higher quality images and video, the need still exists for better image and video processing techniques including despeckle filtering. Toward this direction, it is anticipated that the effective use of despeckle filtering (by exploiting the filters and algorithms documented in this book) will greatly help in producing images with higher quality. These images that would be not only easier to visualize and to extract useful information but would also enable the development of more robust image preprocessing and segmentation algorithms, minimizing routine manual image analysis and facilitating more accurate automated measurements of both industrially and clinically relevant parameters.

References

[1] C.P. Loizou, C.S. Pattichis, "Despeckle filtering for ultrasound imaging and video, Volume I: Algorithms and software," 2nd Ed., Synthesis lectures on algorithms and software in engineering, Ed. Morgran & Claypool Publishers, San Rafael, CA, vol. 7, no. 1, pp. 1–180, Apr. 2015. ISBN: 9781627056687.

[2] C.P. Loizou, C.S. Pattichis, "Despeckle filtering for ultrasound imaging and video, Vol. II: Selected applications," Synthesis lectures on algorithms and software in engineering, Ed. Morgan & Claypool Publishers, San Rafael, CA, vol. 7, no. 2, pp. 1–180, Aug. 2015, ISBN-9781627058148.

[3] C.P. Loizou, C. Theofanous, M. Pantziaris, T. Kasparis, "Despeckle filtering software toolbox for ultrasound imaging of the common carotid artery," Comput. Methods Programs Biomed., vol. 114, no. 1, pp. 109–124, 2014.

[4] C.P. Loizou, C. Theofanous, M. Pantziaris, *et al.*, "Despeckle filtering toolbox for medical ultrasound video," Int. J. Monit. Surveill. Technol. Res. (IJMSTR): Special issue Biomed. Monitor. Technol., vol. 4, no. 1, pp. 61–79, 2013.

[5] C.P. Loizou, C.S. Pattichis, C.I. Christodoulou, R.S.H. Istepanian, M. Pantziaris, A. Nicolaides, "Comparative evaluation of despeckle filtering in

ultrasound imaging of the carotid artery," IEEE Trans. Ultrason. Ferroelectr. Freq. Control, vol. 52, no. 10, pp. 1653–1669, 2005.

[6] C. Christodoulou, C. Pattichis, M. Pantziaris, A. Nicolaides, "Texture-based classification of atherosclerotic carotid plaques," IEEE Trans. Med. Imaging, vol. 22, no. 7, pp. 902–912, 2003.

[7] R.M. Haralick, K. Shanmugam, I. Dinstein, "Texture features for image classification," IEEE Trans. Syst. Man Cybern., vol. SMC-3, pp. 610–621, Nov. 1973.

[8] J.S Weszka., C.R. Dyer, A. Rosenfield, "A comparative study of texture measures for terrain classification," IEEE Trans. Syst. Man Cybern., vol. SMC-6, pp. 269–285, Apr. 1976.

[9] M. Amadasun, R. King, "Textural features corresponding to textural properties," IEEE Trans. Syst. Man Cybern., vol. 19, no. 5, pp. 1264–1274, 1989.

[10] C.M. Wu, Y.C. Chen, K.-S. Hsieh, "Texture features for classification of ultrasonic images," IEEE Trans. Med. Imaging, vol. 11, pp. 141–152, 1992.

[11] E. Trouve, Y. Chambenoit, N. Classeau, P. Bolon, "Statistical and operational performance assessment of multi-temporal SAR image filtering," IEEE Trans. Geosci. Remote Sens., vol. 41, no. 11, pp. 2519–2539, 2003.

[12] F. Rakebrandt, D.C. Crawford, D. Havard, D. Coleman, J.P. Woodcock, "Relation between ultrasound texture classification images and histology of atherosclerotic plaque," J. Ultrasound Med. Biol., vol. 26, no. 9, pp. 1393–1402, 2000.

[13] M. Pattichis, C. Pattichis, M. Avraam, A. Bovik, K. Kyriakou, "AM-FM texture segmentation in electron microscopic muscle imaging," IEEE Trans. Med. Imaging, vol. 19, no. 12, pp. 1253–1258, 2000.

[14] N. Mudigonda, R. Rangayyan, J. Desautels, "Detection of breast masses in mammograms by density slicing and texture flow-field analysis," IEEE Trans. Med. Imaging, vol. 20, no. 12, pp. 121–1227, 2001.

[15] C.I. Christodoulou, S.C. Michaelides, C.S. Pattichis, "Multi-feature texture analysis for the classification of clouds in satellite imagery," IEEE Trans. Geosci. Remote Sens., vol. 41, no. 11, pp. 2662–2668, Nov. 2003.

[16] S. Solbo, T. Eltoft, "Homomorphic wavelet based-statistical despeckling of SAR images," IEEE Trans. Geosci. Remote Sens., vol. 42, no. 4, pp. 711–721, 2004.

[17] S.M. Ali, R.E. Burge, "New automatic techniques for smoothing and segmenting SAR images," Signal Process., North-Holland, vol. 14, pp. 335–346, 1988.

[18] C.K. Zarins, C. Xu, S. Glagov, "Atherosclerotic enlargement of the human abdominal aorta," Atherosclerosis, vol. 155, no. 1, pp. 157–164, 2001.

[19] Y. Yongjian, S.T. Acton, "Speckle reducing anisotropic diffusion," IEEE Trans. Image Process., vol. 11, no. 11, pp. 1260–1270, 2002.

[20] S. Jin, Y. Wang, J. Hiller, "An adaptive non-linear diffusion algorithm for filtering medical images," IEEE Trans. Inf. Technol. Biomed., vol. 4, no. 4, pp. 298–305, Dec. 2000.

[21] K. Abd-Elmoniem, A.-B. Youssef, Y. Kadah, "Real-time speckle reduction and coherence enhancement in ultrasound imaging via nonlinear anisotropic diffusion," IEEE Trans. Biomed. Eng., vol. 49, no. 9, pp. 997–1014, Sep. 2002.

[22] X. Hao, S. Gao, X. Gao, "A novel multiscale nonlinear thresholding method for ultrasonic speckle suppressing," IEEE Trans. Med. Imaging, vol. 18, no. 9, pp. 787–794, 1999.

[23] A. Baraldi, F. Pannigianni, "A refined gamma MAP SAR speckle filter with improved geometrical adaptivity," IEEE Trans. Geosci. Remote Sens., vol. 33, no. 5, pp. 1245–1257, Sep. 1995.

[24] M. Karaman, M. A. Kutay, G. Bozdagi, "An adaptive speckle suppression filter for medical ultrasonic imaging," IEEE Trans. Med. Imaging, vol. 14, no. 2, pp. 283–292, 1995.

[25] A. Achim, A. Bezerianos, P. Tsakalides, "Novel Bayesian multiscale method for speckle removal in medical ultrasound images," IEEE Trans. Med. Imaging, vol. 20, no. 8, pp. 772–783, 2001.

[26] X. Zong, A. Laine, E. Geiser, "Speckle reduction and contrast enhancement of echocardiograms via multiscale nonlinear processing," IEEE Trans. Med. Imaging, vol. 17, no. 4, pp. 532–540, 1998.

[27] N. Rougon, F. Preteux, "Controlled anisotropic diffusion," Conference on Nonlinear Image Processing VI, IS&T/SPIE Symposium on Electronic Imaging, Science and Technology, San Jose, California, pp. 1–12, 5–10 Feb. 1995.

[28] A.M. Wink, J.B.T.M. Roerdink, "Denoising functional MR images: A comparison of wavelet denoising and Gaussian smoothing," IEEE Trans. Med. Imaging, vol. 23, no. 3, pp. 374–387, 2004.

[29] H.-L. Eng, K.-K. Ma, "Noise adaptive soft-switching median filter," IEEE Trans. Image Process., vol. 10, no. 2, pp. 242–251, 2001.

[30] H.R. Sheikh, A.C. Bovik, G. de Veciana, "An information fidelity criterion for image quality assessment using natural scene statistics," IEEE Trans. Image Process., vol. 14, no. 12, pp. 2117–2128, Dec. 2005.

[31] D.L. Donoho, "Denoising by soft thresholding," IEEE Trans. Inf. Theory, vol. 41, pp. 613–627, 1995.

[32] J.S. Lee, "Digital image enhancement and noise filtering by using local statistics," IEEE Trans. Pattern Anal. Mach. Intell., vol. PAMI-2, no. 2, pp. 165–168, 1980.

[33] M. Black, G. Sapiro, D. Marimont, D. Heeger, "Robust anisotropic diffusion," IEEE Trans. Image Process., vol. 7, no. 3, pp. 421–432, Mar. 1998.

[34] D. Schilling, P.C. Cosman, "Image quality evaluation based on recognition times for fast browsing image applications," IEEE Trans. Multimedia, vol. 4, no. 3, pp. 320–331, Sep. 2002.

[35] A. Pommert, K. Hoehne, "Evaluation of image quality in medical volume visualization: The state of the art," Takeyoshi Dohi, Ron Kikinis (eds.): Medical image computing and computer-assisted intervention, Proc.,

MICCAI, 2002, Part II, Lecture Notes in Computer Science, 2489, pp. 598–605, Springer Verlag, Berlin 2002.

[36] Z. Wang, A. Bovik, H. Sheikh, E. Simoncelli, "Image quality assessment: From error measurement to structural similarity," IEEE Trans. Image Process., vol. 13, no. 4, pp. 600–612, 2004.

[37] C.P. Loizou, C.S. Pattichis, M. Pantziaris, T. Tyllis, A. Nicolaides, "Quantitative quality evaluation of ultrasound imaging in the carotid artery," Med. Biol. Eng. Comput., vol. 44, no. 5, pp. 414–426, 2006.

[38] C.P. Loizou, C.S. Pattichis, M. Pantziaris, T. Tyllis, A. Nicolaides, "Snakes based segmentation of the common carotid artery intima media," Med. Biol. Eng. Comput., vol. 45, no. 1, pp. 35–49, Jan. 2007.

[39] C.P. Loizou, C.S. Pattichis, M. Pantziaris, A. Nicolaides, "An integrated system for the segmentation of atherosclerotic carotid plaque," IEEE Trans. Inform. Techn. Biomed., vol. 11, no. 5, pp. 661–667, 2007.

[40] J.E. Wilhjelm, M.S. Jensen, S.K. Jespersen, B. Sahl, E. Falk, "Visual and quantitative evaluation of selected image combination schemes in ultrasound spatial compound scanning," IEEE Trans. Med. Imaging, vol. 23, no. 2, pp. 181–190, 2004.

[41] T.J. Chen, K.S. Chuang, J. Wu, S.C. Chen, I.M. Hwang, M.L. Jan, "A novel image quality index using Moran I statistics," Phys. Med. Biol., vol. 48, pp. 131–137, 2003.

[42] M. Eckert, "Perceptual quality metrics applied to still image compression," Canon information systems research, Faculty of Engineering, University of Technology, Sydney, Australia, pp. 1–26, 2002.

[43] J.C. Bamber, C. Daft, "Adaptive filtering for reduction of speckle in ultrasonic pulse-echo images," Ultrasonic, vol. 24, pp. 41–44, 1986.

[44] J.T.M. Verhoeven, J.M. Thijssen, "Improvement of lesion detectability by speckle reduction filtering: A quantitative study," Ultrason. Imaging, vol. 15, pp. 181–204, 1993.

[45] C. Kotropoulos, I. Pitas, "Optimum nonlinear signal detection and estimation in the presence of ultrasonic speckle," Ultrason. Imaging, vol. 14, pp. 249–275, 1992.

[46] E. Brusseau, C.L. De Korte, F. Mastick, J. Schaar, A.F.W. Van der Steen, "Fully automatic luminal contour segmentation in intracoronary ultrasound imaging-A statistical approach," IEEE Trans. Med. Imaging, vol. 23, no. 5, pp. 554–566, 2004.

[47] M.E. Olszewski, A. Wahle, S.C. Vigmostad, M. Sonka, "Multidimensional segmentation of coronary intravascular ultrasound images using knowledge-based methods," Med. Imaging: Image Processing, Proc. SPIE, 5747, pp. 496–504, 2005.

[48] M.R. Cardinal, J. Meunier, G. Soulez, E. Thérasse, G. Cloutier, "Intravascular ultrasound image segmentation: A fast-marching method," Proc., MICCAI, LNCS 2879, pp. 432–439, 2003.

[49] M. Oezkan, A. Erdem, M. Sezan, A. Tekalp, "Efficient multi-frame Wiener restoration of blurred and noisy image sequences," IEEE Trans. Image Process., vol. 1, pp. 453–476, Oct. 1992.

[50] P.M.B. Van Roosmalen, S.J.P Westen, R.L. Lagendijk, J. Biemond, "Noise reduction for image sequences using an oriented pyramid threshold technique," IEEE Int. Conf. Image Process., vol. 1, pp. 375–378, 1996.

[51] M. Vetterli, J. Kovacevic, Wavelets and sub band coding, Englewood Cliffs, NJ: Prentice Hall, 1995.

[52] S. Winkler, "Digital video quality," Vision models and metrics, Chichester, West Sussex: John Wiley & Sons Ltd., 2005.

[53] J.-H. Jung, K. Hong, S. Yang, "Noise reduction using variance characteristics in noisy image sequence," Int. Conf. on Consumer Electronics, pp. 213–214, 8–12 Jan. 2005.

[54] M. Bertalmio, V. Caselles, A. Pardo, "Movie denoising by average of warped lines," IEEE Trans. Image Process., vol. 16, no. 9, pp. 233–2347, 2007.

[55] B. Alp, P. Haavisto, T. Jarske, K. Oestaemoe, Y. Neuro, "Median based algorithms for image sequence processing," SPIE Visual Communications and Image Processing, pp. 122–133, 1990.

[56] V. Zlokolica, W. Philips, D. van de Ville, "Robust non-linear filtering for video processing," *IEEE 14th Int. Conf. Digit. Sign. Process.*, Santorini, Greece, pp. 1–4, 1–3 July 2002.

[57] V. Zlokolica, A. Pizurica, W. Philips, "Recursive temporal denoising and motion estimation of video," Int. Conf. Image Process., vol. 3, no. 3, pp. 1465–1468, 2008.

[58] M. Maggioni, G. Boracchi, A. Foi, K. Engiazarian, "Video denoising, deblocking and enhancement through separable 4-D nonlocal spatiotemporal transforms," IEEE Trans. Image Process., vol. 21, no. 9, pp. 3952–3966, 2012.

[59] C. Lui, W.T. Freeman, "A high-quality video denoising algorithm based on reliable motion estimation," European Conf. on Computer Vision, pp. 706–719, 2010.

[60] T.W. Chan, O.C. Au, T.S. Chong, W.S. Chau, "A novel content-adaptive video denoising filter," IEEE Proc. Vision Image Signal Process., vol. 2, no. 2, pp. 649–652, 2005.

[61] T. Elatrozy, A. Nicolaides, T. Tegos, A. Zarka, M. Griffin, M. Sabetai, "The effect of B-mode ultrasonic image standardization of the echodensity of symptomatic and asymptomatic carotid bifurcation plaque," Int. Angiol., vol. 17, no. 3, pp. 179–186, 1998.

Chapter 11
Summary and future directions

Christos P. Loizou[1]

In this final chapter of Part II, we present the summary findings of the different despeckle filtering algorithms presented in Part II by summarising the results presented in Chapters 5–10. Furthermore, areas of future research directions on despeckle filtering are briefly discussed.

11.1 Summary on despeckle filtering

We have shown in this part that despeckle filtering may be used as an important operation for the enhancement of ultrasound images, and videos not only in the common carotid artery (CCA) but also in many other clinical organ images and/or video acquired by ultrasound. Despeckle filtering may be applied as a preprocessing step in the cases of segmentation, texture analysis, quality evaluation, visual evaluation by the experts and in image and video encoding [1–3]. In this book, a number of despeckle filtering techniques were presented and evaluated on artificial and real ultrasound images and videos.

Chapter 5 introduced the reader into the field of speckle filtering, by emphasising its characteristics that are relevant for every practitioner in the field. The importance of preserving information over drastic filtering was discussed, as well as that different speckle filters may demonstrate a very good performance for one particular application but can miserably fail in other cases.

Chapter 6 provided an introduction and an overview of selected despeckle filtering techniques for ultrasound imaging and video. Chapter 7 provided the basic theoretical background of linear despeckle filtering techniques (first-order statistics filtering, local statistics filtering and homogeneous mask area filtering), together with their algorithmic implementation MATLAB® code for selected filters and practical examples on phantom and real ultrasound images. Despeckle filtering was evaluated for all filters presented in this chapter on phantom ultrasound carotid artery images and real ultrasound images and videos of the CCA. An evaluation and comparison of five linear despeckle filtering algorithms was presented, which was carried out on a phantom image, an artificial image and on real carotid and cardiac ultrasound images. Furthermore, findings on video despeckling are presented.

[1]Department of Electrical and Computer Engineering, University of Cyprus, Cyprus

Chapter 8 presents a review on some of the methods proposed in literature to remove the speckle pattern from ultrasound data based on non-linear processing. For some purposes, a simple multiplicative model will suffice, while for some specific applications, more accurate models must be used. It is concluded that the filtering method must be selected following the specific needs of the problem. There is no all-purpose filter that, with the same configuration parameters, could perform excellently in all situations.

Wavelet despeckle filtering is presented in Chapter 9. The effect of transform features (shift-sensitivity and directional selectivity) has been examined by implementing the homomorphic and non-homomorphic speckle suppressors in three alternative wavelet domains; discrete wavelet transform (DWT), redundant wavelet transform (RDWT) and complex wavelet transform (CWT). The experimental results demonstrated that performance of DWT is worst on all type of images, whereas the performance of RDWT and dual tree complex wavelet transform (DT-CWT) is comparable. It was finally concluded that both DT-CWT and RDWT are equally good for designing wavelet-based denoising applications. However, the low-computational complexity of DT-CWT and the textured nature of medical US images favour the use of DT-CWT in comparison to RDWT for despeckling applications. More work is required to develop shorter length filters for the DT-CWT (e.g. analogous to Haar wavelet), in order to further improve the despeckling performance of the US images.

Chapter 10 presented methods of texture analysis and image-quality evaluation, which may be used to evaluate despeckle filtering on ultrasound imaging and video.

11.2 Future directions

All different despeckle filtering algorithms and the measures which may be used for the qualitative evaluation of the algorithms as introduced in this book can also be applied to other image and video processing application areas. It should be furthermore noted that we have presented and investigated in this part only a small number of despeckle filtering algorithms and image-quality evaluation metrics. Numerous other extensions, additions, improvements and applications can be envisaged.

A lot of work has been reported in the literature on the development of despeckle filtering algorithms for image and lately for video despeckling. Although this is a very well-investigated field and many researchers have been involved in this subject, there is still not an appropriate method proposed or found, which will satisfy both criteria set in this book. These criteria are the visual perception of the image/video and the automated interpretation of image processing and analysis tasks. It should be furthermore noted that it is important to promote and perform more comparative studies of despeckle filtering, where other different filters could be evaluated by using multiple experts. Furthermore, the use of additional image quality and evaluation metrics together with those presented in this chapter may be used for a complete quantitative evaluation of the algorithms.

In the area of video despeckling, there is still a lot of work which remains to be done. This area is currently being investigated by many researchers and new methods which are adapted specifically for video filtering are being investigated and proposed. It is noted, however, that the proposed methods and algorithms as documented in this book may be also investigated in video sequences (by frame filtering). There still are many issues related to video despeckle filtering that remain to be solved. In general, the development of a multiplicative model based on video sequences is required, since most of the models developed for video filtering were for additive noise [4–7]. Furthermore, the adaptation of the algorithm for effectively filtering the consecutive video frames and the tuning of the different despeckle filtering parameters are also important issues, where a solution still needs to be found.

Despeckle filtering algorithms and techniques presented in this book may be also used as a preprocessing step in ultrasound images or videos for other organs. This includes the detection of hyperechoic or hypoechoic lesions in the kidney, lesions or tumours in the liver, estimate the size of the spleen, thyroid including hyperthyroidism or hypothyroidism, kidney injury using texture analysis, echocardiographic images, detect and analyse lesions in ultrasound mammography and other. Despeckle filtering may be increasingly effective when combined with harmonic imaging, in which they both increase tissue contrast. Despeckle filtering may also be found useful in different other applications when trying for example to fuse ultrasound with other imaging technologies such as computed tomography (CT), MRI, positron emission tomography or optical coherence tomography. In a clinical case where an examination has been performed with a CT scan and a lesion is suspected, but it is not very clearly visible, then despeckle filtering may be applied for accentuating subtle details and the borders of the suspected lesion/s, which may be masked by speckle noise. It was also shown, from our group, that speckle reduction filtering maybe used to further enhance the performance in image and video encoding and transmission. More specifically, it was shown in [8] that despeckle filtering may favour the transportation of videos of atherosclerotic carotid plaques over a wireless telemedicine channel, thus reducing the cost of the transmission significantly as well as increasing the optical perception evaluation. Previous surveys of encoding methods in other areas have been reported in [9–12].

There are rapid advancements in ultrasound imaging and video instrumentation which are closely linked with imaging hardware and software technology advancements in the last two decades. Although these advanced instrumentations for imaging and video devices produce higher quality images and video, still the need exists for better image and video processing techniques including despeckle filtering.

We anticipate, therefore, to exploit the effectiveness of the filters and algorithms presented in this book towards the above-mentioned directions. The application of them will greatly help in generating images and videos with higher perceptual quality. The images or videos would be then easier to visualised, interpreted, as well as to be used for further image analysis by extracting useful information in the form of texture features as also document in this book. The despeckle filtering techniques may be furthermore used to enable the development of more robust image preprocessing and segmentation algorithms. Furthermore, they may aid in minimising routine manual image analysis and facilitating more accurate automated measurements of both industrially and clinically relevant parameters.

It should be noted that the processing time of the proposed algorithmic methods presented in Part II could be further reduced by applying despeckle filtering only on selected areas of the image. Furthermore, software optimisation methods (i.e. the MATLAB software optimisation toolbox) could be investigated for increasing the performance of the proposed image despeckle filtering [3] and video despeckle filtering [2] software systems. Finally, it should be noted that the proposed methods could also be applied to other applications, such as echocardiography, but a direct comparison of the results produces with this study will not be possible as different results will be produced with a different database.

In [2], selected applications on despeckle filtering for images and videos were presented, where a more detailed despeckle filtering evaluation protocol, which is based on texture features, image-quality evaluation metrics and multiple observer's evaluation on a large number of images and videos is presented. More specifically, applications of despeckle filtering on ultrasound imaging and video of the intima-media complex, plaque segmentation and texture analysis are in detailed presented. Moreover, the usefulness of despeckle filtering in reducing bandwidth needs in an ultrasound video telemedicine platform is furthermore discussed.

References

[1] C. P. Loizou, C. S. Pattichis, "Despeckle filtering for ultrasound imaging and video, Volume I: Algorithms and software," 2nd Ed., Synthesis lectures on algorithms and software in engineering, Ed. Morgran & Claypool Publishers, San Rafael, CA, vol. 7, no. 1, pp. 1–180, April 2015. ISBN: 9781627056687.

[2] C. P. Loizou, C. S. Pattichis, "Despeckle filtering for ultrasound imaging and video, Vol. II: Selected applications," Synthesis lectures on algorithms and software in engineering, Ed. Morgan & Claypool Publishers, San Rafael, CA, vol. 7, no. 2, pp. 1–180, August 2015, ISBN: 9781627058148.

[3] C. P. Loizou, C. Theofanous, M. Pantziaris, T. Kasparis, "Despeckle filtering software toolbox for ultrasound imaging of the common carotid artery," *Comput. Methods Programs Biomed.*, vol. 114, no. 1, pp. 109–124, 2014.

[4] S. Winkler, "Digital video quality," Vision models and metrics, Chichester, West Sussex: John Wiley & Sons Ltd., 2005.

[5] J.-H. Jung, K. Hong, S. Yang, "Noise reduction using variance characteristics in noisy image sequence," *Int. Conf. Consumer Electronics*, pp. 213–214, 8–12 January 2005.

[6] M. Bertalmio, V. Caselles, A. Pardo, "Movie Denoising by average of warped lines," *IEEE Trans. Image Process.*, vol. 16, no. 9, pp. 233–2347, 2007.

[7] B. Alp, P. Haavisto, T. Jarske, K. Oestaemoe, Y. Neuro, "Median based algorithms for image sequence processing," *Proc. SPIE Visual Commun. Image Process.*, Lausanne, Switzerland, vol. 1360, pp. 122–133, 1990.

[8] A. Panayides, M. S. Pattichis, C. S. Pattichis, C. P. Loizou, M. Pantziaris, A. Pitsillides, "Atherosclerotic plaque ultrasound video encoding, wireless transmission, and quality assessment using H.264," *IEEE Trans. Inf. Technol. Biomed.*, vol. 15, no. 3, pp. 387–397, 2011.

[9] T. Painter, A. S. Spanias, "Perceptual coding of digital audio," *Proc. IEEE*, vol. 88, no. 4, pp. 451–513, 2000.

[10] A. S. Spanias, "Digital signal processing; an interactive approach," 2nd Ed., Textbook with JAVA exercises, Lulu Press On-demand Publishers, Morrisville, NC, 403 pages, May 2014. ISBN: 978–971–4675–9892.

[11] A. S. Spanias, "Speech coding: A tutorial review," *Proc. IEEE*, vol. 82, no. 10, pp. 1441–1582, 1994.

[12] J. Thiagarajan, K. Ramamurthy, P. Turaga, A. Spanias, "Image understanding using sparse representations," Synthesis lectures on image, video, and multimedia processing, Ed. Al Bovik: Morgan & Claypool Publishers, 118 pages, 2014. 978–1627053594.

Part III

Speckle tracking

Chapter 12
Introduction to speckle tracking in ultrasound video

Gijs A.G.M. Hendriks[1], *Stein Fekkes*[1], *Kaj Gijsbertse*[2] *and Chris L. De Korte*[1,3]

Ultrasound imaging is widely used in the medical field since the modality is relatively cheap and can be applied nearly in all clinical environments due to its portability. Static images have been used to assess anatomical and geometrical features, but one of the unique features of ultrasound is its capability of examining dynamic events. In addition to anatomical and echogenicity features, ultrasound can provide information regarding movement of tissues. Quantification of tissue motion will be of interest in fundamental and clinical questions; from the motion, the deformability of the tissue can be quantified. When this deformation is induced by a force applied onto the tissue, the deformation is associated with its mechanical structure and composition. But it can also reveal functional behaviour when the deformation is representing the function of the targeted tissue.

There is a vast amount of ultrasound techniques for the detection of tissue motion (functional imaging). For many years, M-mode imaging played an important role in evaluation of rapid motions because of its high sampling rate. Other techniques based on the Doppler effect or applying block-matching algorithms for tracking tissue motion are available. Nowadays, as a result of rapid developments in ultrafast ultrasound imaging, techniques are available that permit fast and complex motions to be measured more accurately. This chapter will introduce the most commonly used techniques in clinical practice and will provide an overview of past and current developments in functional ultrasound imaging.

12.1 M-mode

Motion-mode (M-mode) imaging provides very high temporal resolution (theoretically up to 10,000 lines per second) of tissue motion along a single ultrasound

[1]Medical UltraSound Imaging Center, Department of Radiology and Nuclear Medicine, Radboud University Medical Center, the Netherlands

[2]Orthopaedic Research Laboratory, Department of Orthopedics, Radboud University Medical Center, the Netherlands

[3]Physics of Fluids Group, MIRA, University of Twente, the Netherlands

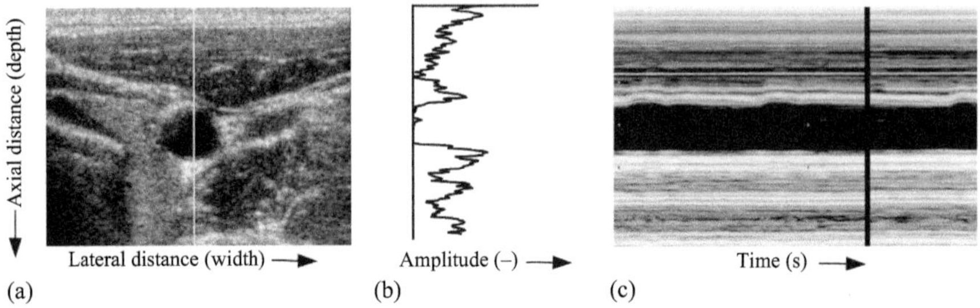

Figure 12.1 *(a) Example of a B-mode ultrasound image of a carotid artery. (b) Single scan line along the white line in image (a). The single scan line as a function of time is called M-mode imaging (c). Figure courtesy of H.H.G Hansen*

beam, and was primarily developed for use in cardiology for diagnostic examinations of the myocardium and heart valves [1–3].

12.1.1 Methods

M-mode ultrasound imaging represents a 1-D view of anatomical structures over time. Initially, a 2-D (B-mode) image is acquired and a single scan line (A-mode) is selected resembling the area of interest. The M-mode shows how the structures intersected by that line move towards or away from the probe and thus also with respect to each other over time as visualized for a carotid artery (Figure 12.1).

12.1.2 Applications

In cardiology, the determination of tissue motion provides a quantitative measure of the cardiac function. M-mode imaging allows determining heart wall motion, thickness change and ventricular volume measurements [1–5]. These parameters deviate in patients with valve stenosis or insufficiency compared to patients with healthy cardiac function. Left ventricle volume measurements allow the estimation of cardiac ejection fraction using Simpson's rule [6,7]. Since there is a clear delineation between tissue and blood due to the different scattering properties, cardiology and vascular diseases are the main fields of application. M-mode ultrasound has been used to estimate arterial stiffness, compliance and distensibility, which provide useful information of atherosclerotic progression [8]. Furthermore, M-mode ultrasound has also been used for non-cardiovascular applications, such as quantification of diaphragmatic motion during respiration [9] and change of diaphragm thickness in relation to contractile activity [10]. Similar work has been performed to study the onset of force transmission in skeletal muscles combining M-mode ultrasound and electromyography [11–13].

For many years, B-mode imaging and M-mode traces of boundary position versus time have been the main clinical tools to study tissue motion. More recently, sophisticated detection and imaging techniques have been developed based on the Doppler effect and on tracking motion in tissue images using speckle tracking.

12.2 Doppler imaging

Ultrasound techniques based on the Doppler principle are the predecessors of many tissue motion imaging methods. This technique has been available to clinicians for nearly 60 years [14,15] and cannot only be used to particularly quantify blood velocity but also to assess tissue motion.

12.2.1 Method

When an acoustic reflector like tissue has a certain speed, the reflected ultrasound signals will not have exactly the same frequency, but the frequency will be shifted (the Doppler frequency). In (12.1), the Doppler equation is presented, where the relation between the Doppler frequency (f_D) and tissue velocity (v) is summarized. In this equation, c is the speed of sound in tissue and blood (normally 1,540 m s^{-1} is taken), θ is the angle between the direction of the motion of the tissue and f_0 the original centre frequency of the ultrasound signal. Tissue moving towards the ultrasound transducer produces positive Doppler-shifted signals and conversely, tissue moving away from the transducer produces negative-shifted Doppler-shifted signals. Doppler imaging techniques provide information regarding the presence, direction and velocity of tissue motion.

$$f_D = \frac{2 \cdot f_0 \cdot v \cdot \cos\theta}{c} \tag{12.1}$$

There are several modalities of this technique to provide more clinical information about the flow in the body. The three standard modalities are continuous wave, pulsed wave, colour and power Doppler. In continuous wave imaging, ultrasound waves are emitted continuously from a transmitting (part of a) transducer while the back-scattered signal is simultaneously received, typically by a different part of the same transducer or a second transducer. Doppler shifts from all tissue moving in the overlap of the transmitted and received beam are observed. By using quadrature demodulation, continuous wave Doppler provides the global direction and intensity of the mean velocity component in the overlapping area. Pulsed wave Doppler uses pulsed ultrasound waves instead of continuous ultrasound. This allows to analyse the Doppler-shifted frequencies from a particular range in time (and therefore, related to the depth along the beam line), thus providing local velocity estimations. Colour flow imaging expands the principle of pulsed wave Doppler along a number of acoustic lines and time ranges. The result is a two-dimensional region with local velocity estimations. Usually the tissue velocity is represented in colour, superimposed on the two-dimensional B-mode image. In power Doppler imaging, the power of the Doppler signal, and not the direction or the value of the Doppler shift is visualized.

In diagnostic ultrasound, these techniques are mainly used to image blood flow, but can also be used to diagnose many cardiovascular conditions, including:

- Heart valve defects and regurgitation;
- Narrowing (stenosis) of an artery;
- A blocked artery (arterial occlusion);
- Blood clots (thrombosis) and
- Varicose veins (venous insufficiency).

The signal amplitude of the back-scattered echoes from blood is relatively low compared to the signal amplitude of the surrounding soft tissues. Therefore, advanced processing is required to detect and separate the blood signals from the surrounding signals, also referred to as clutter filtering. Clutter filters are high-pass filters which filter out the (low) Doppler-shifted frequencies of the surrounding tissue.

12.2.2 Limitations

The Doppler frequency shift is determined by the velocity of the tissue or particles in the direction co-aligned with the ultrasound beam. That implies that when an angle is present between the velocity direction and the ultrasound beam, the projection of the velocity component on the beam determines the frequency shift (see (12.1)). Consequently, additional information about the direction of motion is necessary in order to quantify the magnitude of the velocity vector. The angle dependency is one of the major limitations of the current Doppler techniques since it necessitates an assumption of the flow or motion direction to get a quantitative estimate of the velocity. Especially in complex motion patterns, valid assumptions about the direction of motion are difficult to make since it can vary to a large degree spatially and temporally.

To overcome these limitations, many methods have been suggested to provide an accurate estimate of the full blood/tissue velocity vector. Cross-beam methods, also called vector Doppler [16], utilize multiple 1-D Doppler measurements from different directions to determine the 2-D velocity vector. An alternative technique to estimate the blood velocity, or tissue motion, is the use of speckle tracking techniques [17]. These techniques will be discussed later in this chapter.

12.3 Tissue Doppler imaging

The Doppler principle, explained in the previous section, can be applied to estimate either tissue movement or blood movement. Although the principle is the same, the difference lies in the post-processing. The two main subjects of interest differ in two dominant ways: ultrasound intensity and speed of movement. Mainly, blood has a low intensity and high velocity while the surrounding tissue shows the opposite. Differentiation between blood and tissue is thus a matter of filtering. Tissue Doppler imaging (TDI) is a variation of colour Doppler imaging and can be implemented using a low-pass filter to record low velocities and suppress signals from the movement of blood.

12.3.1 Method

The method to measure tissue movements by low-pass filtering is called TDI [18]. For this, multiple ultrasound excitations with a certain pulse repetition frequency are applied onto the tissue. The received sonographic signal represents the tissue at a certain depth position. When the received signal is compared to the original pulse frequency, the velocity could be estimated by the difference in transmit-to-receive time from the first pulse to the second as the tissue moves through the insonification area. This difference is expressed in terms of a phase shift from which the Doppler frequency is derived as explained earlier. This phase shift representing velocity information can be acquired by an autocorrelation technique correlating the signal with itself at different time points. This information is usually overlaid onto the B-mode image, which is called Duplex ultrasonography and indicates tissue velocity from or towards the transducer. This method can acquire real-time tissue velocities across the whole B-mode image.

12.3.2 Applications

One of the major applications of TDI is the assessment of the cardiac function by measuring physiological information. Aspects like left ventricular diastolic function, filling pressure, temporal evaluation of ventricular systolic contraction or sub-clinical left ventricular dysfunction could be assessed by TDI. Amongst many of these parameters assessed by TDI, the peak systolic and diastolic tissue velocities seems the most simple and robust. Tissue velocities of the myocardium are obtained using 2-D real-time B-mode images (see Figure 12.2), infarcted muscle areas show a loss of normal cyclic wall thickening changes, resulting in decreased velocity or an asynchronous velocity pattern compared to healthy myocardial tissue.

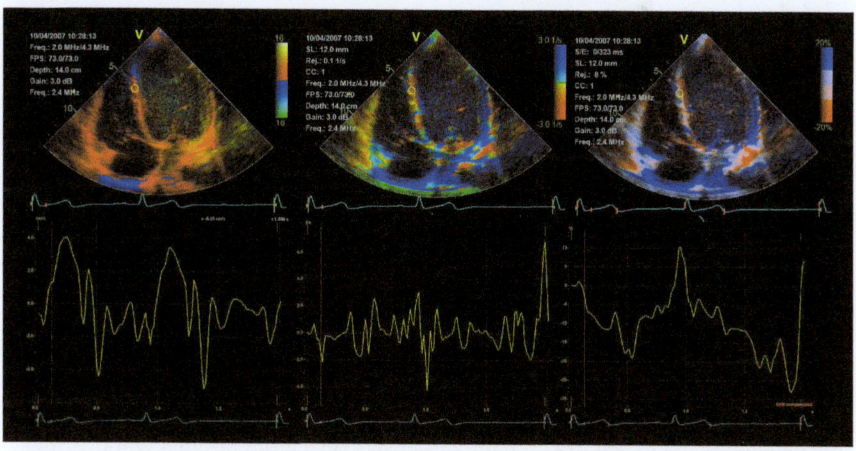

Figure 12.2 (a) TDI applied onto a long-axial view of the heart overlaid with the colour-coded tissue velocities and traces below. (b) The measure of the velocity of deformation of the myocardium is given by Strain Rate Imaging. (c) Integration of the strain rate with respect to time yields the strain, which is the relative shortening and lengthening of the myocardium along the cardiac cycle. Images are composed of sub-images originating from the software package GE EchoPAC version 113.1.3

Other applications of TDI could be found in the area of musculoskeletal ultrasound where it is used for measuring muscle and tendon contractile velocity [11]. In this study, a vector tissue Doppler technique was used to acquire the full 2-D velocity vector using two different ultrasound beams steered at different angles [19]. From the vector muscle and tendon motion, strain rate and strain were obtained during the execution of dynamic tasks.

12.3.3 TDI-based strain (rate) imaging

A more comprehensive assessment of the local myocardial contraction and relaxation, representing regional tissue (dis) function, can be derived from deformation parameters. This has led to the development of a local functional parameter based on tissue motion. Deformation imaging can be based on different underlying motion estimation techniques, like speckle tracking, RF tracking or TDI. The latter method was used to perform strain rate imaging [20] since the strain rate equals the velocity gradient. The strain rate, or in other words, the rate of deformation was calculated by taking the difference between two velocity estimates divided by the distance between them. This yields the difference in tissue velocity per unit length. Heimdal and Stoylen [20] were the first ones to describe this technique. Temporal integration of the strain rate estimates yields the strain curve over the cardiac cycle. TDI-derived strain echocardiography was mainly used for regional myocardial function assessment [21]

12.3.4 Limitations

For TDI-based tissue velocity quantification, as with all Doppler techniques, the direction of the movement should be aligned to the insonification angle as much as possible. Beside this, the main disadvantage of TDI-based velocity estimation is the surrounding of functional contraction tissue around non-contracting tissue. This results in a passive movement of the non-contractile tissue, delivering equal velocity patterns. This is overcome by calculating the strain rate and/or strain form the TDI velocities. However, this technique is a 1-D technique which suffers from angle dependency.

12.4 Ultrasound elastography

A few years after TDI had been introduced, ultrasound elastography was described and developed. Whereas TDI mainly focused on cardiovascular applications as described in the previous section, the initial application of ultrasound elastography was detection of breast cancer. In the clinic, human palpation is one of the most commonly used techniques to detect irregular structures and changes in stiffness in the human body. Clinicians prefer this method as those irregularities and changes are often strong indicators for diseases. For example, stiff and irregular masses in breast are often related to cancers or liver tissue affected by cirrhosis is stiffer compared to healthy tissue. However, human palpation is limited by the accessibility of organs – only superficial organs can be examined like the prostate, liver and breast. Furthermore, palpation is not quantitative and strongly depends on the expertise of the performing clinician and is therefore subject to interpretation.

Ophir *et al.* proposed a new technique to quantify the deformation of tissue [22]. In this way, the two main limitations of palpation, clinician dependency and accessibility, were addressed. Now, deformation can be quantified and visualized, and ultrasound even allows to perform deformation measurements in deeper located organs. Instead of 'feeling' by palpation, a stiff region can now be identified non-invasively as strain will be decreased with respect to its environment. Images of the strain values can be visualized in so-called elastograms (strain maps).

12.4.1 Method

To apply this method, a small force is required to induce tissue deformation. This force can be applied externally or an internal force in the body can be used. For example, the operator can press with the ultrasound transducer on the tissue of interest. As internal body forces, respiration motion or heartbeats can be used as deformation source. This method is often called quasi-static elastography since the rate of deformation is rather slow with respect to the frame rate utilized: ultrasound data sets are obtained pre- and post-deformations and strain as a surrogate measure for stiffness can be estimated from these data sets by block-matching algorithms and some additional post-processing.

In those algorithms, the obtained pre-deformation ultrasound data set is divided in small blocks and these blocks are matched to the most similar part in the post-deformation data. In this way, displacement of these blocks in the post-deformation data can be tracked and strain can be calculated by the gradient of these displacements. Examples of matching strategies are cross-correlation, normalized covariance and hybrid-sign correlation [23]. Note that these so-called blocks can have any arbitrary shape, like lines (1-D), rectangles and parallelograms (2-D) or cubes (3-D). Two variants of block-matching methods are commonly used: speckle tracking and RF-based block matching.

12.4.2 Speckle tracking

In speckle tracking [24,25], speckles and structures are tracked between subsequent B-mode ultrasound images with different states of deformation, for instance, frames during a heart cycle. Speckle patterns are caused by the interference of back-scattered ultrasound waves from structures that are smaller than the wavelength of the ultrasound signal [26]. Speckle tracking is frequently applied in echocardiography [27]. Strain or other mechanical conditions like rotation or torsion of the heart can be estimated by tracking of speckle during the cardiac cycle. The primary application of strain imaging is to identify regions with abnormal function. For instance, areas in the heart wall with reduced strain might indicate the presence of a myocardial infarction. Besides functional properties, haemodynamic parameters can be estimated by the speckle velocities to evaluate cardiac function.

For accurate analysis, the frame rate is crucial. If the frame rate is too low, the speckle pattern will change too much in between two subsequent frames and the tissue cannot be properly tracked anymore. In cardiology, a frame rate in the order of 70 frames per second is considered adequate. The advantage of speckle tracking is that processed B-mode images of the ultrasound scanner, often Digital Imaging and Communications in Medicine (DICOM) format, can be used and is accessible in most commercially available ultrasound scanners. The disadvantage is that only the amplitude information (intensity of signal) can be used for tracking.

12.4.3 RF-based block matching

The second method is RF-based block matching that makes use of both the amplitude and phase information of the ultrasound RF data [28]. RF data are the raw (radio frequency) data originating from the ultrasound probe. It consist of multiple RF lines in the axial direction (along the transmitted beam). The final image shown to the user is an amplitude representation of the RF data and is referred to as Brightness-mode (B-mode) image. The available phase information in RF data enables a ten times more accurate displacement estimation compared to only amplitude information for small strains (up to 5%) between subsequently acquired RF data sets [29]. Similar to speckle tracking, block-matching algorithms are applied to calculate displacements between the different states of deformation. Since phase information is only available in the axial direction, this technique is particularly beneficial for axial strain estimation although the lateral strain estimation is slightly improved [29]. In contrast to DICOM and B-mode images in speckle tracking, RF data are rarely accessible for researchers in commercial ultrasound scanners.

In many block-matching algorithms, an iterative method is implemented, in which coarse displacement estimations are derived from block-matching envelope (B-mode) data and the displacement estimations are refined in the subsequent steps using RF data and smaller block sizes. In this way, speckle tracking and RF-based block matching are combined [29].

12.4.4 Lateral displacements

Ultrasound elastography mainly focuses on axial displacements and strains since deformation (e.g. by the transducer) is often applied in axial direction. Furthermore, lateral (parallel to the transducer surface) displacement estimates are less accurate because speckle size is increased and phase information is not available in lateral direction. As long as the main deformation is expected to occur in the axial direction, this will not be a limitation. Furthermore, since tissue is incompressible, the lateral and elevational deformations are strongly correlated with the axial deformation. For example in breast cancer screening, tissue is deformed in axial direction by the transducer to evaluate tissue and lesion stiffness. However, lateral strain estimates will be of interest for more complex deformations of tissue or organs. For instance, arteries dilate by pulsating blood pressure in radial directions, so the deformations and strains occur not only in axial direction.

A method to overcome the reduced accuracy of lateral displacement estimates might be transverse oscillation [30], in which a pulse echo field with an oscillation is generated in both the axial and transverse (lateral) direction. In this way, a kind of phase information is also available in the lateral direction and so the accuracy of lateral displacement estimates can be improved. This technique is primarily developed for blood velocity imaging [30], but currently also applied for displacement and strain estimation [31–33], and will be elaborated in the next chapter. Another effort to improve lateral accuracy is displacement compounding [34,35], in which ultrasound RF data is collected using multiple beam steering angles in transmit. Consequently, accurate displacements can be calculated in the direction of the steered angle as phase information is available in this transmit direction. These displacements under different angles can be decomposed and combined in axial and lateral components, or other components of interest. An example of this application is plaque detection in the carotid artery, in which the radial strains are obtained by spatial compounding [36] as can be seen in Figure 12.3.

12.4.5 Developments

Next to transverse oscillation and spatial compounding, several studies have been published to improve ultrasound elastography. For instance, the displacement

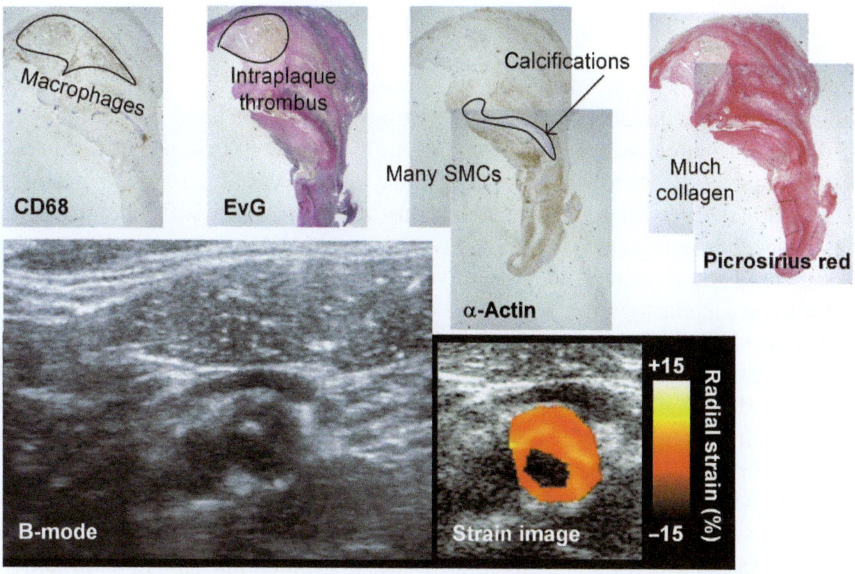

Figure 12.3 Pre-endarterectomy B-mode ultrasound and compound radial strain image and the corresponding post-endarterectomy histology of a fibrous plaque with calcifications. As expected, overall strain values are low, because the plaque is predominantly composed of collagen (purple on Elastin von Gieson (EvG) staining and red on picrosirius red staining), which is relatively stiff. The lowest strains are observed in the calcified region (bright spot on B-mode, purple on the α-actin and CD68 stainings), which is even stiffer material. Figure courtesy of H.H.G Hansen

estimations can be more accurate by improved ultrasound input data for block-matching algorithms in terms of resolution or contrast, or reduced noise levels. In coherent compounding, for instance, lateral resolution is improved and noise reduced by reconstructing and combining ultrasound RF data from multiple steering angles [37]. Also, resolution and contrast of ultrasound data itself can be improved by alternative strategies to reconstruct ultrasound data from the raw element data [38–41]. Obviously, other ways to improve ultrasound elastography are optimization of block-matching strategies or improvement of ultrasound hardware like transducers.

Another development has been the extension of ultrasound elastography to the third dimension since the introduction of 1-D transducers, that are swept or translated in elevational direction, and 2-D matrix array transducers [42–45]. Some examples are 3-D elastography for automated volumetric ultrasound scanner (translating 1-D transducer) in breast screening [46], for imaging of skeletal muscle [47], for carotid plaque detection [48] or for myocardial imaging [49]. Due to the rise of ultrafast ultrasound imaging [50] and increasing computational power, more developments in ultrasound (elastography) can be expected.

12.4.6 Applications in breast

Next to developments in methodology, ultrasound elastography is also validated and implemented in clinical practice. For instance, ultrasound elastography is particularly suitable in breast cancer detection and classification because breast tissue can be easily deformed by the ultrasound transducer or by using the breathing of the patient [51]. Malignant breast lesions are often much stiffer compared to glandular tissue or benign lesion like fibroadenoma [52]. In this way, lesions can be classified by strain: cancers show relatively low strain values compared to benign breast tissues in elastograms. Figures 12.4 and 12.5 show examples of elastograms of benign (fibroadenoma) and malignant (infiltrative ductal carcinoma) lesions, respectively. Sadigh and Carlos [53] concluded, based on a systematic review of clinical studies, that ultrasound elastography has a good diagnostic performance in distinguishing malignant from benign breast lesion, especially in combination with B-mode ultrasound.

A limitation of ultrasound elastography is that it is qualitative, and strain patterns and values in elastograms have to be manually evaluated and scored by clinicians [54]. Furthermore, axial strain values depend on the applied deformation or compression. Therefore, this method is operator-dependent and values can differ between examinations. To overcome this problem, strain ratios can be calculated, in which the mean strain in the lesion is divided by the mean strain in subcutaneous fat [55]. Another way to quantify elastography is by estimating the stiffness (e.g. Young's or shear modulus). Stiffness can be calculated by a strain–stress relation; however, this calculation requires sensors to obtain stress values. Strain ratios and stiffness are two different ways to quantify ultrasound elastography. Finally, the boundary conditions are also of great influence. For example, the presence of a large non-deforming structure on one side of the region of interest precludes

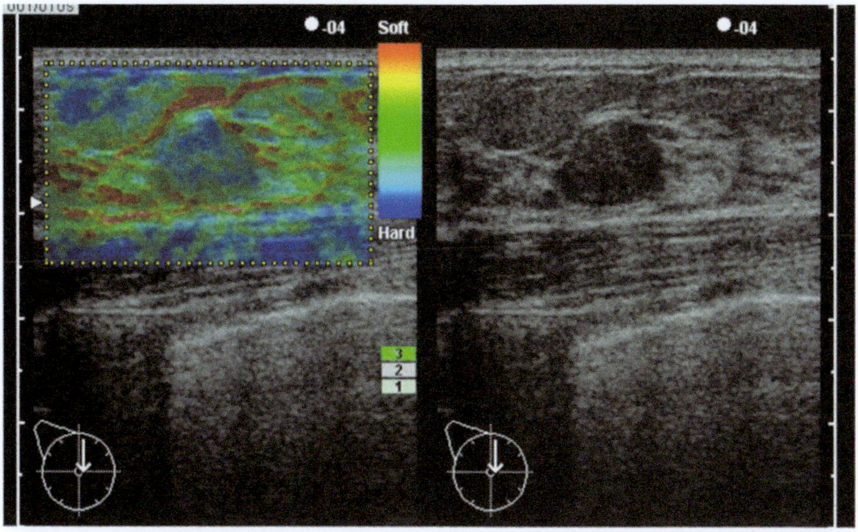

Figure 12.4 *Fibroadenoma: an elastogram overlaying a B-mode image (left) and the corresponding B-mode image (right); blue indicates hard areas (low strain) whereas red, soft areas (high strain). Inside the lesion, the elastogram is green homogeneous, suggesting a benign lesion (fibroadenoma). This image was adapted from Balleyguier and Canale [62]*

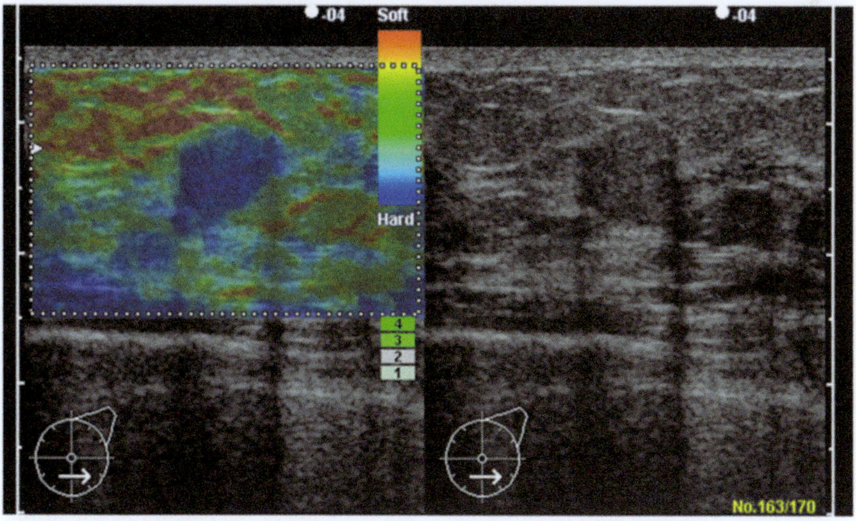

Figure 12.5 *Infiltrative ductal carcinoma (IDC): an elastogram overlaying a B-mode image (left) and the corresponding B-mode image (right); blue indicates hard areas (low strain) whereas red, soft areas (high strain). Inside the lesion, the elastogram is blue with irregular margins, suggesting a malignant lesion (IDC). These images were adapted from Balleyguier and Canale [62]*

lateral motion in this direction. Since tissue is incompressible, this will also affect the axial strain.

12.4.7 Other applications

The methods used in ultrasound elastography, speckle tracking and RF-based tracking, can also be applied to measure blood flow in vessel [56–58]. In this application, ultrasound RF data of vessels is recorded with a very high frame rate up to 10,000 frames per second. The signal of the fast-moving blood cells is relatively low compared to the slow-moving vessel wall and surrounding tissue. These slowly moving surrounding tissues cause slow-moving artefacts to dominate the blood signal. Since displacements and flow have to be estimated by the fast-moving blood signal, the slowly moving signals (clutter) are removed by a so-called clutter filter. Next, displacements can be estimated between each subsequent frame in time by RF-based tracking. Finally, since the frame rate is known, the blood flow can be calculated. As speckle tracking is used, not only the magnitude of the flow but also the direction of the flow can be estimated. When RF-based tracking is utilized, also in this method, the lateral displacement component can be estimated more accurately by using multiple insonification angles and spatial compounding [59]. An example of blood flow estimation can be found in Figure 12.6. The disadvantage of this technique is that high frame rates, and therefore ultrafast imaging strategies, are necessary to track blood velocity, which requires high computational power.

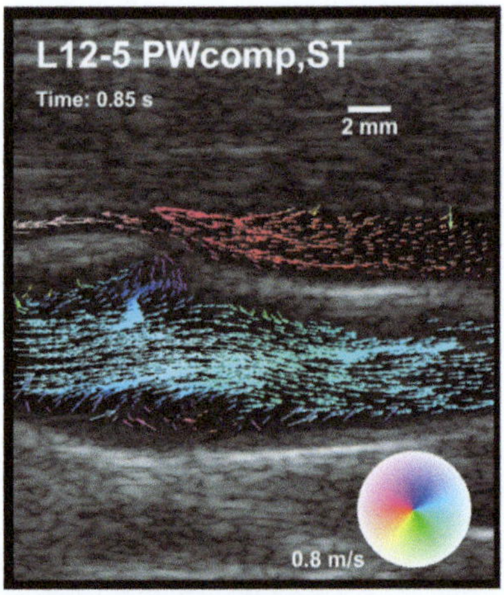

Figure 12.6 Blood flow in carotid artery of a healthy volunteer during systole (ST), the arrows and colour indicate the direction of the flow and brightness represent the velocity: dark (0 m s^{-1}) to light (0.8 m s^{-1}). The flow map overlays the B-mode image of the carotid artery at the bifurcation. The applied method to obtain blood flow velocities was RF-based tracking combined with spatial compounding (comp) of ultrasound data recorded by ultrafast imaging techniques (plane-wave imaging, PW). Figure courtesy of A.E.C.M. Saris

However, the main advantage is that this technique is angle-independent and thus overcomes the main limitation of Doppler ultrasound, in which velocities can only be obtained along the transmitted ultrasound beam as discussed before.

Next to detecting breast cancer and estimating blood flow, ultrasound elastography can be applied to study many other organs. An example is the application for musculoskeletal problems to study healthy and pathological conditions of muscle tissues. The biomechanical properties of soft tissue reflect to some degree the pathophysiology of the musculoskeletal disorder [60,61]. Throughout the years, ultrasound elastography has also been applied in, among others, liver, prostate, heart and lungs, and the number of applications are still rising.

References

[1] Edler I, Hertz CH. The use of the reflectoscope for the continuous recording of the movement of heart walls. Kungliga Fysiografiska Sällskapet I Lund Förhandlingar. 1954;24:40–58.

[2] Anderson T, McDicken WN. Measurement of tissue motion. Proceedings of the Institution of Mechanical Engineers Part H, Journal of Engineering in Medicine. 1999;213(3): 181–91.

[3] Picard MH. M-Mode echocardiography: principles and examination techniques. In: Feigenbaum H, editor. Endocardiology. 5th ed. Philadelphia: Lea and Febiger; 1995. p. 282–301.

[4] Feigenbaum H, Popp RL, Wolfe SB, *et al.* Ultrasound measurements of the left ventricle: a correlative study with angiocardiography. Archives of Internal Medicine. 1972;129(3): 461–7.

[5] Fortuin NJ, Hood WP, Sherman ME, Craige E. Determination of left ventricular volumes by ultrasound. Circulation. 1971;44(4): 575–84.

[6] Pombo JF, Troy BL, Russell RO, Jr. Left ventricular volumes and ejection fraction by echocardiography. Circulation. 1971;43(4): 480–90.

[7] Parisi AF, Moynihan PF, Feldman CL, Folland ED. Approaches to determination of left ventricular volume and ejection fraction by real-time two-dimensional echocardiography. Clinical Cardiology. 1979;2(4): 257–63.

[8] Gamble G, Zorn J, Sanders G, MacMahon S, Sharpe N. Estimation of arterial stiffness, compliance, and distensibility from M-mode ultrasound measurements of the common carotid artery. Stroke. 1994;25(1): 11–6.

[9] Blaney F, English CS, Sawyer T. Sonographic measurement of diaphragmatic displacement during tidal breathing manoeuvres – a reliability study. The Australian Journal of Physiotherapy. 1999;45(1): 41–3.

[10] Wait JL, Nahormek PA, Yost WT, Rochester DP. Diaphragmatic thickness-lung volume relationship in vivo. Journal of Applied Physiology. 1989; 67(4): 1560–8.

[11] Grubb NR, Fleming A, Sutherland GR, Fox KA. Skeletal muscle contraction in healthy volunteers: assessment with Doppler tissue imaging. Radiology. 1995;194(3): 837–42.

[12] Mannion AF, Pulkovski N, Schenk P, *et al.* A new method for the noninvasive determination of abdominal muscle feedforward activity based on tissue velocity information from tissue Doppler imaging. Journal of Applied Physiology. 2008;104(4): 1192–201.

[13] Dieterich AV, Pickard CM, Deshon LE, *et al.* M-mode ultrasound used to detect the onset of deep muscle activity. Journal of Electromyography and Kinesiology: official journal of the International Society of Electrophysiological Kinesiology. 2015;25(2): 224–31.

[14] Satomura S. Ultrasonic Doppler method for the inspection of cardiac functions. The Journal of the Acoustical Society of America. 1957;29(11): 1181–5.

[15] Franklin DL, Schlegel W, Rushmer RF. Blood flow measured by Doppler frequency shift of back-scattered ultrasound. Science. 1961;134(3478): 564–5.

[16] Dunmire B, Beach KW, Labs K, Plett M, Strandness DE, Jr. Cross-beam vector Doppler ultrasound for angle-independent velocity measurements. Ultrasound in Medicine and Biology. 2000;26(8): 1213–35.

[17] Trahey GE, Allison JW, von Ramm OT. Angle independent ultrasonic detection of blood flow. IEEE Transactions on Biomedical Engineering. 1987;34(12): 965–7.

[18] Isaaz K, Thompson A, Ethevenot G, Cloez JL, Brembilla B, Pernot C. Doppler echocardiographic measurement of low velocity motion of the left-ventricular posterior wall. American Journal of Cardiology. 1989;64(1): 66–75.

[19] Eranki A, Cortes N, Ferenček Z, Sikdar S. A novel application of musculoskeletal ultrasound imaging. Journal of Visualized Experiments (79): JoVE. e50595, doi:10.3791/50595; 2013.

[20] Heimdal A, Stoylen A, Torp H, Skaerpe T. Real time strain rate imaging of the left ventricle by ultrasound. Journal of the American Society of Echocardiography. 1998;11:1013–9.

[21] Abraham TP, Dimaano VL, Liang H-Y. Role of tissue Doppler and strain echocardiography in current clinical practice. Circulation. 2007;116(22): 2597–609.

[22] Ophir J, Cespedes I, Ponnekanti H, Yazdi Y, Li X. Elastography: a quantitative method for imaging the elasticity of biological tissues. Ultrason Imaging. 1991;13(2): 111–34.

[23] Viola F, Walker WF, editors. Comparison of time delay estimators in medical ultrasound. 2001 IEEE Ultrasonics Symposium Proceedings an International Symposium (Cat No01CH37263); 2001.

[24] Leitman M, Lysyansky P, Sidenko S, *et al.* Two-dimensional strain-a novel software for real-time quantitative echocardiographic assessment of myocardial function. Journal of the American Society of Echocardiography: Official Publication of the American Society of Echocardiography. 2004; 17(10): 1021–9.

[25] Reisner SA, Lysyansky P, Agmon Y, Mutlak D, Lessick J, Friedman Z. Global longitudinal strain: a novel index of left ventricular systolic function.

Journal of the American Society of Echocardiography: Official Publication of the American Society of Echocardiography. 2004;17(6): 630–3.

[26] Burckhardt CB. Speckle in ultrasound B-mode scans. IEEE Transactions on Sonics and Ultrasonics. 1978;25(1): 1–6.

[27] Blessberger H, Binder T. Non-invasive imaging: two dimensional speckle tracking echocardiography: basic principles. Heart (British Cardiac Society). 2010;96(9): 716–22.

[28] D'Hooge J, Konofagou E, Jamal F, *et al.* Two-dimensional ultrasonic strain rate measurement of the human heart in vivo. IEEE Transactions on Ultrasonics, Ferroelectrics, and Frequency Control. 2002;49(2): 281–6.

[29] Lopata RG, Nillesen MM, Hansen HH, Gerrits IH, Thijssen JM, de Korte CL. Performance evaluation of methods for two-dimensional displacement and strain estimation using ultrasound radio frequency data. Ultrasound in Medicine & Biology. 2009;35(5): 796–812.

[30] Udesen J, Jensen JA. Investigation of transverse oscillation method. IEEE Transactions on Ultrasonics, Ferroelectrics, and Frequency Control. 2006; 53(5): 959–71.

[31] Heyde B, Bottenus N, D'Hooge J, Trahey GE. Evaluation of the transverse oscillation technique for cardiac phased array imaging: a theoretical study. IEEE Transactions on Ultrasonics, Ferroelectrics, and Frequency Control. 2017;64(2): 320–34.

[32] Salles S, Liebgott H, Garcia D, Vray D. Full 3-D transverse oscillations: a method for tissue motion estimation. IEEE Transactions on Ultrasonics, Ferroelectrics, and Frequency Control. 2015;62(8): 1473–85.

[33] Salles S, Chee AJ, Garcia D, Yu AC, Vray D, Liebgott H. 2-D arterial wall motion imaging using ultrafast ultrasound and transverse oscillations. IEEE Transactions on Ultrasonics, Ferroelectrics, and Frequency Control. 2015; 62(6): 1047–58.

[34] Hansen HH, Lopata RG, Idzenga T, de Korte CL. Full 2D displacement vector and strain tensor estimation for superficial tissue using beam-steered ultrasound imaging. Physics in Medicine and Biology. 2010;55(11): 3201–18.

[35] Tanter M, Bercoff J, Sandrin L, Fink M. Ultrafast compound imaging for 2-D motion vector estimation: application to transient elastography. IEEE Transactions on Ultrasonics, Ferroelectrics, and Frequency Control. 2002;49 (10): 1363–74.

[36] Hansen HH, de Borst GJ, Bots ML, Moll FL, Pasterkamp G, de Korte CL. Validation of noninvasive in vivo compound ultrasound strain imaging using histologic plaque vulnerability features. Stroke. 2016;47(11): 2770–5.

[37] Montaldo G, Tanter M, Bercoff J, Benech N, Fink M. Coherent plane-wave compounding for very high frame rate ultrasonography and transient elastography. IEEE Transactions on Ultrasonics, Ferroelectrics, and Frequency Control. 2009;56(3): 489–506.

[38] Hollander B, Hendriks GA, Mann RM, Hansen HH, de Korte CL. Plane-wave compounding in automated breast volume scanning: a phantom-based study. Ultrasound in Medicine & Biology. 2016;42(10): 2493–503.

[39] Garcia D, Le Tarnec L, Muth S, Montagnon E, Poree J, Cloutier G. Stolt's f-k migration for plane wave ultrasound imaging. IEEE Transactions on Ultrasonics, Ferroelectrics, and Frequency Control. 2013;60(9): 1853–67.

[40] Austeng A, Nilsen CIC, Jensen AC, Näsholm SP, Holm S, editors. Coherent plane-wave compounding and minimum variance beam forming. 2011 IEEE International Ultrasonics Symposium; 18–21 Oct. 2011.

[41] Cheng J, Lu JY. Extended high-frame rate imaging method with limited-diffraction beams. IEEE Transactions on Ultrasonics, Ferroelectrics, and Frequency Control. 2006;53(5): 880–99.

[42] Bharat S, Fisher TG, Varghese T, *et al.* Three-dimensional electrode displacement elastography using the siemens C7F2 four Sight four-dimensional ultrasound transducer. Ultrasound in Medicine & Biology. 2008;34(8): 1307–16.

[43] Fisher TG, Hall TJ, Panda S, *et al.* Volumetric elasticity imaging with a 2-D CMUT array. Ultrasound in Medicine & Biology. 2010;36(6): 978–90.

[44] Lindop JE, Treece GM, Gee AH, Prager RW. 3D elastography using freehand ultrasound. Ultrasound in Medicine & Biology. 2006;32(4): 529–45.

[45] Treece GM, Lindop JE, Gee AH, Prager RW. Freehand ultrasound elastography with a 3-D probe. Ultrasound in Medicine & Biology. 2008;34(3): 463–74.

[46] Hendriks GA, Hollander B, Menssen J, Milkowski A, Hansen HH, de Korte CL. Automated 3D ultrasound elastography of the breast: a phantom validation study. Physics in Medicine and Biology. 2016;61(7): 2665–79.

[47] Gijsbertse K, Sprengers AM, Nillesen MM, *et al.* Three-dimensional ultrasound strain imaging of skeletal muscles. Physics in Medicine and Biology. 2017;62(2): 596–611.

[48] Fekkes S, Swillens AE, Hansen HH, *et al.* 2D versus 3D cross-correlation-based radial and circumferential strain estimation using multiplane 2D ultrafast ultrasound in a 3D atherosclerotic carotid artery model. IEEE Transactions on Ultrasonics, Ferroelectrics, and Frequency Control. 2016; 63(10): 1543–1553.

[49] Jasaityte R, Heyde B, D'Hooge J. Current state of three-dimensional myocardial strain estimation using echocardiography. Journal of the American Society of Echocardiography: Official Publication of the American Society of Echocardiography. 2013;26(1): 15–28.

[50] Tanter M, Fink M. Ultrafast imaging in biomedical ultrasound. IEEE Transactions on Ultrasonics, Ferroelectrics, and Frequency Control. 2014;61 (1): 102–19.

[51] Ricci P, Maggini E, Mancuso E, Lodise P, Cantisani V, Catalano C. Clinical application of breast elastography: state of the art. European Journal of Radiology. 2014;83(3): 429–37.

[52] Krouskop TA, Wheeler TM, Kallel F, Garra BS, Hall T. Elastic moduli of breast and prostate tissues under compression. Ultrason Imaging. 1998; 20(4): 260–74.

[53] Sadigh G, Carlos RC, Neal CH, Dwamena BA. Accuracy of quantitative ultrasound elastography for differentiation of malignant and benign breast

abnormalities: a meta-analysis. Breast Cancer Research and Treatment. 2012;134(3): 923–31.

[54] Itoh A, Ueno E, Tohno E, *et al.* Breast disease: clinical application of US elastography for diagnosis. Radiology. 2006;239(2): 341–50.

[55] Cho N, Moon WK, Kim HY, Chang JM, Park SH, Lyou CY. Sonoelastographic strain index for differentiation of benign and malignant nonpalpable breast masses. Journal of Ultrasound in Medicine: Official Journal of the American Institute of Ultrasound in Medicine. 2010;29(1): 1–7.

[56] Udesen J, Gran F, Hansen KL, Jensen JA, Thomsen C, Nielsen MB. High frame-rate blood vector velocity imaging using plane waves: simulations and preliminary experiments. IEEE Transactions on Ultrasonics, Ferroelectrics, and Frequency Control. 2008;55(8): 1729–43.

[57] Fadnes S, Nyrnes SA, Torp H, Lovstakken L. Shunt flow evaluation in congenital heart disease based on two-dimensional speckle tracking. Ultrasound in Medicine & Biology. 2014;40(10): 2379–91.

[58] Kortbek J, Jensen JA. Estimation of velocity vector angles using the directional cross-correlation method. IEEE Transactions on Ultrasonics, Ferroelectrics, and Frequency Control. 2006;53(11): 2036–49.

[59] Saris A, Hansen H, Fekkes S, Nillesen M, Rutten M, de Korte C. A comparison between compounding techniques using large beam-steered plane wave imaging for blood vector velocity imaging in a carotid artery model. IEEE Transactions on Ultrasonics, Ferroelectrics, and Frequency Control. 2016;63(11):1758–1771.

[60] Klauser AS, Miyamoto H, Bellmann-Weiler R, Feuchtner GM, Wick MC, Jaschke WR. Sonoelastography: musculoskeletal applications. Radiology. 2014;272(3): 622–33.

[61] Drakonaki EE, Allen GM, Wilson DJ. Ultrasound elastography for musculoskeletal applications. The British Journal of Radiology. 2012;85(1019): 1435–45.

[62] Balleyguier C, Canale S, Ben Hassen W, *et al.* Breast elasticity: principles, technique, results: an update and overview of commercially available software. European Journal of Radiology. 2013;82(3): 427–34.

Chapter 13
Principles of speckle tracking

Brecht Heyde[1]

13.1 General principles

When a scattering object is small relative to the incident ultrasound (US) wavelength, i.e., a point scatterer, US waves get scattered uniformly in all directions. This is called diffusive scattering [1]. Tissue is inhomogeneous due to local deviations of density and compressibility and is often modeled as a randomly spaced collection of point scatterers. The returned US echo signal is therefore the result of the interference pattern of all scattered wave fronts from the constituting point scatterers. This gives rise to the characteristic speckle pattern seen in US images. While this is a stochastic process in nature, and while speckle statistics can be described by Gaussian (RF) and Rayleigh (RF envelope) distributions [2], it is important to realize that the resulting images are not random but deterministic in the sense that the same tissue imaged under the same conditions will result in the same speckle pattern. As such, speckle should not be interpreted as noise, but should rather be seen as a fingerprint reflecting the underlying scatter distribution. This feature of speckle is used to track tissue motion.

Speckle tracking is a general term used for those techniques that make use of the fact that this characteristic speckle pattern can be tracked when its appearance varies only slowly when the tissue moves or deforms during acquisition, i.e., when the patterns decorrelate at a slow rate. This holds true when the underlying tissue only undergoes small deformations [3] or alternatively, when an US system can image at a sufficiently high frame rate to warrant the previous assumption. While sometimes considered as negatively affecting other image analysis tasks such as image segmentation, speckle is a desirable property in the context of tissue tracking.

US speckle tracking techniques have many applications in the context of elastography and strain imaging. In elastography (or elasticity imaging), a map of the elastic properties of the tissue is created by inducing a mechanical excitation of the tissue and tracking the local tissue motion response. It is mainly used in diagnosing malignant lesions as those tend to present as stiffer lesions in a softer

[1]Cardiovascular Imaging and Dynamics, KU Leuven, Belgium

background. The excitation force can be generated externally, i.e., from palpation with the US probe in quasistatic elastography [4]; by a naturally occurring physiologic motion, e.g., as in cardiac strain imaging [5] or by pushing the tissue with a focused US beam, i.e., in acoustic radiation force imaging [6], shear wave elasticity imaging [7] and supersonic shear imaging [8]. Examples of where speckle tracking techniques have been used are numerous, and it is beyond the purpose of this chapter to provide an extensive overview. Applications worth mentioning are the detection of breast cancer, thyroid nodules, lymph nodes, liver fibrosis and prostate cancer [9,10]; strain imaging in the heart [11], carotid [12], aorta [13], muscle [14], tendon [15] and the skin [16]; nerve motion tracking [17]; blood flow tracking [18] and intravascular elastography [19].

13.2 Classification of speckle tracking techniques

A vast amount of speckle tracking techniques has been developed to extract tissue motion from a time series of medical US images. The purpose of this chapter is to explore the underlying principles of these techniques while highlighting the methodological variety. This diversity also implies that arguably many different classification schemes could be devised to group them. Furthermore, it is important to realize that labeling techniques belonging to a single category can be further complicated given that some methods are conceptually hybrid approaches that combine the strengths of their individual constituents while mitigating their disadvantages as much as possible. As such, rather than being an exhaustive overview, this chapter should instead be used as a practical guide in the ever-evolving US tracking literature.

Common classification criteria include, for example, the type of input data on which the motion estimators operate, the associated data dimensionality, the temporal tracking strategy and the underlying tracking principles (i.e., the methodology). The latter is the subject of Section 13.3.

13.2.1 Input data type

After transmitting US pulses, the received raw signals undergo a series of processing steps to generate a final US image for display. Speckle tracking algorithms have been developed to work with the specific data types available at each of these stages. Figure 13.1 shows a conceptual overview of these different subsequent stages. More details can be found in general US textbooks, e.g., [1].

US scanners acquire raw radio-frequency (RF) data received by each piezoelectric element of the array (*channel data*), typically at a high sampling frequency (i.e., 25–60 MHz) and high precision resolution (i.e., 12–16 bit). After band-pass filtering is used to remove high frequency noise and select the imaging mode (i.e., fundamental or harmonic imaging), beamforming is performed to reconstruct the image. By properly delaying and summing the individual elements, image lines are reconstructed. The resulting data is typically called *beamformed RF data*. Most scanners however represent the channel data internally more efficiently

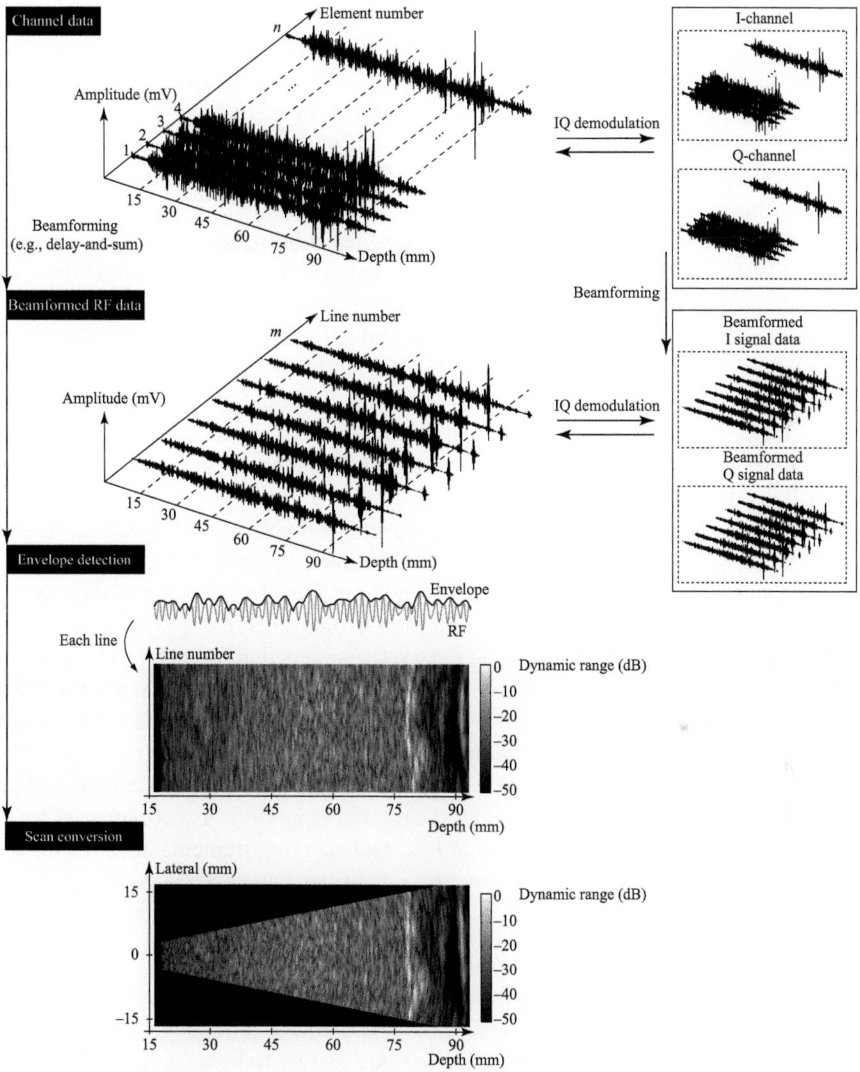

Figure 13.1 Classification of speckle tracking algorithms according to the type of data on which those operate. The object being imaged is a tissue-mimicking phantom acquired with a Verasonics scanner

as a complex signal with the real and imaginary component being the *in-phase and quadrature* (IQ) signal. By performing a quadrature demodulation, the carrier frequency is removed and *baseband signals* are obtained. As such, it allows the data to be sampled at a lower rate (more than half the original rate) without aliasing. This downmixing reduces data requirements down the image processing pipeline. By applying the correct filters and signal processing techniques, one can switch between both representations without loss of information.

As the highly oscillating signal is not useful for image display, the *signal envelope* or *detected signal* is used instead. Envelope detection is performed by taking the magnitude of the complex IQ signal or by taking the magnitude of the Hilbert transform of the RF data. Depending on the geometry of the transducer (phased, curvilinear or convex array), an additional *scan-conversion* or sector reconstruction step is required to interpolate the data unto a Cartesian visualization. Data is finally log-compressed and time gain compensated. This *B-mode* (brightness) image is represented as a series of unsigned 8-bit grayscale values.

It can be seen that the intrinsic data content and tracking potential is different depending on what stage the speckle tracking algorithm is applied. Evidently, there is a relationship between computation time and data amount/precision, with a fully sampled RF image requiring more computational demand compared to the low(er) resolution B-mode image. On the other hand, several studies have shown that due to the higher axial frequency content of RF images signals, more accurate subpixel motion estimates can be obtained compared to B-mode images if interframe motion is sufficiently small, e.g., [20,21].

From the point of view of algorithm design, it therefore seems logical to start from the most complete dataset, i.e., fully sampled channel data, as all the subsequent steps in the data transfer process tend to reduce the amount of data, through filtering, downsampling or data representation. However, some data (channel, RF or IQ) are accessible only from high-end research scanners that provide a platform with an open architecture. More widespread are commercially available scanners. However, due to the proprietary nature of these scanners, typically only B-mode images can be exported, either as grayscale images at a predetermined image resolution (i.e., the pixel/voxel size), or sometimes even with embedded (hard-coded) patient metadata overlaid. Although not optimal for tracking from a theoretical point of view, their widespread availability and low data size requirements have meant that algorithms working within these boundary conditions have been popular.

13.2.2 Data dimensionality

Algorithms can also be classified according to the dimensionality of the data on which the motion estimators operate (either space and/or time). A difference can be made between the dimensionality of the speckle feature to be tracked (in the source image), the dimensionality of the data where that speckle feature is to be searched (in the target image) and the dimensionality of the resulting motion estimate. Figure 13.2 gives an overview of different options, each with an example application/reference.

The first generation of speckle tracking techniques was based on the Doppler effect and was only able to assess the tissue motion component along the US insonification direction (Figure 13.2(a)). It has been widely used in the context of blood flow imaging [22,23] and tissue Doppler imaging [24]. Improvements could be made by combining measurements from different angles by either moving the transducer around the tissue of interest or by electronic beamsteering [25], but one remains limited by the maximum steering angle (Figure 13.2(b)).

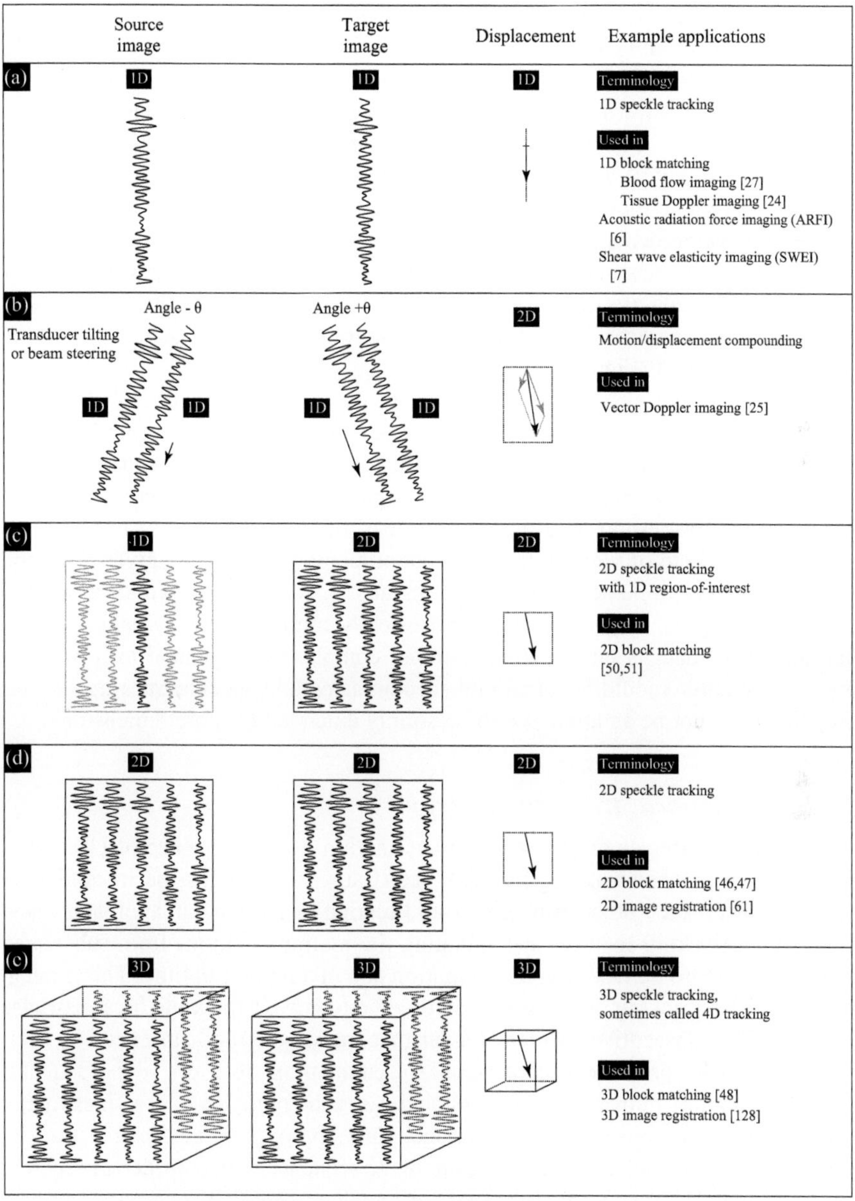

Figure 13.2 Classification of speckle tracking algorithms between a source and target image according to the dimensionality of the input data and the dimensionality of the resulting motion estimate. Note that for illustrational purposes, the ultrasound images were represented in RF space, but a similar classification can be made for the other data representations

As tissue motion and deformation is not limited to a single dimension, the necessity for extending speckle tracking techniques to 2D (and 3D) is evident. By not only tracking the 1D speckle patterns along the US line, but also by extending the search space toward neighboring (or even interpolated) US lines, 2D motion estimates could be obtained (Figure 13.2(c)). At a later stage, 2D speckle patterns were tracked directly. While more motion components could be extracted, errors due to out-of-plane motion still existed (Figure 13.2(d)).

With developments in US transducer technology, microelectronic techniques and both hardware and software computing, systems capable of acquiring real-time full volumetric data are now widely available [11]. These new opportunities have further sparked research interest and have led to a true 3D translation of speckle tracking algorithms (Figure 13.2(e)).

It is worth noting that several challenges exist when translating algorithms to 2D and 3D. First of all, because US images are highly anisotropic, estimates perpendicular to the US insonification (i.e., in the transversal and elevational direction) are intrinsically more difficult compared to the axial direction due to the lower image resolution and low transverse frequency content. Furthermore, increasing the field of view comes at a cost of temporal resolution given that more image lines have to be acquired and reconstructed. As such, speckle decorrelation tends to be higher, making tracking intrinsically more difficult. Finally, because the amount of data is larger, computational complexity in general also becomes higher. The latter should be taken into account as certain speckle tracking families may therefore not be as attractive to be simply extended to more dimensions.

13.2.3 Temporal tracking strategy

A number of strategies exist to track tissue motion over a sequence of US images (i.e., frames) as shown in Figure 13.3. Interframe motions can be tracked independently from each other using either an Eulerian or Lagrangian approach (panel a). Eulerian tracking requires accumulating the motion solutions from subsequent images in order to extract total tissue motion at a given point in time. This strategy is also called tracking with progressive referencing or tracking in a pairwise, sequential or consecutive fashion. Given that tracking errors can occur in every frame, it can be prone to a considerable accumulation of errors if the sequence consists of a lot of frames. Lagrangian tracking, on the other hand, describes motion with respect to a chosen reference image. This approach is also called tracking with fixed referencing. When tracking an image sequence with considerable motion, this strategy tends to be prone to tracking errors due to speckle decorrelation.

Rather than considering each unknown interframe motion as a separate problem, it has also been proposed to solve all interframe tracking problems in a joint fashion. The idea being that any given interframe displacement can help improve accuracy for the other interframe displacements as those all originate from imaging the same tissue.

When imaging tissue is subject to a cyclical motion (e.g., in a cardiac or carotid setting), and when assuming that the US probe has not physically moved

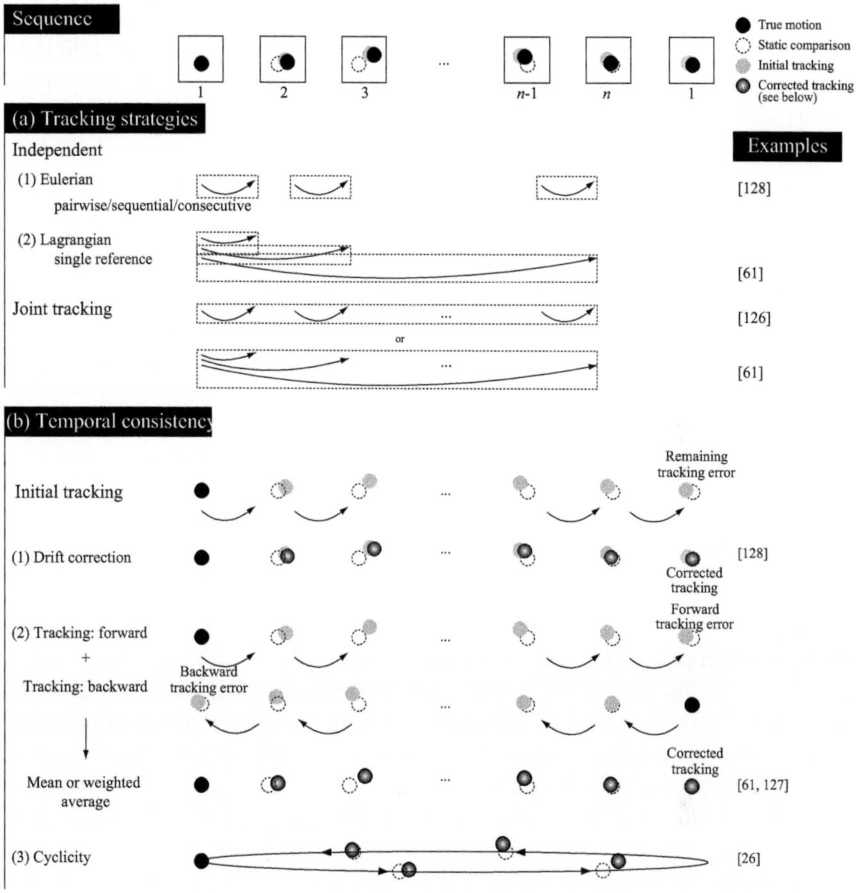

Figure 13.3 Classification of speckle tracking algorithms according to (a) their strategy in tracking a temporal sequence of ultrasound images with (b) the optional use of temporal consistency

during acquisition, then it is preferential to obtain tracked tissue trajectories that are temporally consistent, i.e., which return to the initial undeformed state after tracking (Figure 13.3(b)). However, due to the accumulation of errors as mentioned previously, this is rarely the case. The most straightforward solution is to perform a drift correction step after tracking. This typically involves subtracting the displacement offset uniformly over the remainder of the tracked displacement curve. Other alternatives could involve a weighted distribution of errors related to the confidence of each motion estimate.

A second strategy to enforce temporal continuity is to perform the tracking twice, in the forward and backward direction of the sequence. The final displacements are then found by taking the mean of the individual displacements, or by performing a weighted average depending on the elapsed time of the tracked forward and backward sequence. This further minimizes error accumulation.

Both strategies were based on the fact that interframe displacements were estimated independently. A third strategy would be to explicitly impose cyclicity as a boundary condition in the speckle tracking algorithm, e.g., by representing the velocity field as a diffeomorphism [26].

13.3 Overview of speckle tracking techniques

Traditionally, US-based motion estimators were based on the Doppler technique. Non-Doppler-based methods emerged later and can be divided in several categories as proposed in Figure 13.4. The first category of techniques, based on optical flow (OF), has been popular in the US engineering community. In particular, a subgroup of solutions, termed block matching, has received widespread attention and deserves a separate detailed treatment in Chapter 14. On the other hand, image registration techniques, popular in the image processing society, have also been suggested to assess motion. This will be the topic of Chapter 15. Other generic categories worth mentioning are statistical models, biomechanical models and segmentation-based models.

13.3.1 Doppler-based methods and 1D motion estimators

Due to thc Doppler effect, the frequency of the returned US signals is shifted proportional to the velocity of the insonified tissue. Doppler-based methods are intrinsically 1D methods as only the velocity component along the US beam can be measured. Three different US modalities exist, which exploit this phenomenon to measure velocity (and thus, displacement).

By transmitting a continuous US signal, and by computing the spectrum of the received signal (as in continuous wave Doppler), this frequency shift can be directly estimated. However, it is evident that this technique does not contain spatial information about the velocity distribution. Pulsed wave Doppler imaging, on the other hand, repetitively fires short US pulses and takes samples of the echoes at a fixed time point after transmit, i.e., at the range gate. It follows that the frequency of this sampled signal is equal to the Doppler frequency. As such, this results in a local tissue velocity estimate. Measuring tissue velocities at different locations requires adjusting the range gate.

In order to measure velocities from multiple locations simultaneously, color Doppler imaging was developed. In this method, for a given imaging line, only a few short US pulses (in practice 3 to 8) are sent at a constant pulse repetition frequency. Afterwards, this process is repeated for the other imaging lines until a full image is generated. This method was originally developed to estimate blood flow, typically called color flow mapping [27]. By filtering the high velocity components of the blood and retaining those that originate from tissue, it was later adopted for tracking cardiac tissue motion, termed color tissue Doppler imaging or Doppler myocardial imaging [24]. Often, an interleaving scheme is adopted to generate the corresponding B-mode image to facilitate navigation.

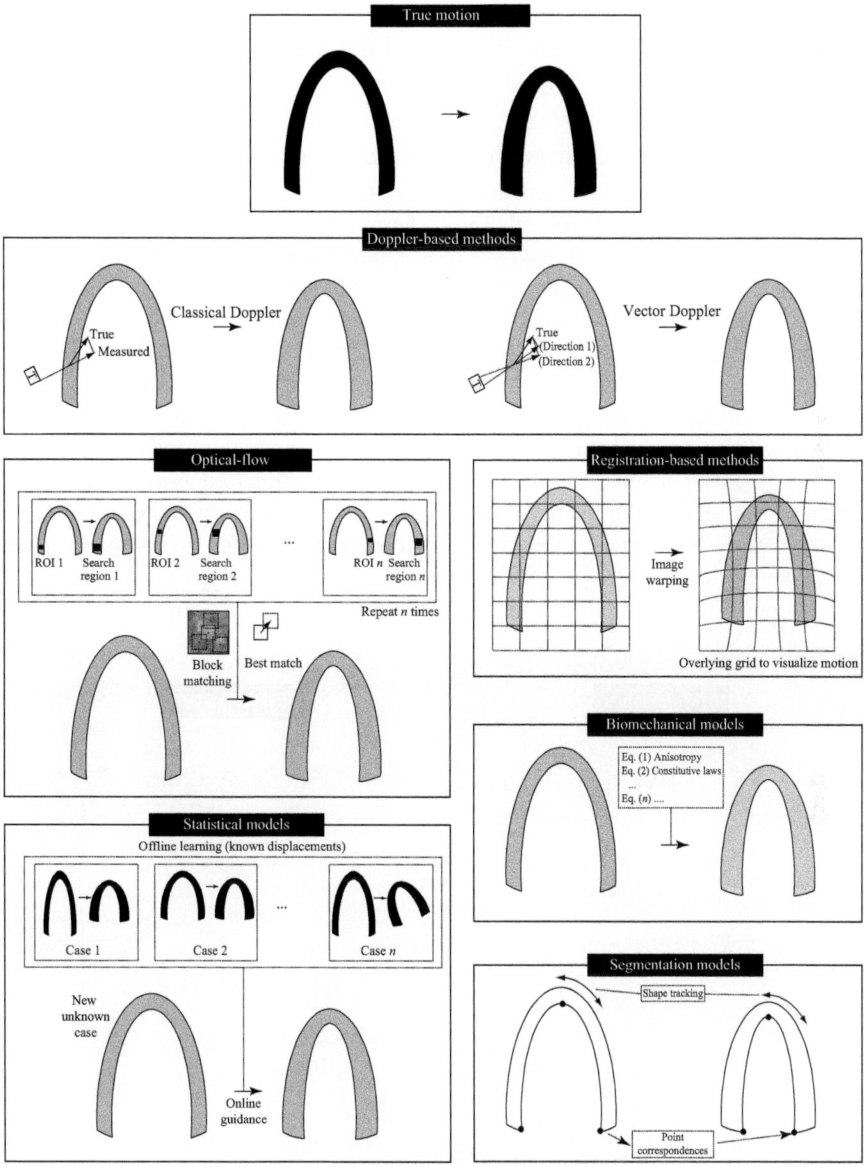

Figure 13.4 Classification of speckle tracking algorithms according to the underlying methodology. The shape to be tracked represents the left ventricle in a cardiac setting. A similar classification scheme can be made for other applications

Two groups of methods exist to estimate motion from the returned echo pulses: time-shift methods and phase-shift methods. In both cases, it is assumed that the reflected echo signal is a scaled, delayed replica of the transmitted pulse [5].

Many of these 1D motion estimators were originally developed in the context of blood flow imaging, but were later adopted for other applications as well, e.g., in the context of ARFI and SWEI [28,29].

13.3.1.1 Time-shift (or time-delay) estimators

The most popular time-shift estimator is the normalized cross-correlation function between two subsequent RF signals [30]. The maximum of this function indicates the point at which the two signals are most similar to each other and can thus be used to determine the displacement (see Figure 13.5(a)). To obtain regional motion estimates, the original RF signal is divided into several shorter RF patterns (sometimes called the region of interest (ROI), kernel or window), which are then searched for in the subsequent RF signal (i.e., the search region). Other similarity measures include, for example, the sum of squared differences and sum of absolute differences [30]. To obtain subsample resolution, the peak of the similarity measure is typically interpolated [31]. In contrast to the phase-based estimators, these techniques do not suffer from aliasing when tissues move at a high velocity. However, those tend to be more computationally demanding. A comprehensive review can be found in [32].

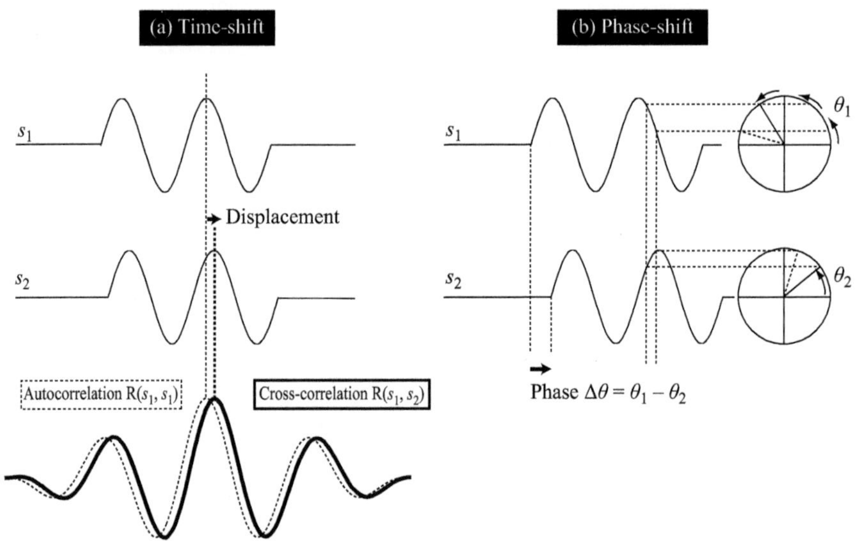

Figure 13.5 The 1D motion estimators assume that the signal s_2 is a delayed (and scaled) replica of signal s_1. Those are typically classified as either (a) time-shift estimators in which the peak of the cross-correlation indicates the intersignal displacement or as (b) phase-shift estimators which estimate motion from the observed phase shift

13.3.1.2 Phase-shift estimators

The displacement between two subsequent RF signals can also be expressed as a phase shift. The most straightforward implementation is shown in Figure 13.5(b). Two samples taken less than a quarter wavelength apart from each other determine the phase of a signal. A second pair of samples taken at the same locations in the delayed signal can therefore be used to determine the local phase shift, and thus the intersignal motion.

A more efficient real-time phase-shift estimator using beamformed IQ data instead of RF data has been proposed by Kasai *et al.*, widely known as the 1D autocorrelator [33]. It can be shown that the phase shift at a given axial position can be determined by taking the angle of the complex autocorrelation function between the original RF signal and its delayed version at that axial position. In theory, this phase shift could be determined from two subsequent signals, but in practice, several signals fired in the same direction are used to temporally average these estimates and reduce its variance. For the same reason, the computed phases at different spatial locations are typically spatially smoothed by convolving it with a rectangular window. Of note, this algorithm is prone to aliasing as it can only extract phase information between $\pm\pi/2$.

The Loupas 2D autocorrelator is another popular phase-shift algorithm [34], and is a direct extension of the Kasai 1D autocorrelator, in the sense that it takes depth samples within a certain axial range into account during motion. It should be noted that the output of this algorithm remains a 1D estimate, even though its dimensionality is labeled as being 2D. This is because of the input of the autocorrelation function (taking axial by temporal samples). The main difference with Kasai is that it no longer assumes a constant carrier frequency as it computes a shift at every axial location. It has been shown to be more accurate than the Kasai autocorrelator [28].

A third popular approach is the algorithm of Pesavento *et al.* [35]. It is based on the observation that the phase of the complex correlation function between the reference and delayed IQ signal has a root at the time delay between both signals. By considering the phase to vary linearly around this root, an efficient iterative root-seeking algorithm was proposed.

13.3.2 Optical flow methods

OF is a general term used to describe the apparent motion of brightness patterns due to the relative motion between the image and the observer. The concept of OF can be translated to US imaging as the motion (and decorrelation) of speckle patterns caused by underlying tissue motion. OF methods can be divided into the following categories depending on how those approach the assessment of tissue motion: differential methods, region-based methods or phase-based methods [36,37].

Differential methods

By making the assumption that the intensity of a particular point in a moving pattern does not change over the image sequence, the well-known OF equation is obtained, see e.g., [36]. In its classical form, this OF equation consists of spatiotemporal derivatives of image intensities, and is therefore also called the gradient constraint equation. However, this single equation is insufficient to be solved given that there are at least two motion components. This is known as the aperture problem. Two families of differential or gradient-based techniques exist depending on the additional constraints used to solve this underdetermined problem.

The Horn–Schunck algorithm estimates flow globally by enforcing the flow field to be smooth across the whole image [38], and it has been adopted for US in e.g., [39]. The Lucas–Kanade approach, on the other hand, operates regionally and constraints the solution space by assuming the flow to be constant within small image regions [40]. It has been popular in US imaging, e.g., [41,42]. The Lucas–Kanade OF formulation also served as the driving force for a family of "demon" algorithms applied on US, e.g., [43,44].

Region-based methods (i.e., block matching)

The numerical differentiation operation required in the gradient-based OF methods may be impractical due to the presence of noise. Region-based methods do not require this operation and find the motion of a small speckle pattern (i.e., the ROI) by searching for the location of the best matching speckle pattern in the next frame. Finding the best match translates into computing a similarity measure between both blocks, e.g., the normalized cross-correlation or the sum of squared differences [45]. The maximum of this measure indicates the amount of tissue motion. For this reason, these techniques are sometimes also called block matching techniques. It is evident that the main underlying assumption is that of a stable speckle pattern between subsequent frames. Block matching techniques have been applied on both B-mode and RF data.

The application of B-mode block matching has been popular due to its conceptual simplicity. Trahey *et al.* were the first to successfully apply it for 2D blood flow tracking [46], later followed by Bohs *et al.* in the context of 2D tissue motion tracking [47]. A straightforward extension to 3D is challenging mainly due to the increased processing time [48]. Not only does the amount of tracking points increase significantly but the search space does as well.

As an alternative, RF block matching has been described by several groups, e.g., [49–51]. While being more computationally demanding, those were shown to be more accurate than B-mode block matching, provided that the image sequences were acquired at a sufficiently high frame rate to ensure acceptable interframe speckle correlation [20]. An extension to 3D is therefore challenging, given the relatively low volumetric frame rates [52].

Importantly, block matching techniques often require an additional regularization step since the initial motion estimates tend to be noisy, e.g., simply by median filtering [53] or using more advanced filtering operations such as wavelet denoising [54]. It should also be noted that in order to obtain subpixel motion estimates, the similarity measure requires interpolating, e.g., by fitting a parabole or cosine near its peak [31].

Phase-based methods

Rather than solving the OF equation with speckle intensity as input, some authors have proposed to reformulate the OF equation as the conservation of image phase with motion [55]. They argued that phase information could be less sensitive to brightness fluctuations and more strictly related to image structure. Compared to intensity-based tissue tracking, phase-based tracking could be helpful in those scenarios with a lower frame rate and the associated speckle decorrelation (such as in volumetric US) or where echo strength varies temporally due to changes in the US reflection angles (such as in myocardial imaging where the angle of the myocardial fiber and the main propagation angle changes). Examples can be found in [56] in which phase was extracted using a set of quadrature filters in several directions, or in [57] in which image phase was extracted without requiring a specific direction, but by computing the phase of the monogenic signal instead.

13.3.3 Registration-based methods

An alternative approach to assess motion between US images is based on image registration, also called image warping. The optimal displacement field is typically found in an iterative fashion by minimizing a cost function describing (dis) similarity between US images in combination with physical penalties to constrain the solutions to remain physiologically realistic. The fundamental difference between image registration and block matching is that image registration is a global approach not requiring an a posteriori regularization step as it is intrinsically embedded during the motion estimation approach.

The displacement field is typically represented by a set of basis functions [58]. By adjusting the coefficients of these functions, a wide variety of displacement fields can be efficiently represented. For US imaging, B-spline free-form deformation (FFD) model and radial basis functions (RBF) have seen most popularity [59,60]. B-spline FFDs are defined on a regular grid and have local support. The latter means that modifying a coefficient only has a local effect on the representation of the displacement field. RBF, on the other hand, express the displacement of a given point as a function to its distance with the center of every basis function, implying that RBFs have a global support. Their main advantage is that these center points can be placed anywhere in the image.

In the field of echocardiography, B-spline FFD models were first applied to 2D US imaging by Ledesma-Carbayo *et al.* [61] and were adopted later to 3D imaging by different groups, e.g., [26,62–64]. Thin-plate RBFs have also been used to extract 3D motion, e.g., in [65].

13.3.4 Biomechanical models

Biomechanical models incorporate our knowledge about the active and passive tissue properties and adopt appropriate constitutive models to mimic the observed tissue properties and motion/deformation behavior. While linear elastic and isotropic models are the easiest to adopt and solve, nonlinear and viscoelastic models more closely model tissue, but come at an increased computational complexity.

Biomechanical models have been used to track US tissue motion. For example, in cardiology by modeling the myocardium as a transversely isotropic linear elastic model, a dense displacement field could be computed starting from a sparse set of motion estimates at the myocardial borders [66]. Other authors have also included the electromechanical behavior of the myocardium in a model to estimate deformation starting from the myocardial boundaries [67]. Alternatively, in the field of elastography, rather than defining a constitutive model, an empirical model was proposed. This empirical model was generated by a sparse displacement/force inputs in a finite element model, combined with an artificial neural network to predict tissue motion response under stress [68].

13.3.5 Statistical models

The family of speckle tracking algorithms based on statistical models employ machine learning techniques to extract motion from a given US dataset. In a first step, a large annotated database with reference motion/deformation curves is used to learn motion patterns offline. Motion in a new dataset is then found by online guidance of the statistical model. During the learning stage, it is critical that the set of images used is representative for the expected range of deformations in the population that it aims to analyze later. The advantage of statistical models is their ability to reduce computational complexity while achieving a robust performance.

Many examples exist where statistical models are used in the context of speckle tracking. Those can be used to regularize OF results by first training a motion model [69]. Those can be used to fuse tracking input from different cues such as speckle tracking, image segmentation and motion statistics, e.g., [70]. Those help in the analysis of the output of speckle tracking techniques by classifying the motion patterns [71]. Those can also be used to handle image areas where speckle tracking results are missing or are of low quality due to image artifacts, e.g., [72,73].

13.3.6 Segmentation-based methods

Although segmentation-based methods are typically not classified under the family of speckle tracking algorithms, those are nevertheless worth mentioning in this context. Providing an extensive review regarding US-based image segmentation is beyond the scope of this section. For a more in-depth treatment of this topic, the reader is referred to other reviews, e.g., [74].

Segmentation-based methods are primarily used to further automate speckle tracking algorithms, e.g., to indicate the ROI for speckle tracking [75]; to automate the interpretation of its output [76] and to improve speckle tracking robustness, e.g., by including segmentation-based energies in the cost function of image registration [77] or in block matching [65].

Rather than tracking the speckle patterns of the organ of interest, these algorithms have also been used for purely tracking the borders over a temporal sequence, e.g., to dynamically track the myocardium from 3D US [78,79]. These algorithms allow estimating global function [80] or provide an indication of global deformation in elastography applications. However, it is typically not possible to obtain regional displacement/deformation estimates at the borders, or within the segmented area, given that no point-to-point correspondences exist between consecutive segmentations, unless an interpolation strategy is used, e.g., by using shape tracking as proposed in [66].

13.4 Determinants of speckle tracking performance

All speckle tracking algorithms rely on temporally stable speckle patterns as a function of tissue motion. This stability can be measured by the speckle decorrelation rate [20]. The major challenge of all tracking algorithms will therefore be signal decorrelation due to off-axis motion, out-of-plane motion, large displacements, poor signal-to-noise ratios, poor spatial resolution, image artifacts and other effects. Some of these issues will be discussed more in detail in the next sections.

13.4.1 Spatial resolution

The spatial resolution of the US imaging system will determine the average speckle size and will thus directly affect speckle tracking performance. For example, by recalling the principles of block matching, if the average speckle size is large, then the search correlation curve will be relatively flat. As such, the exact location of the maximum becomes more difficult to determine, which will affect tracking performance.

13.4.1.1 Point-spread function

The axial resolution is determined by the pulse length, or in other words, by the bandwidth of the transducer. The larger the bandwidth, the easier it is to generate short pulses. The lateral and elevational resolution is determined by the US beam width. It can be improved by increasing the effective size of the transmitting aperture to allow better focusing or by increasing the central frequency of the transmitted pulse. The latter comes at the cost of a lower penetration depth due to signal attenuation.

Given that US images are highly anisotropic with the lateral (and elevational) resolution being lower compared to the axial resolution, it is evident that performance in these directions will be different. Indeed, Ramamurthy *et al.* reported an improved performance in the axial direction over the lateral direction [20]. Similarly, they found substantial improvements in both directions when RF data was used over envelope-detected signals. This can be explained by the fact that the autocorrelation of RF signals exhibits a smaller full width at half maximum, making the correlation search perform better. The high RF frequency component, which gets lost in envelope detection, increases the uniqueness of the speckle patterns, therefore improving performance.

It should also be noted that the point-spread function varies spatially. This affects the appearance of the speckle patterns across the extent of the image. For example, for focused imaging systems, tracking performance is generally better at the focus.

13.4.1.2 Sampling criteria

The most important requirement upon reconstructing the image from channel data is that the Nyquist–Shannon sampling theorem must be satisfied, i.e., the (axial) sampling frequency must be at least twice the total bandwidth of the received signal. In the context of block matching, the sampling frequency determines the smallest axial steps in which signals may be correlated. It has been suggested by Parrilla *et al.* to even sample at least five times the central frequency [81] to ensure reliable correlation computations. Care should also be taken to ensure that images are reconstructed with sufficient line density to satisfy the Nyquist criterion for the lateral spatial frequency, otherwise lateral motion estimates may be prone to aliasing (i.e., peak hopping in block matching). For conventional focused imaging, transmit beam spacing should be at least twice the two-way beam width [82].

13.4.1.3 High frequency imaging

Interrogating tissue with higher US frequencies leads to a better image resolution and has been shown to improve tracking performance in the axial and lateral resolution, e.g., [12,20]. The use of high frequency US is limited to specific applications due to the shallow penetration depth. For example, they are used in small animal settings [83], vascular elasticity imaging [12] or intravascular blood flow tracking [84].

13.4.1.4 Transverse oscillations beamforming

In order to facilitate lateral motion estimation, several techniques have been proposed to also generate oscillations in the lateral direction [85]. Transverse oscillations (TOs) can be introduced during the beamforming process by choosing the appropriate apodization functions during one-way (in either transmit or receive) or two-way beamforming [86]. As an alternative, TOs can also be generated after the beamforming process, i.e., synthetically without the use of dedicated beamformers, either by performing signal manipulations in the frequency domain [87,88] or by image filtering in the frequency domain [89]. TO beamforming has been applied on linear, phased and convex array geometries in the context of tissue imaging and blood flow imaging [86,90,91].

Phase-based methods based on complex autocorrelators have seen most popularity to assess motion from these 2D oscillating fields. Those estimate the phase shift between sampled spatial quadrature (SQ) signal pairs created by parallel receive beamforming, either by steering two beams symmetrically around the transmit beam [85], or by beamforming in the transmit direction with two different receive apodization functions [92]. Rather than directly operating on sampled SQ signals, it is also possible to first beamform the complete US image (showing 2D TOs) and apply block matching [93] or image registration techniques [85] to assess motion.

13.4.1.5 Directional beamforming

Classical 1D motion estimators find the velocity component along the direction of the US beam. This projection makes it impossible to detect transverse motion.

In directional beamforming, signals are beamformed in the direction of the motion. Afterwards, motion between consecutive signals is found by previously described motion estimators such as cross-correlation. This method assumes that the direction of motion is known. It has been applied in the context of blood flow imaging [94,95] and vascular strain imaging [96].

13.4.1.6 Other beamforming strategies

More advanced beamforming techniques are continuously being developed by the US engineering community. These techniques have the potential to outperform the classical delay-and-sum beamforming approach in terms of contrast and spatial resolution, and therefore also have the potential to further improve the accuracy of existing motion estimators. For example, for plane wave imaging these include, but are not limited to, Fourier beamforming, minimum variance beamforming, sparse regularization and inverse-problem-based beamforming [97].

13.4.2 Temporal resolution

13.4.2.1 Optimal frame rate

Increasing the frame rate can decrease the deteriorating effect of speckle decorrelation on tracking performance. Indeed, smaller frame increments suffer from less decorrelation-related tracking inaccuracies. However, the potential for greater cumulative errors at the end of the sequence also increases, given that more estimates are used. It, therefore, seems plausible that an optimal interframe step must exist that result in the smallest relative errors [98]. The optimal frame rate will primarily be dictated by the displacement magnitude encountered in the specific application. For example, in a cardiac setting, different ranges have been suggested: at least 100 Hz for tissue Doppler imaging [99], 40–70 Hz for 2D speckle tracking [100] and at least 500 Hz to fully capture short-lived cardiac events that may contain important diagnostic information [101]. The optimal frame rate will also vary depending on the used motion estimator as the underlying assumptions may be different. Reporting these optimal working conditions is important to warrant optimal tracking performance, particularly if these techniques are to be applied in clinical practice [102].

In elastography, the above trade-offs are often translated into the concept of a strain filter [103]. The strain filter is a term used to describe that any motion/strain estimator only works optimally for a given range of tissue strain. The upper bound of this range is limited by decorrelation errors in case of large tissue strain whereas its lower bound at small strains is limited by errors due to electronic noise.

13.4.2.2 Intrinsic frame rate trade-offs

Because US imaging is based on the pulse-echo principle, the minimum time it takes to generate a single imaging line is physically limited by the speed of sound through the insonified tissue and the imaging depth, which is determined by the application. The only way to increase the frame rate is to reduce the number of transmit events to generate a single image frame. This can be done by either reducing the field of view (preserving spatial resolution, but limiting the potential clinical applications) or by reducing line density (but lowering spatial resolution). As such a trade-off exists between the field of view, spatial resolution and temporal resolution.

13.4.2.3 Fast imaging sequences

In order to increase frame rate without significantly compromising spatial resolution, several beamforming methods have recently been proposed: multiline acquisition (MLA), multiline transmit (MLT) beamforming and plane wave/diverging wave (PW/DW) imaging. Its many applications and technological foundations are reviewed in, e.g., [101,104].

MLA systems transmit a slightly broadened beam compared to standard focused imaging, and reconstruct multiple neighboring lines in parallel for each given transmit. As such, the number of transmit events can be reduced by the number of MLA lines. Due to the broadened beam configuration, lateral resolution is slightly deteriorated.

MLT beamforming is an alternative to MLA, in which multiple focused beams are transmitted simultaneously. Although cross-talk artifacts could emerge due to the spacing of neighboring transmit beams, it has been shown to result in an image quality comparable to focused imaging systems, but with an increased frame rate equal to the number of MLT beams [105].

By sending an unfocused plane wave or diverging wave, up to 16 parallel lines can be beamformed on receive, significantly improving frame rate [106]. It is also possible to beamform all lines with a single transmit at the expense of spatial resolution [107], unless multiple PW/DWs are compounded coherently [108].

These beamforming techniques have the potential to further improve speckle tracking performance as the reduced spatial resolution may be offset by the additional gain in temporal resolution [109].

13.4.3 Other factors

13.4.3.1 Out-of-plane motion

For 2D motion estimators, out-of-plane motion is one of the major sources of the observed in-plane speckle decorrelation. Several studies have shown that even relatively small motions in the elevational direction already have adverse effects on speckle correlation causing additional tracking difficulties, e.g., [110–112]. This is particularly evident in applications with complex motion patterns, for example, in a cardiac setting. Assessing longitudinal strain from a 2D apical view can be difficult due to the twisting motion of the heart, which causes out-of-plane motion. Indeed, apart from errors due to decorrelation, 2D longitudinal motion would also appear to be larger than its motion in 3D because of the 2D projection. This is in agreement with several studies in which global longitudinal strain obtained from tracking in a 2D apical view is generally larger (i.e., more negative) compared to tracking from a 3D recording [113,114].

13.4.3.2 Image quality

It has been well established that tracking performance generally improves with increasing signal-to-noise ratios [20,81,115]. The same trends are also predicted by the Cramer–Rao lower bound (CRLB) (see next section).

Unfortunately, US images are typically corrupted by a variety of image artifacts such as shadowing, reverberations, spatial distortion and clutter. The latter arguably being the most prevalent one [116]. These artifacts can degrade or bias motion estimation in blood flow imaging and elastography [63,117]. Devising strategies to preprocess or filter images prior to speckle tracking may therefore significantly improve tracking performance. Some examples are the use of singular value decomposition techniques to separate signal originating from clutter and of tissue [118–120] by using a model to first decompose the signal into its scattering sites followed by reconstructing only the signals from the ROI [121] or by 3D Wiener filtering [122].

13.4.3.3 Cramer–Rao lower bound

The CRLB predicts the minimum attainable standard deviation of the jitter of the displacement estimates of an unbiased motion estimator. Jitter can be seen as slight displacements of the true peak of the cross-correlation function caused by inherent uncertainties of the tracking process. These can be attributed to the combined effects of signal decorrelation, noise and the use of finite window lengths and bandwidths during motion estimation. Given that these uncertainties cannot be removed, the CRLB provides a theoretical lower bound on tracking performance. It provides insights into the fundamental tradeoffs between speckle decorrelation, SNR and image frequency content.

CRLB expressions have been derived for 1D and 2D motion estimators, in both the axial and lateral direction, see e.g., [123,124], as well as in the context of TOs [91]. These expressions show that the jitter becomes worse when decorrelation is higher, the SNR is lower or when image frequency content is lower.

13.4.3.4 Tissue type

Chen *et al.* investigated whether tracking performance depended on the imaged tissue type in particular muscle versus fat [115]. It was found that motion estimates were better when tracking muscle compared to fat. While overall speckle characteristics were different, the difference in tracking performance was primarily attributed to the presence of resolvable image structures (caused by the muscle fibers) that were absent in fat tissue.

13.4.3.5 Algorithm parameter tuning

Each motion estimator contains a fair amount of parameters, which can all be chosen differently depending on the application. The choice of parameter values will influence tracking performance and care should be taken to ensure that these values are optimized. Given that many algorithms (even those belonging to the same tracking family) can be implemented in different fashions, it remains difficult to extrapolate parameter choices among algorithms. A critical eye is therefore desired when interpreting the reported parameter sensitivity analyses.

Because of the detailed treatment of block matching and registration in the next chapters, some evident parameters affecting performance are already highlighted in this section. For more details, the reader is referred to the respective chapters.

The most sensitive parameters affecting performance in block matching are the size of the ROI and search region kernel.

In general, a large ROI (e.g., for 1D tracking in the order of ten times the axial resolution) will produce a low amplitude, but well-defined correlation peak with low-amplitude sidelobes. The well-defined peak indicates a high confidence in the motion estimate. This is due to the fact that the ROI consists of enough unique speckle features to be well tracked. However, its low amplitude shows that an exact speckle pattern match is difficult. Having a large ROI, therefore, improves tracking performance although it decreases the spatial resolution of the motion estimates [20].

On the other hand, tracking small ROIs (e.g., for 1D tracking in the order of the system's axial resolution) typically produces a high correlation peak implying a close match. However, those also tend to produce a large number of sidelobes with high amplitude showing that the match is not unique. Smaller ROIs thus appear to be more susceptible to false matches, i.e., peak hopping artifacts [125].

The most sensitive parameters affecting performance for FFD-based image registration algorithms are the grid spacing/topology and the regularization weight.

The resolution of the FFD lattice will influence the smoothness of the retrieved deformations. A coarse control point grid will result in capturing only global and intrinsically smooth deformation patterns whereas lowering the grid spacing allows retrieving more local deformations, but at a higher computational cost and often requiring a higher level of regularization to keep the deformations physiologically relevant. The topology of the control point grid will therefore indirectly dictate the range of deformations that can be modeled. For example, the topology could be adapted to the anatomy that is to be tracked [63].

The influence of the regularizer with respect to the similarity metric is controlled by its weight in the cost function. Its weight should be carefully controlled as a weight too high will result in overconstraining the solution space whereas leaving it a too low value will allow image noise to control the displacement output too much. A sensitivity analysis in a controlled environment where ground truth displacements are known is therefore highly desirable.

References

[1] T. Szabo, Diagnostic ultrasound imaging: inside out, second edition, *Elsevier*, ISBN: 978–970–12–396487–8, 2014.

[2] O. Bernard, B. Touil, J. D'hooge, D. Friboulet, Statistical Modeling of the radio-frequency signal for partially- and fully-developed speckle based on a generalized Gaussian model with application to echocardiography, *IEEE Trans Ultrason Ferroelectr Freq Control*, 54(10): 2189–2194, 2007.

[3] G. Trahey, S. Smith, O. von Ramm, Speckle pattern correlation with lateral aperture translation: experimental results and implications for spatial compounding, *IEEE Trans Ultrason Ferroelectr Freq Control*, 33(3): 257–264, 1986.

[4] J. Greenleaf, M. Fatemi, M. Insana, Selected methods for imaging elastic properties of biological tissues, *Annu Rev Biomed Eng*, 5:57–78, 2013.

[5] J. D'hooge, B. Bijnens, J. Thoen, F. Van de Werf, G. Sutherland, P. Suetens, Echocardiographic strain and strain-rate imaging: a new tool to study regional myocardial function, *IEEE Trans Med Imaging*, 21(9): 1022–1030, 2002.

[6] K. Nightingale, Acoustic radiation force impulse (ARFI) imaging: a review, *Curr Med Imaging*, 7(4): 328–339, 2002.

[7] A. Sarvazyan, O. Rudenko, S. Swanson, J. Fowlkes, S. Emelianov, Shear wave elasticity imaging: a new ultrasonic technology of medical diagnostics, *Ultrasound Med Biol*, 24(9): 1419–1435, 1998.

[8] J. Bercoff, M. Tanter, M. Fink, Supersonic shear imaging: a new technique for soft tissue elasticity mapping, *IEEE Trans Ultrason Ferroelectr Freq Control*, 51(4): 396–409, 2004.

[9] D. Cosgrove, F. Piscaglia, J. Bamber, *et al.*, EFSUMB guidelines and recommendations on the clinical use of ultrasound elastography, part 2: clinical applications, *Ultraschall Med*, 34(3): 238–253, 2013.

[10] J. Gennisson, T. Deffieux, M. Fink, M. Tanter, Ultrasound elastography: principles and techniques, *Diagn Interv Imaging*, 94(5): 487–495, 2013.

[11] R. Jasaityte, B. Heyde, J. D'hooge, Current state of three-dimensional myocardial strain estimation using echocardiography, *J Am Soc Echocardiogr*, 26(1): 15–28, 2013.

[12] M. Larsson, B. Heyde, F. Kremer, L. Brodin, J. D'hooge, Ultrasound speckle tracking for radial, longitudinal and circumferential strain estimation of the carotid artery – an in vitro validation via sonomicrometry using clinical and high-frequency ultrasound, *Ultrasonics*, 56:399–408, 2015.

[13] E. van Disseldorp, N. Petterson, M. Rutten, F. van de Vosse, M. van Sambeek, R. Lopata, Patient specific wall stress analysis and mechanical characterization of abdominal aortic aneurysms using 4D ultrasound, *Eur J Vasc Endovasc Surg*, 52(5): 635–642, 2016.

[14] K. Gijsbertse, A. Sprengers, M. Nillesen, *et al.*, Three-dimensional ultrasound strain imaging of skeletal muscles, *Phys Med Biol*, 62(2): 596–611, 2017.

[15] L. Slane, D. Thelen, The use of 2D ultrasound elastography for measuring tendon motion and strain, *J Biomech*, 47(3): 750–754, 2014.

[16] M. Vogt, H. Ermert, Development and evaluation of a high-frequency ultrasound-based system for in vivo strain imaging of the skin, *IEEE Trans Ultrason Ferroelectr Freq Control*, 52(3): 375–385, 2005.

[17] A. Dilley, J. Greening, B. Lynn, R. Leary, V. Morris, The use of cross-correlation analysis between high-frequency ultrasound images to measure longitudinal median nerve movement, *Ultrasound Med Biol*, 27 (9): 1211–1218, 2001.

[18] D. Evans, J. Jensen, M. Nielsen, Ultrasonic colour Doppler Imaging, *Interface Focus*, 1(4): 490–502, 2011.
[19] R. Maurice, M. Daronat, J. Ohayon, E. Stoyanova, S. Foster, G. Cloutier, Noninvasive high-frequency vascular ultrasound elastography, *Phys Med Biol*, 50(7): 1611–1628, 2005.
[20] B. Ramamurthy, G. Trahey, Potential and limitations of angle-independent flow detection algorithms using radio-frequency and detected echo signals, *Ultrason Imaging*, 13(3): 252–268, 1991.
[21] W. Yu, P. Yan, A. Sinusas, K. Thiele, J. Duncan, Towards pointwise motion tracking in echocardiographic image sequences – comparing the reliability of different features for speckle tracking, *Med Image Anal.*, 10(4): 495–508, 2006.
[22] J. Jensen, P. Munk, A new method for estimation of velocity vectors, *IEEE Trans Ultrason Ferroelectr Freq Control*, 45(3): 837–851, 1998.
[23] H. Liebgott, A. Basarab, P. Gueth, D. Friboulet, P. Delachartre, Transverse oscillations for tissue motion estimation, *Ultrasonics*, 50(6): 548–555, 2010.
[24] G. Sutherland, L. Hatle, P. Claus, J. D'Hooge, B. Bijnens, Doppler myocardial imaging: a textbook, *Published by BSWK bvba*, ISBN-10: 9081059211, ISBN-13: 978–9081059213, 2006.
[25] B. Dunmire, W. Beach, K. Labs, M. Plett, D. Strandness, Cross-beam vector Doppler ultrasound for angle-independent velocity measurements, *Ultrasound Med Biol*, 26(8): 1213–1235, 2000.
[26] M. De Craene, P. Allain, H. Gao, *et al.*, Computational and physical phantom setups for the second cardiac motion analysis challenge (cMAC2), In *STACOM – Statistical Atlases and Computational Models of the Heart*, 7746:125–133, 2012.
[27] J. Jensen, Estimation of blood velocities using ultrasound: a signal processing approach, *Cambridge University Press*, ISBN: 9780521464840, 1998.
[28] G. Pinton, J. Dahl, G. Trahey, Rapid tracking of small displacements with ultrasound, *IEEE Trans Ultras Ferroelectr Freq Control*, 53(6): 1103–1117, 2006.
[29] Y. Deng, N. Rouze, M. Palmeri, K. Nightingale, Ultrasonic shear wave elasticity imaging sequencing and data processing using a Verasonics research scanner, *IEEE Trans Ultrason Ferroelectr Freq Control*, 64(1): 164–176, 2017.
[30] F. Viola, W. Walker, A comparison of the performance of time-delay estimators in medical ultrasound, *IEEE Trans Ultrason Ferroelectr Freq Control*, 50(4): 392–401, 2003.
[31] I. Céspedes, Y. Huang, J. Ophir, S. Spratt, Methods for estimation of subsample time delays of digitized echo signals, *Ultrason Imaging*, 17(2): 142–171, 1995.
[32] I. Hein, W. O'Brien, Current time-domain methods for assessing tissue motion by analysis of reflected ultrasound echoes – a review, *IEEE Trans Ultrason Ferroelect Freq Control*, 40(2): 84–102, 1993.

[33] C. Kasai, N. Koroku, A. Koyano, R. Omoto, Real-time two-dimensional blood flow imaging using an autocorrelation technique, *IEEE Trans Ultrason Ferroelectr Freq Control*, 32(3): 458–464, 1985.

[34] T. Loupas, J. Powers, R. Gill, An axial velocity estimator for ultrasound blood flow imaging, based on a full evaluation of the Doppler equation by means of a two-dimensional autocorrelation approach, *IEEE Trans Ultrason Ferroelectr Freq Control*, 42(4): 672–688, 1995.

[35] A. Pesavento, C. Perrey, M. Krueger, H. Ermert, A time-efficient and accurate strain estimation concept for ultrasonic elastography using iterative phase zero estimation, *IEEE Trans Ultrason Ferroelect Freq. Control*, 46(5): 1057–1067,1999.

[36] J. Barron, D. Fleet, S. Beauchemin, Performance of optical flow techniques, *Int J Comput Vision*, 12(1): 43–77, 1994.

[37] E. Angelini, O. Gerard, Review of myocardial motion estimation methods from optical flow tracking on ultrasound data, In *IEEE EMBS Annual Int Conf*, 1537–1540, 2006.

[38] B. Horn, B. Schunck, Determining optical flow, *Artif Intell*, 17(1–3): 185–203, 1981.

[39] R. Mukherjee, C. Sprouse, A. Pinheiro, T. Abraham, P. Burlina, Computing myocardial motion in 4-dimensional echoardiography, *Ultrasound Med Biol*, 38(7): 1284–1297, 2012.

[40] B. Lucas, T. Kanade, An iterative image registration technique with an application to stereo vision, In *DARPA Image Understanding Workshop*, 121–130, 1981.

[41] Y. Chunke, K. Terada, S. Oe, Motion analysis of echocardiograph using optical flow method, In *IEEE Int Conf Systems Man and Cybernetics*, 1:672–677, 1996.

[42] M. Suhling, M. Arigovindan, C. Jansen, P. Hunziker, M. Unser, Myocardial motion analysis from B-mode echocardiograms, *IEEE Trans Image Process*, 14(4): 525–536, 2005.

[43] A. Curiale, G. Vegas-Sánchez-Ferrero, J. Bosch, S. Aja-Fernández, A maximum likelihood approach to diffeomorphic speckle tracking for 3D strain estimation in echocardiography, *Med Image Anal*, 24(1): 90–105, 2015.

[44] O. Somphone, M. De Craene, R. Ardon, *et al.*, Fast myocardial motion and strain estimation in 3D cardiac ultrasound with sparse demons, In *ISBI – Int Symp on Biomedical Imaging*, 1182–1185, 2013.

[45] B. Friemel, L. Bohs, G. Trahey, Relative performance of two-dimensional speckle tracking techniques: normalized correlation, non-normalized correlation and sum-absolute-difference, In *IEEE Int Ultrasonics Symposium*, 1481–1484, 1995.

[46] G. Trahey, J. Allison, O. Von Ramm, Angle independent ultrasonic detection of blood flow, *IEEE Trans Biomed Eng*, 34(12): 965–967, 1987.

[47] L. Bohs, B. Geiman, M. Anderson, S. Gebhart, G. Trahey, Speckle tracking for multi-dimensional flow estimation, *Ultrasonics*, 38(1–8):369–375, 2000.

[48] J. Crosby, B. Amundsen, T. Hergum, E. Remme, S. Langeland, H. Torp, 3-D speckle tracking for assessment of regional left ventricular function, *Ultrasound Med Biol*, 35(3): 458–471, 2009.
[49] M. Lubinski, S. Emelianov, M. O'Donnell, Speckle tracking methods for ultrasonic elasticity imaging using short-time correlation, *IEEE Trans Ultrason Ferroelectr Freq Control*, 46(1): 82–96, 1999.
[50] E. Konofagou, J. Ophir, A new elastographic method for estimation and imaging of lateral displacements, lateral strains, corrected axial strains and Poisson's ratios in tissues, *Ultrasound Med Biol*, 24(8): 1183–1199, 1998.
[51] R. Lopata, M. Nillesen, I. Gerrits, J. Thijssen, L. Kapusta, F. van de Vosse, C. de Korte, Performance evaluation of methods for two-dimensional displacement and strain estimation using ultrasound radio frequency data, *Ultrasound Med Biol*, 35(5): 796–812, 2009.
[52] R. Lopata, M. Nillesen, J. Thijssen, L. Kapusta, C. de Korte, Three-dimensional cardiac strain imaging in healthy children using RF-data, *Ultrasound Med Biol*, 37(9): 1399–1408, 2011.
[53] S. Srinivasan, T. Krouskop, J. Ophir, Comparing elastographic strain images with modulus images obtained using nanoidentation: preliminary results using phantoms and tissue samples, *Ultrasound Med Biol*, 30(4): 329–343, 2004.
[54] N. Bachner-Hinenzon, O. Ertracht, M. Lysiansky, O. Binah, D. Adam, Layer-specific assessment of left ventricular function by utilizing wavelet denoising: a validation study, *Med Biol Eng Comput*, 49(1): 3–13, 2011.
[55] D. Boukerroui, A. Noble, M. Brady, Velocity estimation in ultrasound images: a block matching approach, In *IPMI – Information Processing in Medical Imaging*, 18:586–598, 2003.
[56] L. Tautz, A. Hennemuth, H. Peitgan, Quadrature filter based motion analysis for 3D ultrasound sequences, In *STACOM – Statistical Atlases and Computational Models of the Heart*, 169–177, 2012.
[57] M. Alessandrini, A. Basarab, H. Liebgott, O. Bernard, Myocardial motion estimation from medical images using the monogenic signal, *IEEE Trans Image Process*, 22(3): 1084–1095, 2013.
[58] M. Holden, A review of geometric transformations for nonrigid body registration, *IEEE Trans Med Imaging*, 27(1):111–128, 2008.
[59] M. Buhmann, Radial basis functions, *Acta Numerica*, 9:1–38, 2000.
[60] D. Rueckert, L. Sonoda, D. Hill, M. Leach, D. Hawkes, Nonrigid registration using free-form deformations: application to breast MR images, *IEEE Trans Med Imaging*, 18(8): 712–721, 1999.
[61] M. Ledesma-Carbayo, J. Kybic, M. Desco, *et al.*, Spatio-temporal nonrigid registration for ultrasound cardiac motion estimation, *IEEE Trans Med Imaging*, 24(9): 1113–1126, 2005.
[62] B. Heyde, S. Bouchez, S. Thieren, *et al.*, Elastic image registration to quantify 3D regional myocardial deformation from volumetric ultrasound: experimental validation in an animal model, *Ultrasound Med Biol*, 39(9): 1688–1697, 2013.

[63] B. Heyde, M. Alessandrini, J. Hermans, D. Barbosa, P. Claus, J. D'hooge, Anatomical image registration using volume conservation to assess cardiac deformation from 3D ultrasound recordings, *IEEE Trans Med Imaging*, 35 (2): 501–511, 2015.

[64] Z. Zhang, M. Ashraf, D. Sahn, X. Song, Temporally diffeomorphic cardiac motion estimation from three-dimensional echocardiography by minimization of intensity consistency error, *Med Phys*, 41(5): 052902, 2014.

[65] C. Compas, E. Wong, X. Huang, *et al.*, Radial basis functions for combining shape and speckle tracking in 4D echocardiography, *IEEE Trans Med Imaging*, 33(6): 1275–1289, 2014.

[66] X. Papademetris, A. Sinusas, D. Dione, T. Constable, J. Duncan, Estimation of 3-D left ventricular deformation from medical images using biomechanical models, *IEEE Trans Med Imaging*, 21(7): 786–800, 2002.

[67] M. Sermesant, H. Delingette, N. Ayache, An electromechanical model of the heart for image analysis and simulation, *Med Image Analysis*, 25(5): 612–625, 2006.

[68] C. Hoerig, J. Ghaboussi, M. Insana, An information-based machine learning approach to elasticity imaging, *Biomech Model Mechanobiol*, in press, 2016.

[69] E. Leung, M. Danilouchkine, M. van Stralen, N. de Jong, A. van der Steen, J. Bosch, Left ventricular border tracking using cardiac motion models and optical flow, *Ultrasound Med Biol*, 37(4): 605–616, 2011.

[70] Y. Wang, B. Georgescu, H. Houle, D. Comaniciu, Volumetric myocardial mechanics from 3D+t ultrasound data with multi-modal tracking, In *STACOM – Statistical Atlases and Computational Models of the Heart*, 6364:184–193, 2010.

[71] N. Duchateau, A. Doltra, E. Silva, *et al.*, Atlas-based quantification of myocardial motion abnormalities: added-value for understanding the effect of cardiac resynchronization therapy, *Ultrasound Med Biol*, 38(12): 2186–2197, 2012.

[72] A. Lu, M. Zontak, N. Parajuli, *et al.*, Dictionary learning-based spatiotemporal regularization for 3D dense speckle tracking, In *SPIE Medical Imaging*, vol. 10139, paper 04, 2017. Available from https://www.spiedigitallibrary.org/conference-proceedings-of-spie/10139/1/Dictionary-learning-based-spatiotemporal-regularization-for-3D-dense-speckle-tracking/10.1117/12.2250695.short?SSO=1 for details.

[73] M. Tabassian, M. Alessandrini, R. Jasaityte, L. De Marchi, G. Masetti, J. D'hooge, Handling missing strain (rate) curves using K-nearest neighbor imputation, In *IEEE Int Ultrason Symp*, 1–4, 2016.

[74] J. Noble, D. Boukerroui, Ultrasound image segmentation: a survey, *IEEE Trans Med Imaging*, 25(8): 987–1010, 2006.

[75] B. Heyde, D. Barbosa, A. Daraban, *et al.*, An automated pipeline for regional cardiac strain estimation from volumetric ultrasound data, In *IEEE Int Ultrasonics Symposium*, 1248–1251, 2013.

[76] W. Liu, J. Zagzebski, T. Varghese, C. Dyer, U. Techavipoo, T. Hall, Segmentation of elastographic images using a coarse-to-fine active contour model, *Ultrasound Med Biol*, 32(3): 397–408, 2006.

[77] A. Myronenko, X. Song, D. Sahn, LV motion tracking from 3D echocardiography using textural and structural information, In *MICCAI – Medical Image Computing and Computer-Assisted Intervention*, 4792: 428–435, 2007.

[78] D. Barbosa, B. Heyde, T. Dietenbeck, D. Friboulet, J. D'hooge, O. Bernard, Fast left ventricle tracking in 3D echocardiographic data using anatomical affine optical flow, In *FIMH – Functional Imaging and Modelling of the Heart*, LNCS 7945:191–199, 2013.

[79] F. Orderud, J. Hånsgard, S. Rabben, Real-time tracking of the left ventricle in 3D echocardiography using a state estimation approach, In *MICCAI – Medical Image Computing and Computer-Assisted Intervention*, 4791: 858–865, 2007.

[80] J. Hansegård, S. Urheim, K. Lunde, S. Malm, S. Rabben, Semi-automated quantification of left ventricular volumes and ejection fraction by real-time three-dimensional echocardiography, *Cardiovasc Ultrasound*, 7:18, 2009.

[81] M. Parrilla, J. Anaya, C. Fritsch, Digital signal processing techniques for high accuracy ultrasonic range measurements, *IEEE Trans Instrum Meas*, 40(4);759–763, 1991.

[82] J. Wright, Image formation in diagnostic ultrasound, In *IEEE Int Ultrasonics Symposium*, Short Course, 1997.

[83] V. Ferferieva, A. Van den Bergh, P. Claus, *et al.*, Assessment of strain and strain rate by two-dimensional speckle tracking in mice: comparison with tissue Doppler echocardiography and conductance catheter measurements, *Eur Heart J – Cardiovasc Imaging*, 14(8): 765–773, 2013.

[84] W. Aoudi, H. Liebgott, A. Needles, V. Yang, S. Foster, D. Vray, Estimation methods for flow imaging with high frequency ultrasound, *Ultrasonics*, 44(1): e135–e140, 2006.

[85] B. Heyde, N. Bottenus, G. Trahey, J. D'hooge, Impact of beamforming strategies and regularisation on ultrasound displacement estimation using RF-based image registration, In *Int Symposium on Biomed Imaging*, 16(3): 805–822, 2017.

[86] H. Liebgott, A. Basarab, P. Gueth, D. Friboulet, P. Delachartre, Transverse oscillations for tissue motion estimation, *Ultrasonics*, 50(6): 548–555, 2010.

[87] X. Chen, M. Zohdy, S. Emelianov, M. O'Donnell, Lateral speckle tracking using synthetic lateral phase, *IEEE Trans Ultrason Ferroelectr Freq Control*, 51(5): 540–550, 2004.

[88] H. Liebgott, Fourier domain beamforming for transverse-oscillations, In *IEEE Ultrason Symp*, 1755–1758, 2010.

[89] F. Varray, H. Liebgott, An alternative method to classical beamforming for transverse oscillation images: application to elastography, In *ISBI – Int Symp on Biomedical Imaging*, 716–719, 2013.

[90] J. Jensen, New developments in vector velocity imaging using the transverse oscillation approach, *SPIE Medical Imaging*, 8675:8675F, 2013.

[91] B. Heyde, N. Bottenus, J. D'hooge, G. Trahey, Evaluation of the transverse oscillation technique for cardiac phased array imaging: a theoretical study, *IEEE Trans Ultrason Ferroelectr Freq Control*, 64(2): 320–334, 2017.

[92] M. Anderson, Multi-dimensional velocity estimation with ultrasound using spatial quadrature, *IEEE Trans Ultrason Ferroelectr Freq Control*, 45(3): 852–861, 1998.

[93] A. Basarab, P. Gueth, H. Liebgott, P. Delachartre, Phase-based block matching applied to motion estimation with unconventional beamforming strategies, *IEEE Trans Ultrason Ferroelect Freq Control*, 56(5): 945–957, 2009.

[94] J. Jensen, Directional velocity estimation using focusing along the flow direction I: theory and simulation, *IEEE Trans Ultrason Ferroelectr Freq Control*, 50(7): 857–872, 2003.

[95] J. Jensen, N. Oddershede, Estimation of velocity vectors in synthetic aperture ultrasound imaging, *IEEE Trans Med Imaging*, 25(12): 1637–1644, 2006.

[96] H. Hansen, M. Stuart, C. Hoyos, J. Jensen, C. de Korte, Performance evaluation of compounding and directional beamforming techniques for carotid strain imaging using plane wave transmissions, In *IEEE Int Ultrasonics Symp*, 1814–1818, 2014.

[97] H. Liebgott, A. Rodriguez-Molares, F. Cervenansky, J. Jensen, O. Bernard, Plane-wave imaging challenge in medical ultrasound, In *IEEE Ultrason Symp*, 2016.

[98] J. Ha, W. Walker, J. Hossack, Determination of an optimal image frame interval for frame-to-frame ultrasound image motion tracking, *IEEE Trans Ultrason Ferroelectr Freq Control*, 52(3): 386–396, 2005.

[99] B. Lind, J. Nowak, J. Dorph, J. van der Linden, L. Brodin, Analysis of temporal requirements for myocardial tissue velocity imaging, *Eur J Echocardiogr*, 3(3): 214–219, 2002.

[100] T. Yingchoncharoen, S. Agarwal, Z. Popovic, T. Marwick, Normal ranges of left ventricular strain: a meta-analysis, *J Am Soc Echocardiogr*, 26(2): 185–191, 2013.

[101] M. Cikes, L. Tong, G. Sutherland, J. D'hooge, Ultrafast cardiac ultrasound imaging: technical principles, applications, and clinical benefits, *JACC Cardiovasc Imaging*, 7(8): 812–823, 2014.

[102] J. Voigt, G. Pedrizzetti, P. Lysyansky, *et al.*, Definitions for a common standard for 2D speckle tracking echocardiography: consensus document of the EACVI/ASE/Industry Task Force to standardize deformation imaging, *J Am Soc Echocardiogr*, 28(2): 183–193, 2015.

[103] T. Varghese, J. Ophir, A theoretical framework for performance characterization of elastography: the strain filter, *IEEE Trans Ultrason Ferroelectr Freq Control*, 44(1): 164–172, 1997.

[104] M. Tanter, M. Fink, Ultrafast imaging in biomedical ultrasound, *IEEE Trans Ultrason Ferroelectr Freq Control*, 61(1): 102–119, 2014.

[105] L. Tong, H. Gao, J. D'hooge, Multi-transmit beam forming for fast cardiac imaging – a simulation study, *IEEE Trans Ultrason Ferroelectr Freq Control*, 60(8): 1719–1731, 2013.

[106] H. Hasegawa, H. Kanai, High-frame-rate echocardiography using diverging transmit beams and parallel receive beam forming, *J Med Ultrasonics*, 38(3): 129–140, 2011.

[107] C. Papadacci, M. Pernot, M. Couade, M. Fink, M. Tanter, High-contrast ultrasound imaging of the heart, *IEEE Trans Ultrason Ferroelectr Freq Control*, 61(2): 288–301, 2014.

[108] G. Montaldo, M. Tanter, J. Bercoff, N. Benech, M. Fink, Coherent plane-wave compounding for very high-frame rate ultrasonography and transient elastography, *IEEE Trans Ultrason Ferroelectr Freq Control*, 56(3): 489–506, 2009.

[109] M. Alessandrini, B. Heyde, L. Tong, O. Bernard, J. D'hooge, Tracking quality in plane-wave versus conventional cardiac ultrasound: a preliminary evaluation insilico based on a state-of-the-art simulation pipeline, In *IEEE Int Ultrasonics Symposium*, 390, 2015.

[110] J. Chen, B. Fowlkes, P. Carson, M. Rubin, Determination of scan-plane motion using speckle decorrelation: theoretical considerations and initial test, *Int J Imaging Sys Tech* 8(1): 38–44, 1997.

[111] J. Hossack, Influence of elevational motion on the degradation of 2d image frame matching, In *IEEE Int Ultrason Symp*, 1713–1716, 2000.

[112] P. Li, C. Li, W. Yeh, Tissue motion and elevational speckle decorrelation in freehand 3d ultrasound, *Ultrason Imaging*, 24(1): 1–12,2002.

[113] R. Jasaityte, B. Heyde, V. Ferferieva, *et al.*, Comparison of a new methodology for the assessment of 3D myocardial strain from volumetric ultrasound with 2D speckle tracking, *Int J Cardiovasc Imaging*, 28(5): 1049–1060, 2012.

[114] K. Saito, H. Okura, N. Watanabe, *et al.*, Comprehensive evaluation of left ventricular strain using speckle tracking echocardiography in normal adults: comparison of three-dimensional and two-dimensional approaches, *J Am Soc Echocardiogr*, 22(9): 1025–1030, 2009.

[115] E. Chen, W. Jenkins, W. O'Brien, The impact of various imaging parameters on ultrasonic displacement and velocity estimates, *IEEE Trans Ultrason Ferroelectr Freq Control*, 41(3): 293–301, 1994.

[116] M. Lediju, M. Pihl, J. Dahl, G. Trahey, Quantitative assessment of the magnitude, impact, and spatial extent of ultrasonic clutter, *Ultrason Imaging*, 30(3): 151–168, 2008.

[117] K. Leung, M. Danilouchkine, M. van Stralen, N. de Jong, A. F. W. van der Steen, J. Bosch, Probabilistic framework for tracking in artifact-prone 3D echocardiograms, *Med Image Anal*, 14(6): 750–758, 2010.

[118] C. Demené, T. Deffieux, M. Pernot, *et al.*, Spatiotemporal clutter filtering of ultrafast ultrasound data highly increases Doppler and ultrasound sensitivity, *IEEE Trans Med Imaging*, 34(11): 2271–2285, 2015.

[119] F. Mauldin, D. Lin, J. Hossack, The singular value filter: a general filter design strategy for PCA-based signal separation in medical ultrasound imaging, *IEEE Trans Med Imaging*, 30(11): 1951–1964, 2011.

[120] A. Yu, L. Lovstakken, Eigen-based clutter filter design for ultrasound color flow imaging: a review, *IEEE Trans Ultrason Ferroelectr Freq Control*, 57(5): 1096–1111, 2010.

[121] B. Byram, K. Dei, J. Tierney, D. Dumont, A model and regularization scheme for ultrasonic beamforming clutter reduction, *IEEE Trans Ultrason Ferroelectr Freq Control*, 62(11): 1913–1927, 2015.

[122] N. Bylund, M. Andersson, H. Knuttson, Interactive 3D filter design for ultrasound artifact reduction, In *ICIP – Int Conference on Image Processing*, 1–4, 2005.

[123] W. Walker, G. Trahey, A fundamental limit on the performance of correlation based phase correction and flow estimation techniques, *IEEE Trans Ultrason Ferroelectr Freq Control*, 41(5): 644–654, 1994.

[124] W. Walker, G. Trahey, A fundamental limit on delay estimation using partially correlated speckle signals, *IEEE Trans Ultrason Ferroelectr Freq Control*, 42(2): 301–308, 1995.

[125] S. Foster, P. Embree, W. O'Brien, Flow velocity profile via time-domain correlation: error analysis and computer simulation, *IEEE Trans Ultrason Ferroelectr Freq Control*, 37(3): 164–175, 1990.

[126] C. Metz, S. Klein, M. Schaap, T. van Walsum, W. Niessen, Nonrigid registration of dynamic medical imaging data using nD + t B-splines and a groupwise optimization approach, *Med Image Anal*, 15(2): 238–249, 2011.

[127] A. Elen, H. Choi, D. Loeckx, *et al.*, Three-dimensional cardiac strain estimation using spatio-temporal elastic registration of ultrasound images: a feasibility study, *IEEE Trans Med Imaging*, 27(11): 1580–1591, 2008.

[128] B. Heyde, S. Cygan, H.F. Choi, *et al.*, Regional cardiac motion and strain estimation in three-dimensional echocardiography: a validation study in thick-walled univentricular phantoms, *IEEE Trans Ultrason Ferroelectr Freq Control*, 59(4): 668–682, 2012.

Chapter 14
Techniques for speckle tracking: block matching

R.G.P. Lopata[1]

14.1 Introduction

The clinical need for in vivo motion and deformation quantification and the many applications have been clearly explained in the previous chapters. In general, we distinguish between (1) quasi-static elastography: speckle tracking during compression or palpation of tissue to estimate local strains and elasticity and (2) dynamic elastography, where speckle tracking on actively deforming tissue such as the heart, arteries and skeletal muscles is performed, see Figure 14.1. The third class, where motion of the tissue is induced with a vibrational device or a push by the transducer (ARFI, shear wave imaging) is not dealt with in this chapter. We will elaborate on a sub-set of speckle tracking and/or strain imaging techniques, which are based on the so-called **block-matching** techniques. Hence, Doppler-based techniques will not be discussed.

14.1.1 Strain imaging: an overview

An overview of the total pipeline from ultrasound (US) data to strain quantification is shown in Figure 14.2. Starting point is US acquisition in the organ of interest. Here, the heart was chosen as an example, which has been extensively studied (Heimdal *et al.*, 1998; D'hooge, 2000; Konofagou *et al.*, 2002; Lopata *et al.*, 2011). However, block-matching-based techniques have been demonstrated in many other applications, including breast imaging (Cespedes *et al.*, 1993), tumour detection (Ophir *et al.*, 1999; Garra *et al.*, 1997), skeletomuscular applications (Kallel *et al.*, 1998; Deffieux *et al.*, 2008), abdominal applications (Emelianov *et al.*, 1995; Krouskop *et al.*, 1998), vascular imaging (De Korte *et al.*, 1998), etc.

Data can be acquired in several ways. In summary, the different data types that can be used are:

- **RF data:** radio-frequency data, digitized and stored prior to any post-processing. RF data are however pre-amplified, time or lateral gain

[1]Cardiovascular Biomechanics, Department of Biomedical Engineering, Eindhoven University of Technology, The Netherlands

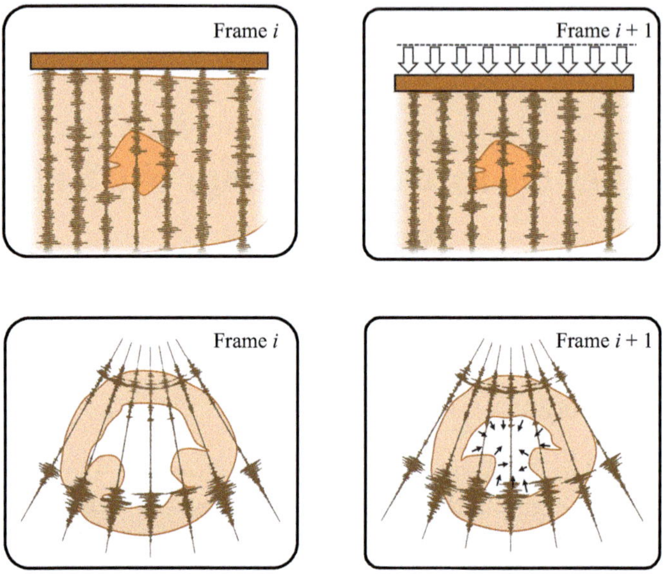

Figure 14.1 Quasi-static vs. dynamic strain imaging

compensated and alternatively based on multiple transmit and/or receive foci. An example is shown in Figure 14.4.

- **Analytical signals/data:** generated by applying the Hilbert transform to the raw RF data.
- **Envelope or amplitude data:** detected signal amplitude, obtained by calculating the modulus of the analytical signal, see also Figure 14.4.
- **Intensity or grey value data:** brightness values obtained after log compression. In case DICOM or other image/movie files are used, the data have also been subjected to post-processing such as persistence filtering, spatial filtering, image enhancement, etc.

In recent years, so-called **channel data** are also acquired and used for speckle tracking, which is basically the RF data pre-beamforming for each channel. For a 128 line-by-line scan, the dimensions of an RF frame are the number of samples in the axial direction N_{ax} (depending on the depth) × the number of lines, N_{lat}, in this case 128. For a single frame, the channel data set will be $N_{ax} \times N_{lat} \times N_c$, with N_c the number of channels. In DICOM data, each frame is 800 (width) by 600 (depth) pixels by three colour channels Red – Green – Blue (RGB).

The second step is processing of the data to estimate the local displacement of the tissue. This is executed by comparing segments of the data in consecutive images, i.e. **block matching**. This is repeated for the entire image, typically in a sliding window fashion, resulting in one-, two- or three-dimensional **displacement images** (u), depending on the data used.

The resulting displacement data need to be regularized to remove outliers and possibly filter the displacement data before strain calculation (see Section 14.5). Next, the strain can be calculated instantly or after tracking. If one calculates the

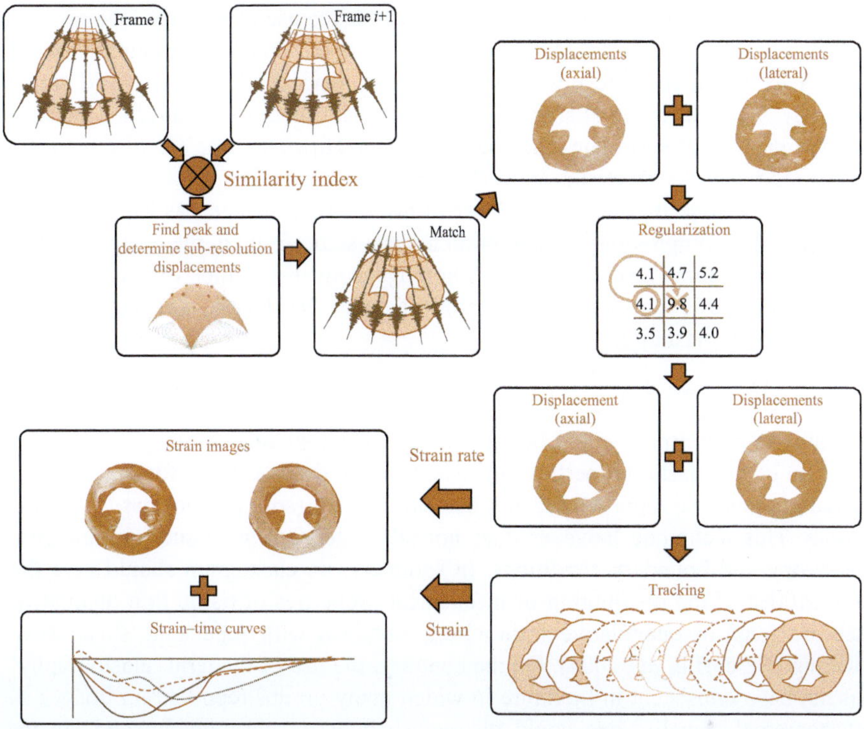

Figure 14.2 The basic steps of a block-matching algorithm, from RF data to strain images

frame-to-frame strain, we obtain the **strain rate** ($\dot{\varepsilon}$). However, if one tracks the tissue of interest, i.e. updating the tissue location by accumulating displacements over time, one can calculate the **cumulative strain** (ε) for a pre-defined grid of points within our region of interest (ROI) (see also Figure 14.2). Once we have obtained the strain rate or cumulative strain images, analysis of the strain–time curves or sectorical analysis of the strain images can be performed. All these steps will be discussed in the upcoming sections. However, before going into detail, it is important to understand the differences between widely used terminology and their actual meaning.

14.1.2 Terminology

Often, **speckle tracking** is used to indicate motion and strain estimation based on series of grey-scale images, i.e. B-mode images: we are 'tracking the speckles', thereby assuming an optical flow (see previous chapter) of the grey values. However, one could argue that tracking of speckles is also performed when analysing the other signal types that are available. The nomenclature has a more historical reason since first block-matching algorithms were based on A-mode (Yagi and Nakayama, 1988), M-mode (Adler *et al.*, 1990) and B-mode data (Trahey *et al.*, 1988) only. In summary, speckle tracking provides you with motion, similar to Tissue Doppler Imaging (TDI), which can be converted into strains in post-processing.

In literature, **strain imaging** typically denotes the use of RF data. The original paper by Ophir *et al.* (1991) presented high-precision and high-resolution **strain images** by processing the raw RF signal rather than the log-compressed signal envelope, which has several advantages (see the next section). As a result, the term 'strain imaging' often implies the use of RF data. However, one can also estimate global (and even local) strains from B-mode or envelope data.

The technique introduced by Ophir in his landmark paper was baptized **elastography**. By compressing a phantom in a quasi-static fashion, the resulting strain data (or strain image) were inverted. A homogeneous distribution of stress (σ) was assumed (stress is constant as a function of depth: $\overline{\sigma}$). Hence, obeying Hooke's simple law for elasticity,

$$\sigma = E\varepsilon \quad \rightarrow \quad E = \frac{\bar{\sigma}}{\varepsilon} = \bar{\sigma}\varepsilon^{-1} \tag{14.1}$$

the inverse strain image could be regarded an '**elastogram**': an image of the distribution of the elastic properties in tissue. Quantitative measures for the Young's modulus cannot be reported, but mechanical contrast (soft vs. hard tissue) is now visible. This technique however does not take into account tissue non-linearity, anisotropy and boundary conditions. In summary, an elastogram should give the user an idea of the distribution of mechanical properties of tissue in a qualitative (see previous) or quantitative fashion, e.g. obtained with supersonic shear wave imaging (Bercoff *et al.*, 2004). On the contrary, the use of the term 'elastography' has not been consistent in literature in which many groups report strain images as 'elastograms'. Finally, one could distinguish between elastography and **elastometry**. The latter involves estimating a single number for the stiffness of an artery or the elasticity of the liver (see also Chapter 22).

14.2 1-D speckle tracking and strain imaging

In block matching, the data are processed 'block by block' (see also Figures 14.2 and 14.3). A ROI is considered in which the organ is situated. Next, within this

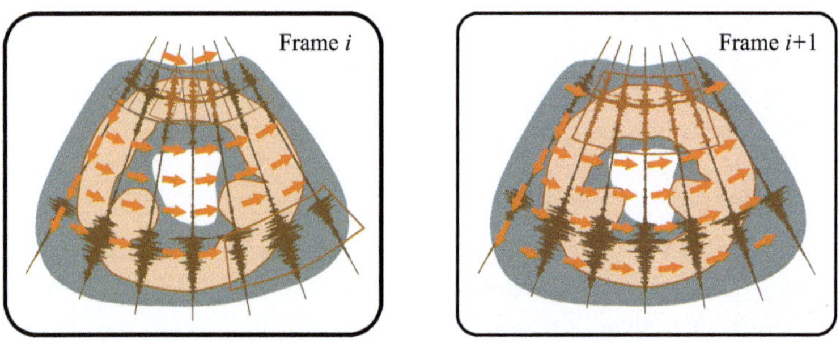

Figure 14.3 A region of interest (grey area) is defined. Next, a template is selected in frame i (see left) in a sliding window fashion. For each template, a search area is defined in the next frame i + 1 that is larger in size

ROI, a segment or 'window' of data is selected in frame i. This is the **template**, **T**. Please note that kernel, segment and window are all names for the sub-set of data pixels that will be used for displacement estimation. The term 'window' is most likely derived from 'sliding window operations', which is traditionally used for displacement estimation.

Next, in the subsequent frame $(i+1)$, a typically larger segment or 'window' is selected that is centred around T, which is basically the **search area, SA**. The size of SA ranges from (1) the same size as T up to (2) the entire image I.

The data in T and SA are compared by calculating a similarity measure. Next, the spatial co-ordinate of maximum similarity ($\vec{r}_{\max}$) with respect to the centre point of the T (and thus, SA), $\vec{r}_0$, is determined. The distance between these co-ordinates is a measure for the displacement $\vec{u}$: $\vec{u} = \vec{r}_{\max} - \vec{r}_0$. In case of one-dimensional (1-D) data, $u = u_{ax}$, whereas for 2-D data, $\vec{u} = u_{ax}\vec{e}_{ax} + u_{lat}\vec{e}_{lat}$.

Several considerations need to be made

- Use of amplitude data (envelope, grey values) or radio-frequent data (RF, analytical data).
- Use of 1-D or multi-dimensional (N-D) kernel sizes.
- Choice of similarity measure and possible refinement.
- Choice of regularization.

These will be dealt with in the following (sub)sections.

14.2.1 Data types

Figure 14.4 shows the RF signals (*solid*) and respective amplitude (*dashed*) for two consecutive images, obtained at the same lateral location, i.e. the same RF line/US beam. Please note that data sets obtained at different time points are often referred to as **frames**. When comparing the signals for frames i and $i+1$, we see that both the RF and envelope are slightly displaced at certain axial positions, which is the result of tissue motion.

This brings us to an important notion in speckle tracking: Tissue motion will cause echogenic scatterers to move, thereby altering the image. By tracking the details in the image (edges, speckles, etc.), we can estimate tissue motion. However, the speckle pattern will not deform and displace linearly with scatter movement. The speckle pattern is different for a different US system/transducer or when imaging from a different position. Second and most importantly, at high levels of compression, scatterers that first could be distinguished as separate objects may now fall within a single resolution cell and appear as one speckle and vice versa. Hence, speckle tracking does impose restrictions on the rate of deformation and the (minimum) frame rate used.

The presence of phase in the RF data is an important feature for strain imaging, since local strains require high-resolution and high-precision displacement data. Envelope data reveal tissue motion but due to the lack of phase has limited resolution. This can easily be depicted from Figure 14.4. Analysis of RF data can be performed on segments of data of only several wavelengths, at a scale

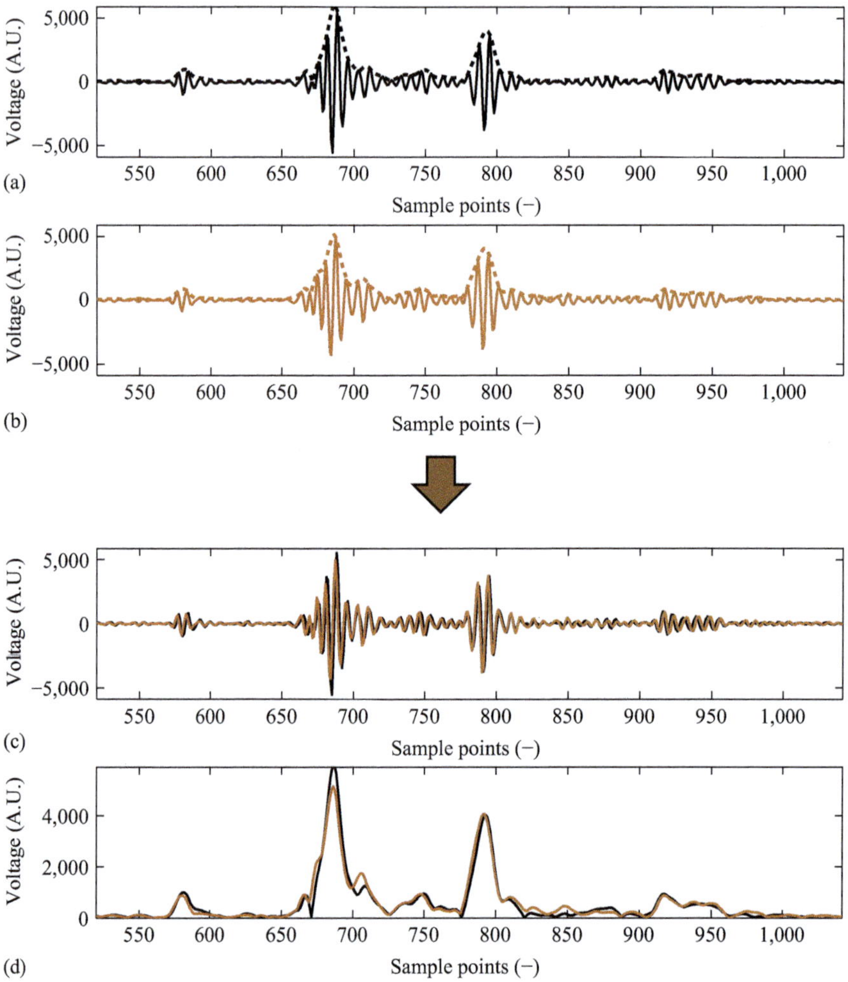

Figure 14.4 (a) RF data (solid) and corresponding envelope signal (dashed) for frame i; (b) RF-data (solid) and envelope (dashed) for frame i + 1; (c) comparison of the two RF signals from frame i (black) and frame i + 1 (brown); (d) same but now for envelope. One can clearly see small shifts and changes in amplitude as a result of tissue motion

of 100–1,000 μm (<mm range). In the envelope data, such a segment should be at least a significant part of each peak, i.e. at least contain one or more speckles (>mm range). As a result, envelope data are not suitable to measure small displacements.

So why not always use RF? The aforementioned problem of deformation vs. changes in backscattered echo signal will be more predominant in RF data, since large deformation will cause the appearance of the signal to change (local scatterers have moved), but the central frequency of the signal hasn't. Hence, this causes signals to **de-correlate**. Hence, the following trade-off in envelope vs. RF data is found:

- Envelope/B-mode: robust and less frame rate dependent, widely available.
- RF: susceptible to large deformation, not widely available.

vs.

- Envelope/B-mode: low resolution, precision and sensitivity: cannot measure local/low strains.
- RF: high resolution, precision and sensitivity: assessment of local and/or low strains feasible.

Choices on window size and further processing will be discussed, but first we introduce widely used similarity measures used for displacement estimation.

14.2.2 Similarity measures

In the Ophir study, RF data were processed line-by-line, dividing each RF line in segments of w_{ax} data samples. In that study, the **normalized cross-correlation** (CC) was used. This is illustrated in Figure 14.5. The CC of two continuous signals f and g is given by

$$\mathrm{CC}(\tau) = f \otimes g = \int_{-\infty}^{\infty} f^*(t) g(t+\tau) dt \tag{14.2}$$

with f^* the complex conjugate of f and τ the time lag. Essentially, g is slid over f, calculating the multiplication of these two functions in the overlapping region and calculating the area under the resulting curve. Signal amplitude in images is typically not complex (except for analytical signals), so f^* can be replaced by f.

In our case, where data are sampled and thus discrete, the CC becomes

$$\mathrm{CC}_d[n] = f \otimes_d g = \sum_{m=-\infty}^{\infty} f^*[m] g[m+n]. \tag{14.3}$$

A comparison between RF and envelope is found in Figure 14.6 for a 1-D segment of RF data. The CC was calculated for the raw RF and the signal envelope. The lag of the peak resembles the relative motion of the RF line in frame i and frame $i+1$. Zooming in on the peak (Figure 14.6, *right*) clearly demonstrates the difference in axial resolution between RF and envelope-based displacement estimation.

In the case of (2-D) data with two spatial dimensions x and y, the CC is given by

$$\mathrm{CC}_d[u,v] = (f) \otimes_{\mathrm{2D}} (g) = \sum_{u=-\infty}^{\infty} \sum_{v=-\infty}^{\infty} f^*[x,y] g[x+u, y+v] \tag{14.4}$$

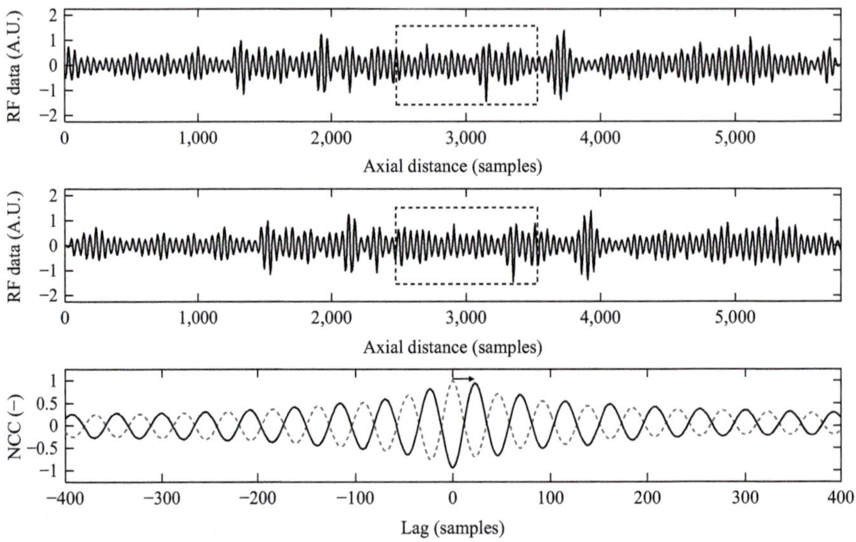

Figure 14.5 A single RF line for frame i (top), frame i + 1 (middle) and the corresponding normalized cross-correlation or cross-correlation function (bottom, black solid) and autocorrelation function (bottom, dashed grey). One can appreciate the movement of the peak of the NCC due to tissue motion (bottom, arrow)

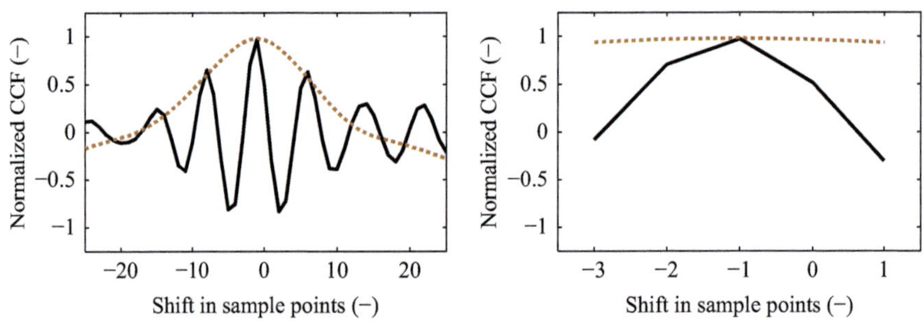

Figure 14.6 The normalized cross-correlation function (left) for the RF signal (solid) and the signal envelope (dashed). One can appreciate the increase in displacement tracking precision due to the use of RF data, especially when zooming in on the peak (right)

We distinguish between the two signals. Here f is the total image or large SA, whereas g is the T. Moreover, the signal may vary considerably in amplitude for different regions. Therefore, the normalized CC function (CCF) is used

$$\mathrm{NCC}_d[u,v] = \frac{\sum_{x=-\infty}^{\infty}\sum_{y=-\infty}^{\infty}\left[f[x,y]-\bar{f}_{u,v}\right]\left[g[x+u,y+v]-\bar{g}\right]}{\sqrt{\left(\sum_{x=-\infty}^{\infty}\sum_{y=-\infty}^{\infty}\left[f[x,y]-\bar{f}_{u,v}\right]^2\sum_{x=-\infty}^{\infty}\sum_{y=-\infty}^{\infty}\left[g[x+u,y+v]-\bar{g}\right]^2\right)}} \tag{14.5}$$

with $\bar{f}_{u,v}$, the mean of the image or signal in the overlapping region with the T and $\bar{g}$ the mean of the T. Hence, the local CC is calculated in the numerator and divided by the local sums found in the denominator. The latter can be sped up significantly by calculating running sum tables. In the resulting function, the maximum value $\mathrm{NCC}_{\max}$ is detected and the corresponding lag is assumed to be the tissue motion for that T.

An alternative similarity measure is the sum of absolute differences (SAD):

$$\mathrm{SAD}[u,v] = \sum_{x=-\infty}^{\infty}\sum_{y=-\infty}^{\infty}|f[x,y]-g[x+u,y+v]| \tag{14.6}$$

which assesses the similarity in grey value more directly. Closely related is the sum of squared differences (SSD)

$$\mathrm{SAD}[u,v] = \sum_{x=-\infty}^{\infty}\sum_{y=-\infty}^{\infty}(f[x,y]-g[x+u,y+v])^2. \tag{14.7}$$

Opposed to finding a peak, a minimum value is sought for when using the SAD or SAD measure of similarity (Langeland *et al.*, 2003). Other methods include mutual information, hybrid-sign or polarity-coincidence correlation, normalized covariance, etc.

14.2.3 Sub-sample displacement estimation

For strain estimation, integer displacement values result in unrealistic strain estimates, especially when motion is small. If a row of displacement values is given by (0.2, 0.4, 0.6, 0.8, 1.0) mm, with a spacing of $\Delta x = 1$ mm, a uniform strain of 20% is present. However, the estimated displacement values (in integers) would be [0 0 1 1 1], resulting in strain values of [0 1 0 0 0 0]. Hence, sub-sample displacement estimates are needed. There are two different strategies: data upsampling and NCC peak fitting, which can also be combined.

Data upsampling has been demonstrated and used in both the axial and lateral direction. However, to improve the axial displacement estimate, this method is computationally intensive. For lateral displacement estimation, i.e. interpolating more lines, this method is indeed useful in improving the overall definition of the NCC peak (see Section 14.3.1). NCC peak fitting requires an analytical function that describes the shape of the NCC peak, i.e. NCC ($\vec{r}$) for a domain $\vec{r}$ centred around the peak at $\vec{r}_{\max}$. The most popular fitting functions are a parabolic and

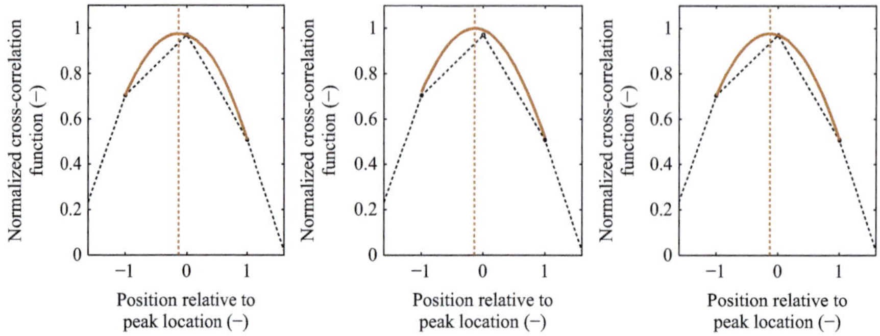

Figure 14.7 Interpolation of the cross-correlation peak for sub-resolution displacement estimation: parabolic interpolation (left), cosine interpolation (middle) and spline interpolation (right). Measured cross-correlation function values are indicated by the dashed black line and dots, whereas the interpolated curve is shown as a green solid. The green dashed vertical line indicates the interpolated peak location

cosine function, see Figure 14.7. A second option is the use of an interpolant, such as a cubic, spline or other interpolation scheme, which may yield similar or slightly better results, but is more time-consuming (Céspedes *et al.*, 1995; Lopata *et al.*, 2009). Typically, a fast approach is required for real-time block-matching capability.

To fit a quadratic or parabolic function, one can instantly calculate the lag in one dimension using

$$x_{\text{sub}} = \frac{\text{NCC}(x_{\max} - 1) - \text{NCC}(x_{\max} + 1)}{2\text{NCC}(x_{\max} - 1) - 4\text{NCC}(x_{\max}) + 2\text{NCC}(x_{\max} + 1)} \tag{14.8}$$

with x_{ax} the position of the peak (integer). The resulting displacement is then

$$x_{\text{tot}} = x_{\max} + x_{\text{sub}}. \tag{14.9}$$

The interpolated maximum value of the NCC can be calculated using the analytical solution of the parabolic function as well. A parabolic function may also include more data points, but typically three is sufficient. Any higher order polynome is possible, but will require more data points.

The cosine fit consists of two parts. First, the 'fundamental frequency' is estimated

$$\omega_0 = \arccos\left(\frac{(\text{NCC}(x_{\max} - 1) + \text{NCC}(x_{\max} + 1))}{2\text{NCC}(x_{\max})}\right). \tag{14.10}$$

Next, the phase shift is calculated

$$\theta = \arctan\left(\frac{\mathrm{NCC}(x_{\max} - 1) - \mathrm{NCC}(x_{\max} + 1)}{2\mathrm{NCC}(x_{\max})\sin(\omega_0)}\right) \tag{14.11}$$

which yields the sub-samples lag

$$x_{\text{sub}} = -\frac{\theta}{\omega_0} \rightarrow \quad x_{\text{tot}} = x_{\max} + x_{\text{sub}}. \tag{14.12}$$

An efficient, two-step method is the phase-zero crossing method that uses the analytical signal rather than the normal RF data. The analytical signal segments are cross-correlated, hence the CCF is complex. Next, the magnitude of the CCF is detected by calculating the modulus of the complex CCF, see Figure 14.8. The peak of the modulus is detected to find the integer-valued shift (lag) $x_{\max}$. Next, the phase of the CCF is determined by calculating the argument of the complex-valued CCF. The change in phase is linear and the phase at the true maximum should be equal to zero. Hence, one can calculate the zero crossing in the region of $x_{\max}$ using simple linear interpolation, which is both accurate and time-efficient. Other methods include spline fitting, grid slopes, iterative fitting and many others.

14.2.4 Window size

Window size is far from an arbitrary choice in displacement estimation. In this section, we focus on 1-D displacement estimation using CC. In literature, the T is often referred to as the pre-compression kernel, whilst the SA is called the post-compression kernel. This nomenclature originates from the original papers on quasi-static elastography that typically involved compression/palpation of soft tissue.

T size: The T or pre-compression kernel size $w_{\text{ax},i}$ depends on the deformation of the tissue. In case there is no strain, the displacement error is inversely proportional to the kernel size or 'observation time'. Hence, larger kernels will always be preferred. In case there is strain present, there is a general inverse relation between window size and maximum strain

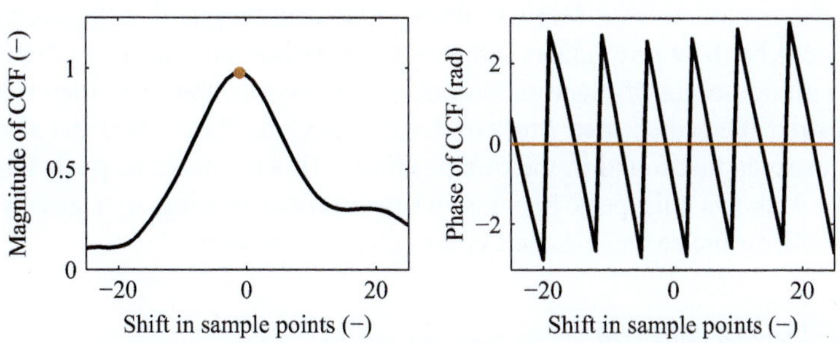

Figure 14.8 Magnitude of the cross-correlation function based on analytical signals (left) and the corresponding phase (right)

$$|\varepsilon| T_{\mathrm{ax}\,fc} = \frac{1}{2} \tag{14.13}$$

with ε the strain, T_{ax} the axial window size in (s) and f_c the centre frequency of the US transducer used. The axial window size in pixels is given by $w_{ax} = T_{ax} f_s$. One can depict from this simple relation that for a larger window size, a lower maximum strain can be measured accurately. Moreover, higher strains can be measured at lower frequencies. Vice versa, using shorter windows will allow higher strains to occur and be measured. The concept of using small windows to estimate high strains accurately is also used in the phase lag method introduced in the previous section.

Varghese and Ophir (1997b) provided a theoretical framework to examine the performance of strain SNR for different transducer settings, called the **strain filter**. It used the lower bound on motion tracking as reported by Walker and Trahey in 1995, but also provided the upper bound, allowing the calculation of measureable strain ranges for a certain transducer and algorithm setting. For instance, for a 5 MHz probe with 60% bandwidth, strains can be measured accurately between 0.1% and 5.0%, with considerable increases in SNR for higher bandwidths. Follow-up studies showed the influence of window size, centre frequency, beam width, etc., and the expected contrast in lesion detection. A formula that gives an estimate of the optimal kernel size is

$$T_{ax} \approx \frac{3B}{2\varepsilon f_c^2} \tag{14.14}$$

with B the bandwidth of the transducer.

Hence, the window size of the T depends on the expected strain value. A larger window size will result in a more robust and well defined CCF, but will only work at lower levels of strain, whereas a smaller window will enable the estimation of higher strain values. Figure 14.9 shows the effect of decreasing window size. The diagonal shows a CC based on the same amount of data points, but for decreasing T and SA size (top-left to bottom-right). At higher strains, the shorter T size yields a better CCF.

SA size: The size of the SA or post-compression kernel basically depends on the total tissue motion from frame to frame. One could argue that the SA by definition should be the entire image, allowing all possible translations in the field of view, assuming no out-of-plane motion occurs. However, the most important reason to restrict the search area i to avoid erroneous matches, where the similarity measure exceeds that found in the true positions. This is known as **peak-hopping**. Figure 14.9 shows this peak-hopping when cross-correlating a relatively short signal T with an increasing SA (left column, top to bottom).

14.2.5 De-correlation

During line (or block) matching, different factors will cause the envelope or RF data to correlate with maximum NCC values <1. This can be caused by

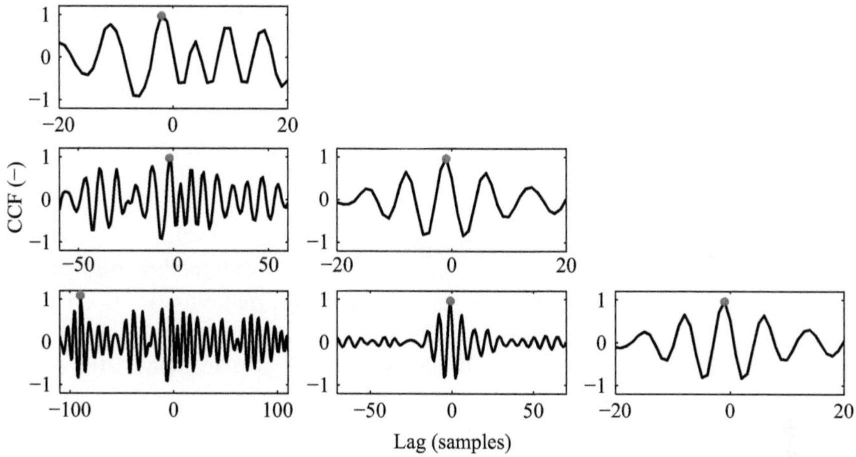

Figure 14.9 Cross-correlation for a window of 201 (top), 101 (middle) and 21 samples (bottom row) that is correlated with a window of 241 (left), 141 (middle) and 61 samples (right). The maximum value of the cross-correlation function is indicated with the brown circle

- Motion of tissue vs. physics of US: If a tissue moves to a different location, the angle and distance between transducer and tissue may change, resulting in a different appearance in the image not only due to refraction, diffraction and different speckle appearance, but also attenuation and acoustic shadowing.
- Rotational movement: see also previous item. Rotation leads to significant de-correlation due to the nature of US images and the underlying physics of speckle appearance.
- Out-of-plane motion: tissue simply moves out of the field of view. This can be solved by using 3-D US.
- High level of deformation: see the previous sub-section.
- Sub-sample displacements: tissue motion translates into to sub-sample lags. In other words, the 'true' peak of the NCC is missed.
- Electronic noise.

14.2.6 Re-correlation

The aforementioned problem of de-correlation is especially predominant in RF data. Several techniques have been proposed to improve the correlation when high de-correlation was encountered, which is sometimes referred to as 're-correlation'.

14.2.6.1 Regularization of cross-correlation functions

One can regularize the displacement estimates by filtering the CCF to enforce continuity. Lubinski *et al.* (1999) introduced a technique where the CCF of kernel $j-2$ to $j+2$ was averaged using a Gaussian weighting function. The result was a more robust CCF for kernel j, which reduced peak-hopping and displacement errors in general. The downside is the smoothing nature of this technique that will reduce accuracy and the ability to measure large steps in strain.

In 2009, Petrank et al. reported on a dynamic programming approach, where a Viterbi algorithm was employed to find the most likely path in a time sequence of events to reduce peak-hopping at large strain (Petrank *et al.*, 2009).

14.2.6.2 Iterative approaches

Several groups have worked on so-called hybrid, coarse-to-fine or multi-level displacement estimation algorithms. One of the first algorithms that used multiple steps of block matching to enhance displacement estimation was the first 2-D algorithm by Konofagou and Ophir in 1998 (see Section 14.3 and Konofagou and Ophir, 1998). In an iterative or multi-step approach, displacement estimates are used as input in a second iteration of the displacement estimation by selecting either a pre-compression window that is corrected for the displacement measured or by redefining the SA using a similar correction (with opposite sign). This is already a form of re-correlation, since translational movement is corrected, which increases the overlap of the pre- and post-compression windows and thus the similarity.

Chen and Varghese (2009) proposed a multi-step approach that first estimates the large displacements in a robust fashion using envelope. Then, in a second iteration, the algorithm change to RF data and uses the initial displacements to re-locate the kernels before CC and displacement estimation.

Lopata *et al.* (2009) published a method that combined the principles introduced so far, but with an additional feature: the window size was decreased by each step (Figure 14.10). This strategy has the advantage of measuring the large translational movement using large windows of envelope data, but gaining precision when switching to smaller kernels of RF data. For each iteration, the window is systematically decreased, thereby increasing the strain level that can be measured.

One doesn't always need multiple iterations to get displacement or strain images. Zhu and Hall (2002) used a priori knowledge, i.e. the displacement estimate of window j as input for window $j+1$ when analysing quasi-static deformation, i.e. compressing tissue with a plate, see Figure 14.11. This method works, since the displacement will increase monotonically: displacements near the plate are low and increase for larger depths. However, as in all these methods, error propagation can cause difficulties. In this approach, errors at an early stage may ruin the displacement estimation for the entire line.

An attractive approach is the diamond search approach introduced by Chen *et al.* (2009), which has later been extended by Jiang and Hall (2011). This block-matching technique starts with a 'seeding phase' where a random number of Ts are cross-correlated with corresponding SAs in the next frame. The seeds with highest CC are selected. Next, using a diamond search, see Figure 14.11, the four neighbouring Ts are processed, using the displacement of the seed as input, which is similar to the multi-step approaches described above. Next, the following ring of neighbouring Ts are processed and so on. If the CC operation results in a low maximum NCC, the result is rejected. These classes of algorithms

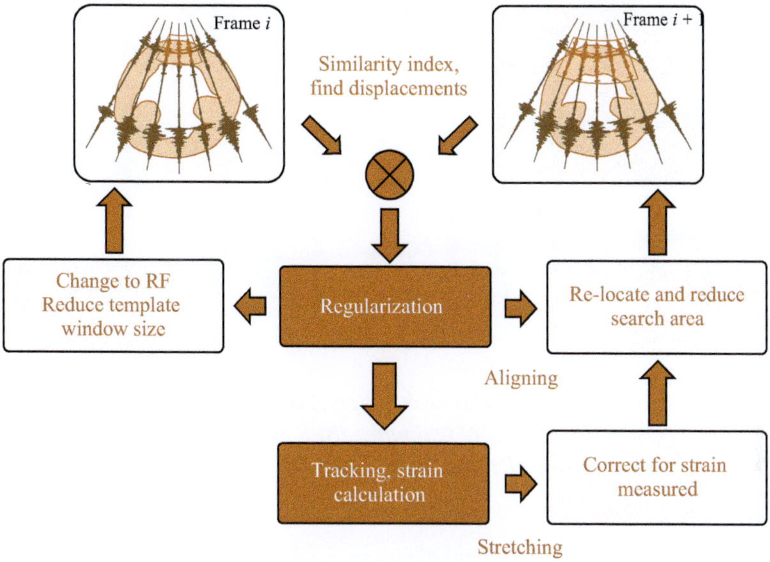

Figure 14.10 Schematic overview of an iterative, multi-level displacement estimation algorithm

require dynamic programming but have the advantage of imposing continuity on the displacement fields.

14.2.6.3 Sub-sample alignment

At a window position x_{ax}, the displacement is found to be $\Delta x_{tot} = \Delta x_{max} + \Delta x_{sub}$. Next, the data are selected at position $x'_{ax} = x_{ax} + \Delta x_{max}$ (see the previous section). Sub-sample alignment is achieved by interpolating the RF data for $x^{al}_{ax} = x'_{ax} + \Delta x_{sub}$, see Figure 14.12.

Especially in cases where the sub-sample resolution is near 0.3 sample points, the bias in displacement estimates is large (Céspedes *et al.*, 1995). Using sub-sample alignment improves these displacement values considerably and results in a more continuous strain image or elastogram.

14.2.6.4 Strain-based stretching

Temporal stretching, i.e. stretching of the RF line in the axial direction, has been introduced by Varghese and Ophir (1997a). This operation influences 'stretching' of the window of RF data based on a priori knowledge of the strain in this region or a previous strain estimate. Basically, interpolation of the data is performed to stretch or compress the RF data within w_{ax} using an altered axial axis

$$\begin{aligned} x^{st}_{ax} &= (1-\varepsilon)\left(x_{ax} - x_{ax,c}\right) + x_{ax,c} \\ \mathrm{RF}^{st}(x_{ax}) &= \mathrm{RF}\left(x^{st}_{ax}\right) \end{aligned} \tag{14.15}$$

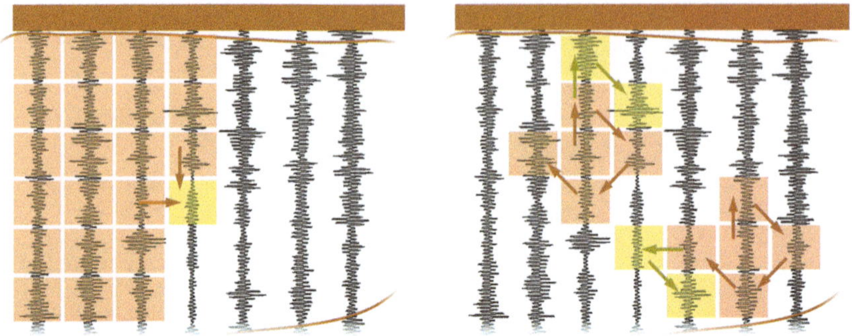

(a) (b)

Figure 14.11 *(a) a line-by-line search scheme, using neighbouring displacement estimates as initial estimate; (b) a diamond search scheme using a seeding initialization step*

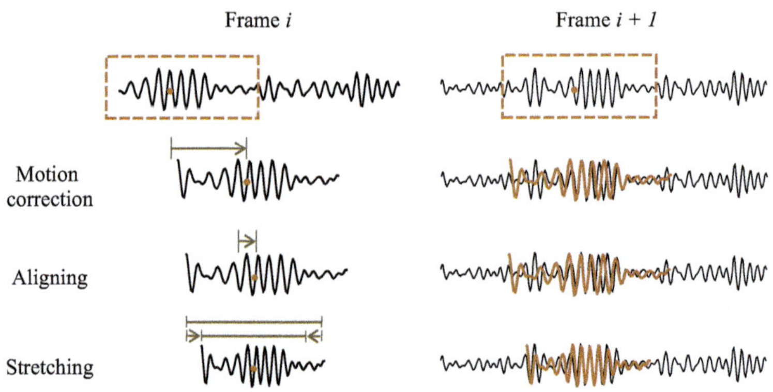

Figure 14.12 *Re-correlation in three steps (top to bottom): after the first estimation of the shift, the re-selection of the template will lead to improved correlation and enables the use of a smaller kernel size. Next, one can perform sub-sample alignment and stretching, improving similarity and thus correlation*

resulting in a stretched version in case of elongational strain ($\varepsilon > 0$) and a compressed version for $\varepsilon < 0$. Please note that the axial axis is here denoted in axial spatial co-ordinates, which can have unit (m), but can also be unitless (in case of sample points). In literature, the RF line x-axis is also often denoted as time in (s).

This process can be applied to the entire image line. One could think of a quasi-static compression experiment where the total amount of strain applied is known. However, in in vivo applications, it is more suitable to use a local strain estimate (from a previous image or iteration) to stretch the pre- or post-compression window.

Srinivasan *et al.* (2002) presented a different approach that uses the same principle but with a different approach. Here, strain was estimated by stretching the RF kernel for several strain values within an expected range. Strain was estimated by selecting the strain value for which the highest maximum CC value was found.

The stretching of kernel data seems intuitively more valid for envelope/grey value data as used in image registration techniques (see the next chapter). For large strains, this operation in fact alters the centre frequency f_c of the RF data by $\varepsilon \cdot 100\%$. However, it also alters distinct patterns that were altered due to scatterer compression, which improves similarity thereby leading to 're-correlation'. The merit actually is more significant than the possible side effects. In fact, signal frequency content changes by depth due to attenuation and thus varies not only with depth, but also with large strains. It must be stressed though, that these techniques (see also Section 14.2.6.3) will only lead to enhancement if the available strain information or estimates are sufficiently accurate.

14.3 Multi-dimensional displacement estimation

The previous sections have dealt mostly with 1-D displacement estimation methods. However, in many cases, one is interested in the 2-D (or even 3-D) displacement and/or deformation field. In terms of block matching, one can also process two-dimensional data kernels to obtain the full displacement vector and strain tensor.

14.3.1 From line to block matching

Several approaches are available for 2-D or 3-D displacement estimation. 2-D TDI (McDicken *et al.*, 1992) was used but lacked accuracy and suffered from angle dependency. Heimdal *et al.* (1998) was the first to convert 1-D TDI data into strain rate imaging (Figure 14.13). Two-dimensional speckle tracking was first introduced by Bohs and Trahey (1991), with several studies to follow (Chaturvedi *et al.*, 1998; Ramamurthy and Trahey, 1991; Chen *et al.*, 2004). Now, angle-independent estimates could be estimated (Leitman *et al.*, 2004). Typically, one selects a T with one to several speckles and a SA that is sufficiently large for the displacements to be tracked between frames. Once 3-D US systems were commercially available, the first studies on 3-D block matching were reported (Chen *et al.*, 2005; Crosby *et al.*, 2009; Jia *et al.*, 2007; Saito *et al.*, 2009). Other techniques such as optical flow (see the previous chapter) and image registration (Elen *et al.*, 2008), see next chapter, have also been extensively studied in literature.

After RF-based displacement and strain imaging became more popular, Konofagou and Ophir (1998) reported on a technique to measure the lateral displacement. A 1-D T with size $w_{ax} \times 1$ was selected and cross-correlated with a 2-D SA, see Figures 14.13 and 14.14. Additional interpolation of RF lines was conducted to measure sub-sample lateral displacement estimates using a weighted interpolation scheme. In later years, 2-D kernels of linear and phased array data were used (Figures 14.13 and 14.14) by Langeland *et al.* (2006) and Lopata *et al.* (2009), etc., yielding

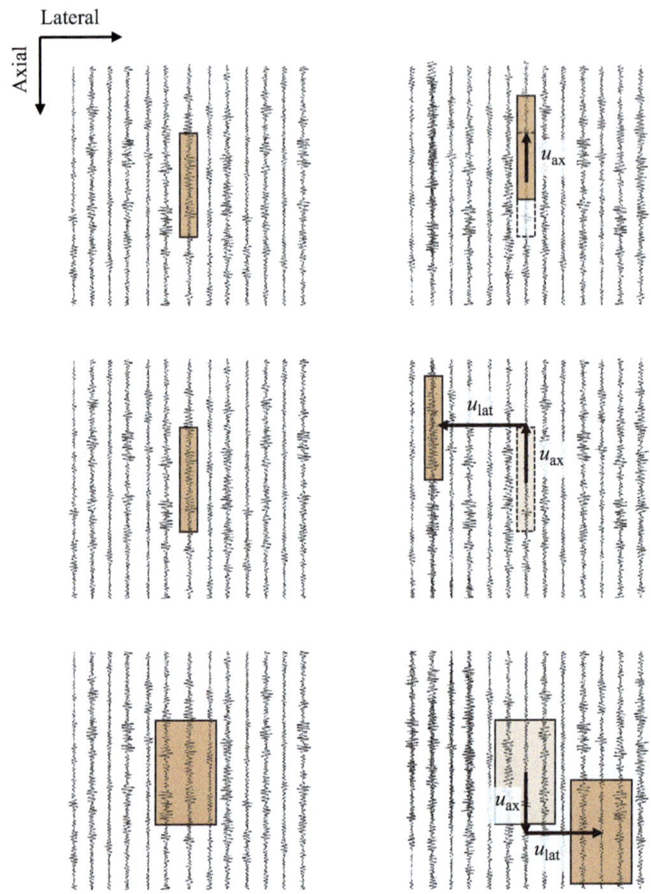

Figure 14.13 RF lines of frame i (left) with a pre-compression kernel (orange) in 1-D (top, middle) and 2-D (bottom) and the corresponding match found in frame i + 1 (right) for a 1-D search (top) and 2-D search (middle, bottom)

good results, even when kernels of diverging lines were used. Not only does 2-D block matching yield the 2-D displacement vector, but it also improves the overall robustness and the precision of the axial displacement estimates. The use of RF data for 3-D tracking was sparse due to the low frame rates involved. The first studies showed mostly preliminary results (Lindop *et al.*, 2006; Said *et al.*, 2006; Patil *et al.*, 2007; Lopata *et al.*, 2011). Current advances in ultrafast imaging are dealing with these issues (Gennisson *et al.*, 2015; Papadacci *et al.*, 2017).

14.3.2 Multi-dimensional cross-correlation

Similarity measures such as the NCC, SAD and SSD can be expanded to 2-D and 3-D. The overall computation time increases due to the second dimension in

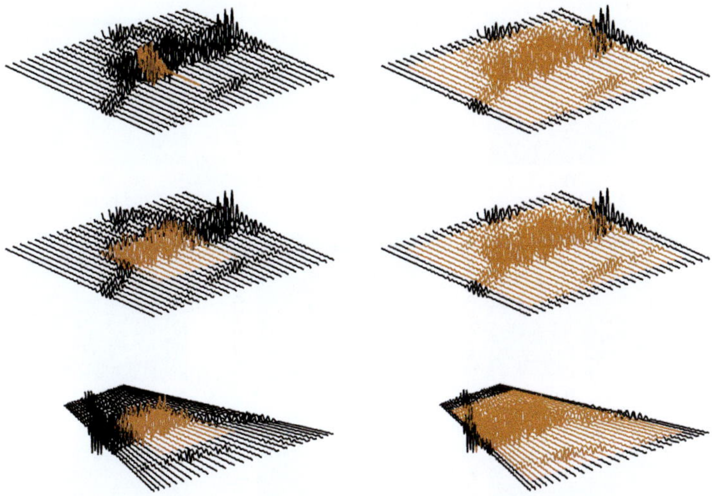

Figure 14.14 RF lines (black) of frame i (left) with a pre-compression kernel (brown) and corresponding SA (orange) in frame i + 1 (right) for a 1-D template (top left), 2-D template (middle left) and 2-D template of diverging lines (bottom left)

the running sum tables. Depending on the size, a Fourier-approach can be faster (especially in 3-D). Fast implementations have been reported (Luo and Konofagou, 2010).

Besides interpolation, similar methods for peak fitting have been applied to obtain sub-sample lateral displacement estimates. One could repeat the fit function in two or three directions, thereby assuming separability of NCC, i.e. $\mathrm{NCC}(x,y) = \mathrm{NCC}(x)\ \mathrm{NCC}(y)$ or $\mathrm{NCC}(x,y,z) = \mathrm{NCC}(x)\mathrm{NCC}(y)\mathrm{NCC}(z)$. In case of the parabolic function, one could also expand to a multi-variable (2-D or 3-D) function or 2-D–3-D splines.

An extension of the zero-phase crossing method as shown in Section 14.2.4 was introduced by Chen *et al.* (2004). They introduced a method that was able to improve lateral displacement estimates using synthetic lateral phase. Current developments in transverse oscillations actually yield RF data with phase in both directions (Liebgott *et al.*, 2010).

14.3.3 2-D window sizes

An example of the CCF in 2-D is shown for DICOM, envelope and RF data in Figure 14.15. One can appreciate again the high-resolution definition of the peak in the axial direction when using RF data, which has been extensively discussed in the previous sections. One can also see the difference in peak width between the axial and lateral direction, most strikingly in the RF data.

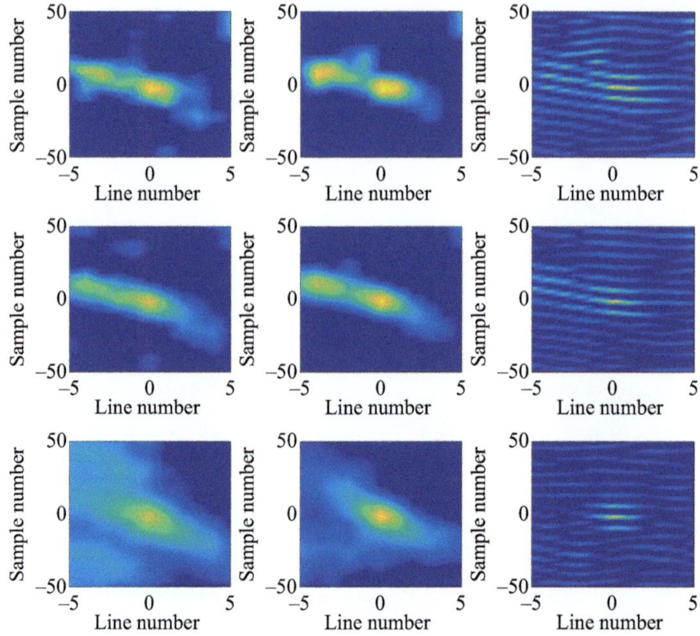

Figure 14.15 2-D-cross correlation (colourbar ranges from 0 to 1) calculated for a window of DICOM (left), envelope (middle) and RF data (right). The dimensions of the window at frame i are 101 data points × 1 line (top), 101 data points × 3 lines (middle) and 101 data points × 11 lines (bottom). The corresponding window at frame i + 1 is 201 data points × 21 lines and shares the same centre point as the window corresponding to frame i

The difference between DICOM and signal envelope is not too high, as expected. One can easily reconstruct the signal envelope from DICOM data, although the sampling will differ. Increasing the lateral window size results in a more distinct peak in the centre (Figure 14.15, bottom) whilst the other peaks are suppressed (in all cases). However, one can also depict smoothing of the actual peak (becomes wider), which will reduce precision.

There are no true rules in choosing lateral window size. Beam width increases width depth and even sampling in case of a phased or curved array transducer. Lopata *et al.* (2009) showed that depending on the application and strain level, an optimal kernel size of three to five lines should be chosen. In cardiac applications, often 1-D Ts are correlated in a 2-D SA, although 2-D Ts can be (and have been) used quite commonly as well (Langeland *et al.*, 2006; Lopata *et al.*, 2010).

Similar to the multi-level or iterative approaches discussed in Section 14.2, an iterative approach can be used to improve on axial and lateral strain when using 2-D kernels. Both axial and lateral displacements are used as input, although the lateral displacements typically require more smoothing. If convergent, the resulting axial and lateral strain images improve in both SNR and CNR (Lopata *et al.*, 2009).

14.3.3.1 Re-correlation approaches

Similar to the 1-D approaches, re-correlation or 'companding' techniques can be employed in 2-D. The latter was already shown in the Konofagou and Ophir paper, where the sub-sample lateral search improved the axial displacement and strain estimates and the overall correlation. Lopata *et al.* (2009) showed the use of sub-sample alignment in both axial and lateral direction improved both axial and lateral strain estimates using both 1-D and 2-D kernels of envelope and RF data.

In terms of stretching, one of the first papers in 2-D is that by Chaturvedi *et al.* (1998). They already divided 2-D data sets into kernels and performed both global and local stretching in two dimensions. In the iterative 2-D block-matching scheme of Lopata *et al.* (2009), stretching was only performed in one dimension, since initial strain estimates were used (no prior knowledge), which rendered the use of lateral strains inadequate. Later papers included the use of linear elastic registration methods that deformed the entire image to match the next one, thereby estimating the total displacement field, see next the chapter or Elen *et al.* (2008) and Heyde *et al.* (2013).

14.4 Resolution

The resolution of the displacement and strain images depends on the sampling of the US data and the frequency used. In the **axial** direction, the resolution of the strain images depends on the axial resolution of the US (= wavelength, pulse length), the axial window size and the overlap used (see below).

Overlap: To increase the resolution of the displacement and/or strain data, one can perform the correlation technique or block matching for overlapping windows. Instead of sliding the window to the next segment of equal shape, one can shift the window by a number of pixels s_{ax} that $<w_{ax}$. The overlap percentage can be calculated from the shift used:

$$\%\,\text{overlap} = (1 - s_{ax/}w_{ax}) * 100\% \qquad (14.16)$$

Hence, the sampling distance between two displacement or strain values is therefore equal to s_{ax} (samples) or $s_{ax}\frac{c_0}{2f_s}$ in (m) with f_s the sampling frequency of the RF data [in (Hz)] and c_0 the speed of sound [in (m/s)]. The lateral resolution of displacement and strain data depends on the beam width and the use of a linear array or a phased/curved array (whose diverging lines lead to a larger sampling distance with depth). However, the amount of strain pixels in the lateral direction is normally equal to the number of RF lines. Hence, there is always overlap in case kernels are used with a lateral window size >1.

14.5 Regularization

The final displacement fields need to be regularized to reduce measurement errors such as peakhopping, drift, etc. Simple approaches usually use a smoothing kernel such as a median filter or a Gaussian smoothing kernel. The median filter is especially useful in removing outliers, whereas Gaussian or averaging kernels help in smoothing the data. One can also fit multi-variable functions or smoothen the motion fields by minimizing procedures that trigger on higher order derivatives in the motion data. Opposed to smoothing the displacement field, one can also perform regularization by imposing a certain shape to the object being tracked (Kremer *et al.*, 2010) or by prescribing a continuum constraint (Guo *et al.*, 2015), which has been used to smooth lateral displacement estimates (or derive these from axial estimates all together). There exists no ground truth or rule of thumb. It is important though, to increase SNR, remove outliers but preserve gradients in motion or strain to ensure tracking and strain contrast. Regularization at strain level will be discussed in the next section.

14.6 Strain estimation

14.6.1 Strain measures

In biomechanics and engineering, several definitions for strain are available. In speckle tracking and strain imaging literature, the linear strain is typically used:

$$\varepsilon = \frac{l - l_0}{l_0} = \frac{l}{l_0} = \lambda - 1 \tag{14.17}$$

with l_0 and l the original and deformed length of the object, respectively and λ the stretch. Hence, after determining the 1-D displacement field, the axial strain can be estimated by computing the spatial gradient of the axial displacement:

$$\varepsilon = \frac{du_{\mathrm{ax}}}{dx_{\mathrm{ax}}} \tag{14.18}$$

In the first papers, this gradient was calculated using a simple numerical differentiator, see Figure 14.16. However, in 1997, Kallel and Ophir introduced a low-pass differentiator that fits a linear curve through the displacement data along a line using a least-squares fitting procedure and takes the tangent of the curve as strain estimate

$$u_{\mathrm{ax}}(x_{\mathrm{ax}}) = \varepsilon x_{\mathrm{ax}} + u_{\mathrm{ax},0} \tag{14.19}$$

This **least-squares strain estimator**, or LSQSE in short, has been widely used since in numerous studies, see Figure 14.16 (Kallel and Ophir, 1997). For an N-point LSQSE, the strain can be calculated in a computationally efficient manner:

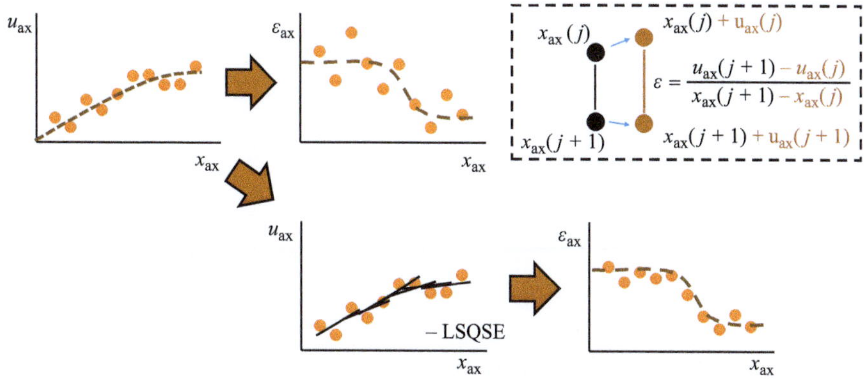

Figure 14.16 Top row: displacements and strain estimation using a simple differentiators. Bottom row: least-squares strain estimation (LSQSE), resulting in less dispersion in the strain estimates

$$\begin{aligned} A &= \begin{bmatrix} 1 & 2 & \dots & N \\ 1 & 1 & \dots & 1 \end{bmatrix} \\ p &= \left[A^T \cdot (A \cdot A^T)^{-1}\right]^T u_{ax}(x_{ax} - N/2 : x_{ax} + N/2) \\ \varepsilon(x_{ax}) &= p(1) \end{aligned} \tag{14.20}$$

One can expand the number of points used in the linear fit to reduce noise and increase strain SNR, but at the cost of strain resolution. The downside is smoothing of large gradients in strains in tissue fractures or at tissue–tissue interfaces. Other fitting functions or low-pass filters are available, including other low-pass differentiators, combinations with smoothing kernels, multi-variable fitting functions (including 2-D/3-D LSQSE for *N*-D strain estimation) and PDE regularization.

14.6.1.1 Strain vs. strain rate: the need for tracking

In case of quasi-static elastography, often a constant rate of deformation is applied. The results are averaged over all the frames. To avoid de-correlation, typical block matching involves processing of frame i and $i+1$, yielding the frame-to-frame displacements and strains. For cardiovascular or musculoskeletal applications, these values as a function of time are the incremental strain or **strain rate**, whereas the total strain is often desired.

To obtain the cumulative strain, there are two well-known strategies:

- Perform correlation analysis for all frames i with respect to frame 1. This yields the total, cumulative strain. The downside of this approach is the fundamental limit imposed by de-correlation and the occurrence of propagating errors.
- Track a pre-defined grid of tracking points using the displacements measured, see Figure 14.17. Next, calculate the strains based on the updated co-ordinates.

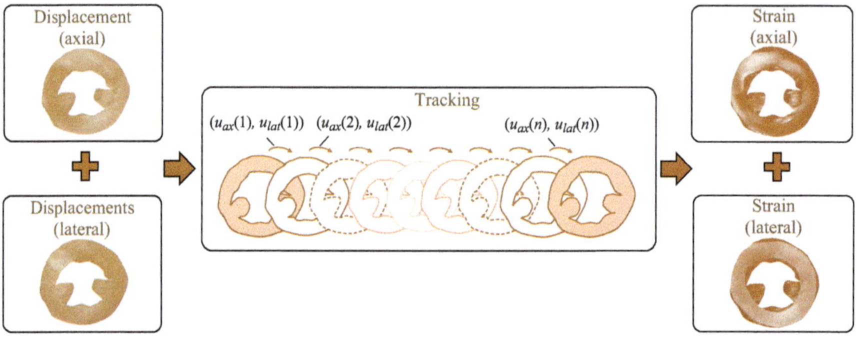

Figure 14.17 Schematic overview of tracking for strain accumulation: based on the measured displacements, the initial ROI or grid of reference points is translated and deformed over type. Based on the updated co-ordinates, strain images are obtained

Error propagation due to tracking inaccuracies will be the major source of error again.

Tracking is commonly used in cardiovascular applications since strains are too high for the former. One can track over the entire cardiac cycle, or from systole to diastole (both sides) or over several cycles. The total or cumulative strain is estimated by either (1) determining the strain rate at the updated location and sum all strain rates over time or by (2) calculating the strain from the updated co-ordinates.

However, due to the aforementioned error propagation, drift occurs. The latter is often reduced by a **re-set** of the tracking algorithm to the original segmentation, or to a newly obtained segmentation, when for instance the updated shape deviates too much from a parallel running segmentation algorithm [this is used on arteries in the ArtLAB system (Esaote, NL)]. Popular methods include **drift correction**, which is basically a de-trending step on the resulting strain curves. A priori knowledge on tissue motion (based on a shape-model or finite-element analysis) can also be used to regularize displacements and thus tracking.

14.6.2 Strain vs. local strain

The strains found with speckle tracking are either the Cartesian strains in *z*-, *x–z* or *x–y–z* directions, or the axial, axial-lateral or axial-lateral-elevational strains in case the US-line data were available. Transformation of the strains from axial-lateral to *x–z* directions is straightforward and depends on the transducer geometry. For tumour or other palpation-like applications, this normally suffices.

However, in tissue that actively deforms due to contraction (heart, muscle) or due to blood pressure pulsation (arteries, veins), the local strain co-ordinates are of interest. Early studies converted axial/lateral displacements into radial and circumferential displacements, from which the strains were estimated. Alternatively, strains in the axial and lateral direction were calculated and then transformed to their polar directions. In healthy arteries and to some extent the heart, this is a valid approach, although the resulting directions are depended on the centroid defined in the artery or heart (Zervantonakis *et al.*, 2007). One can also perform principal component analysis on the strain data and associate the strains to the radial or circumferential direction, depending on their principal direction.

In pathological tissue such as hypertrophic hearts, congenital heart disease related malformations, stenosed arteries or aneurysmatic aortas, or in non-standard imaging views, one needs to find the local strains. This can be achieved by defining a local co-ordinate system and then project the measured strains into the local normal and tangent directions.

14.7 In vivo challenges

After discussing all theoretical, physical and practical considerations for block matching, a good impression of the do's and don'ts should have been obtained. First of all, the image quality and sensitivity of the US system is crucial in obtaining high-resolution motion tracking and strain estimates. Garbage in = garbage out. Several other factors have been discussed earlier, such as bandwidth, US resolution, field of view and frame rate. However, there are several challenges to be encountered once using these methods *in vivo*.

14.7.1 Mismatch between US propagation direction and tissue strain

Depending on the insonification angle and echo window, and the transducer used, local or desired strain measurements do not align with the propagation direction of the US. In general, measurements in the axial direction are preferred using RF data, since this will yield the highest precision and resolution. Beam steering can help to measure strains in a $\pm 45°$ sector with loss of field of view. However, in case of for example cardiac strain imaging, the mismatch between the direction of sound propagation and strain can depend on location and image view, see Figure 14.18. Hence, strains can be accurately measured in a certain part of the heart in for instance the long-axis parasternal view, but not in the apical view. Similar problems are found not only in arteries, but also in skeletal muscle where large deformations are mostly in the direction orthogonal to the sound propagation.

14.7.2 Anistropy and non-linearity

Most biological tissue is anisotropic, i.e. material properties differ in the three major directions. Moreover, tissue can be loosely bounded or firmly bounded. Furthermore, tissue may react differently for varying strain levels due to non-linear mechanical behaviour. All these factors make strain images difficult to interpret and standardization cumbersome.

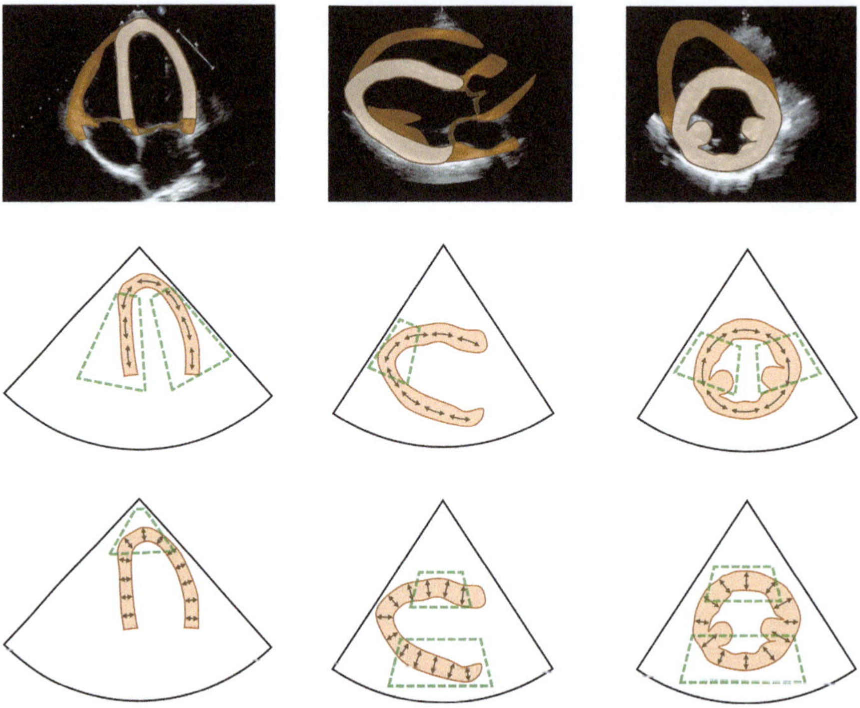

Figure 14.18 Top row: Apical four-chamber view (left); parasternal long axis (middle) and corresponding short axis view of the heart (right). The left ventricle is indicated in (light brown); The middle row shows the longitudinal (left, middle) and circumferential strain directions (right) vs. the areas of high strain precision (green dashed). The radial strain direction is shown in the lower figures for all views

14.8 Elastography

As stated earlier, 'elastography' should not be confused with strain imaging. Elastography means providing the user with an image that shows differences in material properties or better yet: a quantitative map of the material properties.

In case of palpation, an inverse strain image can indicate differences in elasticity, since soft tissue will correspond to large strains, and more stiffer regions to low strains. This requires, however, a high SNR and CNR of the strain images or elastograms. In arterial tissue, strain has been correlated to plaque rupture potential (De Korte *et al.*, 2000). However, the strains measured are the result of the complex and heterogeneous tissue morphology and the load applied. High strains means softer tissue does not apply here. The same goes for the heart, where contraction is an active process and tissue elasticity consists of a passive and active component. However, in cardiac applications, contractility is more of interest than (passive) elasticity, hence strain measurements are potentially more interesting than pure elastographic measurements.

Current developments in elastography aim at a direct quantification of the tissue elasticity rather than the deformation. To this end, shear wave elastography, ARFI and model-based approaches have been developed and research is ongoing.

References

R. S. Adler, J. M. Rubin, P. H. Bland, and P. L. Carson. Quantitative tissue motion analysis of digitized M-mode images: gestational differences of fetal lung. *Ultrasound in Medicine & Biology*, 16 (6): 561–569, 1990. ISSN 0301-5629.

J. Bercoff, M. Tanter, and M. Fink. Supersonic shear imaging: a new technique for soft tissue elasticity mapping. *IEEE Transactions on Ultrasonics, Ferroelectrics, and Frequency Control*, 51 (4): 396–409, Apr. 2004. ISSN 0885-3010.

L. N. Bohs and G. E. Trahey. A novel method for angle independent ultrasonic imaging of blood flow and tissue motion. *IEEE Transactions on Bio-medical Engineering*, 38 (3): 280–286, Mar. 1991. ISSN 0018-9294. doi: 10.1109/10.133210.

E. I. Céspedes, Y. Huang, J. Ophir, and S. Spratt. Methods for estimation of subsample time delays of digitized echo signals. *Ultrasonic Imaging*, 170 (2): 142–171, 1995. URL http://uix.sagepub.com/content/17/2/142.short.

I. Céspedes, J. Ophir, H. Ponnekanti, and N. Maklad. Elastography: elasticity imaging using ultrasound with application to muscle and breast in vivo. *Ultrasonic Imaging*, 15 (2): 73–88, 1993. URL http://uix.sagepub.com/content/15/2/73.short.

P. Chaturvedi, M. F. Insana, and T. J. Hall. 2-D companding for noise reduction in strain imaging. *IEEE Transactions on Ultrasonics, Ferroelectrics, and Frequency Control*, 45 (1): 179–191, 1998. ISSN 0885-3010. doi: 10.1109/58.646923.

H. Chen and T. Varghese. Multilevel hybrid 2d strain imaging algorithm for ultrasound sector/phased arrays. *Medical Physics*, 36 (6): 2098–2106, Jun. 2009. ISSN 0094-2405. doi: 10.1118/1.3121426.

L. Chen, G. M. Treece, J. E. Lindop, A. H. Gee, and R. W. Prager. A quality-guided displacement tracking algorithm for ultrasonic elasticity imaging. *Medical Image Analysis*, 13 (2): 286–296, Apr. 2009. ISSN 13618415. doi: 10.1016/j.media.2008.10.007. URL http://linkinghub.elsevier.com/retrieve/pii/S1361841508001187.

X. Chen, M. J. Zohdy, S. Y. Emelianov, and M. O'Donell. Lateral speckle tracking using synthetic lateral phase. *IEEE Transactions on Ultrasonics, Ferroelectrics, and Frequency Control*, 51 (5): 540–550, May 2004. ISSN 0885-3010.

X. Chen, H. Xie, R. Erkamp, K. Kim, C. Jia, J. M. Rubin, and M. O'Donnell. 3-D correlation-based speckle tracking. *Ultrasonic Imaging*, 27 (1): 21–36, Jan. 2005. ISSN 0161-7346. doi: 10.1177/016173460502700102.

J. Crosby, B. H. Amundsen, T. Hergum, E. W. Remme, S. Langeland, and H. Torp. 3-D speckle tracking for assessment of regional left ventricular function. *Ultrasound in Medicine & Biology*, 35 (3): 458–471, Mar. 2009. ISSN 03015629. doi: 10.1016/j.ultrasmedbio.2008.09.011. URL http://linkinghub.elsevier.com/retrieve/pii/S030156290800433X.

C. L. De Korte, E. I. Cespedes, A. F. Van Der Steen, G. Pasterkamp, and N. Bom. Intravascular ultrasound elastography: assessment and imaging of elastic properties of diseased arteries and vulnerable plaque. *European Journal of Ultrasound*, 70 (3): 219–224, 1998. URL http://www.sciencedirect.com/science/article/pii/S0929826698000433.

C. L. De Korte, A. F. Van Der Steen, E. I. Cspedes, *et al.* Characterization of plaque components and vulnerability with intravascular ultrasound elastography. *Physics in Medicine and Biology*, 45 (6): 1465, 2000. URL http://iopscience.iop.org/0031-9155/45/6/305.

T. Deffieux, J.-L. Gennisson, M. Tanter, and M. Fink. Assessment of the mechanical properties of the musculoskeletal system using 2-D and 3-D very high frame rate ultrasound. *IEEE Transactions on Ultrasonics, Ferroelectrics, and Frequency Control*, 55 (10): 2177–2190, Oct. 2008. ISSN 1525-8955. doi: 10.1109/TUFFC.917.

J. D'hooge. Regional strain and strain rate measurements by cardiac ultrasound: principles, implementation and limitations. *European Journal of Echocardiography*, 1 (3): 154–170, Sep. 2000. ISSN 15252167. doi: 10.1053/euje.2000.0031. URL http://ehjcimaging.oxfordjournals.org/cgi/doi/10.1053/euje.2000.0031.

A. Elen, H. F. Choi, D. Loeckx, *et al.* Three-dimensional cardiac strain estimation using spatio temporal elastic registration of ultrasound images: a feasibility study. *IEEE Transactions on Medical Imaging*, 27 (11): 1580–1591, Nov. 2008. ISSN 0278-0062, 1558–254X. doi: 10.1109/TMI.2008.2004420. URL http://ieeexplore.ieee.org/document/4601464/.

S. Y. Emelianov, M. A. Lubinski, W. F. Weitzel, R. C. Wiggins, A. R. Skovoroda, and M. O'Donnell. Elasticity imaging for early detection of renal pathology. *Ultrasound in Medicine & Biology*, 21 (7): 871–883, 1995. ISSN 0301-5629.

B. S. Garra, E. I. Cespedes, J. Ophir, *et al.* Elastography of breast lesions: initial clinical results. *Radiology*, 202 (1): 79–86, 1997. URL http://radiology.rsna.org/content/202/1/79.short.

J.-L. Gennisson, J. Provost, T. Deffieux, *et al.* 4-D ultrafast shear-wave imaging. *IEEE Transactions on Ultrasonics, Ferroelectrics, and Frequency Control*, 62 (6): 1059–1065, Jun. 2015. ISSN 1525-8955. doi: 10.1109/TUFFC.2014.006936.

L. Guo, Y. Xu, Z. Xu, and J. Jiang. A PDE-based regularization algorithm toward reducing speckle tracking noise: a feasibility study for ultrasound breast elastography. *Ultrasonic Imaging*, 370 (4): 277–293, Oct. 2015. ISSN 0161-7346, 1096-0910. doi: 10.1177/0161734614561128. URL http://journals.sagepub.com/doi/10.1177/0161734614561128.

A. Heimdal, A. Stylen, H. Torp, and T. Skjaerpe. Real-time strain rate imaging of the left ventricle by ultrasound. *Journal of the American Society of Echocardiography: Official Publication of the American Society of Echocardiography*, 11 (11): 1013–1019, Nov. 1998. ISSN 0894-7317.

B. Heyde, R. Jasaityte, D. Barbosa, *et al.* Elastic image registration versus speckle tracking for 2-D myocardial motion estimation: a direct comparison in vivo. *IEEE Transactions on Medical Imaging*, 32 (2): 449–459, Feb. 2013. ISSN 0278-0062, 1558-254X. doi: 10.1109/TMI.2012.2230114. URL http://ieeexplore.ieee.org/document/6362224/.

C. Jia, K. Kim, T. J. Kolias, *et al.* 10b-5 4d elasticity imaging of PVA LV phantom integrated with pulsatile circulation system using 2d phased array. pages 876–879. IEEE, Oct. 2007. ISBN 978-1-4244-1383-6 978-1-4244-1384-3. doi: 10.1109/ULTSYM.2007.224. URL http://ieeexplore.ieee.org/document/4409797/.

J. Luo and E. E. Konofagou. A fast normalized cross-correlation calculation method for motion estimation. *IEEE Transactions on Ultrasonics, Ferroelectrics and Frequency Control*, 57 (6): 1347–1357, Jun. 2010. ISSN 0885-3010. doi: 10.1109/TUFFC.2010.1554. URL http://ieeexplore.ieee.org/document/5480177/.

J. Jiang and T. J. Hall. A fast hybrid algorithm combining regularized motion tracking and predictive search for reducing the occurrence of large displacement errors. *IEEE Transactions on Ultrasonics, Ferroelectrics and Frequency Control*, 58 (4): 730–736, Apr. 2011. ISSN 0885-3010. doi: 10.1109/TUFFC.2011.1865. URL http://ieeexplore.ieee.org/document/5750094/.

F. Kallel and J. Ophir. A least-squares strain estimator for elastography. *Ultrasonic Imaging*, 19 (3): 195–208, 1997. URL http://uix.sagepub.com/content/19/3/195.short.

F. Kallel, J. Ophir, K. Magee, and T. Krouskop. Elastographic imaging of low-contrast elastic modulus distributions in tissue. *Ultrasound in Medicine & Biology*, 24 (3): 409–425, 1998. URL http://www.sciencedirect.com/science/article/pii/S0301562997002871.

E. E. Konofagou and J. Ophir. A new elastographic method for estimation and imaging of lateral displacements, lateral strains, corrected axial strains and Poisson's ratios in tissues. *Ultrasound in Medicine & Biology*, 24 (8): 1183–1199, 1998. URL http://www.sciencedirect.com/science/article/pii/S0301562998001094.

E. E. Konofagou, J. D'hooge, and J. Ophir. Myocardial elastography A feasibility study in vivo. *Ultrasound in Medicine & Biology*, 28 (4): 475–482, 2002. URL http://www.sciencedirect.com/science/article/pii/S030156290200488X.

F. Kremer, H. F. Choi, S. Langeland, E. D'Agostino, P. Claus, and J. D'hooge. Geometric regularization for 2-D myocardial strain quantification in mice: an in-silico study. *Ultrasound in Medicine & Biology*, 36 (7): 1157–1168, Jul. 2010. ISSN 03015629. doi: 10.1016/j. ultrasmedbio.2010.04.009. URL http://linkinghub.elsevier.com/retrieve/pii/S0301562910001870.

T. A. Krouskop, T. M. Wheeler, F. Kallel, B. S. Garra, and T. Hall. Elastic moduli of breast and prostate tissues under compression. *Ultrasonic Imaging*, 20 (4): 260–274, Oct. 1998. ISSN 0161-7346. doi: 10.1177/016173469802000403.

S. Langeland, J. D'hooge, H. Torp, B. Bijnens, and P. Suetens. Comparison of time-domain displacement estimators for two-dimensional RF tracking. *Ultrasound in Medicine & Biology*, 29 (8): 1177–1186, Aug. 2003. ISSN 0301-5629.

S. Langeland, P. F. Wouters, P. Claus, *et al.* Experimental assessment of a new research tool for the estimation of two-dimensional myocardial strain. *Ultrasound in Medicine & Biology*, 32 (10): 1509–1513, 2006. URL http://www.sciencedirect.com/science/article/pii/S0301562906017078.

M. Leitman, P. Lysyansky, S. Sidenko, *et al.* Two-dimensional strain-a novel software for real-time quantitative echocardiographic assessment of myocardial function. *Journal of the American Society of Echocardiography: Official Publication of the American Society of Echocardiography*, 17 (10): 1021–1029, Oct. 2004. ISSN 0894-7317. doi: 10.1016/j.echo.2004.06.019.

H. Liebgott, A. Basarab, P. Gueth, D. Friboulet, and P. Delachartre. Transverse oscillations for tissue motion estimation. *Physics Procedia*, 3 (1): 235–244, Jan. 2010. ISSN 18753892. doi: 10.1016/j.phpro.2010.01.032 . URL http://linkinghub.elsevier.com/retrieve/pii/S1875389210000337.

J. E. Lindop, G. M. Treece, A. H. Gee, and R. W. Prager. 3d elastography using freehand ultrasound. *Ultrasound in Medicine & Biology*, 32 (4): 529–545, Apr. 2006. ISSN 0301-5629. doi: 10.1016/j. ultrasmedbio.2005.11.018.

R. Lopata, M. M. Nillesen, H. H. Hansen, I. Gerrits, J. Thijssen, and C. L. De Korte. Performance evaluation of methods for two-dimensional displacement and strain estimation using ultrasound radio frequency data. *Ultrasound in Medicine & Biology*, 35 (5): 796–812, 2009. URL http://www.sciencedirect.com/science/article/pii/S0301562908005310.

R. Lopata, M. Nillesen, C. Verrijp, *et al.* Cardiac biplane strain imaging: initial in vivo experience. *Physics in Medicine and Biology*, 55 (4): 963, 2010. URL http://iopscience.iop.org/0031-9155/55/4/004.

R. Lopata, M. M. Nillesen, J. Thijssen, L. Kapusta, and C. L. De Korte. Three-dimensional cardiac strain imaging in healthy children using RF-data. *Ultrasound in Medicine & Biology*, 37 (9): 1399–1408, 2011. URL http://www.sciencedirect.com/science/article/pii/S0301562911011288.

M. A. Lubinski, S. Y. Emelianov, and M. O'Donnell. Speckle tracking methods for ultrasonic elasticity imaging using short-time correlation. *IEEE Transactions on Ultrasonics, Ferroelectrics, and Frequency Control*, 46 (1): 82–96, 1999. ISSN 0885-3010. doi: 10.1109/58.741427.

W. N. McDicken, G. R. Sutherland, C. M. Moran, and L. N. Gordon. Colour Doppler velocity imaging of the myocardium. *Ultrasound in Medicine & Biology*, 18 (6–7): 651–654, 1992. ISSN 0301-5629.

J. Ophir, E. Cespedes, H. Ponnekanti, Y. Yazdi, and X. Li. Elastography: a quantitative method for imaging the elasticity of biological tissues. *Ultrasonic*

Imaging, 13 (2): 111–134, 1991. URL http://www.sciencedirect.com/science/article/pii/016173469190079W.

J. Ophir, S. Alam, B. Garra, *et al.* Elastography: ultrasonic estimation and imaging of the elastic properties of tissues. *Proceedings of the Institution of Mechanical Engineers, Part H: Journal of Engineering in Medicine*, 213 (3): 203–233, 1999. URL http://pih.sagepub.com/content/213/3/203.short.

C. Papadacci, E. A. Bunting, E. Y. Wan, P. Nauleau, and E. E. Konofagou. 3d myocardial elastography in vivo. *IEEE Transactions on Medical Imaging*, 36 (2): 618–627, Feb. 2017. ISSN 1558-254X. doi: 10.1109/TMI.2016.2623636.

A. V. Patil, C. D. Garson, and J. A. Hossack. 3d prostate elastography: algorithm, simulations and experiments. *Physics in Medicine and Biology*, 52 (12): 3643–3663, Jun. 2007. ISSN 0031-9155. doi: 10.1088/0031–9155/52/12/019.

Y. Petrank, L. Huang, and M. O'Donnell. Reduced peak-hopping artifacts in ultrasonic strain estimation using the Viterbi algorithm. *IEEE Transactions on Ultrasonics, Ferroelectrics and Frequency Control*, 56 (7): 1359–1367, Jul. 2009. ISSN 0885-3010. doi: 10.1109/TUFFC.2009.1192. URL http://ieeexplore.ieee.org/document/5116862/.

B. S. Ramamurthy and G. E. Trahey. Potential and limitations of angle-independent flow detection algorithms using radio-frequency and detected echo signals. *Ultrasonic Imaging*, 13 (3): 252–268, Jul. 1991. ISSN 0161-7346. doi: 10.1177/016173469101300303.

G. Said, O. Basset, J. M. Mari, C. Cachard, E. Brusseau, and D. Vray. Experimental three dimensional strain estimation from ultrasonic sectorial data. *Ultrasonics*, 44 Suppl 1: e189–e193, Dec. 2006. ISSN 1874-9968. doi: 10.1016/j.ultras.2006.06.051.

K. Saito, H. Okura, N. Watanabe, *et al.* Comprehensive evaluation of left ventricular strain using speckle tracking echocardiography in normal adults: comparison of three-dimensional and two-dimensional approaches. *Journal of the American Society of Echocardiography: Official Publication of the American Society of Echocardiography*, 22 (9): 1025–1030, Sep. 2009. ISSN 1097-6795. doi: 10.1016/j.echo.2009.05.021.

S. Srinivasan, F. Kallel, R. Souchon, and J. Ophir. Analysis of an adaptive strain estimation technique in elastography. *Ultrasonic Imaging*, 24 (2): 109–118, 2002. URL http://uix.sagepub.com/content/24/2/109.short.

G. E. Trahey, S. M. Hubbard, and O. T. von Ramm. Angle independent ultrasonic blood flow detection by frame-to-frame correlation of B-mode images. *Ultrasonics*, 26 (5): 271–276, Sep. 1988. ISSN 0041-624X.

T. Varghese and J. Ophir. Enhancement of echo-signal correlation in elastography using temporal stretching. *IEEE Transactions on Ultrasonics, Ferroelectrics, and Frequency Control*, 44 (1): 173–180, 1997a. ISSN 0885-3010. doi: 10.1109/58.585213.

T. Varghese and J. Ophir. A theoretical framework for performance characterization of elastography: the strain filter. *IEEE Transactions on Ultrasonics, Ferroelectrics and Frequency Control*, 44 (1): 164–172, 1997b.

S. Yagi and K. Nakayama. Local displacement analysis of inhomogeneous soft tissue by spatial correlation of RF echo signals. In *Proceedings, World Federation for Ultrasound in Medicine & Biology meeting*, page 113, Washington, DC, USA, 1988.

I. K. Zervantonakis, S. D. Fung-Kee-Fung, W.-N. Lee, and E. E. Konofagou. A novel, view-independent method for strain mapping in myocardial elastography: eliminating angle and centroid dependence. *Physics in Medicine and Biology*, 52 (14): 4063–4080, Jul. 2007. ISSN 0031-9155. doi: 10.1088/0031-9155/52/14/004.

Y. Zhu and T. J. Hall. A modified block matching method for real-time freehand strain imaging. *Ultrasonic Imaging*, 24 (3): 161–176, Jul. 2002. ISSN 0161-7346. doi: 10.1177/016173460202400303.

Chapter 15
Techniques for tracking: image registration

Ariel Hernán Curiale[1,2,3], *Gonzalo Vegas-Sánchez-Ferrero*[4,5] *and Santiago Aja-Fernández*[6]

15.1 Ultrasound image registration: speckle tracking

The process of finding a suitable deformation to align two or more images is a process known as image registration, image fusion, matching or warping. Image registration is the keystone in many image analysis tasks, especially important in those methods that involve the combination of various data sources, like in image fusion (functional and structural information), change detection (motion, velocity and deformation) and multichannel image restoration. As introduced in Chapter 13, such image registration techniques can also be used for ultrasound-based motion estimation, i.e., "speckle tracking," which will be elaborated in this chapter.

In general, the term *Speckle Tracking* refers to all those techniques that analyze motion by tracking the intensity or the interference patterns of the US data, known as *speckle*, throughout the temporal sequences. Since this pattern remains stable under the same acquisition conditions and exhibits an inherent relationship with the tissue structure, it can be tracked to estimate the motion of the tissue [1,2] as it is depicted in Figure 15.1. In what follows, we will use the term Speckle Tracking (ST) in a global sense to denote all those methods that estimate the motion by tracking the speckle pattern in the B-mode envelope, extracted from the RF signal.

This chapter is focused on those image registration techniques that estimate the motion and strain by tracking the speckle pattern directly from the intensity of the B-mode US images assuming a temporal relationship between images. The fixed and moving images are noted as I_t and I_{t-1} with t meaning a specific time.

[1]Consejo Nacional de Investigaciones Científicas y Técnicas (CONICET), Argentina
[2]FCEN – Universidad Nacional de Cuyo, Mendoza, Argentina
[3]Departamento de Física Médica, Centro Atómico Bariloche, Argentina
[4]Applied Chest Imaging Laboratory (ACIL), Brigham and Women's Hospital, Harvard Medical School, USA
[5]Biomedical Image Technologies Laboratory (BIT), ETSI Telecomunicación, Universidad Politécnica de Madrid, and CIBER-BBN, Spain
[6]Laboratorio de Procesado de Imagen (LPI), ETSI Telecomunicación, Universidad de Valladolid, Spain

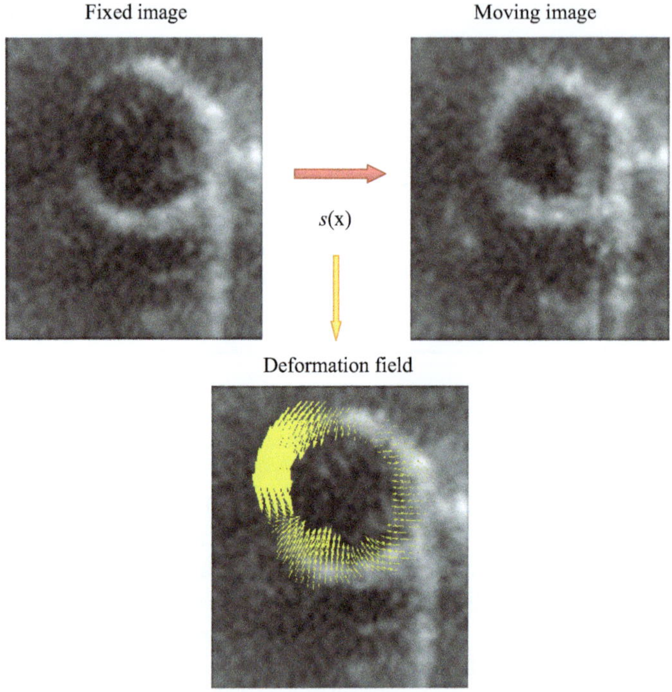

Figure 15.1 Speckle tracking technique for myocardial motion estimation

Historically, image registration is classified according to the nature of deformation to be modeled as [3–6]:

- **Rigid:** Only translations and rotations are allowed. However, affine and projective deformation are commonly included in this category due to the simplicity of the transformation model. In general, in this classification, deformations occur in a global sense.
- **Nonrigid:** Lines can be mapped to curves and most of the time the deformation is not global.

Despite the nature of the deformation and the classification used for describing the image registration method, one can easily distinguish three necessary and interrelated parts within a generic ST approach (see Figure 15.2):

1. **Similarity model:** Necessary to establish the correspondence between images along the time sequence. A common strategy used in ST is to take advantage of speckle characterization in ultrasound images. A complete description of different similarity measure is carried out in Section 15.2. Also, it is discussed, the relation between image intensity assumed by each of the similarity measures such as the sum of squared difference, cross correlation (CC) and mutual information (MI).

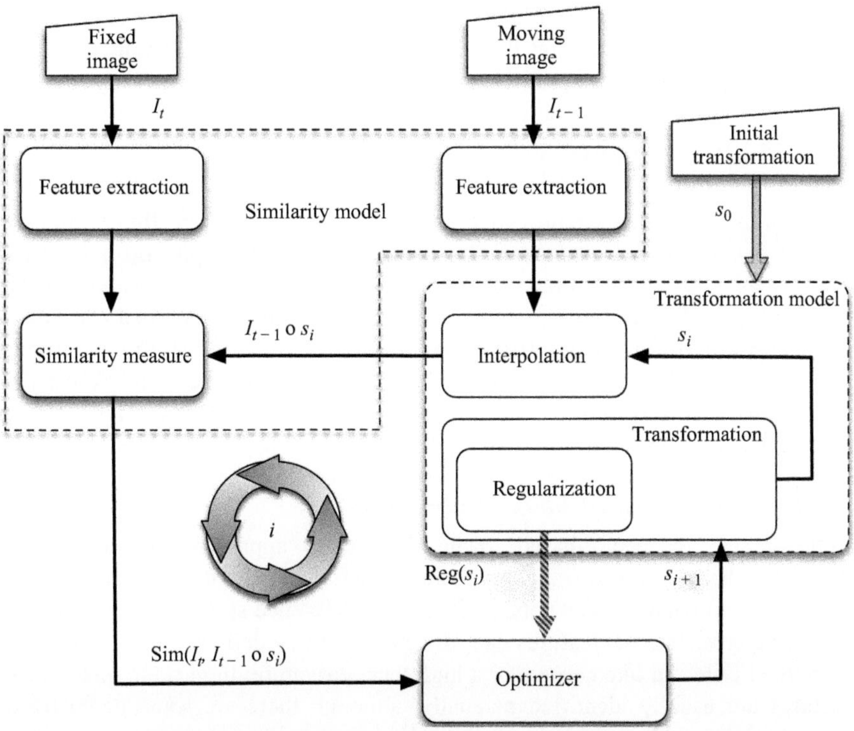

Figure 15.2 Generic image registration approach where I_t and s_i denote a particular image and transformation, respectively. The warped image is represented by the composition operator $I_{t-1} \circ s_i = I_{t-1}(s(\mathbf{x}))$

2. **Transformation model:** It specifies the type of deformation considered between images and the way the similarity measure is introduced into the motion estimation. A wide range of different transformation models are introduced in Section 15.3. In particular, they are introduced, the nonrigid transformation models which includes the transformation models derived from the interpolation theory [radial basis function (RBF), thin plate splines (TPS) and B-spline], and those derived from physical models (elastic, flow, optical flow and diffusion). Also, in this section, it is discussed, the necessity of a regularization which can be implicit (transformation models derived of the interpolation theory) or explicit (most of the transformation models derived from physical models). Finally, it is covered, the main idea and limitations of the diffeomorphism.
3. **Optimization strategy:** It defines a strategy for optimizing the transformation model according to the similarity model. In Section 15.4, the optimization strategies are discussed by distinguishing between the methods for optimizing parametric transformation such as B-splines and the methods used for directly optimizing the deformation field (elastic, flow, optical flow, diffusion and finite element).

Finally, the relations between the different components involved into a ST approach (see Figure 15.2) and the interdependence between different strategies chosen in each component are discussed in Section 15.5.

15.2 Similarity model

The similarity model defines the feature space in which the similarity between two or more images can be compared. For example, the similarity of two images can be established by comparing just the structure and not the intensity levels. More complex similarity measures can be described according to the purpose of the registration methodology. These registration methods are commonly referred to as featured-based registration methods. When the feature space is reduced to the intensity of each pixel, they are known as intensity-based methods.

15.2.1 Feature-based image registration

A crucial step in feature-based image registration approaches is the feature extraction. There is a wide range of features that can be used in a feature-based registration approach such as dots, lines, curves, reference surfaces or even anatomical structures. Indeed, features can also be structures defined with a particular geometrical criterion like corners or a high local curvature. In general, anatomical structures are usually identified manually, although there are some geometrical structures that can be identified automatically [4].

Once the features are detected, i.e., segmented, a similarity measure is defined to establish a degree of similarity between the features of the images. For example, a simple similarity measure that can be defined is the spatial distance between a pair of features by using the ℓ_1-norm or ℓ_2-norm [7]. Finally, is important to point out that the registration accuracy strongly depends on the feature extraction step which, in general, is quite complex. However, feature-based image registration methods are commonly faster than intensity-based approaches due to the reduced number of features used compared with the image dimension.

15.2.2 Intensity-based image registration

If the feature space is confined to the image intensity, i.e., the feature extraction step is trivial, the image registration approach becomes an intensity-based image registration. In a general sense, the speckle tracking approaches are intensity-based image registration methods because the deformation is estimated by tracking the speckle pattern intensity. This makes easier to estimate a dense deformation, although it also implies a higher computational cost.

The most simple similarity measures that can be considered in an ST approach are those derived from the ℓ_1-norm and ℓ_2-norm, for example, the sum of absolute differences (SAD) and the sum of squared differences (SSD), respectively, [4]

$$\varphi_{\text{SAD}}(I_t, I_{t-1} \circ s) = \frac{1}{N} \sum_{\mathbf{x} \in \Omega_x}^{N} |I_t(\mathbf{x}) - I_{t-1} \circ s(\mathbf{x})|, \tag{15.1}$$

$$\varphi_{\text{SSD}}(I_t, I_{t-1} \circ s) = \frac{1}{N} \sum_{\mathbf{x} \in \Omega_x}^{N} (I_t(\mathbf{x}) - I_{t-1} \circ s(\mathbf{x}))^2, \tag{15.2}$$

where the displacement of voxels from t and $t-1$ are defined by the transformation s: $\mathbf{x} \rightarrow \mathbf{x} + \mathbf{s}(\mathbf{x})$ with $\mathbf{x} \in X_t$ and $\mathbf{x} + \mathbf{s}(\mathbf{x}) \in X_{t-1}$. Besides, $N = |\Omega_x|$ refers to the number of overlapped voxels in the images I_t e $I_{t-1} \circ s$, and the warped images is represented by the composition operator, as follows: $I_{t-1} \circ s = I_{t-1}(\mathrm{s}(\mathbf{x}))$.

Similarity measures derived from the ℓ_1-norm are widely used in many different areas like machine learning, image processing and statistical as they are simple and robust. Nevertheless, the SAD can only be used into simple image registration approaches due to the lack of differentiability. Therefore, a natural substitute of this similarity measure is the SSD. However, SAD is more robust to noise than SSD.

The main limitation of SAD and SSD is the underlying assumption about the intensities relation between images. Specifically, both similarity measures assume the same image intensity for registering images with the exception of an additive Gaussian noise. Depending on the application, this assumption may not be appropriate, for instance image fusion from different modalities that may show different intensity levels per tissues and different noise characteristics.

CC and normalized CC (NCC) are the most basic statistical similarity measures used in image registration. They are commonly used in techniques such as template matching. Indeed, NCC was the first similarity measure proposed for ST [8–10] and was defined as follows:

$$\varphi_{\text{NCC}}(I_t, I_{t-1} \circ s) = \frac{\sum_{\mathbf{x} \in \Omega_x} (I_t(\mathbf{x}) - \bar{I}_t)(I_{t-1} \circ s(\mathbf{x}) - \bar{I}_{t-1})}{\sqrt{\sum_{\mathbf{x} \in \Omega_x} (I_t(\mathbf{x}) - \bar{I}_t)^2 \sum_{\mathbf{x} \in \Omega_x} (I_{t-1} \circ s(\mathbf{x}) - \bar{I}_{t-1})^2}}, \tag{15.3}$$

where $\bar{I}_t$ and $\bar{I}_{t-1}$ are the mean intensities of the images $I_t = \{I_t(\mathbf{x})\}_{\mathbf{x} \in \Omega_x}$ and $I_{t-1} = \{I_{t-1}(\mathbf{x})\}_{\mathbf{x} \in \Omega_x}$, respectively. In contrast to SAD and SSD, the CC similarity measures assume a linear intensity relation between images instead of the same intensity, which makes this similarity measure more versatile [3]. However, if the images are taken from different sources such as ultrasound and computed tomography, an assumption of linearity between images intensities will introduce an important error in the deformation estimation.

To avoid this problem, more suitable measures have been proposed. The most common measure used for multimodal image registration or image fusion is *MI*, originally proposed by Shannon, which only assumes a likelihood relationship between image intensities. This way, when the MI is maximized, the redundant or duplicated information (i.e., the joint entropy, $H(I_t, I_{t-1} \circ s)$) is reduced. On the other hand, its maximization tends to increase the marginal information of the images $H(I_t)$ and $H(I_{t-1} \circ s)$ (i.e., the image information). According to Shannon's original proposal, the MI is defined as follows:

$$\varphi_{\mathrm{MI}}(I_t, I_{t-1} \circ s) = H(I_t) + H(I_{t-1} \circ s) - H(I_t, I_{t-1} \circ s)$$
$$= \sum_i \sum_j p(i,j) \log \frac{p(i,j)}{p(i)p(j)}, \qquad (15.4)$$

where $p(i, j)$ is the joint likelihood of the images intensity and $p(i)$ and $p(j)$ are the marginal likelihoods for each image intensity, respectively (i.e., $i = I_t(\mathbf{x})$ and $j = I_{t-1} \circ s(\mathbf{x})$ para $\mathbf{x} \in \Omega_x$). The joint and marginal likelihoods are commonly estimated by using the image histogram [4]. Since the MI is strongly related with the image overlapping, the normalized MI (NMI), a more suitable and robust similarity measure [11], is used instead of the MI:

$$\varphi_{\mathrm{NMI}}(I_t, I_{t-1} \circ s) = \frac{H(I_t) + H(I_{t-1} \circ s)}{H(I_t, I_{t-1} \circ s)}. \qquad (15.5)$$

During the past decades, different similarity measures have been proposed for ST, among them, the more extended are: the NCC [8–10]; the SAD [12,13]; the nonnormalized CC [14]; the SSD [15–22]; the MI [23] and the monogenic phase [24–26].

15.2.3 Maximum likelihood approach

Choosing a suitable similarity measure for image registration approach is not easy and most of the time depends on the application itself. For example, when an ST approach uses the similarity measure SSD, it is assumed that the image intensity to be registered is the same for all the images. If it is used the CC or NCC, a linear intensity relation is considered instead. Nevertheless, the MI or NMI seems to be a more suitable similarity measure for image registration because it is not imposed a particular relationship between images intensity more than a likelihood relation.

In a statistical framework, the minimization of the similarity measure is equivalent to a maximum likelihood estimation [27]. Thus, the optimal deformation between images described by the transformation s, $\hat{s}_{\mathrm{ML}}$, can be estimated by maximizing the following likelihood

$$\hat{s}_{\mathrm{ML}} = \underset{s}{\operatorname{argmax}}\, p(I_{t-1} | I_t, s). \qquad (15.6)$$

Assuming an independent and identically distributed image intensity for each voxel, (15.6) is equivalent to

$$\hat{s}_{\mathrm{ML}} = \underset{s}{\operatorname{argmax}} \prod_{\mathbf{x} \in \Omega_x} p(I_{t-1} \circ s(\mathbf{x}) | I_t(\mathbf{x}), s), \qquad (15.7)$$

and maximize (15.7) is equivalent to minimize the following log-likelihood function when stationarity is assumed, i.e., $p(I_{t-1} \circ s(\mathbf{x})|I_t(\mathbf{x}),s)$ is independent to $\mathbf{x}$:

$$\hat{s}_{\mathrm{ML}} = \underset{s}{\operatorname{argmin}} \sum_{\mathbf{x}\in\Omega_x} -\log(p(I_{t-1} \circ s(\mathbf{x})|I_t(\mathbf{x}), s))$$

$$= \underset{s}{\operatorname{argmin}} \frac{1}{N} \sum_{\mathbf{x}\in\Omega_x} \varphi_{\mathbf{x}}(I_t, I_{t-1} \circ s). \tag{15.8}$$

Following this idea, the maximum likelihood approach provides a general theoretical framework to introduce different relationships between the image intensities. For example, if it is assumed that a scene, I_t, is described as an unknown intensity function of the moving image, $f(I_{t-1} \circ s(\mathbf{x}))$, corrupted by an additive Gaussian noise with zero mean as follows:

$$I_t(\mathbf{x}) = f(I_{t-1} \circ s(\mathbf{x})) + \eta(\mathbf{x}). \tag{15.9}$$

In this case, a tissue class characterized with an average intensity level j will have an average response value $f(j) = f_j$ and the set of locations in the scene I_t, for each jth tissue class is denoted as $\Omega_{\mathbf{x}}^j = \{\mathbf{x} \in \Omega_{\mathbf{x}} : I_{t-1} \circ s^{-1}(\mathbf{x}) = j\}$. So, for each tissue class, the conditional density distribution is reduced to

$$P(I_t = i|j) = \frac{1}{2\sqrt{\pi}\sigma} e^{\frac{i-f_j}{2\sigma^2}} \tag{15.10}$$

The maximization with respect the parameter vector $(f_0, f_1, \ldots, \sigma)$ gives rise to a variance estimate $\hat{\sigma}^2 = \frac{1}{N}\Sigma_j\Sigma_{\Omega_{\mathbf{x}}^j}(I_t(\mathbf{x}) - \hat{f}_j)^2$, where $\hat{f}_j = \frac{1}{N_j}\Sigma_{\Omega_{\mathbf{x}}^j} I_t(\mathbf{x})$ and the cardinals of each set are $N = |\Omega_{\mathbf{x}}|$ and $N_j = |\Omega_{\mathbf{x}}^j|$. On the other hand, the transformation $s{:}\Omega_{t-1} \to \Omega_t$ can be obtained by minimizing the registration energy from the log-likelihood:

$$U(s) = \frac{N}{2}\log\left(2\pi e \frac{1}{N}\sum_j \sum_{x\in\Omega_{\mathbf{x}}^j} \left(I_t(\mathbf{x}) - \hat{f}_j\right)^2\right) \tag{15.11}$$

The energy function shown in (15.11) is minimized when the sum of squares decreases. Thus, according to the function f_j adopted for each tissue class, one can adopt different similarity measures. In the case of $f(j) = j$, the formulation is equivalent to the similarity measure SSD, whereas for a linear relationship $f(j) = \alpha j + \beta$, the maximum likelihood becomes equivalent to the CC. Finally, if the only assumption on $f(.)$ is its stationarity, the similarity measure derived from the maximum likelihood approach is equivalent to MI [28]. The reader is referred to [27] for a detailed derivation of these similarity measures by using the maximum likelihood approach.

Some authors proposed the use of alternative statistical models to provide a better characterization of speckle pattern such as Gaussian [29], Rayleigh [29–31], Gamma [32], bivariate Nakagami [33] and bivariate Generalized Gamma [34].

In this case, the similarity measures based on a statistical characterization of speckle are assuming that the deformation does not change the statistics of speckle, though the intensity values of the image may vary. Thus, the measures are intended to provide the most likely transformations according to the statistical characterization of speckle.

Besides, the metrics proposed by [33,34] also considered a temporal correlation within the statistical model that accounts for correlation between speckle patterns throughout the deformation.

Other hybrid similarity measures such as the SSD combined with structural information [35] or the SSD combined with Rayleigh model [21] have been proposed in order to jointly consider the statistical characterization of speckle and some local structural information.

15.3 Transformation model

The transformation model defines the sort of transformation allowed for the ST technique and the way the similarity measure is evaluated. This comprises the interpolation used when a point is mapped from one space into another by certain transformation, i.e., image values in noninteger coordinates are computed by the appropriate interpolation technique. In particular, the ST accuracy and computational time could be affected by the interpolation used. For example, a simple scheme such as nearest neighbor or linear interpolation is usually used for decreasing the computational time. In contrast, more complex interpolation schemes can be used for higher accuracy, among them, cubic, B-spline or *sinc* interpolation functions.

Both the interpolation and the transformation (rigid or nonrigid) change the statistical behavior of speckle. However, most of the methods proposed in the literature assume a negligible effect on the ST accuracy.

The different transformations can be classified in many ways. According to the nature of the transformation: rigid, affine, nonrigid or elastic [4,36]; according to the reference system as affine, projective or curved [3]. The transformation can be also described by a physical model [37], can act in a local or global way [5] or can be parametric or nonparametric [6].

In this chapter, the classification adopted follows the one proposed in [37] with a special emphasis on the theoretical motivation behind the transformation. Usually, the transformations described by physical models are derived from the continuum theory and, in these models, the transformation is implicitly estimated by computing the deformation field, whereas the parametric transformations are derived from the interpolation and approximation theory that explicitly estimates the transformation.

15.3.1 Rigid transformation

A rigid transformation is defined as any transformation preserving the original distance between points, which is usually characterized by six parameters in 3D

(3 translations and 3 rotations). In general, affine transformations are classified as rigid transformations even when they do not preserve the distance between points. This is because affine transformations are global transformations that preserve parallel lines. As rigid transformations, they can be characterized with 12 parameters (three translations, three rotations and three shearing parameters). Figure 15.3 shows the possible deformations allowed by using an affine transformation.

As stated before, rigid transformations are global transformations and they cannot be used to model complex transformation acting at a local level like the one depicted in Figure 15.4. However, they are commonly used as a previous stage in a nonrigid registration approach.

15.3.2 Nonrigid transformation according to the physical model

15.3.2.1 Elastic transformations

Elastic transformations are derived from continuum mechanics for deformable solids. By assuming linear elasticity, which describes a linear relationship between material stress and strain, the elastic deformation can be estimated from the deformation field computed by solving the system of partial differential equations (PDE) of Navier–Cauchy

$$\mu\nabla^2\mathbf{u} + (\mu + \lambda)\nabla(\nabla.\mathbf{u}) + \mathbf{f} = 0, \tag{15.12}$$

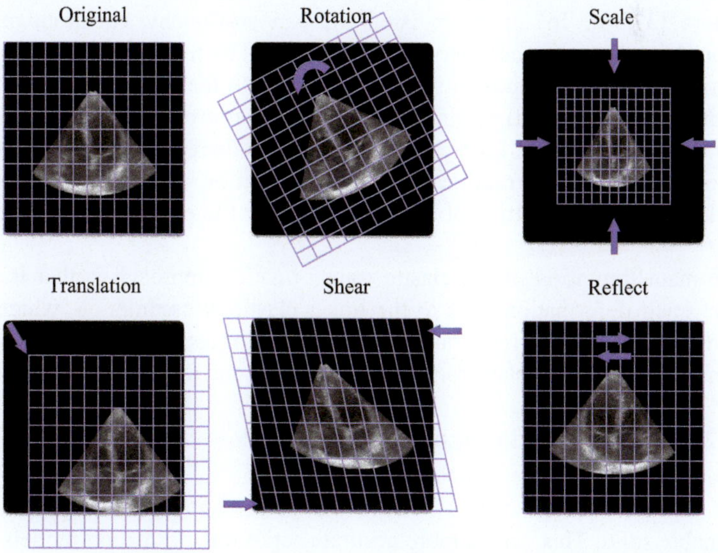

Figure 15.3 Different types of deformation allowed by an affine transformation in a four chamber echocardiography

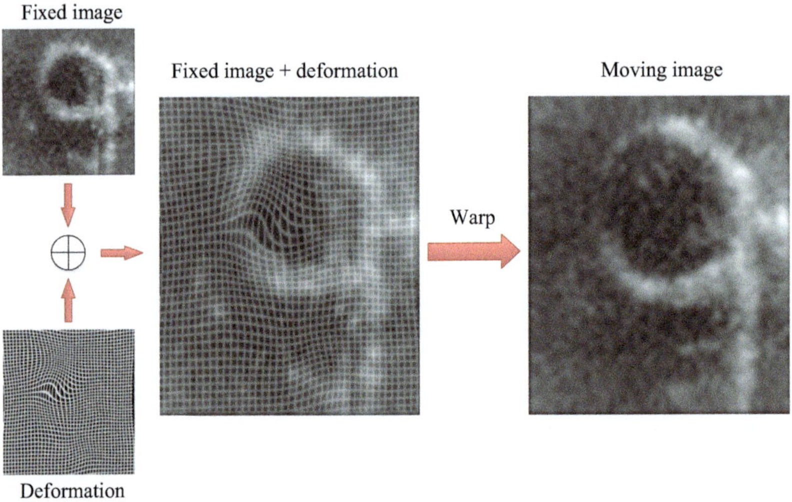

Figure 15.4 The myocardial motion along the cardiac phase presents a highly localized complex deformation which cannot be modeled by means of an affine transformation. Fixed and moving images correspond to the end-diastole and end-systole

where ∇^2 refers to the Laplacian operator and $\nabla\cdot\mathbf{u}$ is the divergence for the displacement vector **u**. The external forces are denoted by **f**; and μ and λ are Lamé parameters [37,38]. In image registration, Navier–Cauchy equations describe the deformation between the external forces imposed by the similarity measure and the internal strains that impose a smooth constraint to the deformation.

Broit proposed the first image registration approach using the Navier–Cauchy equations in [39]. Later, Bajcsy *et al.* introduced a global correction by means of a rigid transformation (translation, rotation and scaling) in [40,41], where they also use a multiresolution approach for the elastic model introduced by Broit.

The main limitation of the elastic transformation approach is that it is only valid for small deformations due to the linear elasticity assumption, which is not usually the case in image registration. Furthermore, most of the biological tissues do not maintain a linear relationship between stress and strain.

15.3.2.2 Transformation models based on flow theory

The main limitation of the elastic models about the assumption of small deformations can be overcome by modeling the deformation as a fluid instead of a deformable solid. This way, a more accurate set of transformation models can be derived from the flow theory that is not limited to small deformations. Among others, the most representatives are the fluid flow, optical flow and the diffusion approach.

15.3.2.3 Fluid flow transformations

Those transformations based on fluid flow are implicitly derived from the Navier–Stokes PDE

$$\mu\nabla^2\mathbf{v} + (\mu+\lambda)\nabla(\nabla.\mathbf{v}) + \mathbf{f} = 0, \tag{15.13}$$

where the incompressibility constant is associated to the term $\mu\nabla^2\mathbf{v}$, while the term $(\mu+\lambda)\nabla(\nabla\cdot\mathbf{v})$ controls the compression and expansion of the fluid. Navier–Stokes PDE (15.13) are almost identical to the Navier–Cauchy (15.12) for elastic deformations. However, Navier–Stokes equations operates on velocity, $\mathbf{v}$, rather than displacement, $\mathbf{u}$. Thus, a numerical integration is required to estimate the deformation.

In fluid flow transformations, as it is for elastic transformations, the deformation is computed iteratively as follows: First, the external forces on the fluid, $\mathbf{f}$, are estimated by using the similarity measure between images and the displacement field $\mathbf{u}$. Then, the Navier–Stokes equations (15.13) are solved to estimate the fluid velocity $\mathbf{v}$. Finally, the displacement or deformation field, $\mathbf{u}$, is computed by means of a numerical integration.

Due to the similarity to Navier–Cauchy equation (15.12), the solutions of linear elasticity can be transformed to fluid flow solutions by means of a numerical integration. Fluid flow is able to model large localized deformations, although it increases the computational cost [37]. The most well-known fluid flow algorithm to solve the Navier–Stokes PDE used in image registration was introduced by Christensen *et al.* in [42–44].

15.3.2.4 Optical flow

According to Gibson [45], optical flow is the relative perception of an observer about a moving object. In particular, the movement is only perceived when a change of the object is represented in the scene as a brightness modification. The relation between optical flow and the real velocity of the object is not entirely straightforward since the optical flow is the apparent velocity of an object in a scene or image [46]. However, there is a link between optical flow and fluid flow [47].

In order to estimate the optical flow from the brightness of an object projected into a scene, it is necessary to introduce some restrictions. In particular, the velocity cannot be estimated only from the brightness information at a single point. Thus, it is necessary to assume that the points within a neighborhood have similar velocities. The brightness reflected by the moving object is also assumed to vary smoothly on the entire object. With this assumption and considering a small movement, the optical flow equation can be derived by using the first order Taylor expansion of the deformed image as follows

$$\mathbf{v}(\mathbf{x})\nabla I_{t-1} \circ s(\mathbf{x}) = I_{t-1} \circ s(\mathbf{x}) - I_t(\mathbf{x}), \tag{15.14}$$

where $s(\mathbf{x}) = \mathbf{x} + \mathbf{v}(\mathbf{x})$ and $\mathbf{v}(\mathbf{x})$ is the displacement in time. In fact, $\mathbf{v}$ is considered the deformation velocity since it represents the displacement in time, i.e., $\mathbf{v}$ is the displacement between two temporal instants. However, it is more natural to consider **v** as the displacement of the deformation.

Optical flow registration is widely used in speckle tracking due to its simplicity and fast computation, and it is usually classified into two general methodologies: block matching methods [8–10,12–16,29,30,48] and variational methods [18,22,24–26,34].

15.3.2.5 Diffusion

In his seminal paper, Thirion [49] introduced the concept of *demons* for estimating the deformation between images in a similar way as Maxwell did for illustrating the Gibbs paradox in thermodynamic in the nineteenth century, in which a semi-permeable membrane contains a set of *demons* that are able to distinguish between two types of particles and allows one kind of particles to diffuse to the other side. In the particular case of image registration, the demons are placed regularly in the image and apply a force on the image to provide a deformation based on the optical flow equation (15.14) [50].

Thirion describes different possible variants for the forces of the demons such as constant magnitude and gradient based. In diffusion models, the transformation is implicitly estimated by means of an iterative update of a composition of the deformation field and the *demons* forces. Then, the deformation field is regularized by convolving it with a Gaussian kernel.

In a posterior work, Vercauteren *et al.* [51] introduced the mathematical foundations to characterize the diffusion model as a classic optimization problem, where a global functional energy is minimized. Furthermore, they introduced a regularization term on the transformation to preserve the topology of objects by proposing the following function energy:

$$E_{\mathbf{x}}(c,s) = \frac{1}{2|\Omega_x|}\sum_{\mathbf{x}\in\Omega_x}\left\|\frac{1}{\sigma_i}(I_t(\mathbf{x}) - I_{t-1}\circ c(\mathbf{x}))\right\|^2 + \frac{1}{\sigma_x^2}\mathrm{dist}(s,c)^2 + \frac{1}{\sigma_T^2}\mathrm{Reg}(s), \tag{15.15}$$

where c and s are two nonparametric spatial transformations, σ_i accounts for the noise on the image intensity, σ_x is the spatial uncertainty on the correspondences and σ_T controls the amount of regularization. However, the topological object preservation in time is not guaranteed by the diffusion approach [37]. The non-parametric spatial transformation, c, is used to decouple the minimization of the nonparametric transformation s into simple and very efficient two steps [52]. Interestingly, depending on the definition of the regularization step, it is possible to find an equivalence between the diffusion and fluid flow models [52]. In a similar way as the fluid flow model, the intensity differences between images act as the similarity measure and can be seen as the external forces, whereas the regularization acts as the internal forces that preserve consistency and restrict the transformation.

15.3.3 Parametric nonrigid transformation

In contrast to transformation models derived from physical models, the parametric transformations are commonly derived from the approximation and interpolation theory [37]. These models define the transformation, s, by a set of parameters or base functions. The most popular parametric nonrigid transformations are the piecewise affine, RBF and B-splines.

The piecewise approach subdivides the image into blocks and for each block is defined an affine deformation [53]. The main advantage of these methods is their simplicity and fast optimization, though they introduce a higher error compared to nonrigid transformations.

15.3.3.1 Radial basis functions

In the RBF approaches, the spatial transformation is defined as a linear combination of radial functions, R, that depends on the distance between the point to be interpolated and certain control points, $\mathbf{x}_i$, as follows:

$$s(\mathbf{x}) = \sum_{i=1}^{N} k_i R(\|\mathbf{x} - \mathbf{x}_i\|), \qquad (15.16)$$

where N is the number of control points and k_i is the weight of the RBF to be estimated. In particular, the RBF can be Gaussian, multiquadratic or TPS. Among different options, the TPS functions are the most used for image registration [54,55].

The TPS functions are derived from the curvature energy minimization of the Euler–Lagrange equation [56,57], where the spatial transformation is defined as a combination of an affine transformation, $\mathbf{Ax} + \mathbf{y}$ and a set of a particular RBF as follows:

$$s(\mathbf{x}) = \mathbf{Ax} + \mathbf{y} + \sum_{i=1}^{N} k_i R(\|\mathbf{x} - \mathbf{x}_i\|), \qquad (15.17)$$

where R for a d-dimensional space is

$$R(r) = \begin{cases} c_0 r^{4-d} \log(r) & \text{if } d \text{ is 2 or 4} \\ c_1 r^{4-d} & \text{otherwise} \end{cases} \qquad (15.18)$$

with c_0 and c_1 constants. For instance, $R(r) = r^2 \log(r)$ for 2D and $R(r) = r$ for 3D.

The main limitation of this approach is its global behavior; i.e., a change in the weight, k_i, implies a change in the spatial transformation for all points. This global behavior could be an inconvenient when a highly localized transformation is estimated. Besides, the addition of new control points increases significantly the computational complexity.

15.3.3.2 B-splines

B-spline transformations are also known as Free Form Deformation (FFD); however, a more general conception involve different transformation models that are not strictly parametric such as diffusion or optical flow. So, the term of FFD will be put into context when it corresponds to B-splines FFD.

Unlike RBF, B-splines are defined into a neighborhood of the control point. This way, a modification of the control point has a local behavior in the spatial transformation. Due to the small number of control points required to model complex deformations, B-splines FFD are widely used in image registration and speckle tracking [17,19–21,31–33,35].

In B-splines FFD, the spatial transformation, s, is defined by the tensorial product of 1-dimensional B-spline functions. For the 3D case, the transformation of a cubic B-spline is defined by $n_x \times n_y \times n_z$ control points, $p_{i,j,k}$, uniformly distributed in the image domain as follows:

$$s(\mathbf{x}, p) = \sum_{l=0}^{3}\sum_{m=0}^{3}\sum_{n=0}^{3} B_1(u_x)B_m(u_y)B_n(u_z)p_{i+l,j+m,k+n}, \tag{15.19}$$

where $\mathbf{x} = (x,y,z)$, $i = \lfloor x/n_x \rfloor$, $j = \lfloor y/n_y \rfloor$ and $k = \lfloor z/n_z \rfloor$, while $u_x = x/n_x - i$, $u_y = y/n_y - j$, $u_z = z/n_z - k$ and $B_{q\in[1,3]}$ refers to the base B-spline function defined as (see Figure 15.5):

$$B_0(v) = (1-v)^3/6 \qquad B_1(v) = (3v^3 - 6v^2 + 4)/6$$
$$B_2(v) = (-3v^3 + 3v^2 + 3v + 1)/6 \quad B_3(v) = v^3/6$$

The local behavior of the B-splines functions allows to model very complex and highly localized deformation. Furthermore, the spatial transformation is two times differentiable at the control points. Figure 15.6 shows the local behavior of a cubic

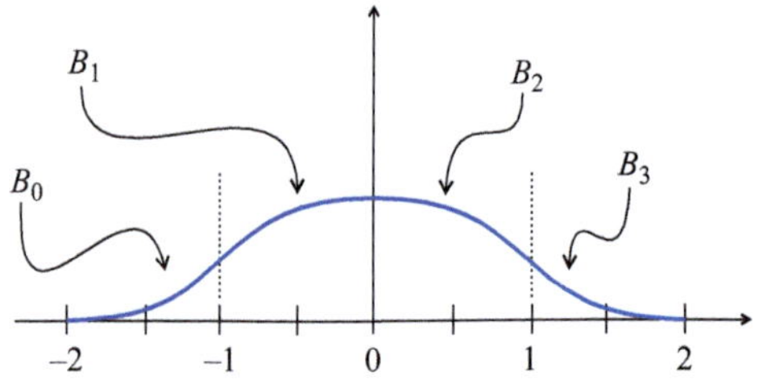

Figure 15.5 Third order 1D B-spline

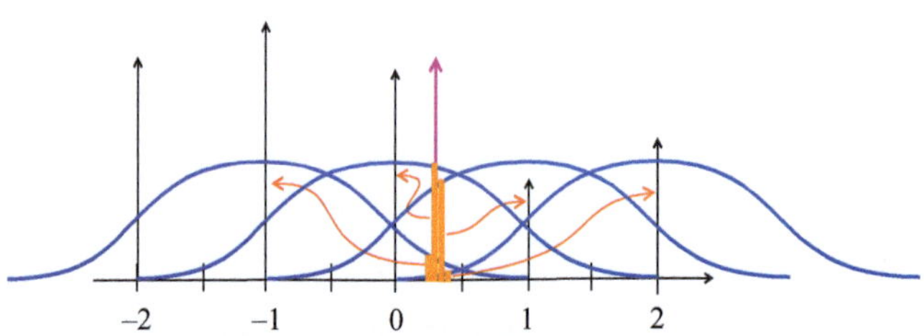

Figure 15.6 Third order 1D B-spline interpolation

B-spline interpolation where the interpolated value is computed as a contribution of the control points within the neighborhood of the point to be interpolated.

A powerful extension of B-splines is nonuniform rational B-splines (NURBS). NURBS are essentially B-splines in homogeneous coordinates. Like B-splines, they are defined by their order and a set of control points, but unlike classic B-splines, each control point is weighted.

15.3.4 Regularization

According to Hadamard's definition [58], a problem is *well-posed* when it has a unique solution and the solution changes continuously with the initial conditions. Consequently, image registration is by definition an *ill-posed* problem since many transformations can be applied to map an image onto the other.

The best way to solve an ill-posed problem is to incorporate prior information to restrict the transformation model to transform the whole problem into a well-posed one. The type of prior information used to regularize the transformation model is highly dependent on the problem itself. However, one of the most common priors is based on the smoothness of the solutions. A classical approach for the regularization is to introduce an explicit penalization term or regularization into the global energy function as follows [59]:

$$E(s) = \text{Sim}(s) + \lambda \text{Reg}(s), \tag{15.20}$$

where Reg(s) corresponds to the regularization term, λ accounts the regularization contribution and Sim(s) is an objective function, which in speckle tracking or image registration is the similarity measure.

In general, parametric transformations incorporate an implicit regularization term restricting the possible deformations to a set of valid deformations. For example, rigid transformations constrain the valid deformation to rotations and translations. On the other hand, in parametric nonrigid models, the deformation smoothness is given by the base function or B-spline. Furthermore, in these cases, the allowed deformations are restricted by the number of control points. Other regularization methodologies consist on constraining the transformation space by means of using a more regular transformation space such as the Sobolev space or to include a temporal dependency on the transformation to guarantee a diffeomorphic transformation. The later will be covered in Section 15.3.5.

In elastic and fluid flow transformations, the balance between internal and external forces on the Navier–Cauchy (15.12) and Navier–Strokes (15.13) acts as an implicit regularization term introducing a smoothness on the transformation model by restricting the deformations. In addition, the fluid flow model ensures a diffeomorphism since the deformation field is computed by means of a numerical integration of the velocity of the displacement field (Section 15.3.5).

On the other hand, optical flow and diffusion models make use of an explicit regularization term (15.20) to guarantee a smooth transformation [51,52]. A relationship between implicit and explicit regularization can be derived by using the regularization theory [60].

15.3.5 Diffeomorphic and inverse transformation

If the spatial correspondence between two or more images does not have an inverse transformation, then it is said that the transformation lacks of *physical sense*. In speckle tracking, this is of paramount importance since the deformation modeled by the transformation often corresponds to a physically possible deformation i.e., the deformation has physical sense if it is smooth, has an inverse and is not generating any foldings. According to the transformation model, the smoothness of the transformation is achieved by an implicit or explicit regularization. However, the smoothness of the transformation is a necessary condition for real deformation, though it is not sufficient. For example, an inverse transformation is not ensured or, if an inverse transformation exists, it is not ensured that the resulting deformation has no foldings.

A common strategy to study if a deformation between images is physically possible is to analyze the determinant of the Jacobian matrix for the transformation describing the deformation

$$J(\mathbf{x}) = \det(\nabla s(\mathbf{x})) = \det(\nabla(\mathbf{x} + s(\mathbf{x}))) = \begin{vmatrix} 1 + \dfrac{\partial s_x}{\partial x} & \dfrac{\partial s_x}{\partial y} & \dfrac{\partial s_x}{\partial z} \\ \dfrac{\partial s_y}{\partial x} & 1 + \dfrac{\partial s_y}{\partial x} & \dfrac{\partial s_y}{\partial z} \\ \dfrac{\partial s_z}{\partial x} & \dfrac{\partial s_z}{\partial y} & 1 + \dfrac{\partial s_z}{\partial z} \end{vmatrix}, \tag{15.21}$$

where $s(\cdot)$ accounts for the spatial transformation and $\mathbf{s}(\cdot)$ corresponds to the displacement field.

If the Jacobian, J, is not zero in $\mathbf{x}$, then according to the inverse function theorem, there is a neighborhood of $\mathbf{x}$ where the inverse transformation exists. Indeed, the absolute value of the Jacobian in $\mathbf{x}$ determines if the transformation s expands or contracts its volume in a neighborhood of x. Furthermore, the sign of the Jacobian can be used to find out when foldings occurs, which is physically impossible to happen in speckle tracking. Figure 15.7 shows a schematic

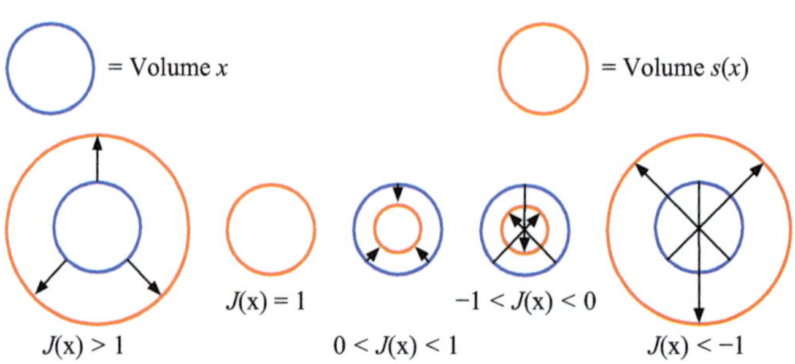

Figure 15.7 Meaning of the Jacobian for the transformation s in a neighborhood of x

representation on how a compression or expansion can be detected by using the Jacobian of the transformation s in a neighborhood of $\mathbf{x}$.

It is important to note that transformations with $J(\mathbf{x}) > 0$ ensure the existence of an inverse transformation and the lack of foldings in a neighborhood of $\mathbf{x}$. Nonetheless, when the transformation is applied into the discrete image domain, it is not possible to ensure the lack of foldings. As an illustration, Figure 15.8 shows a transformation where $J(\mathbf{x}) > 0$, however, once the transformation is applied into a discrete domain, the discrete deformation contains many foldings such as $\overline{P_4P_5}$ and $\overline{P_6P_7}$.

Different strategies can be used to ensure physical transformations; however, as previously stated, not all transformations ensure a physical deformation field. A simple strategy is to reinforce the regularization of the transformation when the evaluation of the Jacobian does not exist or is negative. An alternative strategy is to introduce an additional regularization term to penalize the Jacobian and ensure the incompressibility [61] or invertibility [62].

15.3.5.1 Diffeomorphism by using a variational approach

A different approach is proposed in [63,64], where the transformation is estimated by using a variational approach [65,66]. This way, the space of possible transformations is confined to those that are diffeomorphic. With this approach, the spatial transformation s is obtained at the end point $s = \phi_1$ of the flow defined by the velocity field $\mathbf{v}_t : \Omega \rightarrow \mathbb{R}^n$, $t \in [0,1]$ as follows:

$$\frac{\partial \phi(\mathbf{x}, t)}{\partial t} = \mathbf{v}(\phi_t(\mathbf{x}, t), t). \tag{15.22}$$

Equation (15.22) defines a path $\phi_t : \Omega \rightarrow \mathbb{R}^n$, $t \in [0,1]$ in the transformation space. It starts as the identity $\phi_0(\mathbf{x}) = \mathbf{x}$, $\forall \mathbf{x} \in \Omega$, and ends at $t = 1$ as $s = \phi_1 = \phi_0 + \int_0^1 \mathbf{v}_t(\phi_t)\mathrm{d}t$.

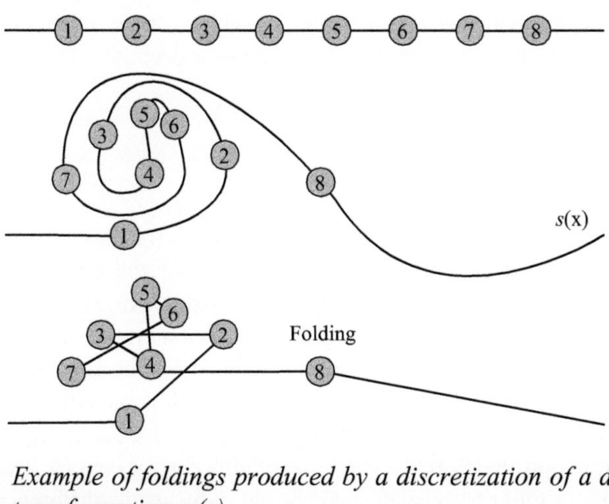

Figure 15.8 Example of foldings produced by a discretization of a diffeomorphic transformation, s(x)

Finally, the spatial transformation is estimated by minimizing a traditional variational approach, that in the smooth velocity field V defined in the domain of the image Ω, is as follows [64]:

$$E(\mathbf{v}) = E_{\text{sim}}(I_t, I_{t-1} \circ s) + \lambda \int_0^1 \|\mathbf{v}_t\|_V^2 \mathrm{d}t, \tag{15.23}$$

where $\|v_t\|_V^2$ corresponds to a Sobolev norm of the velocity field. As it was proved in [65,66], if the velocity field $\mathbf{v}$ is smooth enough, it can be ensured that the transformation s is diffeomorphic. However, the main limitation of this approach is that a numerical integration is required for estimating the deformation field in each iteration [67].

In [51], Vercauteren *et al.* proposed a numerical integration by introducing the variational approach into a Lie group of diffeomorphic transformations that ensures the iterative transformations remain diffeomorphic. The update at iteration $k+1$ is carried out as follows:

$$s_{k+1} = s_k \circ \exp(\mathbf{u}), \tag{15.24}$$

where $s(\mathbf{x}) = \mathbf{x} + \mathbf{s}(\mathbf{x})$ and $\exp(\mathbf{u})$ is computed by means of the so-called *fast vector field exponentials* method also derived in [51].

Following this methodology, Vercauteren *et al.* introduce the diffeomorphism into the diffusion model originally proposed by Thirion in [49]. The main difference with the classic diffusion model is that in the diffeomorphic diffusion approach, $\mathbf{s}$, is considered as a dense velocity field rather than a deformation field. Recently, Curiale *et al.* [34] adapted the diffeomorphic demons method for strain estimation in 3D echocardiography by introducing a Generalized Gamma speckle model into the global energy to be minimized.

There are different approaches to constrain the transformation model with the main goal of improving the ST accuracy. Some authors introduced temporal consistency into the transformation model [17], while others make use of an extra regularization by using the normalized convolution proposed by [68] to constrain the transformation to relevant tissue [18,22,34].

15.4 Optimization strategy

The optimization model defines the strategy to optimize the transformation according to the similarity measure, which is strongly related to the type of transformation (parametric vs. nonparametric). The parameters that maximize the transformation can be computed directly from the data or by means of an iterative search. In the first case, the Procrustes and statistical parametric mapping methods are the most relevant among others [4]. In the second one, an iterative search is usually performed to find the parameters that maximize the similarity measure or global energy.

The iterative optimization approach for minimizing parametric transformations according to the similarity measure can be done by using different optimization approaches. Among them, the most widely used are the Powell's method, the Nelder–Mead method or *downhill simplex*, Levenberg–Marquardt, steepest descent [33,35], conjugate gradient [32] and the Broyden Fletcher Goldfarb Shanno (L-BFGS-B) [17,19–21,31] or the normalized convolution [24,26]. All these methods are well documented in [69]. In a similar way, iterative optimization approaches can be used to estimate the deformation field of nonparametric transformation models by using variational approaches [18,22,25,34]. In particular, this strategy is used in fluid, elastic, diffusion and finite element methods (FEMs):

- **Elastic and fluid flow methods:** The displacement field can be estimated by using different methods such as successive over-relaxation [37,39,43,44,63], full multigrid [6] or by FEM [70].
- **Optical flow:** The displacement field is estimated by using Taylor's first expansion of the moving image (15.14) [46]:

$$\mathbf{u}_k(\mathbf{x}) = \mathbf{u}_{k-1}(\mathbf{x}) - \frac{\nabla^T I_{t-1} \circ \bar{s}_{k-1}(\mathbf{x})}{\|\nabla I_{t-1} \circ \bar{s}_{k-1}(\mathbf{x})\|^2 + \alpha^2}, \tag{15.25}$$

  where k accounts the iteration number, $\bar{s}_{k-1}(\mathbf{x}) = \mathbf{x} + \bar{\mathbf{u}}_{k-1}(\mathbf{x})$ is the spatial transformation and $\bar{\mathbf{u}}_{k-1}(\mathbf{x})$ is the mean displacement field in a neighborhood of $\mathbf{x}$.
- **Diffusion:** The transformation $s(\mathbf{x}) = \mathbf{x} + s(\mathbf{x})$ is optimized by means of the displacement field computation derived from the *demons* force, an explicit regularization step of this field and an update of the transformation, s, as follows:
  - The displacement applied by the *demons* is based on the optical flow equation, hence, the demons displacement field is computed as follows:

$$\mathbf{u} = -\frac{(I_t - I_{t-1} \circ s_{k-1})\nabla I_{t-1} \circ s_{k-1}}{(\nabla I_{t-1} \circ s_{k-1})^2 + (I_t - I_{t-1} \circ s_{k-1})^2}. \tag{15.26}$$

  - Then, the demons displacement field is regularized by using a Gaussian kernel K_{flow} with $\mu = 0$ and σ^2_{flow}

$$\mathbf{u} \leftarrow K_{\text{flow}} \circledast \mathbf{u}. \tag{15.27}$$

    where $\circledast$ is the convolution operator.
  - Next, the transformation, s, is updated as follows

$$s_k \leftarrow s_{k-1} \circ (\mathrm{Id} + \mathbf{u})(\mathbf{x}). \tag{15.28}$$

    In particular, the transformation update (15.28) is carried out by updating the displacement field, $\mathbf{s}$, as follows:

$$\begin{aligned} s_k &= s_{k-1} \circ (\mathrm{Id} + \mathbf{u}) = s_{k-1}(\mathbf{x} + \mathbf{u}(\mathbf{x})) \\ &= \mathbf{x} + \mathbf{u}(\mathbf{x}) + s_{k-1}(\mathbf{x} + \mathbf{u}(\mathbf{x})) \\ &= \mathbf{x} + \mathbf{s}_k(\mathbf{x}) \end{aligned}$$

    where the final deformation field is $s_k(\mathbf{x}) = \mathbf{u}(\mathbf{x}) + s_{k-1}(\mathbf{x}+\mathbf{u}(\mathbf{x}))$.

Finally, the object topology is preserved by doing a new regularization with a Gaussian kernel, K_{diff} with $\mu = 0$ and σ^2_{diff}; but, in contrast to the previous regularization step, it is done on the final displacement field $\mathbf{s}(\mathbf{x})$ [51,52]

$$\mathbf{s}_k \leftarrow K_{\text{diff}} \circledast \mathbf{s}_k. \tag{15.29}$$

- **Diffeomorphic diffusion:** The optimization strategy used by the diffeomorphic diffusion [51] is exactly the same as the one proposed for diffusion with the exception of the transformation update (15.28). In this case, the actualization is done according to the diffeomorphic approach (15.24) as it was described in Section 15.3.5.
- **Finite element:** The FEM is a numerical technique that finds approximate solutions to boundary value problems for PDE. It subdivides a large problem into smaller disjoint parts known as finite elements which act as a domain discretization. Then, the finite elements are optimized by using a variational method from the calculus of variations to approximate a solution by minimizing an associated error function. If the number of finite elements is high, it is possible to solve a differential problem by means of a set of linear equations for each finite element.

This strategy is used in medical image registration due to its simplicity [70–72], although the accuracy of the solution provided strongly depends on the discretization of the domain.

Finally, a widely used strategy for improving the optimization, especially for large deformations, is to use a coarse-to-fine refinement [15–22,24–26,31–33]. This approach is highly recommended for complex deformations such as heart motion in speckle tracking.

15.5 Influence of speckle tracking strategies for motion and strain estimation

Many different approaches to ST can be found in the literature. We have gathered the most representative techniques and some of the recent approaches already introduced in previous sections in Table 15.1. The ST techniques have extensively proven to be powerful tools to provide both quantitative and qualitative information on myocardial deformation, motion and function assessment [73–75]. The clinical relevance of motion estimation in US B-mode images motivates the community to improve the original ST technique pioneered by [8,10] to more complex approaches. New contributions extend the original techniques in different ways such as statistical modeling of speckle, using more complex registration algorithms or applying different optimization algorithms for the ST estimation. It seems clear that modifications in different steps of the process will have a different impact on the results. In addition, the influence of certain methods may obliterate the complexity of previous steps. For instance, the use of certain registration algorithms could make the process highly invariant to the similarity measure used. Thus, it becomes

Table 15.1 Overview of the most representative speckle tracking techniques and a few recent approaches

Author	Similarity model		Transformation model			Optimization model	
	Nonspeckle model	**Speckle model**	**Parametric**	**Nonparametric**	**NC**	**Iterative**	**Multiresolution**
Robinson *et al.* [10]	CC	×	×	OF BM	×	×	×
Trahey *et al.* [8,9]	CC	×	×	OF BM	×	×	×
Bohs and Trahey [12]	SAD	×	×	OF BM	×	×	×
Friemel *et al.* [14]	NCC/CC/SAD	×	×	OF BM	×	×	×
Strintzis and Kokkinidis [30]	×	Rayleigh	×	OF BM	×	×	×
Yeung *et al.* [15]	SSD	×	×	OF BM	×	×	✓
Yeung *et al.* [16]	SSD	×	×	OF BM	×	×	✓
Bohs *et al.* [13]	SAD	×	×	OF BM	×	×	×
Cohen and Dinstein [29]	×	Rayleigh	×	OF BM	×	×	×
Knutsson and Andersson [24]	MP	×	×	OF	×	NC	✓
Myronenko *et al.* [35]	SSD + SI	×	FFD	×	×	Steepest descent	–
Yue *et al.* [31]	×	Rayleigh	FFD	×	×	L-BFGS-B	✓
Myronenko *et al.* [33]	×	Bivariate Nakagami	FFD	×	×	Steepest descent	✓
De Craene *et al.* [17]	SSD	×	FFD	×	×	L-BFGS-B	✓
Curiale *et al.* [32]	×	Gamma	FFD	×	×	Conjugate gradient	✓
Curiale *et al.* [18]	SSD	×	×	Diffusion	✓	Variational	✓
Heyde *et al.* [20]	SSD	×	FFD	×	×	L-BFGS-B	✓
Tautz *et al.* [26]	MP	×	×	OF	×	NC	✓
Heyde *et al.* [19]	SSD	×	FFD	×	×	L-BFGS-B	✓
Somphone *et al.* [22]	SSD	×	×	Diffusion	✓	Steepest descent	✓
Alessandrini *et al.* [25]	MP	×	×	OF with BS	×	Variational	✓
Piella *et al.* [21]	SSD	Rayleigh	FFD	×	×	L-BFGS-B	✓
Curiale *et al.* [34]	×	Bivariate GG	×	Diffusion	✓	Variational	✓

CC: cross-correlation. NCC: nonnormalized cross-correlation. SAD: sum of absolute differences. SSD: sum of squared differences. SI: structural information. MP: monogenic phase. GG: generalized gamma. FFD: free form deformation with b-splines. BS: b-splines. of: optical flow. BM: block matching. NC: normalized convolution.—not specified.

necessary to identify the relevant relations between the different components involved in a ST method in order to clarify which component really improves the accuracy of the estimation of motion and strain, and which ones become redundant. Also, it is necessary to understand the relation between the steps and different choices taken to implement a ST method.

In [76], Curiale *et al.* presented a study to clarify the influence of different techniques that can be used in the stages of any ST method (similarity, transformation and optimization). The specific techniques considered in [76] are the following:

1. Different models for US data representation, some of them assuming an underlying statistical model for the speckle.
2. Different registration philosophies, including the classic block matching based on the optical flow approach and the demons or diffusion approach.
3. Different interpolation schemes such as nearest neighbor, linear and cubic.
4. The use of structural information into the deformation model by using the normalized convolution [68] and a maximum likelihood approach such as the one proposed in [34].
5. The use of different optimization techniques, such as coarse-to-fine refinement or an efficient second-order minimization (ESM).

These techniques were not independently analyzed since the influence of one over the others provides useful insights for the development of novel ST methods.

Due to the extensive number of possible combination of parameters and techniques, in [76] the authors confined the study to the classic block matching and the diffusion approaches since the number of strategies used to optimize the transformation model and the number of free parameters to fix are reduced. The hypotheses assumed in the state of the art are already mentioned in previous sections:

Hypothesis 1. *Similarity measures based on a speckle model characterization are more reliable to real US data and improve the ST accuracy.*
Hypothesis 2. *Speckle models that take into account temporal correlation improve ST accuracy.*
Hypothesis 3. *Although interpolation modifies the statistical model assumed for characterizing the speckle pattern, it has a negligible effect on the ST accuracy.*
Hypothesis 4. *The transformation model has a great influence on the ST accuracy than the similarity measure.*
Hypothesis 5. *Structural information increases the ST accuracy more than just the speckle model.*
Hypothesis 6. *A coarse to fine refinement approach improves significantly the ST accuracy for complex motions.*
Hypothesis 7. *A complex interpolation scheme improves the ST accuracy, regardless of the similarity measure selected.*
Hypothesis 8. *The optimization strategy has more influence in the ST accuracy than the similarity measure.*

In addition to these hypotheses, Curiale *et al.* also provide a complementary analysis of the cross performance of improvements such as a better transformation model with structural information and a coarse to fine refinement. These interrelations are a key factor for an efficient and accurate ST pipeline.

The similarity measures studied comprised the SSD and other metrics based on speckle characterization summarized in Table 15.2. These measures are classified according to the relationship imposed on the intensity levels of images (difference or ratio).

The main conclusions obtained from the analysis of similarity measures are the following:

Conclusion 1. *Similarity measures based on a speckle statistical model show more accurate motion and strain estimation. The more detailed the modeling (including spatial and temporal correlation), the more accurate the results. However, the influence of the similarity measures is reduced when the regularization schemes are applied in the transformation model. Generally, these differences may have no practical implications when compared to the influence of regularization schemes.*
Conclusion 2. *The improvement of the accuracy due to a transformation model outperforms the improvement due to the similarity measures. Thus, the influence of the transformation model over the ST accuracy is higher than the influence of the speckle model itself. This result is consistent with the main conclusion derived from the study proposed in [77] where it is observed that most recent ST techniques have relatively similar performances.*

Table 15.2 Summary of the similarity measures studied. Constants m and β are shape parameters of the generalized gamma distribution; α is the shape parameter of the gamma distribution and ρ is the correlation between different time frames I_{t-1} and I_t (details on these similarity measures can be found in [34])

Relationship	Similarity measure	References
$z = I_{t-1} - I_t$	$\mathrm{SSD} = \| z \|^2$	Yeung *et al.* [15,16], Myronenko *et al.* [35], Curiale *et al.* [18], Heyde *et al.* [19,20], Piella *et al.* [21], Somphone *et al.* [22]
	$\mathrm{CD2} = \log(\exp(2z+1)) - z$	Strintzis *et al.* [30], Cohen *et al.* [29], Yue *et al.* [31], Piella *et al.* [21]
	$\mathrm{MS2} = (m+0.5)\log(\cosh^2(z) - \rho) - 0.5\log(\cosh^2(z))$	Myronenko *et al.* [33]
	$\mathrm{GGCS} = (m+0.5)\log(\cosh^2(z\beta) - \rho) - 0.5\log(\cosh^2(z\beta))$	Curiale *et al.* [34]
$z = I_{t-1}/I_t$	$\mathrm{GS} = \alpha\log(z + z^{-1} + 2)$	Curiale *et al.* [32]
	$\mathrm{GGS} = (m+0.5)\log((z^{2\beta}+1) - 4\rho z^{2\beta}) - 2\beta m\log(z) - \log(z^{2\beta}+1)$	Curiale *et al.* [34]

Conclusion 3. *There is an interdependency between the influence of the similarity measure and the transformation/optimization model. The regularization schemes strongly influence the performance of metrics. Results show that those similarity measures considering the logarithmic compression into the speckle model are more accurate for motion estimation when an iterative optimization approach is used. The logarithmic compression changes the intensity ratio of the speckle model in an intensity difference making the similarity measure more robust to numerical fluctuations. Note that this fact does not mean that the speckle model is more suitable for real US data but for iterative optimization, which increases the effect of regularization for motion estimation, though the performance of strain estimation is reduced due to biases introduced in the regularization.*

The analysis of the influence of interpolation on similarity measures based on statistical assumptions was considered by studying three different interpolation schemes (nearest neighbor, linear, cubic) in a multiresolution implementation in order to increase its contribution. From this analysis, the following conclusions were extracted:

Conclusion 4. *Although interpolation modifies the statistical model assumed for characterizing the speckle pattern, no reductions of the ST accuracy due to interpolation were observed. On the contrary, linear interpolation in the multi-resolution scheme improves the accuracy of all the metrics and especially those that obtained the best results for strain error. This result not only confirms Hypothesis 3 but also indicates that the way the metrics combine with the transformation model plays an important role.*

Conclusion 5. *ST accuracy improves when higher order interpolation schemes are used instead of the nearest neighborhood interpolation, which confirms the Hypothesis 7. However, cubic interpolation does not provide any further improvement compared to linear interpolation.*

Conclusion 6. *The joint effects between the transformation model and the metric are observed with similarity measures based on ratios (without log-compression), which increased their performance in motion estimation due to the refinements of the multi-resolution approach, while they provide the best strain estimation.*

The inclusion of myocardial structural information by means of normalized convolution was also studied for the different similarity measures and transformation models. The improvement of this technique was shown to be dependent on the transformation philosophy, where iterative transformations are especially recommended. Thus, the main conclusion is:

Conclusion 7. *The use of myocardial structural information in the ST technique significantly improves motion and strain accuracy in iterative approaches like demons due to the iterative error reduction. However, its gain depends on the performance of the probabilistic characterization of tissues.*

The analysis of optimization techniques, such as multiresolution and second order minimization, offers very interesting and counterintuitive results:

Conclusion 8. *Though the multi-resolution scheme highly contributes in simple approaches such as block matching, other transformation models including regularization steps do not significantly improve their performance with metrics based on the difference of intensities. However, metrics based on ratios of intensities improve significantly both the motion and the strain estimation in a multi-resolution approach.*
Conclusion 9. *Metrics based on ratios of intensities are prone to numerical fluctuations that reduce the performance of strain estimations when the ESM methodology is applied. However, the ESM is especially recommendable with metrics based on the difference of intensities.*

Finally, the performance of the complete ST pipeline was studied to provide some insights to the interrelations between different combinations of components:

Conclusion 10. *Results showed that the block matching approach is greatly improved due to the multi-resolution scheme. Conversely, the inclusion of structural information does not play a relevant role. However, regarding the strain analysis, the overall results evidence that simple transformation models that do not effectively deal with the circumferential estimation of motion (and thus, strain), are not recommended for strain estimation.*
Conclusion 11. *Similarity measures based on intensity ratios are more sensitive to structural information and its performance depends on the regularization methodology. Thus, multi-resolution is more recommendable than ESM for these metrics.*
Conclusion 12. *Metrics based on intensity differences improve their performance with the use of the ESM.*
Conclusion 13. *The use of the myocardial structural information also improves significantly the ST accuracy regardless the similarity measure used.*

The results and conclusions obtained in [76] clearly showed that the election of certain methods along the pipeline must take into account the choices previously made. Methods that independently achieve the best results are not necessarily optimal when combined together. In fact, the selection of the methodologies to use should not be based just on their individual performance, but on their performance as part of a complete system where all the parts are interconnected. The selection of a particular step must be based on the choices done for previous and following steps. The goodness of a particular method cannot be guaranteed inside an ST system unless it is tested for the whole pipeline.

All these conclusions lead to some recommendations to be considered when developing an ST method:

1. The inclusion of too elaborated similarity measures based on statistics of speckle do not improve significantly the results. The most relevant factor that affects to its performance is the final relationship between intensities, which is a result of considering or not the log-compression in the statistical model.
2. If we are interested just in motion estimation, any similarity measure can be applied with good results, where the most recommended due to its simplicity is

the SSD. However, it is important to consider that those metrics based on ratios of intensities should avoid the use of the ESM optimization technique, since it is prone to numerical fluctuations that decrease their performance.

3. If we are interested in strain estimation, metrics without considering log-compression (GS or GGS) are especially recommended when a multi-resolution scheme regularized with structural information by means of normalized convolution is applied. Those metrics are more sensitive to the structural information and provide a better overall estimation of strain.
4. The regularization step in iterative approaches is of great importance since its numerical stability and a proper inclusion of statistical models can cause unexpected results that may undermine the final results.
5. A linear interpolation scheme is recommended, rather than higher order schemes that do not contribute significantly.
6. The regularization by means of normalized convolution is highly recommended for all similarity measures, especially for those highly sensitive to structural information such as (GS and GGS).

Acknowledgments

This work was partially supported by Consejo Nacional de Investigaciones Científicas y Técnicas (CONICET) and by grants M028-2016 SECTyP, Universidad Nacional de Cuyo, Argentina; PICT 2016-0091, Agencia Nacional de Promoción Científica y Tecnológica, Argentina; Ministerio de Ciencia e Innovación (Spain) with research grant TEC2013-44194-P; Consejería de Educación, Juventud y Deporte of Comunidad de Madrid and the People Programme (Marie Curie Actions) of the European Union's Seventh Framework Programme (FP7/2007-2013) for REA grant agreement no. 291820.

References

[1] Trahey GE, Smith SW, von Ramm OT. Speckle pattern correlation with lateral aperture translation: experimental results and implications for spatial compounding. IEEE Trans Ultrason, Ferroelectr Freq Control. 1986 May; 33(3): 257–264.

[2] Burckhardt CB. Speckle in ultrasound B-mode scans. IEEE Trans Sonics Ultrason. 1978 Jan;25(1): 1–6.

[3] Maintz JBA, Viergever MA. A survey of medical image registration. Med Image Anal. 1998 Mar;2(1): 1–36.

[4] Hill DLG, Batchelor PG, Holden M, Hawkes DJ. Medical image registration. Phys Med Biol. 2001 Mar;46(3): R1–R45.

[5] Zitová B, Flusser J. Image registration methods: a survey. Imag Vision Comp. 2003 Oct;21(11): 977–1000.

[6] Crum WR, Hartkens T, Hill DLG. Non-rigid image registration: theory and practice. Br J Radiol. 2004 Dec;77(suppl 2):S140–S153. PMID: 15677356.

[7] Besl PJ, McKay ND. A method for registration of 3D shapes. IEEE Trans Pattern Anal Mach Intell. 1992 Apr;14(2): 239–256.

[8] Trahey GE, Hubbard SM, von Ramm OT. Angle independent ultrasonic blood flow detection by frame-to-frame correlation of B-mode images. Ultrasonics. 1988 Sep;26(5): 271–276.

[9] Trahey GE, Allison JW, von Ramm OT. Angle independent ultrasonic detection of blood flow. IEEE Trans Biomed Eng. 1987 Dec;BME-34(12): 965–967.

[10] Robinson DE, Chen F, Wilson LS. Measurement of velocity of propagation from ultrasonic pulse-echo data. Ultrasound Med Biol. 1982 Dec;8(4): 413–420.

[11] Studholme C, Hill DLG, Hawkes DJ. An overlap invariant entropy measure of 3D medical image alignment. Pattern Recognit. 1999 Jan;32(1): 71–86.

[12] Bohs LN, Trahey GE. A novel method for angle independent ultrasonic imaging of blood flow and tissue motion. IEEE Trans Biomed Eng. 1991 Mar;38(3): 280–286.

[13] Bohs LN, Geiman BJ, Anderson ME, Gebhart SC, Trahey GE. Speckle tracking for multidimensional flow estimation. Ultrasonics. 2000 Mar; 38(1–8):369–375.

[14] Friemel BH, Bohs LN, Trahey GE. Relative performance of two-dimensional speckle-tracking techniques: normalized correlation, non-normalized correlation and sum-absolute-difference. In: Ultrasonics Symposium, 1995. Proceedings, 1995 IEEE. vol. 2; 1995. p. 1481–1484 vol.2.

[15] Yeung F, Levinson SF, Fu D, Parker KJ. Feature-adaptive motion tracking of ultrasound image sequences using a deformable mesh. IEEE Trans Med Imag. 1998 Dec;17(6): 945–956.

[16] Yeung F, Levinson SF, Parker KJ. Multilevel and motion model-based ultrasonic speckle tracking algorithms. Ultrasound Med Biol. 1998 Mar; 24(3): 427–441.

[17] De Craene M, Piella G, Camara O, *et al.* Temporal diffeomorphic free-form deformation: application to motion and strain estimation from 3D echocardiography. Med Image Anal. 2012;16(2): 427–450.

[18] Curiale AH, Vegas-Sanchez-Ferrero G, Perez-Sanz T, Aja-Fernandez S. Strain rate tensor estimation from echocardiography for quantitative assessment of functional mitral regurgitation. In: Biomedical Imaging (ISBI), 2013 IEEE 10th International Symposium on; 2013. p. 788–791.

[19] Heyde B, Barbosa D, Claus P, Maes F, D'hooge J. Three-dimensional cardiac motion estimation based on non-rigid image registration using a novel transformation model adapted to the heart. In: Camara O, Mansi T, Pop M, Rhode K, Sermesant M, Young A, editors. Statistical Atlases and Computational Models of the Heart. Imaging and Modelling Challenges. vol. 7746 of Lecture Notes in Computer Science. Springer Berlin Heidelberg; 2013. p. 142–150.

[20] Heyde B, Jasaityte R, Barbosa D, *et al.* Elastic image registration versus speckle tracking for 2D myocardial motion estimation: a direct comparison in vivo. IEEE Trans Med Imag. 2013 Feb;32(2): 449–459.

[21] Piella G, Porras A, De Craene M, Duchateau N, Frangi A. Temporal diffeomorphic free form deformation to quantify changes induced by left and right bundle branch block and pacing. In: Camara O, Mansi T, Pop M, Rhode K, Sermesant M, Young A, editors. Statistical Atlases and Computational Models of the Heart. Imaging and Modelling Challenges. vol. 7746 of Lecture Notes in Computer Science. Springer Berlin Heidelberg; 2013. p. 134–141.

[22] Somphone O, Dufour C, Mory B, *et al.* Motion estimation in 3D echocardiography using smooth field registration. In: Camara O, Mansi T, Pop M, Rhode K, Sermesant M, Young A, editors. Statistical Atlases and Computational Models of the Heart. Imaging and Modelling Challenges. Lecture Notes in Computer Science. Springer Berlin Heidelberg; 2013. p. 151–158.

[23] Elen A, Choi HF, Loeckx D, *et al.* Three-dimensional cardiac strain estimation using spatio-temporal elastic registration of ultrasound images: a feasibility study. IEEE Trans Med Imag. 2008 Nov;27(11): 1580–1591.

[24] Knutsson H, Andersson M. Morphons: paint on priors and elastic canvas for segmentation and registration. In: Kalviainen H, Parkkinen J, Kaarna A, editors. Image Analysis. vol. 3540 of Lecture Notes in Computer Science. Springer Berlin Heidelberg; 2005. p. 292–301.

[25] Alessandrini M, Liebgott H, Barbosa D, Bernard O. Monogenic phase based optical flow computation for myocardial motion analysis in 3D echocardiography. In: Camara O, Mansi T, Pop M, Rhode K, Sermesant M, Young A, editors. Statistical Atlases and Computational Models of the Heart. Imaging and Modelling Challenges. vol. 7746 of Lecture Notes in Computer Science. Springer Berlin Heidelberg; 2013. p. 159–168.

[26] Tautz L, Hennemuth A, Peitgen HO. Quadrature filter based motion analysis for 3D ultrasound sequences. In: Camara O, Mansi T, Pop M, Rhode K, Sermesant M, Young A, editors. Statistical Atlases and Computational Models of the Heart. Imaging and Modelling Challenges. vol. 7746 of Lecture Notes in Computer Science. Springer Berlin Heidelberg; 2013. p. 169–177.

[27] Roche A, Malandain G, Ayache N. Unifying maximum likelihood approaches in medical image registration. Int J Imag Syst Technol: Special Issue 3D Imag. 2000 Jul;11(1): 71–80.

[28] Viola P, Wells III W. Alignment by maximization of mutual information. Int J Comput Vision. 1997 Sep;24(2): 137–154.

[29] Cohen B, Dinstein I. New maximum likelihood motion estimation schemes for noisy ultrasound images. Pattern Recognit. 2002 Feb;35(2): 455–463.

[30] Strintzis MG, Kokkinidis I. Maximum likelihood motion estimation in ultrasound image sequences. IEEE Signal Process Lett. 1997 Jun;4(6): 156–157.

[31] Yue Y, Clark JW, Khoury DS. Speckle tracking in intracardiac echocardiography for the assessment of myocardial deformation. IEEE Trans Biomed Eng. 2009 Feb;56(2): 416–425.

[32] Curiale AH, Vegas-Sánchez-Ferrero G, Aja-Fernández S. Speckle tracking in interpolated echocardiography to estimate heart motion. In: Ourselin S,

Rueckert D, Smith N, editors. Functional Imaging and Modeling of the Heart. vol. 7945 of Lecture Notes in Computer Science. Springer Berlin Heidelberg; 2013. p. 325–333.

[33] Myronenko A, Song X, Sahn D. Maximum likelihood motion estimation in 3D echocardiography through non-rigid registration in spherical coordinates. In: Ayache N, Delingette H, Sermesant M, editors. Functional Imaging and Modeling of the Heart. vol. 5528 of Lecture Notes in Computer Science. Springer Berlin Heidelberg; 2009. p. 427–436.

[34] Curiale AH, Vegas-Sanchez-Ferrero G, Bosch JG, Aja-Fernández S. A maximum likelihood approach to diffeomorphic speckle tracking for 3D strain estimation in echocar-diography. Med Image Anal. 2015 Aug;24(1): 90–105.

[35] Myronenko A, Song X, Sahn DJ. LV Motion Tracking from 3D echocardiography using textural and structural information. In: Medical Image Computing and Computer-Assisted Intervention MICCAI. vol. 4792 of Lecture Notes in Computer Science. Springer; 2007. p. 428–435.

[36] Brown LG. A survey of image registration techniques. ACM Comput Surv. 1992 Dec;24(4): 325–376.

[37] Holden M. A review of geometric transformations for nonrigid body registration. IEEE Trans Med Imag. 2008 Jan;27(1): 111–128.

[38] Lester H, Arridge SR. A survey of hierarchical non-linear medical image registration. Pattern Recognit. 1999 Jan;32(1): 129–149.

[39] Broit C. Optimal registration of deformed images [PhD Thesis]. Dept. Comput. Inf. Sci., University of Pennsylvania, Philadelphia; 1981.

[40] Bajcsy R, Lieberson R, Reivich M. A computerized system for the elastic matching of deformed radiographic images to idealized atlas images. J Comput Assist Tomogr. 1983 Aug;7(4): 618–625.

[41] Bajcsy R, Kovačič S. Multiresolution elastic matching. Comput Vision GraphicsImage Proces. 1989 Apr;46(1): 1–21.

[42] Christensen GE, Joshi SC, Miller MI. Volumetric transformation of brain anatomy. IEEE Trans Med Imag. 1997 Dec;16(6): 864–877.

[43] Christensen GE, Rabbitt RD, Miller MI. 3D brain mapping using a deformable neuroanatomy. Phys Med Biol. 1994 Mar;39(3): 609–618.

[44] Christensen GE, Rabbitt RD, Miller MI. Deformable templates using large deformation kinematics. IEEE Trans Med Imag. 1996 Oct;5(10): 1435–1447.

[45] Gibson JJ. The perception of the visual world. Oxford, England: Houghton Mifflin; 1950.

[46] Horn BKP, Schunck BG. Determining optical flow. Artif Intell. 1981 Aug; 17(1–3):185–203.

[47] Liu T, Shen L. Fluid flow and optical flow. J Fluid Mech. 2008 Oct;614: 253–291.

[48] Leitman M, Lysyansky P, Sidenko S, *et al.* Two-dimensional strain – a novel software for real-time quantitative echocardiographic assessment of myocardial function. J Am Soc Echocardiogr. 2004 Oct;17(10): 1021–1029.

[49] Thirion JP. Image matching as a diffusion process: an analogy with Maxwell's demons. Med Image Anal. 1998 Sep;2(3): 243–260.

[50] Barron JL, Fleet DJ, Beauchemin SS. Performance of optical flow techniques. Int J Comput Vision. 1994 Feb;12(1): 43–77.

[51] Vercauteren T, Pennec X, Perchant A, Ayache N. Diffeomorphic demons: efficient non-parametric image registration. NeuroImage. 2009 Oct; 45(1, Supplement 1): S61–S72.

[52] Cachier P, Bardinet E, Dormont D, Pennec X, Ayache N. Iconic feature based nonrigid registration: the PASHA algorithm. Comput Vision Image Understanding. 2003 Feb;89(2–3): 272–298.

[53] Pitiot A, Bardinet E, Thompson PM, Malandain G. Piecewise affine registration of biological images for volume reconstruction. Med Image Anal. 2006 Jun;10(3): 465–483. Special Issue on The Second International Workshop on Biomedical Image Registration (WBIR'03).

[54] Meyer CR, Boes JL, Kim B, *et al.* Demonstration of accuracy and clinical versatility of mutual information for automatic multimodality image fusion using affine and thin-plate spline warped geometric deformations. Med Image Anal. 1997 Apr;1(3): 195–206.

[55] Rohr K, Stiehl HS, Sprengel R, Buzug TM, Weese J, Kuhn MH. Landmark-based elastic registration using approximating thin-plate splines. IEEE Trans Med Imag. 2001 Jun;20(6): 526–534.

[56] Grimson WEL. From Images to Surfaces: A Computational Study of The Human Early Visual System. Cambridge, MA: MIT Press; 1981.

[57] Terzopoulos D. Multiresolution computation of visible-surface representations [PhD Thesis]. Massachusetts Institute of Technology; 1984.

[58] Poggio T, Torre V, Koch C. Computational vision and regularization theory. Nature. 1985 Sep;317(6035): 314–319.

[59] Tikhonov AN, Arsenin VY. Solutions of ill-posed problems. Winston Washington, DC; 1977.

[60] Chen Z, Haykin S. On different facets of regularization theory. Neural Comput. 2002 Dec;14(12): 2791–2846.

[61] Rohlfing T, Maurer JCR, Bluemke DA, Jacobs MA. Volume-preserving nonrigid registration of MR breast images using free-form deformation with an incompressibility constraint. IEEE Trans Med Imag. 203 Jun;22(6): 730–741.

[62] Kybic J, Thevenaz P, Nirkko A, Unser M. Unwarping of unidirectionally distorted EPI images. IEEE Trans Med Imag. 2000 Feb;19(2): 80–93.

[63] Miller MI, Joshi SC, Christensen GE. Large deformation fluid diffeomorphisms for landmark and image matching. In: Toga AW, editor. Brain Warping. Elsevier; 1998. p. 115–131.

[64] Beg MF, Miller M, Trouvé A., Younes L. Computing large deformation metric mappings via geodesic flows of diffeomorphisms. Int J Comput Vision. 2005 Feb;61(2): 139–157.

[65] Dupuis P, Grenander U, Miller MI. Variational problems on flows of diffeomorphisms for image matching. Q Appl Math. 1998;56(3): 587–600.

[66] Trouvé A. An infinite dimensional group approach for physics based models in pattern recognition. Preprint. 1995. Available from: http://www.cis.jhu.edu/publications/papers_in_database/alain/trouve1995.pdf (2015)

[67] Trouvé A. Diffeomorphisms groups and pattern matching in image analysis. Int J Comput Vision. 1998 Jul;28(3): 213–221.

[68] Knutsson H, Westin CF. Normalized and differential convolution: methods for interpolation and filtering of incomplete and uncertain data. In: Computer Vision and Pattern Recognition, 1993. Proceedings CVPR '93., 1993 IEEE Computer Society Conference on; 1993. p. 515–523.

[69] Press WH, Teukolsky SA, Vetterling WT, Flannery BP. Numerical Recipes 3rd Edition: The Art of Scientific Computing. Cambridge, England: Cambridge University Press; 2007.

[70] Schnabel JA, Tanner C, Castellano-Smith AD, *et al.* Validation of nonrigid image registration using finite-element methods: application to breast MR images. IEEE Trans Med Imag. 2003 Feb;22(2): 238–247.

[71] Walker J, Ratcliffe M, Zhang P. MRI-based finite-element analysis of left ventricular aneurysm. Am J Physiol Heart Circ Physiol. 2005 Mar;289(2): H692–H700.

[72] Oliveira FPM, Tavares JMRS. Medical image registration: a review. Comput Methods Biomech Biomed Engin. 2014 Mar;17(2): 73–93.

[73] Suffoletto MS, Dohi K, Cannesson M, Saba S, Gorcsan J. Novel speckle-tracking radial strain from routine black-and-white echocardiographic images to quantify dyssynchrony and predict response to cardiac resynchronization therapy. Circulation. 2006 Feb;113(7): 960–968.

[74] Notomi Y, Lysyansky P, Setser RM, *et al.* Measurement of ventricular torsion by two-dimensional ultrasound speckle tracking imaging. J Am Coll Cardiol. 2005 Jun;45(12): 2034–2041.

[75] Helle-Valle T, Crosby J, Edvardsen T, *et al.* New noninvasive method for assessment of left ventricular rotation. Circulation. 2005 Aug;112(20): 3149–3156.

[76] Curiale AH, Vegas-Sanchez-Ferrero G, Aja-Fernández S. Influence of speckle tracking strategies in motion and strain estimation. Med Image Anal. 2016 Apr;32: 184–200.

[77] De Craene M, Marchesseau S, Heyde B, *et al.* 3D strain assessment in ultrasound (Straus): a synthetic comparison of five tracking methodologies. IEEE Trans Med Imag. 2013 May;32(9): 1632–1646.

Chapter 16

Cardiac strain estimation

Hanan Khamis[1] *and Dan Adam*[1]

List of acronyms

LV	left ventricle
3D	three dimensions
SPECT	single-photon emission computed tomography
PET	positron emission tomography
GLS	global longitudinal strain
SNR	signal-to-noise ratio
RF	radio frequency
TDI	tissue Doppler imaging
2D-STE	two-dimensional speckle tracking echocardiography
VVI	vector velocity imaging
ARFI	acoustic radiation force impulse
CMRI	cardiac magnetic resonance imaging
TTE	transthoracic echocardiography
CT	computed tomography
EF	ejection fraction
EACVI	European Association of Cardiovascular Imaging
ASE	American Society of Echocardiography
ED	end diastole
ES	end systole
ROI	region of interest

An important application domain of ultrasound-based motion estimation is the heart which leads to specific challenges and boundary conditions. In this chapter, a more detailed discussion is given on applying speckle tracking algorithms for cardiac applications.

16.1 Myocardial strain imaging: rationale

Evaluation of left ventricle (LV) myocardial function, the well-being of the myocytes, requires the measurement of the distribution of myocardial stresses. These stresses represent the development and decrease of the forces generated by

[1]Lab for Ultrasound Signals and Image Processing and Modeling, Department of Biomedical Engineering, Israel

the myocyte. The current echocardiographic technologies only enable the estimation of the strain during the cardiac cycle (cf. previous chapters). Yet, in order to estimate the stresses from the strains, one needs to know the loadings – the LV intra-cavity pressures, the preload and afterload, the passive properties of the extracellular matrix, the external changing pressures (e.g. during respiration) and more. Currently, there are no known methods of performing these measurements non-invasively. There is, though, a growing body of clinical evidence that correlates the time-dependent LV strain distribution, with the different pathologies, providing sufficient support for clinical assessments and decision-making, even though the stresses are unknown.

Assessment of myocardial deformation, the local wall thickening and thinning characteristics, has brought a better analysis of regional myocardial function. However, these characteristics are not necessarily directly related to the true myocardial tissue motion since they do not represent a three dimensional (3D) myocardial wall deformation. In his paper [1], D'hooge summarized the different techniques/modalities used to provide myocardial motion analysis. Magnetic resonance imaging (MRI), for instance, enables 3D deformation measurements. It allows quantification and mapping of regional LV wall thickness using the 3D geometry of the heart [2]. Yet, due to the smoothness of the myocardial tissue as imaged by MRI, it is nearly impossible to measure deformations within the walls. Tagged MRI utilizes non-invasive markers (or tags) that are imposed on the myocardium at the end-diastolic frame, to measure deformations even within the cardiac walls. Using a combination of perpendicular tagged images of long and short axis views, 3D deformation analysis can be obtained [3–6]. Nevertheless, this approach never became clinically relevant. Other modalities such as computed tomography (CT) and gated single-photon emission CT/positron emission tomography were introduced to allow a 3D acquisition of wall thinning and thickening [7,8] and to make myocardial infarction diagnosis more feasible. Two main drawbacks of the aforementioned modalities are the low temporal resolution, which may cause missing of important myocardial mechanical events, and the cost and lack of availability of these large systems. As an alternative modality, ultrasound is found to be the most favourable modality to be used in practice for cardiac functional analysis.

The conventional clinical quantification of global and regional myocardial function combines the measurements of wall thickening and shortening with the visual analysis of wall motion, while focusing mainly on the subendocardium. As recommended by European Association of Cardiovascular Imaging/American Society of Echocardiography (EACVI/ASE) in [9], visual assessment is translated to semi-quantitative wall motion score. The scoring system assigns grade '1' for normal (or hyperkinetic), grade '2' for hypokinetic, '3' for akinetic and '4' for dyskinetic movement of each segment. It is also recommended that the segmental analysis should be performed individually for the multiple views, and then the scores should be averaged to a final segmental motion assessment. However, since the myocardial motion may also be produced by tethering of the adjacent segments/layers or even the overall myocardial displacement, one must be aware that passive deformation will not be able to accurately reflect myocardial contraction. Velocity and motion are measured relative to the transducer and are consequently dependent on the tethering and overall cardiac motion. Thus, it is preferable to use deformation parameters, such as strain and strain rate, for a better myocardial functional analysis and quantification.

16.2 Myocardial strain: definitions

Strain is a mechanical measure of deformation that represents the displacement between two points in an object, relative to a reference length. In other words, it defines the ratio of the total deformation of an object to its initial shape. A 1D object may only be shortened or lengthened.

Recalling the strain definitions as described in [1], the engineering normal strain, 'ε', which is a dimensionless measure usually expressed in per cent, defines the change in the object length relative to its original length and is written as

$$\varepsilon = \frac{l - l_0}{l_0} \tag{16.1}$$

where l_0 is the initial length of the object and l is the length of the object after deformation. If the strain is instantaneous, i.e. the length of the object is also known during the deformation, then a *Lagrangian* strain is defined:

$$\varepsilon(t) = \frac{l(t) - l(t_0)}{l(t_0)} \tag{16.2}$$

where t and t_0 represent the time and initial time of deformation, respectively, and $l(t)$ is the length at time instance t. Notice that $l(t_0) = l_0$.

Similarly, the deformation can be defined as a function of a previous time instance, representing a deformation occurring during an infinitesimally small time interval dt. In this case, an infinitesimally amount of deformation, $d\varepsilon(t)$, can be described as follows:

$$d\varepsilon_N(t) = \frac{l(t + dt) - l(t)}{l(t)} \tag{16.3}$$

The total amount of strain, termed '*natural*' strain, can be calculated as the integral over $d\varepsilon(t)$:

$$\varepsilon(t) = \int_{t_0}^{t} d\varepsilon_N(t) \tag{16.4}$$

The non-linear relationship between *Lagrangian* strain and *natural* strain that was introduced by Mirsky [10], is then given by:

$$\varepsilon_N(t) = \ln(1 + \varepsilon(t)) \tag{16.5}$$

It is clear that for deformations smaller than 10 per cent both *Lagrangian* and natural strains are approximately equal, while for larger deformations significant differences may be estimated. During the cardiac function, such as cardiac rapid filling and ejection, deformation reaches large values. Hence, it is recommended to measure the *natural* rather than the *Lagrangian* strain in order to obtain measurements that are less dependent on the initial length l_0.

Given a 2D object, two types of deformation occur. The first one is known as the normal strain, ε_x and ε_y, where the motion is normal to the borders x and y of the object, respectively. The second type is known as shear strain, ε_{xy} and ε_{yx}, where the motion is parallel to the borders of the object. These four strains compose the matrix strain tensor, as follows:

$$\begin{pmatrix} \varepsilon_x = \dfrac{\Delta x}{x} & \varepsilon_y = \dfrac{\Delta y}{y} \\ \varepsilon_{xy} = \dfrac{\Delta x}{y} & \varepsilon_{yx} = \dfrac{\Delta y}{x} \end{pmatrix} \tag{16.6}$$

Similarly, for a 3D object, such as the myocardium, the strain tensor matrix is defined as follows:

$$\begin{pmatrix} \varepsilon_{xx} & \varepsilon_{xy} & \varepsilon_{xz} \\ \varepsilon_{yx} & \varepsilon_{yy} & \varepsilon_{yz} \\ \varepsilon_{zx} & \varepsilon_{zy} & \varepsilon_{zz} \end{pmatrix} \tag{16.7}$$

where ε_{xx}, ε_{yy} and ε_{zz} are the normal strain components, while the remaining components are shear strains.

Equivalent to the distance-velocity relationship, one can define the instantaneous natural strain rate to be

$$\dot{\varepsilon}_N(t) = \frac{l'(t)}{l(t)} \tag{16.8}$$

where $l'(t)$ is the deformation rate and $l(t)$ is the instantaneous length of the object.

16.2.1 Myocardial strain

Myocardial wall thickening is defined as the change in myocardial wall thickness at end-diastolic and end-systolic phases divided by the end-diastolic thickness:

$$\mathrm{WT} = \frac{T_{\mathrm{ES}} - T_{\mathrm{ED}}}{T_{\mathrm{ED}}} \tag{16.9}$$

where WT is the myocardial wall thickening (%), T_{ES} and T_{ED} are the myocardial wall thickness at the end-systolic and end-diastolic phases, along one heart cycle, respectively. This relationship is identical to the 1D *Lagrangian* strain relation as in (16.1), measured across the LV wall. Similarly, the rate of the myocardial thickening is defined as in (16.8), where $\dot{\varepsilon}_N(t) \rightarrow \dot{\mathrm{W}}\mathrm{T}(t)$ and $l(t) \rightarrow T(t)$. Given that the myocardial motion and deformation are 3D, a 3D strain tensor is measured. Moreover, a 3D cardiac-adapted coordinate system is used commonly composed of the radial, longitudinal and circumferential axis. The radial axis, which is perpendicular to the epicardium, commonly points outward of the cavity, as depicted in Figure 16.1(a). The longitudinal axis is in a direction tangent to the epicardial layer, i.e. perpendicular to the radial axis, as can been seen in Figure 16.1(b). The circumferential axis is perpendicular to both the longitudinal and radial axis.

The aforementioned multidimensional unitless measures of deformation describe the myocardial strains. These strain parameters are affected by the global forces such as cardiac preload and afterload, by the myocardial local contractility, and by the extracellular matrix. Consequently, they represent the shortening or lengthening of the tissue of the myocardial wall, during the cardiac cycle. During systole the ventricular myocardium shortens in both the longitudinal and circumferential orientations while it thickens in the radial orientation. During diastole, reciprocal changes occur to allow active and passive ventricular filling. Shortening and thickening are indicated by negative and positive strain values, respectively.

Today, global and local strain measurements are performed. The global strain provides an overall functionality assessment where the overall shortening of the myocardial wall is measured. Only the measurement of the global longitudinal strain (GLS) is currently recommended, by the EACVI/ASE guidelines, to be used in the clinical practice. As for the local strain measurement, the myocardium is divided into six equal segments, as recommended by the EACVI/ASE guidelines [9]. Segmental measurements allow a better detection and location of regional

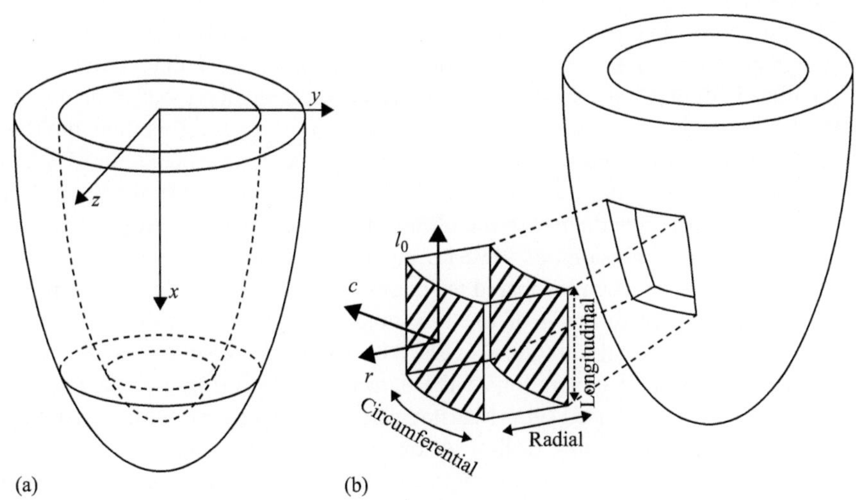

Figure 16.1 A global Cartesian coordinate system (a) and a local heart coordinate system (b). © 2016, Reprinted, [1]

pathology. Some studies have also demonstrated the usefulness of layer-specific strain analysis, where the myocardial wall is divided into its three layers: subendocardium, myocardium (midwall) and subepicardium and the strain are calculated for each one of these layers [11–15].

16.3 Cardiac strain estimation in practice

In previous chapters, the various methods towards ultrasound-based motion estimation were extensively covered. Two dimensional (2D) speckle tracking echocardiography (STE) is considered one of the most widely used techniques for cardiac strain estimation. It is commercially available for research use in the clinics by the different vendors, in order to push it as an alternative or additional technique for reliable cardiac function assessment, **based on strain and strain rate estimation**.

Although motion and strain estimation using STE and Tissue Doppler imaging (TDI) were reported to be comparable, STE was proven to provide slightly more accurate results than TDI, since TDI is angle dependent and prone to underestimating motion, when the ultrasound beam is not parallel to the motion direction [9]. Hence, in the apical views, STE allows longitudinal and transversal strain measurements, while for the parasternal views radial and circumferential strain measurements are also allowed. In addition, ventricular twisting and rotation can be easily extracted as well, providing additional parameters for functionality estimation. The ease of usage and the ability to measure strain throughout the whole LV myocardium from the acquisition of one heart cycle (versus multiple measurements required for TDI estimation) have won STE for many devotees.

Most commercial products for estimating 2D-STE employ a lot of smoothing and regularization (as explained in Section 16.4), much more than employed when estimating TDI, thus it is usually less sensitive to detect small regions of pathology. Beam drop-out is also problematic as well as stationary reverberation interfere with frame-by-frame tracking, resulting in drift or incorrect calculation of strain. Additionally, since spatial resolution in the transverse direction is relatively low, a tracking that is perpendicular to the ultrasound beam is less robust [16,17].

The very early versions of 2D-STE algorithms have been shown to exhibit moderate correlation when compared to sonomicrometry, with differences reported mainly due to overestimation of the low range of values, providing inaccurate results for the dyskinetic regions [18]. An improved version was developed [19], which is the first generation of the currently used software packages. This improved approach is based on a two-stage tracking algorithm, with a first stage of frame-by-frame tracking, followed by a second stage of spatio-temporal smoothness. This algorithm was also validated against sonomicrometry showing better agreement [20,21].

This two-stage approach is potentially problematic with noisy data. Despite the weighted-calculation approach that is utilized to avoid noisy velocity fields, the smoothness used to produce the smoothed field of velocity (with artificial

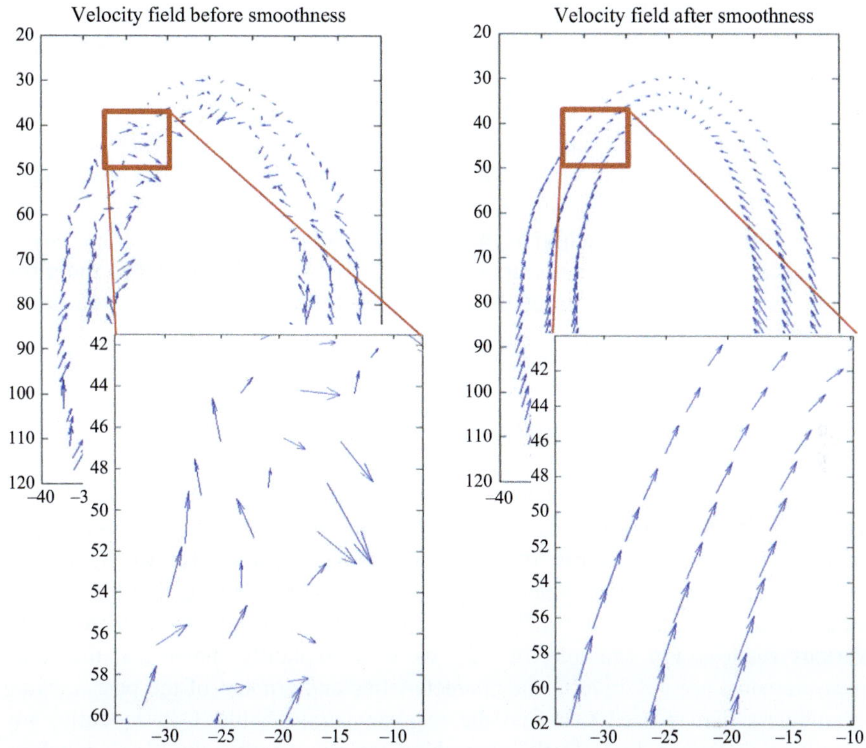

Figure 16.2 *An example of velocity fields (left) before and (right) after smoothness, when applied in the two-stage 2D speckle tracking echocardiography algorithms*

values at the very noisy area), produce over-smoothness of the velocity field, as depicted in Figure 16.2, and potentially causing erroneous strain results [22].

To avoid over-smoothness and erroneous strain results, a new approach was presented [12], which suggests to detect and eliminate outliers during the tracking process in each frame. The elimination is performed by additional round of tracking, in which a new matching block is found. This new matching block should guarantee the more naturally smoothed field of velocity, associated with a local uniformity. The results of this approach are promising, thus it is recommended to adopt this approach in the commercial software packages.

Recently, vector velocity imaging (VVI) was introduced as a new alternative echocardiographic technique that is based on 2D B-mode images. VVI, unlike the conventional TDI, is angle independent, which allows global and regional cardiac function quantification in the longitudinal, transversal, radial and circumferential directions [23–27]. VVI combines speckle tracking, mitral annulus motion, periodicity of the cardiac cycle (usually three cycles are recorded) and the border defined between the intracavitary blood and the myocardial tissue. It uses real-time speckle tracking technique to acquire amplitude and phase information of 2D pixels and to measure the motion displacement and velocities, strain and strain rate [28–31].

VVI has been shown to be useful not only for regular transthoracic echocardiography (TTE) but also for myocardial strain measurements in the first trimester fetal echocardiography [32,33]. Despite the aforementioned advantages, similar limitations to those of the conventional speckle tracking must be taken into account [32,34]: the required image quality is between reasonable quality to high quality. Also, when the orientation of the myofibers is parallel to the ultrasound beam it may deteriorate the spatial resolution in the lateral and septal segments.

16.4 The effect of smoothness on strain analysis

The primary source of discordance in the strain measurements among the different vendors, [35–37], has been as associated to the different post-processing algorithms, which smooth the raw displacement measurements performed by speckle tracking [38]. The different smoothing/processing approaches applied to the measurements, may explain the different myocardial strain values obtained by the various vendors. For example, in [22], we have explicitly shown that the strain measurements are sensitive to the characteristics and amount of the post-tracking smoothness that is used to refine the resultant strain fields. Consequently, any modification that is made to the smoothing techniques after the block-matching may cause the expected inter-vendor strain differences. This paper, analyses the principles and specific details of the first generation of two-stage STE algorithms, currently employed by the commercial vendors. For this purpose, an ‘open’ generic algorithm was developed and its tracking and strain results were compared to a commercial product, utilizing both software-based phantom simulations and clinical data. The algorithm is composed of a two-stage approach, where the first stage is the block-matching-based tracking and the second stage is the post-processing smoothness. The second stage involves some trade-off between weighting and smoothing. Consequently, the post-processing smoothed results are usually depending on the weighted smoothness. The reported results of this study show that once the weighting factor is different, the same data set with the same image quality and initial segmentation will provide significantly different strain measurements. This implies that the first generation of STE software packages, which are characterized by two consecutive stages (tracking then smoothness), tend to suffer from inaccuracies and some uncertainties.

Another study [39] has shown that even when the spatial and temporal smoothing are controlled by the user, in different speckle tracking software packages, the smoothing can significantly influence the strain measurements. Although longitudinal strain was shown to be stable under different additional smoothing, controlled by the user, circumferential and radial strain were significantly affected.

16.5 Factors affecting strain estimation

In Chapter 13, factors impacting the accuracy of speckle tracking were already introduced. In this section, we address this problem again specifically in the context of cardiac strain imaging. Indeed,both global and segmental strain measurements were shown [35] to be dependent on many factors affecting their reproducibility. These factors may include:

16.5.1 Image quality

Image quality is a critical factor that affects the performance of any software that measures and estimates myocardial deformation. Many reports have related to the dependence of strain and strain rate calculations on image quality and tracking algorithm. For example, Marwick [40] has stated that strain and strain rate that are measured using either TDI or STE are influenced by image quality and measurement quality of the velocity fields. Hoit [41] and Trache *et al.* [42] have also emphasized that the effect of image quality on speckle tracking performance is significant. Trache *et al.* have shown that limited image quality has a significant impact on the agreement between 3D and 2D numerical strain values, while Brian D.H. has reported that measurement of strain rate (and strain) is influenced by image and signal quality, where a very high image quality is required to produce reasonable strain and strain-rate results.

16.5.2 Modality

Different modalities may provide different strain measurements. Although these differences are sometimes not significant, this should be considered while providing a clinical diagnosis. For example, as reported by Gardner [43], cardiac magnetic resonance imaging (CMRI) allows cardiac function assessment, but the estimated values were found to be significantly different from those provided by TTE. Another study, published by Tee [44], shows significant differences in segmental strain measurements obtained by CMRI, CT and TTE.

16.5.3 Vendor software and software version

Recent study, published by the EACVI and ASE [36], was initiated to study the inter-vendor variability of GLS measurements. Seven different vendors participated in this study for the data acquisition and for the strain analysis. In addition, two more software-only vendors have been evaluated. Echocardiography clips were acquired from 62 volunteers, and conventional echocardiographic parameters were measured for comparison. Inter-vendor comparison results have reported significant absolute differences. Although these differences were lower than those for ejection fraction, their significance should be considered as well during a clinical diagnosis. Alongside, a recent joint task force [45] of the EACVI, ASE and the industry was initiated to standardize quantitative functional imaging.

In addition to the inter-vendor variability, one should also pay attention to the inter-software variability of the same vendor. Significant changes in GLS values were reported [35,37] when using different software versions of the same vendor. These results may provide not only different clinical evaluation in general but may also affect a follow-up study of an individual patient. Hence, it is suggested for follow-up studies to use the same 2D-STE software version and ultrasound scanner, both of the same vendors, to avoid inter-vendor and inter-software variability and inconsistency.

One should also notice the differences that are produced due to improper segmentation [22,46]. Segmentation of the endocardium is challenging due the trabecula, in addition to the clutter a noise. Segmentation of the epicardium is difficult, since the border is not clearly visible, especially at the apical region and the lateral wall where in many cases part of the lateral wall is missing. When the segmentation is manually defined or corrected, then inter-user variability may be added to the software-based inaccuracies.

A more essential factor, which may significantly influence strain measurements, is the timing definitions of end diastole (ED) and end systole (ES). Mada *et al.* has reported, in [47,48], that an exact temporal definition of timing has a major impact on the accuracy of the strain measurements. This work also reported that Doppler is found to be the best for the timing of ED and ES for STE analysis. However, the automatic definition of these timing parameters may be different from vendor to vendor, and is dependent on the specific acquisition, for each patient. Some acquisitions may not include Doppler recordings. If an automatic detection is not an option, or cannot be used due to missing data, a manual detection will be required. Consequently, an inter-user variability will then influence the reliability and accuracy of the results.

16.5.4 Methodology of estimation

Inter-vendor variability occurs mainly due to differences in algorithm implementations, assumptions and constraints. Even if the same approach is adopted, there are no guidelines that guarantee similar implementation. For example, in [22], it is shown that slight changes in some of the implementation parameters, such as smoothness factor, may produce significantly different strain measurements. In addition, the size and shape of the traced block and of the region of search (defined by the tracking algorithm) will produce different measurements. The noisier the image is, the more significant the differences are. Different criteria of similarity of locating the matching block may also add to the differences in performance among the various algorithms. Another implementation factor that may also affect the results is the backward tracking. Some algorithms, e.g. [21,49], perform the tracking in the natural direction (forward tracking, starting from the first frame to the last frame) and in the opposite direction (backward tracking, starting from the last frame to the initial frame). The final strain measurement is a weighted average of the measurements performed in the backward and forward directions. This approach is also used to evaluate the quality of tracking, as it should provide identical results to the forward tracking alone, when the data is without noise. Finally, one may also mention the constraints used by many of the algorithms, such as the maximal and minimal velocities allowed in each direction, the local uniformity expected along and across the myocardium, and the relationship between the myocardial layer that is assumed to provide transmural strain measurements. For example, some algorithms may assume a preset linear or non-linear relationship among the adjacent layers, while other algorithms may provide separate transmural measurements.

16.5.5 Acquisition parameters

The specifications of the data acquisition may have a strong effect on the performance of the tracking algorithm and the strain measurements [50]. Data acquisition may differ due to the following parameters:

1. Sample volume and frame rate: lower frame rate decreases the temporal resolution, which may miss some cardiac events. Higher frame rate is essential for a more accurate strain measurement. Despite the many efforts to provide systems that allow acquisitions at higher frame rates, this is still possible only with a decrease in the spatial resolution. This problem is more critical when considering 4D imaging [51,52].
2. Electrocardiography (ECG) gating: any echocardiographic acquisition should be ECG gated [52,53]. ECG is consistently used to detect timing of the different cardiac phases, to allow accurate timing of start and ES, and timing of strain measurements such as post systolic shortening, for pathology detection.
3. Image sector: the imaging sector must be set wisely: it should be wide enough so that the entire cardiac wall is visible, while it should be sufficiently narrow to achieve maximal frame rate. This trade-off should be optimized to allow fine tracking performance.
4. Contrast, gain, sharpness and angle correction parameters must be set to values that guarantee the best image quality. Noisier images will produce erroneous/artefactual results.
5. Sonographer and scanner: as mentioned above, using different scanners for a follow up study may cause misleading measurements due to the inter-vendor variability, which is caused by both the software and the scanner differences [51,52]. Additionally, it is advisable that the same sonographer will perform the acquisition for the same patient, to avoid inter-sonographer variability.

16.6 How should strain be estimated?

16.6.1 Physiological aspects and concerns

- Most algorithms for estimating strain perform the calculations throughout (along and across) the myocardial wall of the LV, thus the whole cross-section of the LV wall must be contained within the imaged sector, throughout the whole cardiac cycle.
- The standard three long-axis views must be acquired as close as possible to their defined locations. When the apical long-axis views are foreshortened – the apex is usually actually not acquired, as viewed by an exaggerated wall width.

When the angle of the apical long-axis view is not exact – features that should not be included in the imaged cross-section are actually included and distort the 'horse-shoe' shape, producing erroneous strain results.
- The standard three short-axis views must be acquired as close as possible to their defined locations and at right-angle versus the LV long axis. When the location (height between the apex and base) is incorrect, the strain values would be inaccurate. Similarly, when the angle is incorrect, and the myocardial wall cross-section shape becomes oval instead of circular, the results would be inaccurate.
- The movements of the trabeculae are very different from those of the compact muscle, both in the radial orientation and the long-axis orientation. Thus – they should not be included within the segmented walls. When they are unintentionally included – erroneous strain results will be obtained.

16.6.2 Processing aspects and concerns

- The cardiac coordinate system (radial-longitudinal-circumferential axis system) used to define strain tensor is not well defined for the most distal apical point of the ventricle [1]. Consequently, neither the longitudinal nor the circumferential strain can be measured there. Hence, one should take this fact into consideration.
- The ultrasound machine coordinate system is different from the cardiac coordinate system. Once the ultrasonic beam is perpendicular or parallel to the myocardial wall, the longitudinal and radial axis, respectively, will correspond with the ultrasonic beam directions. However, since the acquisition is performed manually, an accurate overlapping of the different axis of the two coordinate systems is hard to achieve, causing the ultrasound beam to reach the myocardial wall in an oblique way, thus the measured strain may be a combination of the longitudinal and radial strain components. Consequently, one should always keep in mind that the measured strain might not be the true strain.
- Proper and reproducible segmentation of the myocardium is critical – since improper segmentation increases the irregularity of the velocity field, by adding discontinuities. Since the mandatory regularization of the velocity field is usually based on smoothing – the inclusion of such discontinuities results in increased inaccuracy. This indicates the high degree of caution that should be exercised in multi-vendor clinics.
- Automatic segmentation of the myocardial wall in echocardiographic 2D LV cross-sections is essential for guarantying reproducibility and objectivity. Automatic segmentation usually produces a proper segmentation.
- The initial automatic segmentation is preferably based on automatic detection of fiducial points – e.g. the epicardial border at the apex and the two basal points, and the tracking of these three points along the cardiac cycle.
- Several iterations of the segmentation, performed after lateral (horizontal and vertical) shifts of the initial segmentation, which is implemented automatically

and in an optimized procedure, may obtain the optimal segmentation (optimal – in the sense of strain estimation with maximal accuracy, reproducibility and objectivity).

16.6.3 Signal to noise aspects and concerns

As detailed earlier above, most algorithms for speckle tracking echocardiography are sensitive to speckle decorrelation noise.

- Filtering and smoothing, as commonly performed, may produce erroneous results. Hence, imposing constraints on the measured data and/or eliminating outliers in the data may improve accuracy (see, e.g. the local uniformity index [12], which has been shown to be useful in fine-tuning the basal regions, specifically in clips that depict complex movements of the myocardial wall versus the mitral ring).
- Block matching, which is commonly used in speckle tracking echocardiography, usually does not provide accurate strain calculations in the apical regions, when measured from 2D long-axis cross-sections. The size of the apical regions, in which strain calculations are inaccurate, may be determined by a local uniformity index.
- The tracking at the mid regions is usually feasible – as demonstrated by the insensitivity of the results to different parameters.
- The accuracy of the strain calculations depends on the quality of the segmentation and the tracking, which are practically dependent on the image quality. A physiological constraint that the displacement field is continuous in some sense, as manifested in [12], could be a good indicator of tracking quality.

16.6.4 Recommendations

In addition to the obvious recommendations that the user should aim for generating the best image quality and ensure that the entire myocardium is inside the image, the following ones should be noted:

- Recommended frame rate should be as high as possible, preferably around 60–70 fps, without compromising line density. More stringent precautions are required when trying to analyse clips acquired at lower frame rates (but definitely not below 40 fps). For high heart rate, even higher frame rates are recommended.
- Due to the dependence of the tracking results (and thus also of the strain results) on the segmentation of the LV myocardium [the region of interest (ROI)], one should confirm utilization of an automatic segmentation, thus ensuring reproducibility. The user should also verify that practically all the myocardial wall is included within the ROI. Automatic segmentation algorithms may vary among the different vendors and thus result in different strain values.
- The apical strain values are less reliable, and the results at these regions depend very much on the weighting parameters of the regularization (smoothing)

method being used. One should therefore employ caution when measuring apical strain by algorithms provided by different vendors.

- When the automatic segmentation of the ROI seems to fail at the apical zone, it is recommended to abort the clip, rather than to adjust it manually.
- Speckle tracking algorithms (or myocardial strain algorithm) have limited accuracy. Automatic tracking quality indices provided by the various vendors may also have limited accuracy (e.g. 2D strain has been reported to have 86 per cent accuracy [34]). It is thus recommended to visually inspect the tracking results, specifically at the base, which has a considerable effect on the global strain.
- Measurement of the exact timing of the different phases of the cardiac cycle are critical. It is recommended to employ Doppler measurements for the timing of the ED and ES instants. Additionally, it is important to synchronize the stain measurements with the ECG signal, where a cycle is defined from peak R-wave to the next peak R-wave, as zero strain should be measured at both times.

16.7 Tracking quality and reliability index

As mentioned previously, many studies have shown the great potential of using the peak strain amplitude and its timing as clinical landmarks for cardiac diagnosis and prognosis. On the other hand, only few studies have suggested utilising the temporal behaviour of the entire strain curve to detect and analyse functional abnormalities [54,55]. Both approaches indeed allow good analysis and diagnosis of cardiac function. However, incorrect or inaccurate strain calculation, due to inadequate segmentation, poor tracking, over smoothness or bad image quality, affects the reliability and the ability to diagnose and provide prognosis.

This, consequently, implies that there is an essential need for a reliable measure of quality of the tracking – the core of the most commonly used strain estimation.

The studies [47,56,60] and many more have related to tracking quality indices that have been employed to determine whether to include or exclude strain measurements. Tracking quality indices provided by the commercial vendors are used as Boolean scoring, designating as 'acceptable' or 'non-acceptable' the segmental strain measurements, with the option of manual corrections. Generally, tracking quality indices should indicate how well the motion of the subendocardial and subepicardial borders is tracked [47]. Any software that does not provide this step may not be reliable enough and should be used in caution, as the expected strain values may be different. Some papers, such as [61], have listed criteria for STE commercial software, on which the tracking quality index should be based. These criteria are (1) adequate tracking is assumed when at the end of the cardiac cycle the speckle coordinates return to baseline; (2) significant differences of tissue velocities between adjacent speckles indicate bad tracking quality and (3) equal strain values are expected at the beginning and at the end of heart cycle, thus a large drift indicates low tracking quality. These software-based tracking quality indices can be either rejected or accepted by the user.

Despite the rationale of the three criteria listed above, these tracking quality indices are not always reliable, since the tracking algorithm may provide 'good' tracking results even if a non-tissue object is being tracked, consequently providing erroneous strain measurements. These indices also do not take into account the temporal behaviour of each strain measure (except for criteria (3) above, which may become useless once over-smoothness is applied). Another tracking quality index is the 'trashogram', [62], which identifies regions of high or low strain magnitude, based on the cross-correlation that is calculated during the speckle tracking process. Yet, since high cross-correlation may be a result of the wavelength, while low correlation may still allow displacement estimation, this trashogram approach may not be sufficiently reliable [63].

Consequently, the development of reliability and tracking quality indexes is essential to allow the acceptance of strain measurements as part of the clinical diagnosis protocol.

16.8 Clinical application of cardiac strain echocardiography

Since many of the cardiac pathologies, such as those caused by reduced local blood supply, inflammation, regional changes in the extracellular matrix construct, and more, produce localized changes in contractility, it is desirable to be able to measure changes in myocardial function locally. Thus, there have been several attempts to study localized, segmental, regional or layer-specific myocardial function. Since tissue Doppler, as implemented on most clinical machines, provides only a local value, it may provide strain values at a point within a segment, region or layer. Yet, the measurement may be too localized, thus may acquire data from a normally functioning tissue within a patchy region, where its neighbouring tissue segments are, e.g. ischemic.

2D Strain imaging, on the other hand, as implemented by the various vendors, may provide regional or layer-specific strain values, but currently due to its inaccuracy and inter-vendor variability, the EACVI/ASE recommends the employment of GLS only [9].

In spite of these recommendations, there have been quite a few reports on measurements of segmental, regional (e.g. [61,64]) and/or layer-specific strain values (e.g. [14,15,65]).

As explained below, due to the high noise level (low signal-to-noise ratio) inherent to echocardiographic clips, most commercial products that calculate myocardial strain employ several levels of noise filtration (e.g. smoothing). Therefore, the strain values calculated for a segment (or a region, or a layer) heavily depends on the values of its neighbours. Thus, for example, in one implementation, the midwall strain is actually the average of the subendocardial strain and the subepicardial strain.

There are, however, reports on 2D strain calculations, in which the longitudinal strain is calculated independently for each layer, and for each segment. In this report, the processing was validated by employing a software-based phantom [12].

Strain has been introduced as a promising clinical index of global and regional myocardial function. Thousands of papers have been published indicating the importance of myocardial strain measurements in providing cardiac functionality quantification and in helping clinical diagnosis. In [66], a study in healthy subjects has shown that strain measurements allow quantification of myocardial deformation. Many similar studies with metadata analysis were performed to provide range of strain values for normal subjects, for example [67,68]. Some other studies also emphasized the benefits of strain rate measurements for the assessment of regional preload dependent changes during diastole [69].

As a diagnostic tool, strain has been shown to measure changes in myocardial mechanics, associated with ischemic LV remodelling [70]. Specifically, longitudinal strain is considered the most commonly used deformation parameter to estimate systolic LV function. For example, GLS measure was found to be related to myocardial infarct size [71] and location [72] in chronic ischemic heart disease and after coronary reperfusion [73], and post-systolic shortening was found to be a good indicator for myocardial ischemia [74,75]. Additionally, regional contractile quantification after infarction was found to be superior to wall thickening in differentiating between infarcted or non-infarcted related myocardial regions [76]. Strain measurements were also used to detect changes in the LV mechanical property changes during acute atrio ventricular synchronous right ventricular pacing in children [77]. Regional and GLS measurements were used to characterize cardiac amyloidosis, as well [54]. Regional myocardial strain mapping during ventricular pacing allowed understanding the effect of pacing on the mechanical properties of the myocardium, while allowing diagnosis of abnormalities in perfusion, metabolism, structure and pump function [55].

It is important to mention that most of these studies have used the strain as single-time parameter extracted from the time–strain curves, which were measured for the whole cardiac cycle. These parameters are called ‘peak strain’, where the minimum strain amplitude (maximal negative value) and its time were extracted. Only very few studies considered the entire time–strain curve pattern to perform a diagnosis [78,79].

Together with this promising functional analysis, based on contractility measurements, it is important to emphasize that functional imaging in general, provides only motion and deformation parameters. These parameters cannot qualify or quantify the loading conditions, such as forces and pressure of the heart. Thus, changes in perfusion and myocardial fiber metabolism will remain invisible unless they affect the contractility of the heart [47].

16.9 Summary

It is well known that the measure needed for proper assessment of LV function is stress – the development and decrease of the forces generated by the myocytes (and thus their well-being). With the current echocardiographic technologies, we are able to assess only the strain development and decrease during the cardiac cycle.

In order to estimate the stresses from the stains, one needs to know the loadings – the LV intra-cavity pressures, the preload and afterload, etc. Currently, there are no methods of performing these measurements non-invasively, and even when invasive measurements are approved and acceptable – it may be possible to perform these measurements just at a few sites, while their distributions remain unknown. The growing body of clinical evidence that correlates with pathology the strain distribution within the LV walls, and the changes that occur with time – may provide sufficient support for clinical assessments and decision-making, even though the stresses are unknown.

It is well known that the subendocardium, in the normal cases, is activated first, and that the mechanical activation follows the electrical activation, as its wave-front propagates from the endocardial layers to the epicardial layers (within ~50 ms). The current generation of echocardiographic machines allow acquisition at frame rates <100 fps, which are not sufficient to sample the mechanical activation propagation at high enough rate. Thus, current strain measurements do not allow assessment whether the endocardium is actively contracting – or passively pushed by the more external layers. With the introduction of ultrafast imaging, where $\times 100$ higher frame rates are expected, it is predicted that future generations of echo machine will allow such clinically vital assessment.

The new generation of echocardiographic imaging systems ('fully digital') allow development of novel beamforming methods and novel signal processing methods, so that with enough computational resources – image quality is improving fast. Yet, the patient population is changing – it is ageing as life expectancy is growing, and unfortunately, in many cases patients are more obese. Thus, as the need for echocardiography imaging is growing, the need for better image quality is also rising. Thus, the need for even better image quality, and for much larger computational resources – will continue to increase. Concurrently, the need for more accurate strain estimation will continue to grow.

The spread of 'point of care' echocardiographic imaging – renders that the image acquisition is expected to be performed under much worse conditions than at an echocardiography lab. It may be expected to be performed under more stressful conditions (e.g. emergencies) and the clips assessed by less experienced readers. Thus, automation of the whole process of strain estimation is needed, and much better tools for tracking quality assessment are mandatory.

There is a need, therefore, for development of novel approaches of automatic strain estimation and accurate tracking quality assessment, to be performed on ultrafast ultrasound imaging systems that are small and hand-carried, and inexpensive.

References

[1] D'hooge, J., Heimdal, A., Jamal, F., *et al.* 'Regional strain and strain rate measurements by cardiac ultrasound: principles, implementation and limitations'. European Heart Journal – Cardiovascular Imaging, 2000; 1(3):154–170.

[2] Beyar, R., Shapiro, E. P., Graves, W. L., *et al.* 'Quantification and validation of left ventricular wall thickening by a three-dimensional volume element magnetic resonance imaging approach'. Circulation, 1990; 81(1):297–307.

[3] Rademakers, F. E., Bogaert, J. 'Left ventricular myocardial tagging'. The International Journal of Cardiac Imaging, 1997; 13(3):233–245.

[4] Park, J., Metaxas, D., Young, A. A., Axel, L. 'Deformable models with parameter functions for cardiac motion analysis from tagged MRI data'. IEEE Transactions on Medical Imaging, 1996; 15(3):278–289.

[5] Petitjean, C., Rougon, N., Cluzel, P. 'Assessment of myocardial function: a review of quantification methods and results using tagged MRI'. Journal of Cardiovascular Magnetic Resonance, 2005; 7(2):501–516.

[6] McVeigh, E. R. 'MRI of myocardial function: motion tracking techniques'. Magnetic Resonance Imaging, 1996; 14(2):137–150.

[7] Schmermund, A., Gerber, T., Behrenbeck, T., *et al.* 'Measurement of myocardial infarct size by electron beam computed tomography: a comparison with 99mTc sestamibi'. Investigative Radiology, 1998; 33(6):313–321.

[8] Shen, M. Y., Liu, Y. H., Sinusas, A. J., *et al.* 'Quantification of regional myocardial wall thickening on electrocardiogram-gated SPECT imaging'. Journal of Nuclear Cardiology, 1999; 6(6):583–595.

[9] Lang, R. M., Badano, L. P., Mor-Avi, V., *et al.* 'Recommendations for cardiac chamber quantification by echocardiography in adults: an update from the American Society of Echocardiography and the European Association of Cardiovascular Imaging'. Journal of the American Society of Echocardiography, 2015; 28(1): 1–39.

[10] Mirsky, I. 'Review of various theories for the evaluation of left ventricular wall stresses'. Cardiac mechanics: Physiological, clinical, and mathematical considerations. (A 74-39626 20-05) New York, John Wiley and Sons, Inc., 1974, 381–409.

[11] Michael, L., Noa, B. H., Hanan, K., *et al.* 'Measurements of transmural strain variations by two dimensional ultrasound speckle tracking'. Journal of Biomedical Graphics and Computing, 2012; 2(1): 15.

[12] Khamis, H., Shimoni, S., Hagendorff, A., Smirin, N., Friedman, Z., Adam, D. 'Optimization-based speckle tracking algorithm for left ventricle strain estimation: a feasibility study'. *IEEE Transactions on Ultrasonics, Ferroelectrics, and Frequency Control*, 2016; 63(8): 1093–1106.

[13] Bachner-Hinenzon, N., Ertracht, O., Leitman, M., *et al.* 'Layer-specific strain analysis by speckle tracking echocardiography reveals differences in left ventricular function between rats and humans'. American Journal of Physiology-Heart and Circulatory Physiology, 2010; 299(3): H664–H672.

[14] Bachner-Hinenzon, N., Ertracht, O., Malka, A., *et al.* 'Layer-specific strain analysis: investigation of regional deformations in a rat model of acute versus chronic myocardial infarction'. American Journal of Physiology-Heart and Circulatory Physiology, 2012; 303(5):H549–H558.

[15] Sarvari, S. I., Haugaa, K. H., Zahid, W., *et al.* 'Layer-specific quantification of myocardial deformation by strain echocardiography may reveal significant CAD in patients with non-ST-segment elevation acute coronary syndrome'. Journal of the American College of Cardiology: Cardiovascular Imaging, 2013; 6(5):535–544.

[16] Teske, A. J., De Boeck, B. W., Melman, P. G., Sieswerda, G. T., Doevendans, P. A., Cramer, M. J. 'Echocardiographic quantification of myocardial function using tissue deformation imaging, a guide to image acquisition and analysis using tissue Doppler and speckle tracking'. Cardiovascular Ultrasound, 2007; 5(1):1–19.

[17] Amundsen, B. H., Crosby, J., Steen, P. A., Torp, H., Slørdahl, S. A., Støylen, A. 'Regional myocardial long-axis strain and strain rate measured by different tissue Doppler and speckle tracking echocardiography methods: a comparison with tagged magnetic resonance imaging'. European Heart Journal – Cardiovascular Imaging, 2009; 10(2):229–237.

[18] Korinek, J., Wang, J., Sengupta, P. P., *et al.* 'Two-dimensional strain – a Doppler-independent ultrasound method for quantitation of regional deformation: validation in vitro and in vivo'. Journal of the American Society of Echocardiography, 2005; 18(12):1247–1253.

[19] Leitman, M., Lysyansky, P., Sidenko, S., *et al.* 'Two-dimensional strain – a novel software for real-time quantitative echocardiographic assessment of myocardial function'. Journal of the American Society of Echocardiography, 2004; 17(10):1021–1029.

[20] Korinek, J., Kjaergaard, J., Sengupta, P. P., *et al.* 'High spatial resolution speckle tracking improves accuracy of 2-dimensional strain measurements: an update on a new method in functional echocardiography'. Journal of the American Society of Echocardiography, 2007; 20(2):165–170.

[21] Amundsen, B. H., Helle-Valle, T., Edvardsen, T., *et al.* 'Noninvasive myocardial strain measurement by speckle tracking echocardiography: validation against sonomicrometry and tagged magnetic resonance imaging'. Journal of the American College of Cardiology, 2006; 47(4):789–793.

[22] Khamis, H., Shimoni, S., Hagendorff, A., Smirin, N., Friedman, Z., Adam, D. 'Feasibility of reproducible vendor independent estimation of cardiac function based on first generation speckle tracking echocardiography'. Journal of Biomedical Engineering and Informatics, 2015; 2(2): 57.

[23] Vannan, M. A., Pedrizzetti, G., Li, P., *et al.* 'Case reports: effect of cardiac resynchronization therapy on longitudinal and circumferential left ventricular mechanics by velocity vector imaging: description and initial clinical application of a novel method using high-frame rate B-mode echocardiographic images'. Echocardiography, 2005; 22(10):826–830.

[24] Chen, J., Cao, T., Duan, Y., Yuan, L., Wang, Z. 'Velocity vector imaging in assessing myocardial systolic function of hypertensive patients with left ventricular hypertrophy'. Canadian Journal of Cardiology, 2007; 23(12): 957–961.

[25] Wang, C. H., Wang, Y. H., Niu, N. N., Xie, Y. X., Wang, L. 'Evaluation of the asynchronization and function of the left ventricle in patients with chronic pulmonary hypertension by velocity vector imaging'. Chinese Medical Journal, 2013; 126(23):4457–4462.

[26] Aminian, F., Esmaeilzadeh, M., Moladoust, H., *et al.* 'Does accessory pathway significantly alter left ventricular twist/torsion? A study in Wolff-Parkinson-White syndrome by velocity vector imaging'. Echocardiography, 2014; 31(7):872–878.

[27] Parameswaran, A. C., Purushottam, B., Amanullah, A., Figueredo, V. M. 'Distribution of dyssynchrony in subjects with no known cardiac disease and comparison of velocity vector imaging to color-coded tissue Doppler imaging'. Echocardiography, 2013; 30(2):180–189.

[28] Zhou, J., Pu, D. R., Tian, L. Q., *et al.* 'Noninvasive assessment of myocardial mechanics of the left ventricle in rabbits using velocity vector imaging'. Medical Science Monitor Basic Research, 2015; 21:109–115.

[29] Zeng, S., Zhou, Q. C., Peng, Q. H., *et al.* 'Assessment of regional myocardial function in patients with dilated cardiomyopathy by velocity vector imaging'. Echocardiography, 2009; 26(2):163–170.

[30] Yang, Z. R., Zhou, Q. C., Lee, L., *et al.* 'Quantitative assessment of left ventricular systolic function in patients with coronary heart disease by velocity vector imaging'. Echocardiography, 2012; 29(3):340–345.

[31] Wei, Z., Zhang, H., Su, H., Zhu, T., Zhu, Y., Zhang, J. 'Correlation between myocardial dysfunction and perfusion impairment in diabetic rats with velocity vector imaging and myocardial contrast echocardiography'. Echocardiography, 2012; 29(10):1247–1255.

[32] Chelliah, A., Dham, N., Frank, L. H., Donofrio, M., Krishnan, A. 'Myocardial strain can be measured from first trimester fetal echocardiography using velocity vector imaging'. Prenatal Diagnosis, 2016; 36(5):483–488.

[33] Pu, D. R., Zhou, Q. C., Zhang, M., Peng, Q. H., Zeng, S., Xu, G. Q. 'Assessment of regional right ventricular longitudinal functions in fetus using velocity vector imaging technology'. Prenatal Diagnosis, 2010; 30(11):1057–1063.

[34] Zeng, S., Jiang, T., Zhou, Q. C., Yuan, L., Zhou, J. W., Cao, D. M. 'Time-course changes in left ventricular myocardial deformation in STZ-induced rabbits on velocity vector imaging'. Cardiovascular Ultrasound, 2014; 12(1):1–9.

[35] Castel, A. L., Menet, A., Ennezat, P. V., *et al.* 'Global longitudinal strain software upgrade: implications for intervendor consistency and longitudinal imaging studies'. Archives of Cardiovascular Diseases, 2016; 109(1):22–30.

[36] Farsalinos, K. E., Daraban, A. M., Ünlü, S., Thomas, J. D., Badano, L. P., Voigt, J. U. 'Head-to-head comparison of global longitudinal strain measurements among nine different vendors: the EACVI/ASE inter-vendor comparison study'. Journal of the American Society of Echocardiography, 2015; 28(10):1171–1181.

[37] Nagata, Y., Takeuchi, M., Mizukoshi, K., *et al.* 'Intervendor variability of two-dimensional strain using vendor-specific and vendor-independent software'. Journal of the American Society of Echocardiography, 2015; 28(6):630–641.

[38] Negishi, K., Lucas, S., Negishi, T., Hamilton, J., Marwick, T. H. 'What is the primary source of discordance in strain measurement between vendors: imaging or analysis?'. Ultrasound in Medicine and Biology, 2013; 39(4): 714–720.

[39] Moen, C. A., Salminen, P. R., Dahle, G. O., Hjertaas, J. J., Grong, K., Matre, K. 'Is strain by speckle tracking echocardiography dependent on user controlled spatial and temporal smoothing? An experimental porcine study'. Cardiovascular Ultrasound, 2013; 11(1):1–14.

[40] Marwick, T. H. 'Measurement of strain and strain rate by echocardiography: ready for prime time?'. Journal of the American College of Cardiology, 2006; 47(7):1313–1327.

[41] Hoit, B. D. 'Strain and strain rate echocardiography and coronary artery disease'. Circulation: Cardiovascular Imaging, 2011; 4(2):179–190.

[42] Trache, T., Stöbe, S., Tarr, A., Pfeiffer, D., Hagendorff, A. 'The agreement between 3D, standard 2D and triplane 2D speckle tracking: effects of image quality and 3D volume rate'. Echo Research and Practice, 2014; 1(2):71–83.

[43] Gardner, B. I., Bingham, S. E., Allen, M. R., Blatter, D. D., Anderson, J. L. 'Cardiac magnetic resonance versus transthoracic echocardiography for the assessment of cardiac volumes and regional function after myocardial infarction: an intrasubject comparison using simultaneous intrasubject recordings'. Cardiovascular Ultrasound, 2009; 7(1):1–7.

[44] Tee, M., Noble, J. A., Bluemke, D. A. 'Imaging techniques for cardiac strain and deformation: comparison of echocardiography, cardiac magnetic resonance and cardiac computed tomography'. Expert Review of Cardiovascular Therapy, 2013; 11(2):221–231.

[45] Voigt, J. U., Pedrizzetti, G., Lysyansky, P., *et al.* 'Definitions for a common standard for 2D speckle tracking echocardiography: consensus document of the EACVI/ASE/Industry Task Force to standardize deformation imaging'. European Heart Journal – Cardiovascular Imaging, 2014; 28(2):183–193.

[46] Marwick, T. H., Leano, R. L., Brown, J., *et al.* 'Myocardial strain measurement with 2-dimensional speckle-tracking echocardiography: definition of normal range'. Journal of the American College ofCardiology: Cardiovascular Imaging, 2009; 2(1): 80–84.

[47] Mada, R. O., Duchenne, J., Voigt, J. U. 'Tissue Doppler, strain and strain rate in ischemic heart disease "How I do it". Cardiovascular Ultrasound, 2014; 12(1):1.

[48] Mada, R. O., Lysyansky, P., Daraban, A. M., Duchenne, J., Voigt, J. U. 'How to define end-diastole and end-systole?: impact of timing on strain measurements'. Journal of the American College of Cardiology: Cardiovascular Imaging, 2015; 8(2):148–157.

[49] Amundsen, B. H., Crosby, J., Steen, P. A., Torp, H., Slordahl, S. A., Stoylen, A. 'Regional myocardial long- axis strain and strain rate measured by different tissue Doppler and speckle tracking echocardiography methods: a comparison with tagged magnetic resonance imaging'. European Heart Journal – Cardiovascular Imaging, 2009; 10(2):229–237.

[50] Kuecherer, H. F., Kee, L. L., Modin, G., Cheitlin, M. D., Schiller, N. B. 'Echocardiography in serial evaluation of left ventricular systolic and diastolic function: importance of image acquisition, quantitation, and physiologic variability in clinical and investigational applications'. Journal of the American Society of Echocardiography, 1991; 4(3):203–214.

[51] Lang, R. M., Badano, L. P., Tsang, W., *et al.* 'EAE/ASE recommendations for image acquisition and display using three-dimensional echocardiography'. Journal of the American Society of Echocardiography, 2012; 25(1):3–46.

[52] Lang, R. M., Bierig, M., Devereux, R. B., *et al.* 'Recommendations for chamber quantification: a report from the American Society of Echocardiography's Guidelines and Standards Committee and the Chamber Quantification Writing Group, developed in conjunction with the European Association of Echocardiography, a branch of the European Society of Cardiology'. Journal of the American Society of Echocardiography, 2005; 18(12):1440–1463.

[53] D'hooge, J., Bijnens, B., Thoen, J., Van de Werf, F., Sutherland, G. R., Suetens, P. 'Echocardiographic strain and strain-rate imaging: a new tool to study regional myocardial function'. IEEE Transactions on Medical Imaging, 2002; 21(9):1022–1030.

[54] Koyama, J., Ray-Sequin, P. A., Falk, R. H. 'Longitudinal myocardial function assessed by tissue velocity, strain, and strain rate tissue Doppler echocardiography in patients with AL (primary) cardiac amyloidosis'. Circulation, 2003; 107(19): 2446–2452.

[55] Prinzen, F. W., Hunter, W. C., Wyman, B. T., McVeigh, E. R. 'Mapping of regional myocardial strain and work during ventricular pacing: experimental study using magnetic resonance imaging tagging'. Journal of the American College of Cardiology, 1999; 33(6): 1735–1742.

[56] Cameli, M., Caputo, M., Mondillo, S., *et al.* 'Feasibility and reference values of left atrial longitudinal strain imaging by two-dimensional speckle tracking'. Cardiovascular Ultrasound, 2009; 7(1):1–6.

[57] Di Salvo, G., Russo, M. G., Paladini, D., *et al.* 'Two-dimensional strain to assess regional left and right ventricular longitudinal function in 100 normal foetuses'. European Heart Journal – Cardiovascular Imaging, 2008; 9(6):754–756.

[58] Brown, J., Jenkins, C., Marwick, T. H. 'Use of myocardial strain to assess global left ventricular function: a comparison with cardiac magnetic resonance and 3-dimensional echocardiography'. American Heart Journal, 2009; 157(1):102.e1–102.e5.

[59] Belghiti, H., Brette, S., Lafitte, S., *et al.* 'Automated function imaging: a new operator-independent strain method for assessing left ventricular function'. Archives of Cardiovascular Diseases, 2008; 101(3):163–169.

[60] Becker, M., Bilke, E., Kühl, H., *et al.* 'Analysis of myocardial deformation based on pixel tracking in two dimensional echocardiographic images enables quantitative assessment of regional left ventricular function'. Heart, 2006; 92(8):1102–1108.

[61] Perk, G., Tunick, P. A., Kronzon, I. 'Non-Doppler two-dimensional strain imaging by echocardiography – from technical considerations to clinical applications'. Journal of the American Society of Echocardiography, 2007; 20(3): 234–243.

[62] Kaluzynski, K., Chen, X., Emelianov, S. Y., Skovoroda, A. R., O'Donnell, M. 'Strain rate imaging using two-dimensional speckle tracking. IEEE Transactions on Ultrasonics, Ferroelectrics, and Frequency Control, 2001; 48(4):1111–1123.

[63] Hall, T. J., Jiang, J. 'Motion tracking for palpation imaging'. IEEE International Symposium on Biomedical Imaging: Nano to Macro; 2004. pp. 45–48.

[64] Serri, K., Reant, P., Lafitte, M., *et al.* 'Global and regional myocardial function quantification by two-dimensional strain: application in hypertrophic cardiomyopathy'. Journal of the American College of Cardiology, 2006; 47(6): 1175–1181.

[65] Koos, R., Altiok, E., Doetsch, J., *et al.* 'Layer-specific strain-encoded MRI for the evaluation of left ventricular function and infarct transmurality in patients with chronic coronary artery disease'. International Journal of Cardiology, 2013; 166(1): 85–89.

[66] Kowalski, M., Kukulski, T., Jamal, F., *et al.* 'Can natural strain and strain rate quantify regional myocardial deformation? A study in healthy subjects'. Ultrasound in Medicine and Biology, 2001; 27(8): 1087–1097.

[67] Yingchoncharoen, T., Agarwal, S., Popovic, Z. B., Marwick, T. H. 'Normal ranges of left ventricular strain: a meta-analysis'. Journal of the American Society of Echocardiography, 2013; 26(2): 185–191.

[68] Caballero, L., Kou, S., Dulgheru, R., *et al.* 'Echocardiographic reference ranges for normal cardiac Doppler data: results from the NORRE Study'. European Heart Journal Cardiovascular Imaging, 2005; 16(9): 1031–1041.

[69] Voigt, J. U., Lindenmeier, G., Werner, D., *et al.* 'Strain rate imaging for the assessment of preload-dependent changes in regional left ventricular diastolic longitudinal function'. Journal of the American Society of Echocardiography, 2002; 15(1):13–19.

[70] D'Elia, N., D'hooge, J., Marwick, T. H. 'Association between myocardial mechanics and ischemic LV remodelling'. Journal of the American College of Cardiology: Cardiovascular Imaging, 2015; 8(12), 1430–1443.

[71] Gjesdal, O., Hopp, E., Vartdal, T., *et al.* 'Global longitudinal strain measured by two-dimensional speckle tracking echocardiography is closely related to

myocardial infarct size in chronic ischaemic heart disease'. Clinical Science, 2007; 113(6): 287–296.

[72] Steelant, B., Stankovic, I., Roijakkers, I., *et al.* 'The impact of infarct location and extent on LV motion patterns: implications for dyssynchrony assessment'. Journal of the American College of Cardiology: Cardiovascular Imaging, 2016; 9(6): 655–664.

[73] Vartdal, T., Brunvand, H., Pettersen, E., *et al.* 'Early prediction of infarct size by strain Doppler echocardiography after coronary reperfusion'. Journal of the American College of Cardiology, 2007; 49(16): 1715–1721.

[74] Asanuma, T., Nakatani, S. 'Myocardial ischaemia and post-systolic shortening'. Heart, 2015; 101(7): 509–516.

[75] Braunwald, E., Kloner, R. A. 'The stunned myocardium: prolonged, post-ischemic ventricular dysfunction'. Circulation, 1982; 66(6):1146–1149.

[76] Götte, M. J., van Rossum, A. C., Twisk, J. W., Kuijer, J. P., Marcus, J. T., Visser, C. A. 'Quantification of regional contractile function after infarction: strain analysis superior to wall thickening analysis in discriminating infarct from remote myocardium'. Journal of the American College of Cardiology, 2001; 37(3): 808–817.

[77] Tejman-Yarden, S., Bratincsak, A., Bachner-Hinenzon, N., *et al.* 'Left ventricular mechanical property changes during acute AV synchronous right ventricular pacing in children'. Pediatric Cardiology, 2016; 37(1): 106–111.

[78] Tabassian, M., Alessandrini, M., De Marchi, L., *et al.* 'Principal component analysis for the classification of cardiac motion abnormalities based on echocardiographic strain and strain rate imaging'. International Conference on Functional Imaging and Modeling of the Heart, 2015; 201: 83–90.

[79] Tabassian, M., Alessandrini, M., Herbots, L., *et al.* 'Automatic detection of ischemic myocardium by spatio-temporal analysis of echocardiographic strain and strain rate curves'. IEEE International Ultrasonics Symposium (IUS); Sep 2015. pp. 1–4.

Chapter 17
Combined techniques of filtering and speckle tracking

Martino Alessandrini[1]

Abstract

Speckle tracking allows estimating tissue motion with ultrasound. Since tracking quality directly depends on image quality, several preprocessing techniques have been used to improve image quality and ease the tracking problem. The objective of this chapter is therefore to review such techniques and to provide some qualitative guidelines as to in which conditions they should and should not be employed.

17.1 Introduction

Speckle tracking techniques allow the automatic quantification of mechanical tissue properties (displacements/deformation/strain) with ultrasound. The basic principle exploited is that, at least roughly, the motion of speckle patterns correlates with the motion of the underlying tissue. As discussed in this book, there are several design choices in the development of a speckle tracking algorithm, which are synthetized in Figure 17.1. The first choice is whether using raw radiofrequency (RF) signals (if available) or B-mode pixel/voxel data. Data preprocessing can be employed to ease the following tracking problem. A further choice is what similarity metric to employ. A motion model could be used to regularize the displacement estimates (e.g. rigid motion, affine motion and b-spline parameterization). The resulting error metric will be optimized with a certain numerical solver. Finally, the motion field can be regularized, e.g. to remove outliers. Of note, these are only conceptual blocks which are not, at least not necessarily, applied sequentially. For instance, image smoothing and filtering of the displacement field can be both part of a coarse-to-fine elastic registration framework [1].

This chapter will focus on the preprocessing step, denoted by the red block in Figure 17.1. We note that, although image preprocessing, e.g. by edge-enhancing speckle removal, is widely used to improve segmentation, the use of preprocessing

[1]Department of Electrical, Electronic and Information Engineering, University of Bologna, Italy

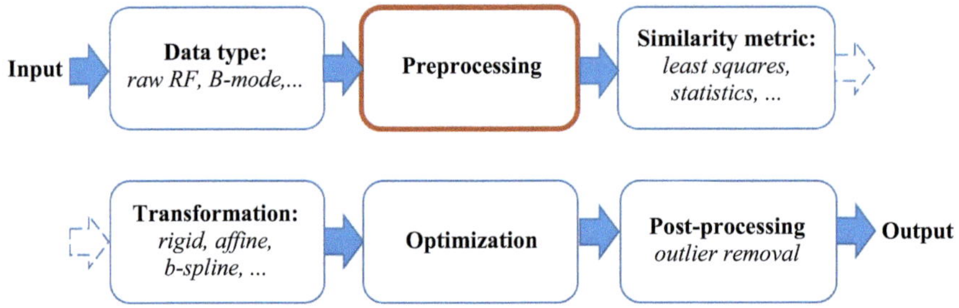

Figure 17.1 Basic building blocks of a speckle tracking algorithm

for speckle tracking should be done with caution and requires a careful consideration of the problem at hand. For instance, image de-speckling should not be applied if speckle-specific properties are used for tracking. Hereto, we note that many successful tracking techniques, some of which are reviewed in the recent comparison studies [2,3], work directly on native speckle images and do not apply a preprocessing step.

Existing preprocessing techniques can be grouped into five principal families:

- Techniques for *speckle removal*, or de-speckling, i.e. aiming to suppress speckle and preserve larger scale intensity variations, as due to the transitions between different tissues.
- Techniques for *feature tracking* [4]. Feature tracking is different from speckle tracking in that the tracking problem is limited to a discrete set of landmark points. A preprocessing step is therefore used to enhance and detect the salient image features to be tracked.
- Techniques to construct *parametric images* which, in turn, can be used for tracking in place of the native speckle images. We include in this family techniques making use of advanced feature representations, mostly coming from computer vision, such as image phase [5] and scale-invariant feature transform (SIFT) [6].
- *Deconvolution* techniques. Although yet unexplored in the context of speckle tracking, deconvolution could be employed to improve the estimation of small displacements and to mitigate the motion decorrelation problem.
- *Beamforming* techniques, aiming to improve speckle tractability by acting directly in the beam space, i.e. at the image formation stage.

Figure 17.2 provides a visual comparison between the five families of techniques considered on a common synthetic image. The figure shows obvious differences between the kinds of output produced.

A quantitative comparison of existing image preprocessing techniques is impossible. On one side, preprocessing is often presented as a constitutive part of an algorithm and not analysed separately. On the other, there is no comparison of existing techniques on common data. Hopefully, the recent efforts towards the creation of open access ultrasound datasets will help in this sense [2,3,7].

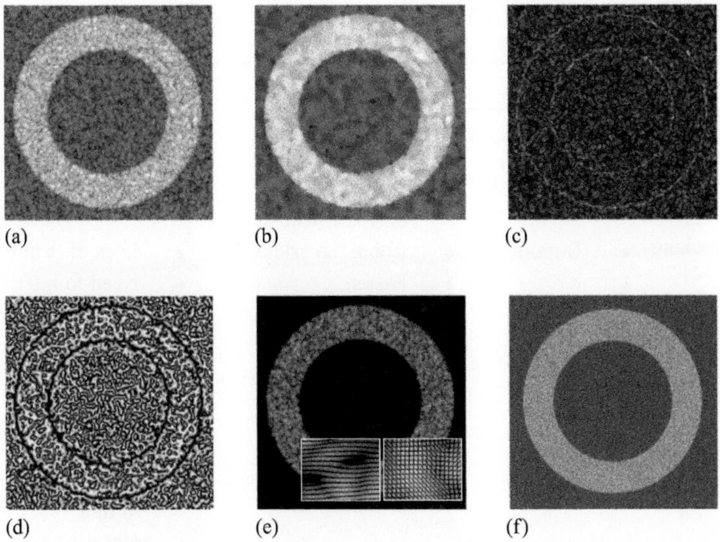

Figure 17.2 Visual comparison between the five families of techniques considered in this chapter when applied to a common synthetic image. (a) Simulated ultrasound image obtained by convolving a matrix of random numbers, representing the tissue response, with a synthetic point-spread function (cf. e.g. [26]). (b) De-speckled image by using speckle reducing anisotropic diffusion [27] and implemented in the 'despeckle filtering software toolbox' [28]. (c) Feature image used for feature tracking. Magnitude of the image gradient is used, as in [14]. (d) Parametric image of monogenic phase, computed as in [18]. Example of beamforming using transverse oscillations [24]. The two smaller subfigures illustrate the different speckle patterns (standard beamforming on the left, transverse oscillations on the right) on a 1 × 1 cm^2 zoom. Output of the deconvolution technique in [29], log-compressed to a 60 dB range to optimize visualization

In this context, the objectives of this chapter are:

- To review existing preprocessing techniques for speckle tracking and provide the references to the key papers. Hereto, the classification in five families presented above will be used.
- Given the apparent differences between the different techniques (cf. Figure 17.2), to establish some qualitative guidelines as to in which conditions each technique should and should not be employed. Such guidelines are also summarized in Table 17.1.

The chapter proceeds as follows: Section 17.2 discusses de-speckling techniques; feature tracking techniques are discussed in Section 17.3; parametric images are presented in Section 17.4; deconvolution techniques are discussed in Section 17.5

Table 17.1 Preprocessing techniques considered in the chapter

Technique	Data type	Pros	Cons
De-speckling [8–10]	• B-mode	• Matching of large structures • Regular displacement field	• Speckle coherency is lost • Loss of detail
Feature tracking [4, 11–16]	• B-mode • RF	• Robust to artefacts • Faster	• Loss of detail • Need to interpolate • Result depends on features used
Parametric images [6, 17–20]	• B-mode • RF	• Robust to artefacts	• Result depends on features used
Deconvolution	• RF • (B-mode)	• Can improve estimation of small displacements	• Heavy computation • Many parameters to tune • Not yet tested
Beamforming [20–25]	• RF • (B-mode)	• Can improve speckle trackability	• Requires costly research systems

and beamforming is discussed in Section 17.6. Discussions and concluding remarks are left to Section 17.7.

17.2 De-speckling

Speckle reduction is a common topic in medical ultrasound [30]. De-speckled images are assessed more easily by the clinician. Therefore, most commercial ultrasound systems apply image despeckling internally before display. Edge-enhancing speckle reduction can also improve automatic quantification by easing image segmentation.

There have been few attempts to apply image de-speckling to improve the performance of speckle tracking. On the one hand, de-speckling should be avoided when speckle specific properties are used for tracking, such as speckle statistics [31,32] and temporal coherency of speckle patterns [16]. On the other, de-speckling can be helpful when more generic intensity based criteria, as used for natural images, are employed, such as in elastic registration based on sum of squared differences [33] and optical flow.

By reducing image details, de-speckling helps match large structures, such as organ boundaries, while it misses the finer details contained in the motion of small speckle patches. Therefore, de-speckling should be avoided when small displacements are addressed, such as in RF tracking. For the same reason, de-speckling might be helpful in the case of large displacements, which reduce temporal correlation and might induce false detections, such as the ‘peak-hopping’ effect in block-matching techniques [34].

In [8], a modified version of Perona-Malik anisotropic diffusion was used to remove speckle noise from 3D echocardiographic recordings. An example output of anisotropic diffusion is given in Figure 17.2(b). Temporal resolution was ~10 frames per cardiac cycle and de-speckling was therefore employed to account for the large inter-frame displacements. Block-matching based on cross-correlation was then used for motion tracking.

In [9], the authors analyse the effects of pre-filtering and of the size of the region of interest in a block-matching algorithm for the estimation on cardiac motion with 2D echocardiography. Three despeckling solutions were considered: nonlinear Gaussian filter chain, adaptive anisotropic diffusion and a linear unsharp filter. The study shows that preprocessing with nonlinear filtration (either by nonlinear Gaussian or anisotropic diffusion) improves tracking only for the case of images with very strong reflectors. Conversely, unsharp masking did not improve the tracking accuracy. In image regions with relatively weak reflectors, the influence of nonlinear filtration was instead not significant.

The very recent [10] implemented a 'data-driven' denoising step, which intrinsically preserve the spatial and temporal correlation of the dataset. This is obtained by computing a *low-rank* approximation of the image time sequence, which is achieved by a singular value decomposition of the associated Casorati matrix, as explained in the paper. Elastic registration with a rigidity constraint was used to estimate cardiac displacement from 2D ultrafast (500 frames/s) echocardiographic recordings. Thanks to the fast matrix factorization techniques employed, this method can de-speckle an entire time series in few seconds and is therefore a computationally effective alternative to heavier solutions, such as anisotropic diffusion. Yet, it might be poorly generalizable to 3D due to the need to store and factorize the full spatio-temporal data matrix.

17.3 Feature tracking

As opposed to common speckle tracking, feature tracking algorithms limit the tracking problem to a set of preselected landmarks, which are more reliable and stable under tissue deformation. Such landmarks are computed by maximizing a given feature image. The global displacement field can then be computed by interpolation of the point estimates.

We note that only a very small number of techniques for feature tracking have been proposed. The common approach in speckle tracking is indeed to use either the full pixel image or a masked version of it, as in image registration, or a set of regularly spaced seed points, as in block matching. The advantage of speckle tracking against feature-tracking techniques is therefore that tissue displacement is assessed with a higher spatial resolution. The disadvantage is that there is often no quantitative measure to assess the reliability of the local displacement estimates, which, instead, is intrinsic of feature tracking approaches. Moreover, by acting on a limited number of points, feature tracking methods are computationally less demanding.

Of note, the problem of extracting corresponding features on image pairs is also proper of ultrasound mosaicking and fusion. Hereto, a number of feature descriptors have been used (see e.g. the recent [35] and the references therein). Since these techniques were not used within a speckle tracking problem, although several analogies exist, they will not be reviewed here.

Feature tracking was used in [11] to compute blood flow from 3D ultrasound RF data. Local maximum was used as image feature and the method was applied to RF data. Feature tracking was contrasted against block matching for 1D blood flow measurements in [12] where the two estimators were found to be comparable in terms of mean error while feature tracking exhibited a smaller error variance.

Other techniques were instead applied to B-mode data. In [4], the feature energy function consisted of a sum of oriented band-passed decompositions of ultrasound images using multichannel Gabor filters. An example of the obtained feature image is provided in Figure 17.3(a). The local maxima of the feature images are then computed and used as nodes of a deformable mesh to track tissue displacement.

In [13], one of the first commercial packages for cardiac strain estimation with 2D echo was evaluated. The algorithm tracks a set of pre-identified 'acoustic markers' (cf. Figure 17.3(b)). Yet, the specific way such markers were computed was not reported.

In [14,15], the feature points are instead selected based on the maximum image gradient (cf. Figure 17.2(c)). These are used within a sparse implementation of the popular Demons registration algorithm called Sparse Demons (cf. Figure 17.3(c)). In [14], Sparse Demons was applied to images of the liver, while in [15], it was used to compute cardiac strain with 3D echocardiograph. In the very recent [16], features were identified by selecting the pixel with largest intensity within a window of assigned size. A minimum distance between the feature points was further imposed. A combinatorial optimization problem (Munkres algorithm) was used to establish point correspondences between frames and therefore estimate displacement [16].

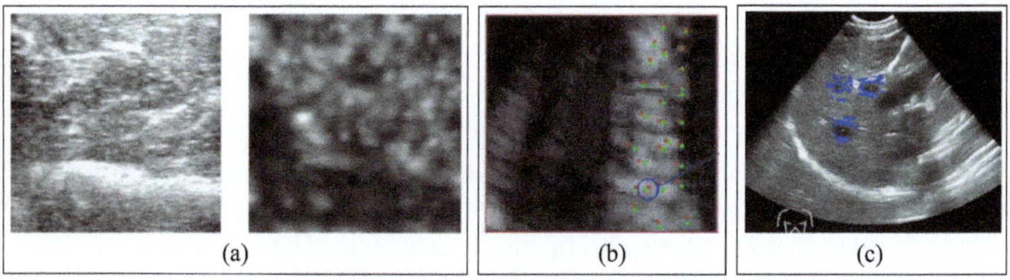

Figure 17.3 (a) Original image (left) and feature image obtained by Gabor filter bank filtering (right), modified from [4]. (b) Acoustical markers used for feature tracking, modified from [13]. (c) Markers used in the Sparse Demons registration of liver images, modified from Reference [14]

17.4 Parametric images

Few studies have based the tracking on parametric images instead of on the native pixel intensity. The rationale is to use features which are robust to common ultrasound artefacts that can bias standard motion estimators. In this sense, image phase has been proposed as a relevant feature for tracking. Image phase is robust to local intensity variations which might be due to shadowing or to the change in the angle between the ultrasound beam and cardiac fibres.

Phase can be used to perform 1D velocity measurements from RF signals, as done in colour Doppler. The principle exploits the fact that a time delay corresponds to a phase shift [21]. Local phase can be easily obtained by means of the Hilbert transform. The technique was extended to estimate 2D displacements from RF images with transverse oscillations (TO) in [20]. In order to do that, an n-D generalization of the Hilbert transform, based on single orthant signals, was used [20]. TO will be discussed in Section 17.5.

Local phase can also be used on B-mode images. Hereto, the original idea applied to natural image sequences, was developed in [36]. Computing image phase requires a generalization of the Hilbert transform to multiple dimensions. One way is to apply the 1D Hilbert transform separately along a given set of directions by using a bank of directional filter. Each direction is therefore decomposed in two components in quadrature with respect to each other, from which the phase can be computed. This approach was used in [17] and used for cardiac strain estimation with 3D ultrasound. The final displacement estimate was obtained by weighting the individual estimates coming from the directional filters.

Another possibility is to compute image phase by using the monogenic signal [5]. This way, image phase is uniquely computed from the response of a single pair of quadrature filters, i.e. not a bank of directional filters. By that, it reduces the computational burden and removes the need to choose specific directions. The quadrature filters used in the monogenic signal are

$$Q_1(\omega_x, \omega_y) = \frac{\omega_x}{\sqrt{\omega_x^2 + \omega_y^2}} B(\omega_x, \omega_y) \quad \text{and} \quad Q_2(\omega_x, \omega_y) = \frac{\omega_y}{\sqrt{\omega_x^2 + \omega_y^2}} B(\omega_x, \omega_y) \tag{17.1}$$

where ω_x and ω_y are the angular frequency components and $B(\omega_x, \omega_y)$ is an even rotationally invariant band-pass kernel. Common choices for B are Log-Gabor and differences of Poisson filters. Image phase can then be computed between the responses to Q_1 and Q_2. A monogenic phase based optic flow algorithm was used for cardiac motion estimation in [18] and extended to 3D in [19]. An image of monogenic phase is provided in Figure 17.2(d).

Recently, there have been noteworthy efforts towards the definition of a multi-resolution monogenic signal using steerable wavelets [37]. The recent framework, available in an open access toolbox[1], could be exploited for the definition of

[1] http://bigwww.epfl.ch/demo/steerable-wavelets/.

coarse-to-fine motion estimation algorithms exploiting different levels of approximation at different scales. Yet, this application remains unexplored.

Within this class of methods, we cite an attempt to use dense SIFT as a parametric image for motion estimation in [6]. The SIFT images were used to estimate liver displacement on images of the liver by using Log-Demons as a registration technique. SIFT is an extremely successful technique in computer vision to enhance distinctive features of images to perform 2D image registration. Yet, as recognized in [6], its application in medical images, and ultrasound in particular, remain largely unexplored. The work in [6] is therefore a noteworthy effort in this direction.

17.5 Deconvolution

Deconvolution aims to restore the acquired data (in our case, the insonified tissue) from the distortion/blur introduced by the measurement system (in our case, the ultrasound transducer). In soft tissues, ultrasound propagation can be assumed linear and the transducer effect can be represented by a linear convolution (hence, the name deconvolution):

$$y = h * x + n \tag{17.2}$$

where y is the beamformed RF signal, h is the impulse response (i.e. the point spread function PSF) of the ultrasound system, x is the tissue response (also called reflectivity function) and n is measurement noise. Deconvolution aimed therefore to estimate the tissue response x given the acquisition of y. In the simplest case, deconvolution can be performed with a linear filter, such as the Wiener filter, which implements a regularized inverse of the PSF h [39]. More advanced techniques aim instead to enforce sparse estimates of x. Physically, sparsity is a realistic assumption which accounts for the presence of few strong reflectors (e.g. the interfaces between tissues) against a background of weak scattering sites (i.e. the speckle). Sparsity constraints typically lead to more complex, sometimes non-convex, optimization problems which must be solved numerically [26,29]. A more methodical review of deconvolution techniques for medical ultrasound is beyond the scope of this manuscript. What's of interest here is that deconvolution could be exploited to improve motion estimation.

On one side, sparser images lead to narrower cross-correlation functions with better localized peaks. This can improve the reliability of the displacement estimate and reduce the susceptibility to local maxima. This is illustrated in Figure 17.4. In Figure 17.4, we considered a simulated B-mode image, in (a), and the result of deconvolution [29], in (c). Tissue reflectivity is used here as an example output of a (perfect) deconvolution algorithm. A translation of 2 pixels along x and y directions was applied to the same block extracted from the two images (the red squares in (a) and (c)) and the cross-correlation was then computed ((b) and (d)). Clearly, peak detection is becoming much easier in the deconvolved case.

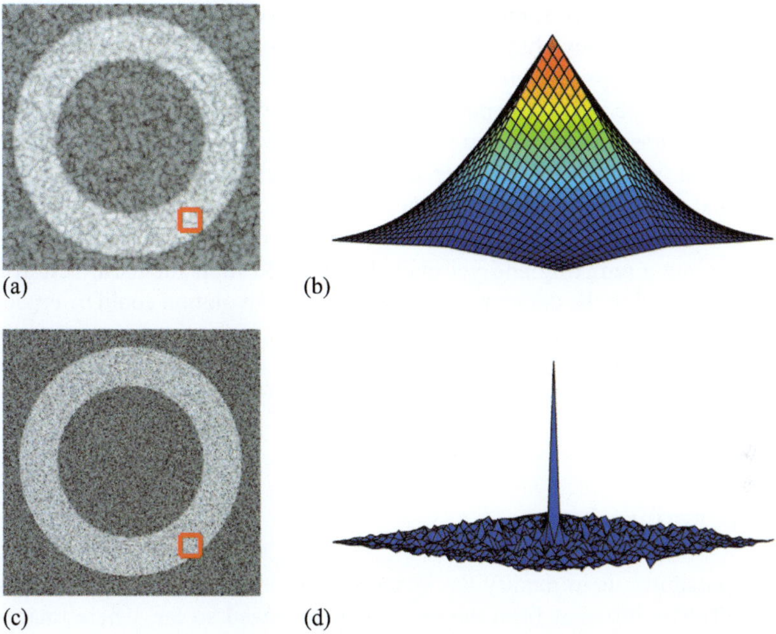

Figure 17.4 (b) Simulated B-mode image. (b) Correlation function between a block of (a) (in red) and its translated version of 2 pixels in each direction. (c) Result of the deconvolution algorithm in [29] (e.g. result of a perfect deconvolution), log compressed for the ease of visualization. (d) Correlation function between a block of (c) (in red) and its translated version of 2 pixels in each direction

Second, deconvolution can be used to mitigate the motion-feature decorrelation problem [40]. Motion-feature decorrelation refers to the possible discrepancy between the tissue motion and the motion of the associated speckle. Motion decorrelation is a consequence of the averaging effect due to the system PSF and therefore, barring very simple motions such as pure translations which are unrealistic in a real scenario, is always present [40]. Motion-feature decorrelation is often neglected in the design of a speckle-tracking algorithm. The main difficulty is that compensating for motion-feature decorrelation would imply knowing the kind of underlying motion (i.e. the amount of rotation and deformation) which is of course unknown beforehand. Deconvolution, ideally, would allow removing this uncertainty by reconstructing images of tissue motion directly, i.e. not based on speckle.

Despite these potential theoretical advantages, the use of deconvolution for motion estimation has remained so far largely unexplored. Apart of [41], where Wiener filtering is used, but its effect is not analysed separately. One main reason is the high computational cost, especially when sparse priors are involved [29,42], which conflicts with the real time capability of ultrasound. Another reason is that deconvolution requires acquiring raw RF signals which are available only in special research dedicated systems. Finally, also for the above reasons, medical ultrasound deconvolution has always had a very moderate appeal on the medical ultrasound community.

Yet, due to the gain in popularity of compressed sensing, and therefore the analysis of sparse signals, we are witnessing a revived interest on ultrasound deconvolution, which has resulted in the development of increasingly better performing and more computationally effective techniques [29,43–45]. Testing the effects on motion estimation, e.g. by using available open access ground truth data [3,46], remains a tempting and yet unexplored application for these new techniques. With respect to the diagram in Figure 17.1, deconvolution could be especially useful to improve the accuracy of RF based motion/strain estimates, e.g. by adding a refinement step on the deconvolved data. Ideally, this would require the development of *ad-hoc* motion estimators taking the sparse nature of deconvolved images into account.

17.6 Beamforming

Another possibility is to modify the image formation itself (i.e. the beamforming process). This is different from the techniques reviewed so far, where image and signal processing concepts are used to elaborate previously acquired (RF or B-mode) data. On the one side, modifying the beamformer requires specific technical knowledge of the ultrasound image formation process, moreover, it requires the availability of, typically expensive, research systems that allow accessing the individual channels. As such, beamforming techniques are typically proposed by laboratories whose focus is the development of the ultrasound technology.

Conventional beamforming consists in reconstructing the image line by line by using focused beams. Yet, designing new beamforming schemes is an active area of research. Hereto, one group of techniques aims to move away from the time resolution limit connected to line-by-line reconstruction in order to allowing for *ultrafast* imaging [47,48]. A second group of techniques aims instead to modify the PSF of the imaging system to improve image quality and quantification. This section will focus therefore on this second class of techniques. In particular, we will review those approaches that have been shown to compare favourably against conventional beamforming for tissue deformation imaging.

The beamforming technique that has been analysed more thoroughly in this sense is probably given by TO beamforming. The PSF, i.e. the image reconstructed from a single point target, of a conventional system can be parameterised as

$$h(x,z) = e^{-\frac{x^2}{\alpha_x}} e^{-\frac{z^2}{\alpha_z}} \cos(2\pi f_0 x) \tag{17.3}$$

where x and z are the axial (i.e. the direction of beam propagation) and lateral coordinates, f_0 is the centre frequency, i.e. the resonating frequency of the piezo-electric crystal, while α_x and α_z depend directly on the transducer's bandwidth and the aperture size, respectively [22,24].

The presence of the axial modulating component implies that motion estimation is intrinsically more accurate in the axial direction than in the lateral one, for two main reasons. First, the PSF's axial width is essentially given by the wavelength $\lambda_0 = (2\pi f_0)^{-1}$, which is smaller than the lateral width, established by α_z. Therefore, the cross-correlation function used for motion estimation will be more narrow in the axial direction. Second, the modulating component allows expressing a displacement as a phase-shift in the Fourier domain, which can be computed analytically with subpixel accuracy.

The goal of TO beamforming is therefore to ease the estimation of lateral displacements by introducing a modulating frequency in the direction perpendicular to the beam direction (cf. Figure 17.2(e)), thereby leading to a PSF of the kind:

$$h(x,z) = e^{-\alpha x^2} e^{-\beta z^2} \cos\left(2\pi f_{0,x} x\right) \cos\left(2\pi f_{0,z} z\right). \tag{17.4}$$

There are several ways to introduce TO. One common approach is to use a bimodal receive anodization function, where the distance between the two lobes defines the lateral oscillation frequency [49].

TO were initially proposed by Jensen *et al.* [21] for blood flow imaging. More recently, they were extended to phased arrays in use in echocardiography by Liebgott *et al.* [49]. The two perpendicular modulating components were exploited in the development of new TO-dedicated motion estimation algorithms based on directional Hilbert analysis [20]. TO were shown to compare favourably against standard beamforming for cardiac motion estimation in [24], where an implementation on the ULA-OP research platform [50] was also presented. The very recent [22] presents a theoretical analysis of motion estimation based on TO versus conventional focused beamforming. Hereto, several possible TO implementations were considered and an expression of the Cramer-Lao lower bound of jitter error was derived. The conclusion of that study was that the benefit of TO is limited to small displacements, while for large displacements such a benefit is overbalanced by an increase in motion decorrelation, which is due to the larger extent of the PSF with TO. TO were also used recently to evaluate lateral deformation of the common carotid artery wall, which was demonstrated by several studies to be associated with the presence of cardiovascular risk factors and to predict cardiovascular outcome in patients with suspected coronary artery disease [23].

Another beamforming sequence that was recently analysed for cardiac motion estimation is the *aperture domain model image reconstruction* (in short, ADMIRE). ADMIRE was proposed by Byram and coll. [51]. Briefly, it is a nonlinear beamforming scheme aimed to reduce image clutter by addressing multipath and off-axis sources. In [52], ADMIRE was applied to a set of synthetic echocardiographic data with assigned levels of diffuse and coherent clutter. Images reconstructed with ADMIRE were shown to improve the estimation of global longitudinal strain as compared to clutter-corrupted images. The motion estimation technique used in [52] was based on elastic registration applied to the B-mode images.

Figure 17.5 illustrates the TO (a, b) and ADMIRE (c, d) schemes against conventional beamforming on experimental acquisitions and simulations, respectively.

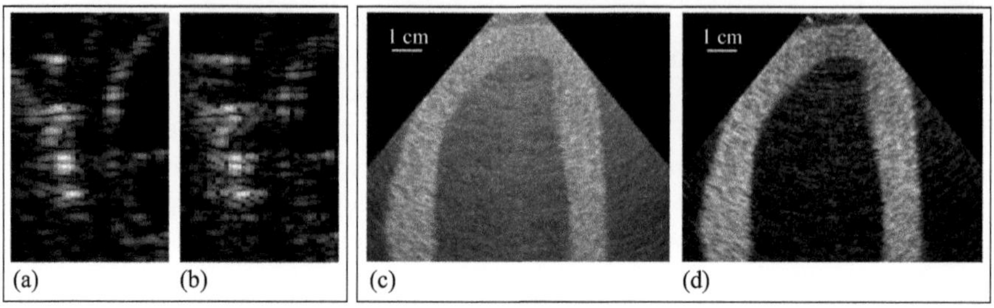

Figure 17.5 Image acquired with the ULA-OP experimental system with conventional beamforming (a) and transverse oscillations (b), modified from [24]. (c) Simulated image with diffuse clutter noise reconstructed with conventional beamforming (c) and with ADMIRE (d), modified from [52]

Finally, spatial coherence imaging [53] was shown to provide better contrast to noise ratio as compared to standard beamforming. This could imply a benefit in terms of deformation imaging. Yet, this specific application remains unexplored.

17.7 Conclusion

We reviewed several possible preprocessing strategies to improve speckle tracking estimates. They were grouped into five conceptually different families: techniques for speckle reduction; techniques to extract salient features for feature tracking; techniques to extract parametric images and deconvolution and beamforming techniques.

Preprocessing is not a necessary choice in speckle tracking and many state-of-the-art solutions don't employ such a step. In particular, a certain preprocessing technique might be relevant in certain conditions but disruptive in others. The goal of this chapter was therefore to review the principal approaches and to give some qualitative guidelines about their usage. The main considerations made are also summarized in Table 17.1.

Acknowledgements

The work of Martino Alessandrini is funded by the European Union's Horizon 2020 research and innovation programme under the Marie Skłodowska-Curie grant agreement No 659082. The author would like to thank Adrian Basarab for the help in generating the examples on image deconvolution.

References

[1] M. J. Ledesma-Carbayo, J. Kybic, M. Desco, *et al.*, "Spatio-temporal nonrigid registration for ultrasound cardiac motion estimation," *IEEE Trans. Med. Imaging*, vol. 24, no. 9, pp. 1113–1126, 2005.

[2] M. Alessandrini, B. Heyde, S. Queirós, *et al.* "Detailed evaluation of five 3D speckle tracking algorithms using synthetic echocardiographic recordings," *IEEE Trans. Med. Imaging*, vol. 62(January), pp. 1–13, 2016.

[3] M. De Craene, S. Marchesseau, B. Heyde, *et al.*, "3D strain assessment in ultrasound (Straus): A synthetic comparison of five tracking methodologies," *IEEE Trans. Med. Imaging*, vol. 32, no. 9, pp. 1632–1646, 2013.

[4] F. Yeung, S. F. Levinson, D. Fu, and K. J. Parker, "Feature-adaptive motion tracking of ultrasound image sequences using a deformable mesh," *IEEE Trans. Med. Imaging*, vol. 17, no. 6, pp. 945–956, 1998.

[5] M. Felsberg and G. Sommer, "The monogenic signal," *IEEE Trans. Signal Process.*, vol. 49, no. 12, pp. 3136–3144, 2001.

[6] A. Hallack, B. W. Papiez, A. Cifor, M. J. Gooding, and J. A. Schnabel, "Robust Liver Ultrasound Tracking using Dense. Distinctive Image Features," *Chall. Liver Ultrasound Track. (CLUST 2015), MICCAI*, 2015.

[7] O. Bernard, J. G. Bosch, B. Heyde, *et al.*, "Standardized evaluation system for left ventricular segmentation algorithms in 3D echocardiography," *IEEE Trans. Med. Imaging*, vol. 62, no. 4, pp. 967–977, April 2016. doi: 10.1109/TMI.2015.2503890.

[8] Q. Duan, E. D. Angelini, S. L. Herz, *et al.*, "Region-based endocardium tracking on real-time three-dimensional ultrasound," *Ultrasound Med. Biol.*, vol. 35, no. 2, pp. 256–265, 2009.

[9] V. Behar, D. Adam, P. Lysyansky, and Z. Friedman, "The combined effect of nonlinear filtration and window size on the accuracy of tissue displacement estimation using detected echo signals," *Ultrasonics*, vol. 41, no. 9, pp. 743–753, 2004.

[10] A. I. Aviles, T. Widlak, A. Casals, M. M. Nillesen, and H. Ammari, "Robust Cardiac Motion Estimation using Ultrafast Ultrasound Data: A Low-Rank-Topology-Preserving Approach," *Phys Med. Biol.*, vol. 62, no. 12, 4831–4851, 2017.

[11] G. R. Bashford and O. T. von Ramm, "Ultrasound three-dimensional velocity measurements by feature tracking," *IEEE Trans. Ultrason. Ferroelectr. Freq. Control*, vol. 43, no. 3, pp. 376–384, 1996.

[12] G. R. Bashford and D. J. Robinson, "Direct comparison of feature tracking and autocorrelation for velocity estimation," *IEEE Trans. Ultrason. Ferroelectr. Freq. Control*, vol. 54, no. 4, pp. 757–767, April 2007.

[13] M. Leitman, P. Lysyansky, S. Sidenko, *et al.*, "Two-dimensional strain – a novel software for real-time quantitative echocardiographic assessment of myocardial function," *J. Am. Soc. Echocardiogr.*, vol. 17, no. 10, pp. 1021–1029, 2004.

[14] O. Somphone, S. Allaire, B. Mory, and C. Dufour, "Live feature tracking in ultrasound liver sequences with sparse demons," *Proc. MICCAI Work. Chall. Liver Ultrasound Track.*, no. August, 2015.

[15] O. Somphone, M. De Craene, R. Ardon, *et al.*, "Fast myocardial motion and strain estimation in 3D cardiac ultrasound with Sparse Demons," 2013 *IEEE*

10th International Symposium on Biomedical Imaging, San Francisco, CA, pp. 1182–1185, 2013.

[16] M. V. Andersen, C. Moore, K. Arges, *et al.*, "High-frame-rate deformation imaging in two dimensions using continuous speckle-feature tracking," *Ultrasound Med. Biol.*, vol. 42, no. 11, pp. 2606–2615, 2016.

[17] L. Tautz, A. Hennemuth, and H.-O. Peitgen, "Quadrature filter based motion analysis for 3D ultrasound sequences," in *Statistical Atlases and Computational Models of the Heart. Imaging and Modelling Challenges: Third International Workshop, STACOM 2012, Held in Conjunction with MICCAI 2012, Nice, France*, October 5, 2012, Revised Selected Papers, O. Camara, T. Mansi, M. Pop, K. Rhode, M. Sermesant, and A. Young, Eds. Berlin, Heidelberg: Springer Berlin Heidelberg, 2013, pp. 169–177.

[18] M. Alessandrini, A. Basarab, H. Liebgott, and O. Bernard, "Myocardial motion estimation from medical images using the monogenic signal," *IEEE Trans. Image Process.*, vol. 22, no. 3, pp. 1084–1095, 2013.

[19] M. Alessandrini, H. Liebgott, D. Barbosa, and O. Bernard, "Monogenic phase based optical flow computation for myocardial motion analysis in 3D echocardiography," *Lect. Notes Comput. Sci. (including Subser. Lect. Notes Artif. Intell. Lect. Notes Bioinformatics)*, vol. 7746 LNCS, pp. 159–168, 2013.

[20] A. Basarab, H. Liebgott, and P. Delachartre, "Analytic estimation of subsample spatial shift using the phases of multidimensional analytic signals," *IEEE Trans. Image Process.*, vol. 18, no. 2, pp. 440–447, February 2009.

[21] J. A. Jensen and P. Munk, "A new method for estimation of velocity vectors," *IEEE Trans. Ultrason. Ferroelectr. Freq. Control*, vol. 45, no. 3, pp. 837–851, 1998.

[22] B. Heyde, N. Bottenus, J. D'hooge, and G. E. Trahey, "Evaluation of the transverse oscillation technique for cardiac phased-array imaging: a theoretical study," *IEEE Trans. Ultrason. Ferroelectr. Freq. Control*, vol. 64, no. 2, pp. 320–334, Feb. 2017.

[23] G. Zahnd, S. Salles, H. Liebgott, D. Vray, A. Sérusclat, and P. Moulin, "Real-time ultrasound-tagging to track the 2D motion of the common carotid artery wall in vivo Real-time ultrasound-tagging to track the 2D motion of the common carotid artery wall in vivo," vol. 820, no. 2, pp. 820–830, 2015.

[24] M. Alessandrini, A. Basarab, L. Boussel, *et al.*, "A new technique for the estimation of cardiac motion in echocardiography based on transverse oscillations: a preliminary evaluation in silico and a feasibility demonstration in vivo," *IEEE Trans. Med. Imaging*, vol. 33, no. 5, pp. 1148–1162, 2014.

[25] B. Heyde and B. Byram, "Non-linear Beamforming with ADMIRE to Facilitate Deformation Imaging in Cluttered Cardiac Ultrasound," *2016 IEEE International Ultrasonics Symposium (IUS)*, Tours, pp. 1–4, 2016.

[26] M. Alessandrini, S. Maggio, J. Porée, *et al.*, "A restoration framework for ultrasonic tissue characterization," *IEEE Trans. Ultrason. Ferroelectr. Freq. Control*, vol. 58, no. 11, pp. 2344–2360, 2011.

[27] Y. Yu and S. T. Acton, "Speckle reducing anisotropic diffusion.," *IEEE Trans. Image Process.*, vol. 11, no. 11, pp. 1260–1270, January 2002.

[28] C. P. Loizou, C. Theofanous, M. Pantziaris, and T. Kasparis, "Despeckle filtering software toolbox for ultrasound imaging of the common carotid artery," *Comput. Methods Programs Biomed.*, vol. 114, no. 1, pp. 109–124, 2014.

[29] N. Zhao, A. Basarab, D. Kouamé, and J. Y. Tourneret, "Joint segmentation and deconvolution of ultrasound images using a hierarchical Bayesian model based on generalized Gaussian priors," *IEEE Trans. Image Process.*, vol. 25, no. 8, pp. 3736–3750, 2016.

[30] C. Loizou and C. Pattichis, *Despeckle Filtering Algorithms and Software for Ultrasound Imaging*. San Rafael, CA: Morgan & Claypool, 2008.

[31] A. Porras, M. Alessandrini, M. De Craene, *et al.*, "Improved myocardial motion estimation combining tissue Doppler and B-mode echocardiographic images," *IEEE Trans. Med. Imaging*, vol. 33, no. 11, pp. 2098–2106, 2014. doi: 10.1109/TMI.2014.2331392.

[32] B. Cohen and I. Dinstein, "New maximum likelihood motion estimation schemes for noisy ultrasound images," *Pattern Recognit.*, vol. 35, no. 2, pp. 455–463, 2002.

[33] D. Rueckert, L. I. Sonoda, C. Hayes, D. L. Hill, M. O. Leach, and D. J. Hawkes, "Nonrigid registration using free-form deformations: application to breast MR images," *IEEE Trans. Med. Imaging*, vol. 18, no. 8, pp. 712–721, August 1999.

[34] M. McCormick, N. Rubert, and T. Varghese, "Bayesian regularization applied to ultrasound strain imaging," *IEEE Trans. Biomed. Eng.*, vol. 58, no. 6, pp. 1612–1620, 2011.

[35] R. J. Schneider, D. P. Perrin, N. V Vasilyev, G. R. Marx, P. J. del Nido, and R. D. Howe, "Real-time image-based rigid registration of three-dimensional ultrasound," *Med. Image Anal.*, vol. 16, no. 2, pp. 402–414, 2012.

[36] D. J. Fleet and A. D. Jepson, "Computation of component image velocity from local phase information," *Int. J. Comput. Vis.*, vol. 5, no. 1, pp. 77–104, 1990.

[37] M. Unser, N. Chenouard, and D. Van De Ville, "Steerable pyramids and tight wavelet frames in L_{2}({BBR}^{d})," *IEEE Trans. Image Process.*, vol. 20, no. 10, pp. 2705–2721, 2011.

[38] M. Unser, D. Sage, and D. Van De Ville, "Multiresolution monogenic signal analysis using the Riesz–Laplace wavelet transform," *IEEE Trans. Image Process.*, vol. 18, no. 11, pp. 2402–2418, Nov. 2009.

[39] T. Taxt, "Three-dimensional blind deconvolution of ultrasound images," *IEEE Trans. Ultrason. Ferroelectr. Freq. Control*, vol. 48, no. 4, pp. 867–871, 2001.

[40] W. Yu, P. Yan, A. J. Sinusas, K. Thiele, and J. S. Duncan, "Towards pointwise motion tracking in echocardiographic image sequences – comparing the reliability of different features for speckle tracking," *Med. Image Anal.*, vol. 10, no. 4, pp. 495–508, 2006.

[41] M. Mischi, N. Kuijsters, F. Sammali, C. Rabotti, and B. Schoot, "Feasibility of uterine speckle tracking for improved embryo implantation," 2015 *IEEE International Ultrasonics Symposium (IUS)*, Taipei, pp. 1–4, 2015.

[42] Z. Chen, A. Basarab, and D. Kouamé, "Compressive deconvolution in medical ultrasound imaging," *IEEE Trans. Med. Imaging*, vol. 35, no. 3, pp. 728–737, 2016.

[43] O. Lorintiu, H. Liebgott, M. Alessandrini, O. Bernard, and D. Friboulet, "Compressed sensing reconstruction of 3D ultrasound data using dictionary learning and line-wise subsampling," *IEEE Trans. Med. Imaging*, vol. 34, no. 12, pp. 2467–2477, 2015.

[44] N. Zhao, Q. Wei, A. Basarab, D. Kouam, and J. Y. Tourneret, "Blind deconvolution of medical ultrasound images using a parametric model for the point spread function," in *2016 IEEE International Ultrasonics Symposium (IUS)*, 2016, pp. 1–4.

[45] Z. Chen, A. Basarab, and D. Kouamé, "Reconstruction of enhanced ultrasound images from compressed measurements using simultaneous direction method of multipliers," *IEEE Trans. Ultrason. Ferroelectr. Freq. Control*, vol. 63, no. 10, pp. 1525–1534, 2016.

[46] M. Alessandrini, M. De Craene, O. Bernard, *et al.*, "A pipeline for the generation of realistic 3D synthetic echocardiographic sequences: methodology and open-access database.," *IEEE Trans. Med. Imaging*, vol. 34, no. 7, pp. 1436–1451, July 2015.

[47] M. Tanter and M. Fink, "Ultrafast imaging in biomedical ultrasound," *IEEE Trans. Ultrason. Ferroelectr. Freq. Control*, vol. 61, no. 1, pp. 102–119, 2014.

[48] M. Cikes, L. Tong, G. R. Sutherland, and J. D'hooge, "Ultrafast cardiac ultrasound imaging: technical principles, applications, and clinical benefits," *JACC Cardiovasc. Imaging*, vol. 7, no. 8, pp. 812–823, 2014.

[49] H. Liebgott, A. Basarab, P. Gueth, D. Friboulet, and P. Delachartre, "Transverse oscillations for tissue motion estimation," *Ultrasonics*, vol. 50, no. 6, pp. 548–555, 2010.

[50] P. Tortoli, L. Bassi, E. Boni, A. Dallai, F. Guidi, and S. Ricci, "ULA-OP: an advanced open platform for ultrasound research," *IEEE Trans. Ultrason. Ferroelectr. Freq. Control*, vol. 56, no. 10, pp. 2207–2216, 2009.

[51] B. Byram and M. Jakovljevic, "Ultrasonic multipath and beamforming clutter reduction: a chirp model approach," *IEEE Trans. Ultrason. Ferroelectr. Freq. Control*, vol. 61, no. 3, pp. 428–440, 2014.

[52] B. Heyde, K. Dei, and B. Byram, "Non-linear beamforming with ADMIRE to facilitate deformation imaging in cluttered cardiac ultrasound," in *2016 IEEE International Ultrasonics Symposium (IUS)*, 2016, pp. 1–4.

[53] G. Pinton, G. Trahey, and J. Dahl, "Spatial coherence in human tissue: implications for imaging and measurement," *IEEE Trans. Ultrason. Ferroelectr. Freq. Control*, vol. 61, no. 12, pp. 1976–1987, 2014.

Chapter 18
Summary and future directions

Jan D'hooge[1,2] and Lasse Lovstakken[2]

Although ultrasound motion estimation has many applications in distinct scientific domains, within the medical field, motion estimation naturally goes hand in hand with cardiac imaging. As such, it is not surprising to see that most practical examples discussed in this part of the book relate to the heart despite the fact the motion estimation methodologies presented are generic.

Myocardial motion and deformation imaging based on echocardiographic recordings was introduced in the late 1990s and was originally based on the Doppler principle [1]. As a result, the technique could only assess the component of the velocity/deformation in the direction of wave propagation (i.e., the direction of the image line), which brought about several disadvantages such as the angle dependency of the measurement as well as a cumbersome and time-consuming analysis process. To tackle some of these pitfalls, speckle tracking was reintroduced in the mid noughties [2] after it had been conceptually demonstrated in the early 1980s. At present, many commercial 2D speckle tracking solutions exist, most of which are based on the block-matching principle applied to the B-mode data (cf. Chapter 14), implying that the motion estimation is done locally in independent windows with a posteriori filtering of the resulting motion field. Moreover, given that 3D systems have become more readily clinically available, extension of speckle tracking to 3D seemed a very logic next step. Indeed, since the late noughties, the state-of-the-art motion/deformation estimation is done in 3D thereby giving access to the complex cardiac mechanics from a single volumetric recording [3]. Also for 3D, the commercially available solutions are mostly based on processing the B-mode data using a block-matching approach.

Although 2D and 3D tracking solutions are often said to be independent of insonation angle (in contrast to Doppler), this is not entirely true. Indeed, ultrasound image resolution is intrinsically anisotropic due to the underlying wave physics (cf. Chapter 1) implying that speckle has a finer structure in the direction along the ultrasound beam than orthogonal to it (cf. Chapter 2). As a result, tracking speckle is intrinsically easier/more accurate along the ultrasound line than

[1]Department of Cardiovascular Sciences, University of Leuven, Belgium
[2]Department of Circulation and Medical Imaging, Norwegian University of Science and Technology (NTNU), Norway

orthogonal to it and, in this sense, it is to be expected that the accuracy and robustness of the motion/deformation estimates do remain dependent on the insonation angle. This theoretical consideration has also been experimentally demonstrated [4]. As such, a more accurate phrasing would be that 2D/3D tracking solutions are *less dependent* on insonation angle compared to Doppler. Because of this intrinsic limitation, it is not surprising to see that in the clinical setting only the use of the motion/deformation component along the ultrasound line is recommended despite the underlying 2D/3D tracking technologies [5]. Potentially, registration-based approaches (as presented in Chapter 15) could mitigate this problem by imposing boundary conditions on the motion/deformation field during the estimation process rather than doing this purely a posteriori (i.e., independent of the image information) as currently done in most commercial solutions. Although this seems attractive and has already been demonstrated to show advantages over block matching in experimental conditions [6], image registration-based approaches cannot overcome the intrinsic nature of ultrasound image formation. Moreover, the computational workload associated with these registration approaches makes their translation to a clinical workflow more challenging although relatively fast solutions have already been presented [7].

Many studies have shown the potential benefit of measuring myocardial mechanical properties for clinical decision-making and patient follow-up. Figure 18.1 gives the number of publications found in PubMed for the past 15 years (data captured November 2014) for each of the available motion/strain modalities. Clearly, the number of Doppler-based motion and deformation imaging publications steadily increased until 2008 after which its numbers went down. This was obviously the result of the introduction of the user friendlier speckle tracking

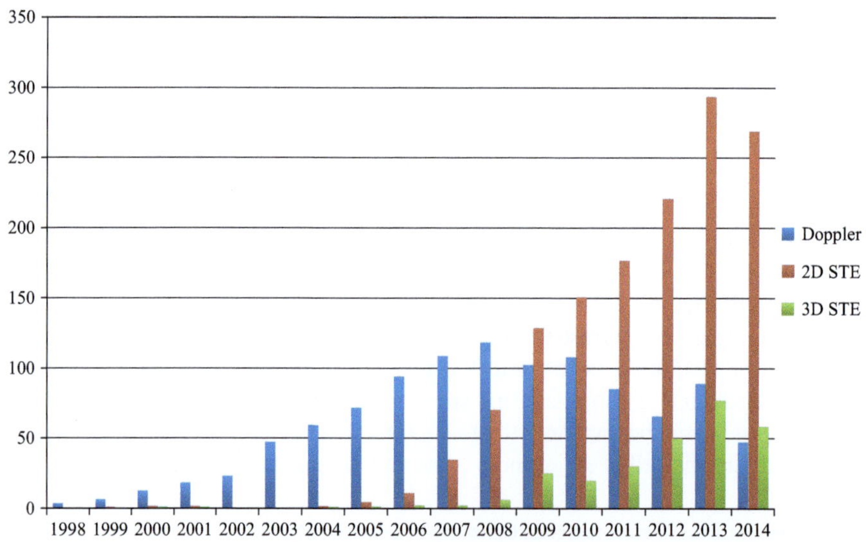

Figure 18.1 Number of publications on echocardiographic motion/deformation imaging over the past 15 years (data captured November 2014)

technique in 2005 that quickly took over literature and started producing about one publication a day. Although 3D speckle tracking was introduced shortly after the 2D technique, it didn't have the same (publication) impact and the number of publications based on 3D tracking is not (yet) catching up with its 2D correlate. This is likely due to the fact that: (i) 3D systems are still not as widely spread as 2D systems; (ii) 3D imaging remains more challenging as is 3D tracking; (iii) 2D remains the cornerstone of clinical echo and (iv) fewer 3D commercial speckle tracking solutions exist. These figures clearly demonstrate that motion/deformation imaging technology draws significant interest that is, likely driven by the clinical need for better (quantitative) descriptors of (regional) cardiac function.

Although 3D motion/deformation estimation may seem the best technology currently available as it gives access to all strain components in the entire left ventricle, this increased field-of-view and 3D velocity/deformation information comes at a cost. Indeed, at present, 3D image quality remains inferior to 2D not only in terms of spatial resolution but also in terms of signal-to-noise ratio and—most importantly—in terms of temporal resolution. As such, all motion/deformation technologies currently available have their intrinsic strengths and weaknesses that are schematically summarized in Table 18.1. Based on this summary, it is clear that all technologies remain relevant, and the best methodology at hand might be application dependent. Indeed, for regional pathology, it may be more relevant to have good spatial resolution (e.g., ischemia) while for others time resolution might be critical (e.g., diagnosis requiring exercise testing) while for yet others sensitivity might be the bottle neck (e.g., monitoring the cardiotoxicity of chemotherapy).

Given these strengths and weaknesses of the different approaches, hybrid solutions combining their strengths while avoiding their weaknesses might be of benefit. In this context, Amundsen *et al.* demonstrated that the combination of Doppler and (block-matching based) speckle tracking might be beneficial [8] while Porras *et al.* entered the Doppler information in the cost function to be optimized for B-mode tracking in an image registration framework [9,10]. However, further work toward optimally combining different approaches is still required.

Despite the current pitfalls of 3D echocardiographic motion/deformation imaging, it can be anticipated that, on the mid-term, this 3D modality will become

Table 18.1 Schematic overview of the strengths and weaknesses of the current motion/deformation imaging approaches

	Spatial resolution	**Temporal resolution**	**SNR**	**Field of view**	**Number of motion/strain components**	**Angle independent**
Doppler-based*	+	++	++	−	−	−−
2D speckle tracking	+	+	+	+	+	+
3D speckle tracking	−−	−−	−	++	++	++

*Assuming narrow-angle acquisitions in order to keep the spatiotemporal resolution adequate.

the standard. Indeed, the pitfalls of lower spatiotemporal resolution and signal-to-noise ratio (SNR) of the volumetric data sets are being challenged by the introduction of better matrix array transducers, new imaging front ends (i.e., systems), and improved imaging techniques and solutions for image quantification. All these combined will ultimately result in large field of view, volumetric data sets of the heart at high spatial and temporal resolution with an excellent SNR.

Although an extensive overview of all technical options currently being explored for high spatiotemporal resolution (volumetric) imaging falls outside the scope of this book, two examples will be given. The reader is referred to recent literature for more information [11,12].

A first option to reduce the acquisition time for a single image or volume is to form several image lines from each emitted pulse, often referred to as multiline acquisition or parallel beamforming [13,14]. In order to exploit this option, broader transmit pulses are used at the expense of lateral image quality as well as SNR. This technique has been used with success for focused imaging, typically increasing the frame rate by 2–4 without significant trade-offs. More recently, this concept has been pushed further, as already briefly mentioned in Chapter 1, by transmitting very broad pulses in order to "illuminate" the whole heart with a single transmission and reconstruct the entire (3D) image from the received echo signals [15]. Although this approach allows going up to 5,000 Hz volumetric imaging, SNR and spatial resolution are compromised unless additional transmits are done for averaging (i.e., compounding). As such, the technique requires finding a compromise between SNR, time and space resolution. As an alternative approach, acquisition time for a single image is reduced by transmitting multiple image lines at once, i.e., multiline transmit imaging. Although this could result in cross talk between the different transmit beams, it has been demonstrated that the image quality obtained remains good when the system is correctly set up. In this way, the feasibility of high spatial resolution 2D imaging at good SNR at a frame rate of 450 Hz for a full field of view of 90-degree sector image was recently demonstrated [16]. These concepts have recently been explored for 3D imaging as well [17]. In summary, however, it is clear that new imaging strategies will be developed over the next years in order to allow for large field-of-view (volumetric) imaging at high spatiotemporal resolution. Realistically, we can expect to obtain an effective time resolution of about 500–1,000 Hz (i.e., 1–2 ms). When imaging the heart at such time resolution, short-lived mechanical cardiac events can be studied in detail, which could bring valuable information on cardiac mechanics and pathophysiology [11].

High frame rate imaging will facilitate accurate motion/deformation estimation in two ways. First, the added temporal information can be used to enable more sophisticated filtering techniques, thereby enhancing the speckle/features to be tracked and hence the accuracy of the estimate (cf. Chapter 17). Second, the improved time information limits decorrelation between subsequent recordings, thereby facilitating the use of RF-based motion estimators that are known to be more sensitive to subtle motion/deformation (cf. Chapters 13 and 14). In fact, in order to ensure sufficient RF correlation between subsequent recordings, current systems make use of a packet-based acquisition scheme in which the acquisition of a given image line is repeated prior to the entire image has been recorded. Such a packet-based approach can clearly also be used with novel beam-forming schemes in order to guarantee sufficient correlation between subsequent recordings to enable RF-based tracking.

Similarly, new methodologies toward improved motion/deformation that require a dedicated acquisition scheme are being developed (cf. Chapters 13 and 17). It can be anticipated that these newer methods will be introduced on commercial systems in the following years thereby making the (3D) assessment of cardiac mechanics more sensitive, accurate and robust. With the ever-increasing power of modern computer architecture, it can also be anticipated that real-time solutions toward motion/deformation imaging will be introduced so that off-line processing is no longer required.

18.1 Automation

Next to better quality motion/deformation information (i.e., robust 3D at high space–time resolution), also the analysis process will be further automated. Indeed, at present, a rather time-consuming and tedious part of the postprocessing is related to (automated) identification of the region of interest, i.e., the myocardium, to be analyzed. Solutions toward fully automatic segmentation of the left ventricular myocardium as well as the whole heart are currently being developed and can be expected to enter the clinics in the following years. This implies that no user interaction will be required in order to generate a bull's eye representation of the mechanical properties of the heart. An example of such an automatically generated bull's eye of the end-systolic strain was proposed in [18] (cf. Figure 18.2). More recently, Philips has commercially released a workflow combining automatic image segmentation with subsequent speckle tracking. It can be anticipated that such an automated analysis will become the standard thereby reducing (and even

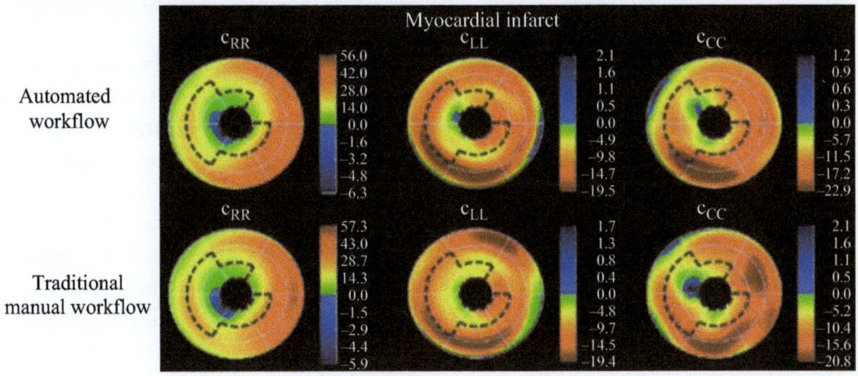

Figure 18.2 Bull's eye plot of the radial (left), longitudinal (middle) and circumferential (right) end-systolic strain of a patient with an apical infarction generated by conventional manual analysis (bottom) and fully automated analysis (top)

eliminating) intra- and interobserver variability as well as processing time. As both these factors are critically important in making a technique viable in the clinical setting, this will thus have a significant impact on daily use of these techniques in the clinical echo lab.

Moreover, it can be anticipated that interpretation of the extracted motion/strain information will be performed in a computer-assisted manner. At present, end-systolic strain and—for the Doppler-based methodology—peak systolic strain rate are typically considered to be (techno)markers of regional myocardial function where specific cutoff values for normality are considered. Of course, it is well known that such cutoffs should take boundary conditions such as ventricular size, blood pressure, gender, etc. into account. For example, to date, the magnitude of the end-systolic strain cannot distinguish increased local loading conditions from a reduced local contractile status (i.e., intrinsic function). This remains a major limitation of the current methodologies.

Two approaches to tackle this problem are being explored. On the one hand, a statistical approach can be taken where normal as well as abnormal motion/strain profiles are "learned" by a computer algorithm in a training phase whereby the operator guides the algorithm in identifying normal and abnormal cases. Subsequently, these algorithms can then identify whether a newly measured motion/strain curve is likely normal or not e.g., [19,20]. Similarly, advanced statistical methods can learn what the impact of e.g., blood pressure or gender on the appearance of the (ab)normal strain curve is and take this into consideration when classifying a given measurement [21]. Interestingly, these methods do not only consider the values at end systole but take the full temporal behavior of the measured curves into account as well as how they spatially relate. The latter can be particularly relevant in picking up subtle changes in regional mechanical properties and how they would interact with equally subtle changes in other segments. Such effect might be very difficult to capture visually but would naturally appear in such machine-learning approaches. An example of a machine learned likelihood of normality for cardiac deformation is given in Figure 18.3.

Alternatively, a more mechanistic approach toward data interpretation can be taken by feeding the echographic mechanical measurements into a biomechanical model. Certain parameters of the model (e.g., regional active contraction force or viscosity) can then be deduced from the mechanical measurements in an integrated and consistent way by optimizing the parameters of the model in order to make the model fit the experimental data at hand [23,24]. This model-based mechanistic approach could not only support interpretation of the measurements but could also provide new (techno)markers for disease that can otherwise not be directly measured [24,25].

Finally, both approaches toward the interpretation of motion/deformation measurements could be used to try to distinguish true measurements from measurement artifacts. Indeed, as for any measuring technique, motion and deformation estimates can contain artifacts which make the clinical use of this information much more cumbersome as clinicians don't know whether they should treat the abnormal behavior of the motion/deformation data as a source of information on pathology or whether they should disregard this information as being corrupted.

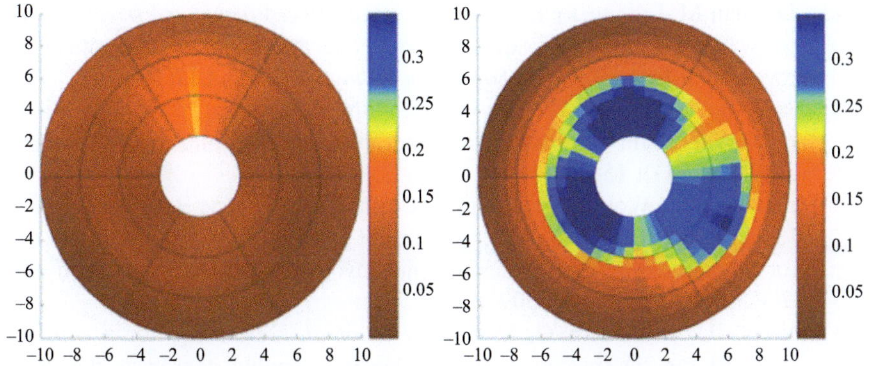

Figure 18.3 Bull's-eye likelihood maps of the regional myocardial strain profile being abnormal for a normal subject (left) and a patient with an apical infarction (right). From [22]

To date, no good quality-assurance mechanism has been proposed although the first steps toward machine-learning-based feedback have been made [26].

In summary, it can thus be anticipated that motion/deformation imaging is going to make major steps forward in the near future by

- Becoming a true 3D imaging modality in which 3D motion and deformation can be assessed reliably and accurately, at a high spatiotemporal resolution.
- Being fully automatic allowing to analyze the acquired images without further user interaction in a matter of seconds or even in real time.
- Supporting data interpretation via advanced statistical analyses and/or biomechanical modeling.

Overall, we can thus envision that, within the next decade, ultrasound characterization of the mechanical properties of organs will become similar to the current electrocardiogram workflow: after the patient has been prepared for data acquisition and data has been captured, subsequent data analysis is done in an automatic manner thereby generating a protocol for the patient that remains to be validated by the physician. In fact, a fully automatic image analysis/interpretation framework in the context of echocardiography was very recently proposed with very promising results [27]. On the longer term, we can envision that similar approaches will be made available on portable, handheld and even wearable systems. These developments combined with cloud computing will allow building huge databases on (normal) biomechanics of organs, thereby continuously improving the power and the accuracy of the automatically generated protocols.

References

[1] Sutherland GR, Stewart MJ, Groundstroem KW, *et al.* Color Doppler myocardial imaging: a new technique for the assessment of myocardial function. *J Am Soc Echocardiogr.* 1994 Sep–Oct;7(5): 441–58.

[2] Leitman M, Lysyansky P, Sidenko S, *et al.* Two-dimensional strain-a novel software for real-time quantitative echocardiographic assessment of myocardial function. *J Am Soc Echocardiogr.* 2004 Oct;17(10): 1021–9.
[3] Jasaityte R, Heyde B, D'hooge J. Current state of three-dimensional myocardial strain estimation using echocardiography. *J Am Soc Echocardiogr.* 2013 Jan;26(1): 15–28.
[4] Langeland S, Wouters PF, Claus P, Leather HA, Bijnens B, Sutherland GR, Rademakers FE, D'hooge J. Experimental assessment of a new research tool for the estimation of two-dimensional myocardial strain. *Ultrasound Med Biol.* 2006 Oct;32(10): 1509–13.
[5] Voigt JU, Pedrizzetti G, Lysyansky P, *et al.* Definitions for a common standard for 2D speckle tracking echocardiography: consensus document of the EACVI/ASE/Industry Task Force to standardize deformation imaging. *J Am Soc Echocardiogr.* 2015 Feb;28(2): 183–93.
[6] Heyde B, Jasaityte R, Barbosa D, *et al.* Elastic image registration versus speckle tracking for 2-D myocardial motion estimation: a direct comparison in vivo. *IEEE Trans Med Imaging.* 2013 Feb;32(2): 449–59.
[7] Somphone O, De Craene M, Ardon R, *et al.* Fast myocardial motion and strain estimation in 3D cardiac ultrasound with Sparse Demons. *IEEE 10th International Symposium on Biomedical Imaging* 2013, p. 1182–1185.
[8] Amundsen BH, Crosby J, Steen PA, Torp H, Slørdahl SA, Støylen A. Regional myocardial long-axis strain and strain rate measured by different tissue Doppler and speckle tracking echocardiography methods: a comparison with tagged magnetic resonance imaging. *Eur J Echocardiogr.* 2009 Mar;10(2): 229–37.
[9] Porras AR, Alessandrini M, De Craene M, *et al.* Improved myocardial motion estimation combining tissue Doppler and B-mode echocardiographic images. *IEEE Trans Med Imaging.* 2014 Nov;33(11): 2098–106.
[10] Porras AR, Alessandrini M, Mirea O, D'hooge J, Frangi AF, Piella G. Integration of multi-plane tissue Doppler and B-mode echocardiographic images for left ventricular motion estimation. *IEEE Trans Med Imaging.* 2016 Jan;35(1): 89–97.
[11] Cikes M, Tong L, Sutherland GR, D'hooge J. Ultrafast cardiac ultrasound imaging: technical principles, applications, and clinical benefits. *JACC Cardiovasc Imaging.* 2014 Aug;7(8): 812–23.
[12] Tanter M, Fink M. Ultrafast imaging in biomedical ultrasound. *IEEE Trans Ultrason Ferroelectr Freq Control.* 2014 Jan;61(1): 102–19.
[13] Shattuck DP, Weinshenker MD, Smith SW, von Ramm OT. Explososcan: a parallel processing technique for high speed ultrasound imaging with linear phased arrays. *J Acoust Soc Am.* 1984 Apr;75(4): 1273–82.
[14] Hergum T, Bjåstad T, Kristoffersen K, Torp H. Parallel beamforming using synthetic transmit beams. *IEEE Trans Ultrason Ferroelectr Freq Control.* 2007 Feb;54(2): 271–80.
[15] Provost J, Papadacci C, Arango JE, *et al.* 3D ultrafast ultrasound imaging in vivo. *Phys Med Biol.* 2014 Oct 7;59(19): L1–L13.

[16] Tong L, Ramalli A, Jasaityte R, Tortoli P, D'hooge J. Multi-transmit beam forming for fast cardiac imaging—experimental validation and in vivo application. *IEEE Trans Med Imaging.* 2014 Jun;33(6): 1205–19.
[17] Ortega A, Provost J, Tong L, *et al.* A comparison of the performance of different multiline transmit setups for fast volumetric cardiac ultrasound. *IEEE Trans Ultrason Ferroelectr Freq Control.* 2016 Dec;63(12): 2082–91.
[18] Heyde B, Barbosa D, Daraban A-M, *et al.* An automated pipeline for regional cardiac strain estimation from volumetric ultrasound data. *Proceedings of the IEEE International Ultrasonics Symposium* 2013, p. 1248–1251.
[19] Tabassian M, Alessandrini M, Herbots L, *et al.* Machine learning of the spatio-temporal characteristics of echocardiographic deformation curves for infarct classification. *Int J Cardiovasc Imaging.* 2017 Aug; 33(8): 1159–1167.
[20] Gatos I, Tsantis S, Spiliopoulos S, *et al.* A machine-learning algorithm toward color analysis for chronic liver disease classification, employing ultrasound shear wave elastography. *Ultrasound Med Biol.* 2017 Jun 17. pii: S0301-5629(17)30197-7.
[21] Khamis H, Claes P, Cauwenberghs N, Adam D, Kuznetsova T, D'hooge J. Machine learning to understand anthropomorphic modulators of spatio-temporal myocardial mechanics. *Proceedings of the IEEE International Ultrasonics Symposium*, 2017 (In Press).
[22] Aoued F, Eroglu E, Herbots, Rademakers F, D'hooge J. A statistical model-based approach for the detection of abnormal cardiac deformation. *Proceedings of the IEEE International Ultrasonics Symposium* 2005, p.512–515.
[23] Le Rolle V, Hernández A, Richard PY, Donal E, Carrault G. Model-based analysis of myocardial strain data acquired by tissue Doppler imaging. *Artif Intell Med.* 2008 Nov;44(3): 201–19.
[24] Langdon JH, Elegbe E, McAleavey SA. Single tracking location acoustic radiation force impulse viscoelasticity estimation (STL-VE): a method for measuring tissue viscoelastic parameters. *IEEE Trans Ultrason Ferroelectr Freq Control.* 2015 Jul;62(7): 1225–44.
[25] Mast TP, Teske AJ, Walmsley J, *et al.* Right ventricular imaging and computer simulation for electromechanical substrate characterization in arrhythmogenic right ventricular cardiomyopathy. *J Am Coll Cardiol.* 2016 Nov 15;68(20): 2185–97.
[26] Khamis H, Yahav A, Friedman Z, D'hooge J, Adam D. Supervised learning approach for tracking quality determination of transmural and segmental strain curves: a feasibility study. *J Biomed Eng Inform*, 2017; 3(2): 43–52.
[27] Deo RC, Zhang J, Hallock LA, *et al.* An end-to-end computer vision pipeline for automated cardiac function assessment by echocardiography. 2017 arXiv:1706.07342.

Part IV

Selected applications

Chapter 19

Segmentation of the carotid artery IMT in ultrasound

Kristen M. Meiburger[1], Cristina Caresio[1], Massimo Salvi[1], U. Rajendra Acharya[2,3,4], and Filippo Molinari[1]

19.1 Introduction

Ultrasound imaging plays a fundamental role as a diagnostic tool in the assessment of the cardiovascular system and the determination of the possible onset of a cardiovascular disease (CVD). Atherosclerosis is the earliest manifestation of CVD and refers to the degeneration of the arterial wall and the deposition of lipids within the wall [1–3]. This therefore causes an increase of the artery intima-media thickness (IMT). The IMT of the common carotid artery is the most widely adopted and validated ultrasound marker for the assessment of atherosclerosis and cardiovascular risk [4–8]. Polak *et al.* recently published a multiethnic study of atherosclerosis and found that an IMT score can be derived from noninvasive measurements of the common and internal carotid artery wall and that this measurement improved the Framingham risk score for predicting coronary heart disease events, even after addition of coronary calcium to the model [9].

The carotid IMT can be computed by measuring the distance between the lumen–intima (LI) interface of the artery from the media–adventitia (MA) boundary. This measurement can be done manually on the ultrasound image, as the operator can place a marker in correspondence of these two interfaces and therefore calculate the arterial wall thickness. However, manual measurements are user-dependent, not fully standardized, subjective, time-consuming, and prone to errors [10]. Much research has been done focusing on the development of semiautomatic or completely automatic techniques to aid the measurement of this important cardiovascular risk factor. Computer methods for segmenting the ultrasound arterial images mainly aim at tracing the LI and MA boundaries. In some studies, the media and intima thicknesses were measured separately [11].

[1]Biolab, Department of Electronics and Telecommunications, Politecnico di Torino, Italy
[2]Department of Electronic & Computer Engineering, Ngee Ann Polytechnic, Singapore
[3]Department of Biomedical Engineering, SIM University, Singapore
[4]Department of Biomedical Imaging, University of Malaya, Malaysia

In clinical practice, ultrasounds offer several advantages such as (i) use of nonionizing radiation, (ii) safe and quick examination of the patient, (iii) absence of documented biological effects, (iv) low-cost equipment (when compared to other medical imaging devices), (v) wide availability of ultrasound scanners, and (vi) effective visualization of the components of the arterial wall.

In this chapter, we will present the most widely used computer techniques for the carotid IMT segmentation from cardiovascular ultrasound images. We will focus on ultrasound image and carotid artery characteristics, and the difference between semiautomatic and completely automatic segmentation methods, also presenting numerous used and established techniques.

19.2 Ultrasound and carotid artery characteristics

19.2.1 Properties of ultrasound images

An important feature for all types of imaging modalities is image resolution. In ultrasound imaging, image resolution is directly related to the transducer frequency. High-frequency ultrasound waves generate images with a higher axial resolution; however, high-frequency waves are attenuated more than lower frequency waves for a given distance. Since the carotid artery is a superficial structure, high frequency transducers (up to 10–15 MHz range) are to be preferably used, since a high resolution helps make the IMT segmentation an easier task.

B-mode ultrasound images are also easily distinguishable from other imaging modalities because of the typical granular appearance that they present, which is known as speckle. Speckle is formed from backscattered echoes of randomly or coherently distributed scatterers in tissue, giving it its random and deterministic nature [12]. Speckle contains important information on scatterer statistics and is fundamental for many techniques that have been developed for the real-time tracking of structures, where a specific speckle pattern is followed in time [13–16]. Still, when considering the localization and segmentation in non-temporal B-mode ultrasound images, such as in the case of IMT segmentation, speckle is generally considered to be an image-degrading characteristic. In fact, much research effort is precisely aimed at developing effective methods of minimizing speckle while maintaining the true detail of the morphology in the image [17]. Loizou *et al.* published a comparative evaluation of despeckle filtering in ultrasound imaging of the carotid artery [17] where they found that a first-order statistics filter gave the best performance.

Despeckling, the act of minimizing speckle in ultrasound images, is often a precursor to many semiautomatic and completely automatic IMT segmentation techniques, as the removal of this granular appearance on the image can help increase the accuracy and robustness of computational methods.

More detail about speckle, speckle tracking, and despeckling techniques can also be found in Chapters 2–4, 5–9, 12–17.

19.2.2 Carotid artery structure and appearance in ultrasound images

The carotid artery geometry is quite well defined and repeatable: it has a circular section, a three-layered wall, and lumen filled with blood. In ultrasound images, blood is anechoic (see Figure 19.1), meaning that the lumen of the artery is theoretically black, since blood does not reflect any portion of the ultrasound beam. The liquid part of the blood (plasma) is anechoic as all liquids are, whereas the erythrocytes (*i.e.*, the corpuscular part) have a dimension much lower than the resolution power of the ultrasound equipment.

The three-layered structure of the arterial wall is neatly observable in ultrasound (US) images. In a longitudinal projection (Figure 19.1(a)), the arterial structure is characterized by a black lumen, which can be roughly considered as a black rectangle, surrounded by two bright stripes, which represent the adventitial layer of the walls. When no calcium deposits are present, the adventitial layers are usually the most hyperechoic structures in an arterial scan, as demonstrated in a previous study [18]. Due to resolution limitations, the intima layer is usually merged with the media layer, leading to the definition of two interfaces: the

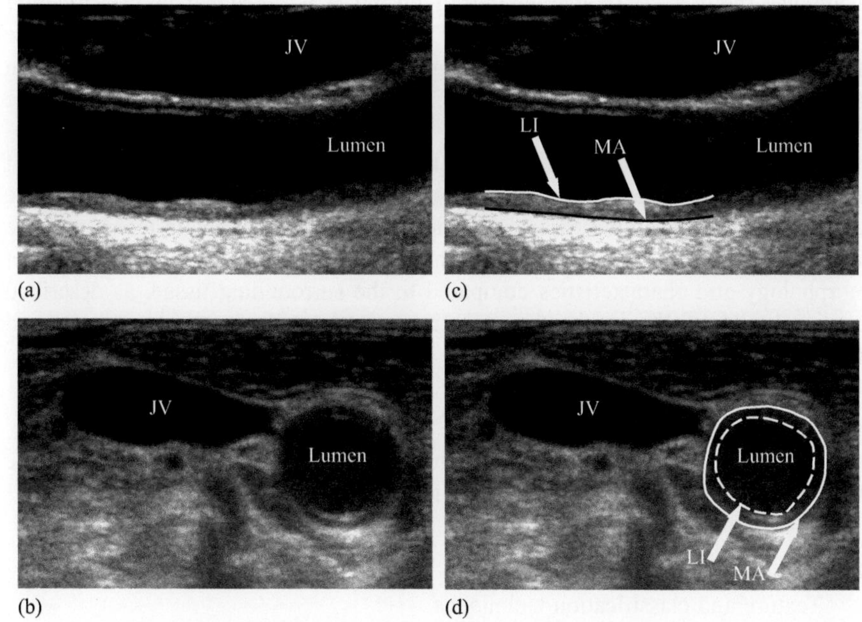

Figure 19.1 Ultrasound image of a common carotid artery in (a) longitudinal; (b) transverse projection; (c) longitudinal projection with manually traced profiles; (d) transverse projection with manually traced profiles. The jugular vein (JV) is also visible in both projections. The vessel lumen is black, since blood is anechoic in ultrasound images. LI – lumen–intima interface. MA – media adventitia interface

LI and the MA interfaces (pictorial tracings of the LI and MA interfaces are reported by Figure 19.1(c)). The arterial wall portion that is found between the LI and MA interfaces is called the "intima-media complex" by some authors [19,20]. In a transverse projection (Figure 19.1(b)), the arteries appear as circular black regions delimited by an upper and a lower bright boundary. The lateral portions of the wall are usually underrepresented, due to a poor reflection of the ultrasound wave. Figure 19.1(d) shows the boundaries of the LI and MA, manually traced by an expert sonologist.

The carotid IMT segmentation is almost always done on the distal wall of the carotid artery from an image acquired with the artery in a longitudinal projection. Further on in this chapter, we will therefore focus only on these specific carotid IMT segmentation techniques.

19.3 Carotid artery recognition

Typically, the first step in any IMT segmentation technique is the initial identification of the carotid artery. This is where the distinction between semiautomatic and completely automatic techniques comes into play. In fact, semiautomatic techniques require user-interaction during this phase, with the manual identification of the carotid artery section where the IMT is to be segmented. Typically, the operator manually crops the image to contain only the section to be examined, but some techniques instead rely on other manual intervention, such as drawing the carotid artery lumen axis.

On the contrary, completely automatic techniques do not require any type of human interaction, operating completely on their own starting directly with the ultrasound image acquired from the device. Completely automatic techniques are made possible thanks to the fact that the carotid artery presents a very distinct morphology and characteristics compared to the surrounding tissue, as described previously. The following section goes more into detail about automatic carotid artery recognition techniques.

19.3.1 Techniques for automatic carotid artery localization

The carotid artery localization can initially be broad, since a more accurate segmentation of the actual IMT is performed in a subsequent step.

These recognition techniques can be divided into the following macro-areas:

- Shape prior techniques
- Texture and classification techniques
- Pixel-intensity and/or local-statistics-based techniques

19.3.1.1 Shape priors

Anatomical shape prior methods are based on the a-priori knowledge of the expected anatomical structure of the carotid artery. These types of techniques can cope very well with suboptimal images; *i.e.*, with images with weak or underrepresented edges or affected by noise. Models are typically built from a large database of training samples to determine the final shape prior.

A major possible drawback of these techniques is pathology. For example, if a shape prior were built on the healthy common carotid artery morphology, it would be difficult to adapt it to the case of a diseased vessel possibly containing a plaque. In other words, shape priors are usually only as good as the training samples.

19.3.1.2 Texture and classification

Texture and classification methods are based on finding the features of the microstructure of the tissue being imaged and consequently classifying the pixels or sections of the image into different regions based on these features. These techniques are typically based on statistical patterns of the pixel intensities, so they are more independent of the physics of the imaging system. Numerous texture techniques rely on the calculation of Haralick's co-occurrence matrices [21]. While they are computationally expensive, these methods have performed well in a number of applications and studies [22–26].

So-called "superpixel" or "graph-based" techniques also fall into this category. These techniques are based on the division of the original image into "superpixels" or patches, which are then labeled as belonging to either the artery or background, using graph cuts [27]. A more detailed example of this technique is available in the work by Rosati *et al.* [28]. In this multi-scale approach, different patches of a pixel's neighborhood were considered and up to 141 features were computed. With this method, pixels were assigned to either the lumen (red), the intima and media layers (blue) or the adventitia (green) layer (see Figure 19.2). The result seen in the figure was obtained after a feature selection and reduction step, followed by a voting classifier. In a first version (Figure 19.2(a)), the authors used three training datasets of 1,500 pixels each, and then (Figure 19.2(b)) three datasets of 1,800 pixels each.

19.3.1.3 Pixel intensity and/or local statistics

These approaches exploit the carotid appearance in ultrasound images. Vessel representation can be thought of as a mixture model with varying intensity distributions. This is because, as discussed in an earlier section,

- pixels belonging to the carotid lumen are characterized by an intensity close to zero and low standard deviation;
- pixels belonging to the adventitia layer of the carotid wall are characterized by a high-intensity and low-standard deviation;
- all remaining pixels should have a different mean intensity and higher standard deviation.

It is therefore possible to explore the neighborhood of a pixel and determine whether the pixel belongs to the lumen, wall, or other structures/tissues based on its intensity value, the mean intensity of its neighborhood, and the standard deviation of its neighborhood.

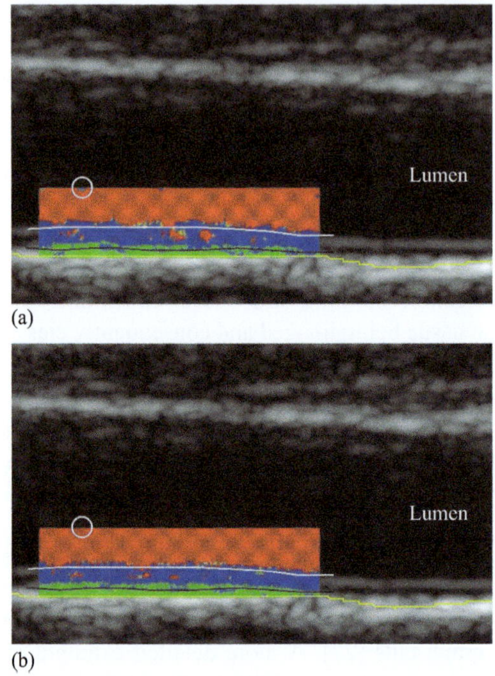

Figure 19.2 *Comparison between the first version of voting classifier, (a) trained with three datasets of 1,500 pixels each and the final voting classifier, (b) trained with three datasets of 1,800 pixels each. Red, blue, and green points mark the pixels classified as belonging to lumen, IM, and adventitia classes, respectively. Pixels not classified by the voting procedure are indicated with yellow points. The white circle highlights an example of pixels zone added to the initial datasets. These pixels are chosen among those pixels resulting in a wrong class from the first voting classification (a) and in the last classifier the same pixels result in correct class (b). The white line corresponds to the lumen–intima (LI) interface, the black line marks out the media–adventitia (MA) interface, and the yellow line delimits the far adventitia layer. Reproduced, with permission, from Reference [28]*

A complete description of such an approach can be found in the works by Molinari *et al.* [24,29,30]. With reference to Figure 19.3, the pixels belonging to the lumen (and, more in general, to the blood) are easily detected because they are characterized by a low-intensity value and low-standard deviation of their neighborhood. It is therefore possible to mark all the pixels possibly corresponding to blood in the image by considering a bidimensional histogram (Figure 19.3(b) and (c)). It is then possible to mark the center of the lumen (L) and the far adventitia wall (Figure 19.3(d)) by using simple conditions on the mask.

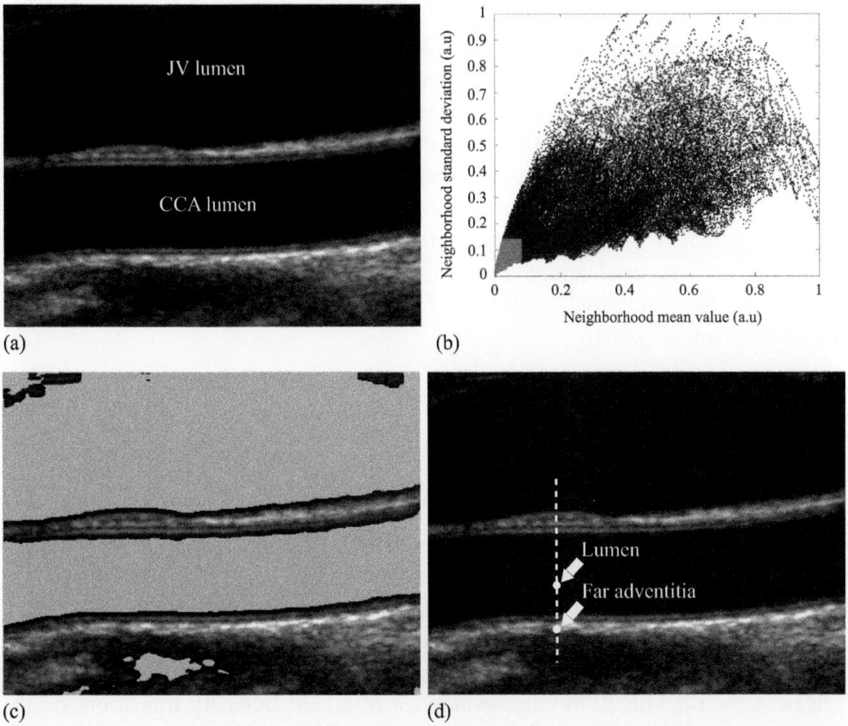

Figure 19.3 Strategy for far wall adventitial tracing. (a) Original image. (b) Bidimensional histogram (2DH). The gray portion of the 2DH denotes the region in which we suppose to find only lumen pixels. (c) Original image with lumen pixels overlaid in gray. (d) Sample processing of one column, with the marker points of the far (ADF) adventitia layer and of the lumen (L)

19.4 Carotid wall and final IMT segmentation

Once the artery has been recognized in the image frame, either automatically or manually, its walls must be then accurately segmented, giving forth the final IMT measurement. Here, we will present various techniques that have been proposed for the automatic delineation of the LI and MA profiles.

19.4.1 Edge-tracking and gradient-based techniques

Pignoli *et al.* were the first to apply a computer-based technique to perform the IMT measurement of the carotid artery [31]. Taking an ultrasound image of the carotid artery in a longitudinal projection, they measured the distal wall IMT by considering the intensity profile of a section of the image when moving from the center of the vessel to the borders. Since the vessel lumen is ideally black (*i.e.*, zero-mean), they tracked the increase in the intensity profile that occurs in proximity of the LI interface [32].

A similar approach was then adopted in 2001 by Liguori *et al.* They proposed a segmentation technique based on edge-detection that used image gradients. They considered the artery as horizontally placed in the B-Mode ultrasound image. For each column of the image they calculated the gradient of the intensity profile. In order to facilitate edge detection, Liguori *et al.* adopted a statistical thresholding to reduce noise before computing the image gradient.

Edge-tracking and gradient-based methods can suffer from the problem of superimposed noise. In fact, noise may preclude the proper detection of the LI and MA interfaces. Faita *et al.* adopted a gradient-based approach which is more robust to noise than the traditional ones [33]. The core of the method is the first-order absolute moment (FOAM):

$$\mathrm{FOAM}(x,y) = \frac{1}{A_\theta}\int_\theta |I_1(x,y) - I_2(x-x',y-y')| * G(x',y',\sigma)dx'dy' \quad (19.1)$$

where $I_1(x,y) = I(x,y) * G_1(x,y,\sigma_1)$ is a Gaussian low-pass filtered version of the input image $I(x,y)$; $I_2(x,y) = I(x,y) * G_2(x,y,\sigma_2)$, is a Gaussian low-pass filtered version of the input image $I(x,y)$ with different standard deviation; and $G(x',y',\sigma)$ is a regularization term, and third version of Gaussian low-pass filter.

This operator computes the average dispersion of the image pixels in a circular domain called A_θ. The FOAM is equal to zero when the image has no intensity changes in the domain θ. In correspondence of a neat intensity transition, on the other hand, the FOAM has a high value. The overall performance of this methodology was very high, showing an IMT measurement error equal to 10.0 ± 38.0 μm. Moreover, the FOAM operator and intelligent procedures to discover maxima ensured a good robustness to noise. This technique is real-time; hence, it is also suitable for clinical application.

19.4.2 Dynamic programming techniques

Dynamic programming techniques were first introduced in the early 1990s in order to reduce the variability in ultrasound measurements [34]. Wendelhag *et al.* first introduced a dynamic programming procedure for the automatic detection of echo interfaces [35]. This technique combined multiple measurements of echo intensity, intensity gradient, and boundary continuity. The system also allowed an optional interactive modification by the human operator, if so desired. An initial set of ultrasound images was first manually segmented by expert operators and served as reference (ground truth). The estimated values of the three boundary features (echo intensity, intensity gradient, and boundary continuity) were then linearly combined to create a cost function. Each image point was associated with a specific cost that in turn correlated with the likelihood of that point being located at the echo interface. In this way, points located at the interfaces between different artery layers were expected to have a low cost, whereas points located far from the interfaces were associated with a high cost. The weights of the linear combination originating the cost function were determined by training the system, considering the ground truth as reference. Dynamic programming was used to reduce the computational cost given by the need of inspecting all the points of the image. The IMT measurement error of this technique was better than 40 ± 36 μm.

Dynamic programming methods can also be applied in a multi-resolution framework: starting from the image in a low-resolution scale, the image features are computed; a refinement procedure is then applied and the features are computed at each step [36]. The artery detection can therefore be obtained in the coarse scale image, whereas the accurate detection of the LI/MA interfaces can be made in the fine scale image.

19.4.3 Active contours (snakes)

Active parametric contours, also known as *snakes*, have been widely used in the segmentation of medical images. The snake can be thought of as a set of vertices connected by line segments, which evolve under the action of different forces. The popularity of the snake-based segmentation methodology relies on the fact that the artery LI and MA boundaries can be well distinguished in the image. Therefore, a straight deformable model could be able to adapt to such interfaces after a proper tuning of its parameters. Most studies adopt the traditional formulation of a snake as proposed by Williams and Shah [37]. A two-dimensional snake is a parametric contour represented by $v(s) = [x(s), y(s)]$, where (x, y) denotes the spatial coordinates of an image and [ ] represents the parametric domain. The snake then adapts by a dynamic process that minimizes a global energy function:

$$E[v(s)] = E_{\text{int}}[v(s)] + E_{\text{ext}}[v(s)] \tag{19.2}$$

where

- $E_{\text{int}}[v(s)]$ is the "internal energy" that constrains the shape of the curve. Usually, this energy term is proportional to the curve derivatives, in order to regularize the curvature and elasticity of the curve. In the case of segmenting the LI/MA interfaces in longitudinal US images, the internal energy is set at a high value, since such interfaces are almost linear.
- $E_{\text{ext}}[v(s)]$ is the "external energy" and drives the curve toward the image intensity edges. Therefore, this energy term is often modeled by image gradients.

The snake points should therefore move toward the features of the image while remaining constrained by the internal forces. The equilibrium condition is met when the internal forces counterbalance the external ones. Therefore, fine-tuning of the snake parameters is fundamental for an accurate segmentation.

A complete and thorough summary of snake performances in carotid segmentation was given in 2007 by Loizou *et al.* [38]. The same research team further improved their snake-based system and made it fully automated [39] and suitable also to the processing of arteries with plaques [40].

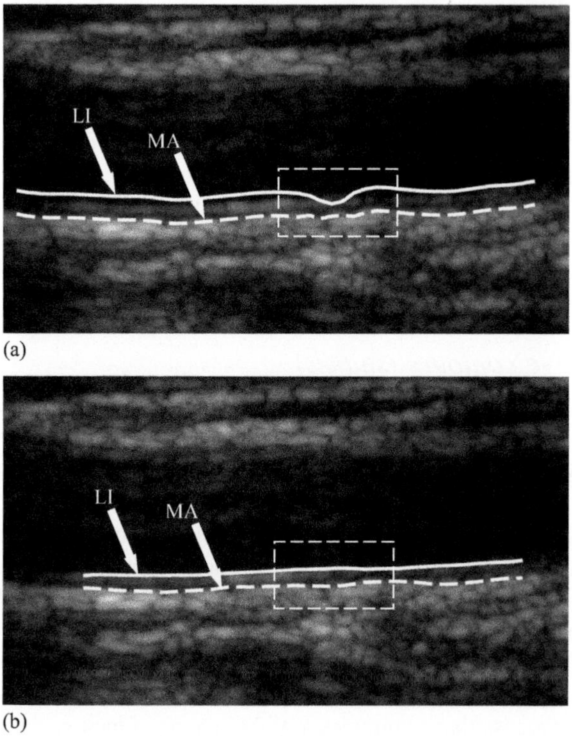

Figure 19.4 Performance difference between unconstrained (panel (a)) and constrained (panel (b)) dual-snake segmentation system. The dashed box in panel (a) indicates an image region in which the unconstrained LI snake is almost collapsed on the MA snake. The constrained snakes are prevented from bleeding or collapsing, hence in panel (b) the inaccuracy is solved

In 2012, Molinari *et al.* proposed a dual-snake system consisting of two different active contours (one for the LI and one for the MA interface) evolving together [41]. A "mutual energy" term was added in this implementation in order to prevent the LI snake from bleeding or collapsing on the MA snake. The authors demonstrated that dual-snake systems have superior performance in IMT measurement compared to conventional snakes (Figure 19.4) [42].

19.4.4 Transform-based and modeling approaches

Often, the layers of the carotid wall can be recognized and accurately segmented by relying on modeling techniques or mathematical transformations.

One of the most used transformation approaches is the Hough transform [43]. This tool allows for an efficient detection of shapes in an image, if a description of the shape is mathematically provided and a scale parameter is selected. The Hough transform is mostly used to detect lines and circles. Golemati *et al.* exploited the properties of the Hough transform and developed an algorithm that could automatically segment both longitudinal and transverse B-Mode images [25,44]. With the Hough transform, it is possible to detect straight lines in longitudinal images (corresponding to the LI/MA interfaces) and circles in transverse images. This method is also fairly robust to small morphological changes of the artery wall, so it can also be used in presence of small atherosclerotic plaques. It was demonstrated that, compared to the pixel classification performed by human tracings, it is possible to segment the carotid artery with a sensitivity of about 96% in longitudinal images and 82% in transverse images, with specificity of about 96% in both cases, when using the Hough transform.

In modeling approaches, the image is considered as the combination of the intensity typical of the artery layers plus noise. Hence, an image region containing a portion of the vessel lumen, the wall, and some surrounding tissues could be characterized by the specific distributions mimicking the intensity distributions of the three components. In vascular ultrasound imaging, the most used models are the Gaussian mixture model and the Nakagami modeling.

The Nakagami distribution proved effective in modeling the radiofrequency ultrasound signal that was scattered by the artery wall layers [45]. Destrempes *et al.* proposed a segmentation strategy based on Nakagami mixture modeling and stochastic optimization [46]. This technique performed very well in the segmentation of the common carotid artery in longitudinal projection: using the mean absolute distance (MAD) metric the authors obtained LI and MA segmentation errors equal to 21.0 ± 13.0 and 0.16 ± 7.0 μm, respectively.

19.4.5 Data mining techniques

Due to the recent growing interest in the fields of data mining and big data analysis, nonlinear and innovative techniques have been applied in the field of vascular ultrasounds. Most of these techniques have the following architecture in common [47]:

- Step 1: feature extraction. The image is analyzed in order to extract as many descriptors (*i.e.*, features) as possible to characterize the image. Some authors stick to conventional and first-order descriptors (*i.e.*, analysis of the gray scale distribution of the image or of a portion of the image) [29,48], whereas others prefer to also include higher order texture descriptors [21,49].
- Step 2: feature reduction/selection. A high number of features are initially extracted and there is therefore the risk of having collinear variables that could lead to an over-constrained system. To avoid this, the features are usually selected and their number is reduced. Collinear and strongly correlated variables are taken out, whereas variables with negligible variance are ignored. Rosati *et al.* recently revised the most performing and widely used reduction and selection techniques for vascular ultrasound images [28].

- Step 3: classification. The features associated to each pixel are then classified to assign the pixel to a specific image component (*i.e.*, the lumen, the intima, the media, the adventitia, etc.). Pixels with borderline conditions are usually kept in an "uncertainty" class or cluster and ignored. Several methods have been used to accomplish this step, even though fuzzy classifiers or artificial neural networks are often used [47].
- Step 4: vessel boundaries refinement. Due to intrinsic data variability and to classification errors, the output of the classifier is usually not accurate enough to be considered as the final segmentation.

This approach has been used not only for IMT measurement and image segmentation but also for the assessment of the cardiovascular risk score based on the analysis of the arterial layer [47], for the assessment of the subjects' vascular age [50], and for the characterization of atherosclerotic plaques [22].

19.5 Performance measurement and comparison

As stated previously, the final IMT measurement is calculated as the distance between the LI and the MA profiles. Since these profiles are made up of a certain number of points, whether calculated manually or semiautomatically or automatically, the issue of how to calculate the distance between the two profiles to give forth the final IMT measurement is quite important. This is especially critical when comparing automated techniques to ground truth manual tracings, as different distance measuring techniques may be more or less sensitive to the number of points making up the boundary.

Commonly used distance metrics for the IMT calculation are:

- The MAD
- The Hausdorff Distance (HD)
- The Polyline Distance Metric (PDM)
- The Centerline Distance Metric (CDM)

For a complete review and definition of these distance measurement techniques, please refer to Molinari *et al.* [51] and see Figure 19.5, which displays how these distances are calculated. The authors Saba *et al.* compared the HD, PDM, and CDM measurement techniques to determine which method performed better when measuring the carotid IMT automatically [52]. From their study, it emerged that the HD was not a suitable metric since it is very sensitive to the number of points in the profile and tends to largely overestimate the IMT. The PDM and CDM measurement methods yielded similar results, where the PDM is to be preferred in presence of a small number of points that make up the boundaries and when the pixel density of the image is low. The CDM is instead to be preferred in presence of curved arteries [52]. It is not advisable to use the MAD when the number of points constituting the LI/MA profiles is low. In fact, similarly to the HD, the MAD tends to considerably overestimate the IMT if the points of the LI profile and the corresponding ones of the MA profile are not vertically aligned.

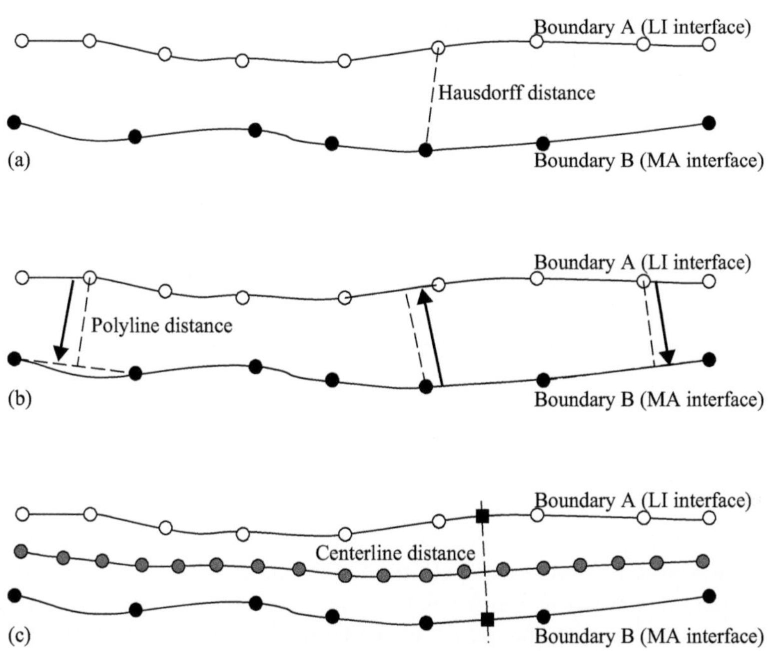

Figure 19.5 (a) Hausdorff distance (HD); (b) Polyline distance metric (PDM); and (c) Centerline distance metrics (CDMs). The HD is defined as the maximum Euclidean distance of a boundary A to the nearest point in the Boundary B. The PDM is the average distance between the points on one boundary and the segments of the other boundary. The arrows in panel (b) indicate that the distance between the LI points (white circles) and the MA (downward arrows) must be calculated and, vice versa, the distance between the MA points (black circles) and the LI (upward arrows). The CDM is calculated by finding and interpolating the centerline profile between the LI and MA profiles and then calculating the average of chord perpendiculars to the two profiles at each centerline point. LI = lumen–intima; MA = media–adventitia

Once the IMT is calculated, there are also numerous techniques that can be used to evaluate the performance of the computer-based segmentation techniques, when comparing it to manual ground truth tracings of the LI and MA borders. The most upfront way to evaluate the performance of computer-based techniques is through calculating the IMT error, which is typically done by simply subtracting the IMT calculated by the automatic technique from the IMT calculated with the manual tracings. An advantage to this simple measurement is that it gives an idea of whether the technique overestimates or underestimates the ground truth IMT value. Along with presenting the numerical IMT error in terms of mean plus or minus the standard deviation, many authors choose to also graphically present the comparison between the computer-based segmentation method and manual segmentations. This is often done using tools such as a correlation plot, a Bland–Altman plot, which is very helpful in determining if there is a bias in the measurements, and error histograms. The IMT absolute error and squared error may also be calculated and give a good idea of the performances of the technique.

Along the same lines, a segmentation error of each individual profile (*i.e.*, LI and MA) can be compared to the ground truth manual tracings. This is done by calculating the distance between the manual profile and the automatic or semiautomatic profile [48]. Since numerous techniques for IMT segmentation have been developed and each technique presents their own biases and merits, it is possible to combine the different results by creating a sort of fusion technique using the manual ground truth tracings as an ideal marker. Molinari *et al.* presented such a method in their study where they developed an Inter-Greedy (IG) approach [53]. Starting from the segmentation method that produced the lowest error, the authors iteratively swapped the vertices of the automated profiles until its overall distance with respect to ground truth was minimized. The final fusion boundary, the IG boundary, provided about an average 30% improvement when compared to the initial best performing technique [53].

Another very usual technique for evaluating a computer-based technique, when numerous manual tracings are available, is the Percent Statistic Test [54,55]. This technique basically tests to see if the computer-generated boundary behaves like a human-generated boundary; if it does, it must have the same probability of falling within the inter-observer range as the manual segmentation.

Now that it is clear how IMT measurements are performed and compared to manual tracings, we will present here a few IMT segmentation algorithms (semiautomatic and completely automatic) that have recently been developed and compare their final performances, in terms of IMT error.

Polak *et al.* recently used a semiautomatic edge detection algorithm in a multiethnic study of atherosclerosis and found that the edge detected IMT has similar if not stronger associations with coronary heart disease outcomes when compared with manually traced IMT [56]. The algorithm weighed gradients between pixels and pixel density values through a dynamic programming process that minimizes cost functions. The algorithm is considered semiautomatic because the it uses manual tracings to determine which section of the common carotid artery should be examined [57]. The IMT error results for two different manual tracings can be seen in the second line of Table 19.1.

Zahnd *et al.* presented a fully automatic contour segmentation method that introduces an augmented dimension to process 2-D images in a 3-D space. The third dimension corresponds to the tentative local thickness of the intima–media complex. The method is based on a dynamic programming scheme that runs in a 3-D space generated with a shape-adapted filter bank. The optimal solution corresponds to a single medial axis representation that fully describes the two anatomical interfaces of the arterial wall [58]. See line three of Table 19.1 for segmentation results.

Table 19.1 Comparison of recent IMT segmentation algorithms

Authors	Technique	Fully automated/ semiautomated	No. images	IMT error (mm)
Polak *et al.*	Dynamic programming	Semiautomated	5,641	0.090 ± 0.160 0.250 ± 0.110
Zahnd *et al.*	Dynamic programming in 3D space	Fully automated	60 – training 184 – validation	0.066 ± 0.090
Ikeda *et al.*	Carotid geometry and pixel classification	Fully automated	649	0.011 ± 0.003
Xiao *et al.*	Markov random field models	Fully automated	80	0.024 ± 0.023
Menchòn-Lara *et al.*	Machine learning and artificial neural networks	Fully automated	67	0.058 ± 0.034

Ikeda *et al.* developed a completely automatic algorithm that detects the carotid bulb edge, a reference marker for measurements of the carotid IMT. The method then automatically calculates segment-based IMT measurements, using 10 mm segments proximal to the bulb edge. The methodology used an integrated approach which combines carotid geometry and pixel-classification paradigms [59].

Xiao *et al.* proposed an automated IMT segmentation method based on Markov random field models. The label field is initialized from line segments generated using the Hough transform, and the iterated conditional modes method is applied to detect the final LI and MA boundaries [60].

Menchòn-Lara *et al.* proposed a technique based on machine learning and artificial neural networks for IMT segmentation. They developed a deep learning strategy to obtain abstract and efficient data representations by means of auto-encoders with multiple hidden layers [61].

19.6 Discussion and final remarks

In this chapter, we discussed carotid IMT segmentation techniques in ultrasound, which are of paramount importance in clinical routine and in research projects.

Ultrasound images have an overall quality that is dependent on the scanner used and on its settings. In fact, ultrasound imaging is a human-dependent scanning technique and so different operators may render the same object in different manners. As mentioned previously, speckle is another obstacle to overcome when developing segmentation methods for ultrasound images.

Another complication in automatic carotid IMT segmentation techniques is given by the high variability in normal vessel morphology and in vessel appearance under pathology. These challenges justify why, currently, the IMT segmentation in ultrasound images is often still an open problem.

Because of the variability caused by physiology and by pathological conditions, it is not possible to pick an "ideal" technique for the IMT segmentation of all carotid artery ultrasound images. However, robustness is certainly a key point for all techniques. When facing the problem of carotid IMT segmentation, it is important to remember that carotid arteries are different for several parameters, including shape, size, orientation, and composition.

References

[1] J. Badimon, B. Ibanez, and G. Cimmino, "Genesis and dynamics of atherosclerotic lesions: implications for early detection," *Cerebrovasc. Dis.*, vol. 27, no. Suppl. 1, pp. 38–47, 2009.

[2] M. Walter, "Interrelationships among HDL metabolism, aging, and atherosclerosis," *Arterioscler. Thromb. Vasc. Biol.*, vol. 29, no. 9, pp. 1244–1250, 2009.

[3] A. Kampoli, D. Tousoulis, and C. Antoniades, "Biomarkers of premature atherosclerosis," *Trends Mol. Med.*, vol. 15, no. 7, pp. 323–332, 2009.

[4] J. U-King-Im, V. Young, and J. Gillard, "Carotid-artery imaging in the diagnosis and management of patients at risk of stroke," *Lancet Neurol.*, vol. 8, no. 6, pp. 569–580, 2009.

[5] J. Kastelein, A. Wiegman, and E. de Groot, "Surrogate markers of atherosclerosis: impact of statins," *Atheroscler. Suppl.*, vol. 4, no. 1, pp. 31–36, 2003.

[6] J. Polak, M. Pencina, D. Herrington, and D. O'Leary, "Associations of edge-detected and manual-traced common carotid intima-media thickness measurements with Framingham risk factors the multi-ethnic study of atherosclerosis," *Stroke*, vol. 42, no. 7, pp. 1912–1916, 2011.

[7] P. Touboul, M. Hennerici, and S. Meairs, "Mannheim intima-media thickness consensus," *Cerebrovasc. Dis.*, vol. 18, no. 4, pp. 346–349, 2004.

[8] P. Touboul, M. Hennerici, and S. Meairs, "Mannheim carotid intima-media thickness consensus (2004–2006)," *Cerebrovasc. Dis.*, vol. 23, no. 1, pp. 75–80, 2007.

[9] J. F. Polak, M. Szklo, and D. H. O'Leary, "Carotid intima-media thickness score, positive coronary artery calcium score, and incident coronary heart disease: the multi-ethnic study of atherosclerosis," *J. Am. Heart Assoc.*, vol. 6, no. 1, p. e004612, 2017.

[10] T. Naqvi, "Ultrasound vascular screening for cardiovascular risk assessment. Why, when and how?," *Minerva Cardioangiol.*, vol. 54, no. 1, pp. 53–67, 2006.

[11] C. P. Loizou, C. S. Pattichis, A. N. Nicolaides, and M. Pantziaris, "Manual and automated media and intima thickness measurements of the common carotid artery," *IEEE Trans. Ultrason. Ferroelectr. Freq. Control*, vol. 56, no. 5, pp. 983–994, 2009.

[12] R. Wagner, S. Smith, and J. Sandrik, "Statistics of speckle in ultrasound B-scans," *IEEE Trans. Sonics Ultrason.*, vol. 30, no. 3, pp. 156–163, 1983.

[13] D. Angelova and L. Mihaylova, "Contour segmentation in 2D ultrasound medical images with particle filtering," *Mach. Vis. Appl.*, vol. 22, no. 3, pp. 551–561, 2011.

[14] A. H. Curiale, G. Vegas-Sánchez-Ferrero, and S. Aja-Fernández, "Influence of ultrasound speckle tracking strategies for motion and strain estimation," *Med. Image Anal.*, vol. 32, pp. 184–200, 2016.

[15] S. Merouche, L. Allard, E. Montagnon, *et al.*, "A robotic ultrasound scanner for automatic vessel tracking and three-dimensional reconstruction of B-mode images," *IEEE Trans. Ultrason. Ferroelectr. Freq. Control*, vol. 63, no. 1, pp. 35–46, 2016.

[16] D. C. Wang, R. Klatzky, B. Wu, *et al.*, "Fully automated common carotid artery and internal jugular vein identification and tracking using B-mode ultrasound," *IEEE Trans. Biomed. Eng.*, vol. 56, no. 6, pp. 1691–1699, 2009.

[17] C. P. Loizou, C. S. Pattichis, C. I. Christodouluo, R. S. H. Istepanian, M. Pantziaris, and A. Nicolaides, "Comparative evaluation of despeckle filtering in ultrasound imaging of the carotid artery," *IEEE Trans. Ultrason. Ferroelectr. Freq. Control*, vol. 52, no. 10, pp. 1653–1669, 2005.

[18] F. Molinari and G. Krishnamurthi, "Hypothesis validation of far-wall brightness in carotid-artery ultrasound for feature-based IMT measurement using a combination of level-set segmentation and registration," *IEEE Trans. Instrum. Meas.*, vol. 61, no. 4, pp. 1054–1063, 2012.

[19] R. Rocha, A. Campilho, J. Silva, E. Azevedo, and R. Santos, "Segmentation of the carotid intima-media region in B-mode ultrasound images," *Image Vis. Comput.*, vol. 28, no. 4, pp. 614–625, 2010.

[20] P. Touboul, M. Hennerici, S. Meairs, and H. Adams, "Mannheim carotid intima-media thickness and plaque consensus (2004–2006–2011)," *Cerebrovascular Dis.*, vol. 34, no. 4, pp. 290–296, 2012.

[21] F. Molinari, C. Caresio, and U. Acharya, "Advances in quantitative muscle ultrasonography using texture analysis of ultrasound images," *Ultrasound Med. Biol.*, vol. 41, no. 9, pp. 2520–2532, 2015.

[22] R. Acharya, O. Faust, A. Alvin, and S. Sree, "Symptomatic vs. asymptomatic plaque classification in carotid ultrasound," *J. Med. Syst.*, vol. 36, no. 3, pp. 1861–1871, 2012.

[23] S. Kakkos, M. Griffin, and A. Nicolaides, "The size of juxtaluminal hypoechoic area in ultrasound images of asymptomatic carotid plaques predicts the occurrence of stroke," *J. Vasc. Surg.*, vol. 57, no. 3, pp. 609–618, 2013.

[24] F. Molinari, K. M. Meiburger, G. Zeng, *et al.*, "Carotid artery recognition system: a comparison of three automated paradigms for ultrasound images," *Med. Phys.*, vol. 39, no. 1, p. 378, Jan. 2012.

[25] S. Golemati, T. J. Tegos, A. Sassano, K. S. Nikita, and A. N. Nicolaides, "Echogenicity of B-mode sonographic images of the carotid

artery: work in progress.," *J. Ultrasound Med.*, vol. 23, no. 5, pp. 659–669, May 2004.

[26] T. Tegos, D. Mavrophoros, and M. Sabetai, "Types of neurovascular symptoms and carotid plaque ultrasonic textural characteristics," *J. Ultrasound Med.*, vol. 20, no. 2, pp. 113–121, 2001.

[27] D. Mahapatra, "Automatic cardiac segmentation using semantic information from random forests.," *J. Digit. Imaging*, vol. 27, no. 6, pp. 794–804, Dec. 2014.

[28] S. Rosati, G. Balestra, F. Molinari, U. Rajendra Acharya, and J. S. Suri, "A selection and reduction approach for the optimization of ultrasound carotid artery images segmentation," in *Machine Learning in Healthcare Informatics SE – 14*, Springer Berlin Heidelberg, 2014, pp. 309–332.

[29] F. Molinari, G. Zeng, and J. Suri, "Intima-media thickness: setting a standard for a completely automated method of ultrasound measurement," *IEEE Trans. Ultrason. Ferroelectr. Freq. Control*, vol. 57, no. 5, pp. 1112–1124, 2010.

[30] F. Molinari, W. Liboni, and P. Giustetto, "Automatic computer-based tracings (ACT) in longitudinal 2-D ultrasound images using different scanners," *J. Mech. Med. Biol.*, vol. 9, no. 4, pp. 481–505, 2009.

[31] P. Pignoli and T. Longo, "Evaluation of atherosclerosis with B-mode ultrasound imaging.," *J. Nucl. Med. Allied Sci.*, vol. 32, no. 3, pp. 166–173, 1988.

[32] F. Molinari, U. Acharya, G. Zeng, and K. Meiburger, "Completely automated robust edge snapper for carotid ultrasound IMT measurement on a multi-institutional database of 300 images," *Med. Biol. Eng. Comput.*, vol. 49, no. 8, pp. 935–945, 2011.

[33] F. Faita, V. Gemignani, E. Bianchini, C. Giannarelli, L. Ghiadoni, and M. Demi, "Real-time measurement system for evaluation of the carotid intima-media thickness with a robust edge operator.," *J. Ultrasound Med.*, vol. 27, no. 9, pp. 1353–1361, Sep. 2008.

[34] I. Wendelhag, T. Gustavsson, M. Suurküla, G. Berglund, and J. Wikstrand, "Ultrasound measurement of wall thickness in the carotid artery: fundamental principles and description of a computerized analysing system," *Clin. Physiol.*, vol. 11, no. 6, pp. 565–577, Nov. 1991.

[35] I. Wendelhag, Q. Liang, T. Gustavsson, and J. Wikstrand, "A new automated computerized analyzing system simplifies readings and reduces the variability in ultrasound measurement of intima-media thickness," *Stroke*, vol. 28, no. 11, pp. 2195–2200, Nov. 1997.

[36] Q. Quan Liang, I. Wendelhag, J. Wikstrand, and T. Gustavsson, "A multiscale dynamic programming procedure for boundary detection in ultrasonic artery images," *IEEE Trans. Med. Imaging*, vol. 19, no. 2, pp. 127–142, Feb. 2000.

[37] D. J. Williams and M. Shah, "A Fast algorithm for active contours and curvature estimation," *CVGIP Image Underst.*, vol. 55, no. 1, pp. 14–26, Jan. 1992.

[38] C. P. Loizou, C. S. Pattichis, M. Pantziaris, T. Tyllis, and A. Nicolaides, "Snakes based segmentation of the common carotid artery intima media," *Med. Biol. Eng. Comput.*, vol. 45, no. 1, pp. 35–49, Jan. 2007.

[39] C. P. Loizou, A. Nicolaides, E. Kyriacou, N. Georghiou, M. Griffin, and C. S. Pattichis, "A comparison of ultrasound intima-media thickness measurements of the left and right common carotid artery," *IEEE J. Transl. Eng. Heal. Med.*, vol. 3, pp. 1–10, 2015.

[40] C. P. Loizou, C. S. Pattichis, M. Pantziaris, and A. Nicolaides, "An integrated system for the segmentation of atherosclerotic carotid plaque," *IEEE Trans. Inf. Technol. Biomed.*, vol. 11, no. 6, pp. 661–667, Nov. 2007.

[41] F. Molinari, K. M. Meiburger, L. Saba, *et al.*, "Fully automated dual-snake formulation for carotid intima-media thickness measurement. A new approach.," *J. Ultrasound Med.*, vol. 31, no. 7, pp. 1123–1136, Jul. 2012.

[42] F. Molinari, K. M. Meiburger, L. Saba, *et al.*, "Constrained snake vs. conventional snake for carotid ultrasound automated IMT measurements on multi-center data sets," *Ultrasonics*, vol. 52, no. 7, pp. 949–961, Sep. 2012.

[43] H. Paul V C, "Method and means for recognizing complex patterns," 1960.

[44] S. Golemati, J. Stoitsis, E. G. Sifakis, T. Balkizas, and K. S. Nikita, "Using the Hough transform to segment ultrasound images of longitudinal and transverse sections of the carotid artery," *Ultrasound Med. Biol.*, vol. 33, no. 12, pp. 1918–1932, 2007.

[45] P. M. Shankar, "A compound scattering pdf for the ultrasonic echo envelope and its relationship to K and Nakagami distributions," *IEEE Trans. Ultrason. Ferroelectr. Freq. Control*, vol. 50, no. 3, pp. 339–343, Mar. 2003.

[46] F. Destrempes, J. Meunier, M.-F. Giroux, G. Soulez, and G. Cloutier, "Segmentation in ultrasonic B-mode images of healthy carotid arteries using mixtures of Nakagami distributions and stochastic optimization," *IEEE Trans. Med. Imaging*, vol. 28, no. 2, pp. 215–229, Feb. 2009.

[47] S. Rosati, K. M. Meiburger, G. Balestra, U. R. Acharya, and F. Molinari, "Carotid wall measurement and assessment based on pixel-based and local texture descriptors," *J. Mech. Med. Biol.*, vol. 16, no. 1, p. 1640006, Feb. 2016.

[48] S. Delsanto, F. Molinari, P. Giustetto, W. Liboni, S. Badalamenti, and J. S. Suri, "Characterization of a completely user-independent algorithm for carotid artery segmentation in 2-D ultrasound images," *IEEE Trans. Instrum. Meas.*, vol. 56, no. 4, pp. 1265–1274, 2007.

[49] D. Pazinato, B. Stein, and W. de Almeida, "Pixel-level tissue classification for ultrasound images," *IEEE J. Biomed. Health Inform.*, vol. 20, no. 1, pp. 256–267, 2016.

[50] K. M. Meiburger, S. Rosati, G. Balestra, U. R. Acharya, and F. Molinari, "Ultrasound B-mode descriptors and their association to age and automated IMT and IMT variability," *J. Mech. Med. Biol.*, vol. 16, no. 1, p. 1640007, Feb. 2016.

[51] F. Molinari, G. Zeng, and J. Suri, "A state of the art review on intima– media thickness (IMT) measurement and wall segmentation techniques for carotid ultrasound," *Comput. Methods Programs Biomed.*, vol. 100, no. 3, pp. 201–221, 2010.

[52] L. Saba, F. Molinari, and K. Meiburger, "What is the correct distance measurement metric when measuring carotid ultrasound intima-media thickness automatically?," *Int. Angiol. a J. Int. Union Angiol.*, vol. 31, no. 5, pp. 483–489, 2012.

[53] F. Molinari, G. Zeng, and J. Suri, "Inter-Greedy technique for fusion of different carotid segmentation boundaries leading to high-performance IMT measurement," *Eng. Med. Biol. Soci. (EMBC), 2010 Annual International Conference of the IEEE*, pp. 4769–4772, 2010.

[54] V. Chalana and Y. Kim, "A methodology for evaluation of boundary detection algorithms on medical images," *IEEE Trans. Med. Imaging*, vol. 16, no. 5, pp. 642–652, 1997.

[55] C. Alberola-Lopez and M. Martín-Fernández, "Comments on: a methodology for evaluation of boundary detection algorithms on medical images," *IEEE Trans. Med. Imaging*, vol. 23, no. 5, pp. 658–660, 2004.

[56] J. F. Polak and D. H. O'Leary, "Edge-detected common carotid artery intima-media thickness and incident coronary heart disease in the multi-ethnic study of atherosclerosis," *J. Am. Heart Assoc.*, vol. 4, no. 6, p. e001492, 2015.

[57] J. F. Polak, M. J. Pencina, D. Herrington, and D. H. O'Leary, "Associations of edge-detected and manual-traced common carotid intima-media thickness measurements with Framingham risk factors," *Stroke*, vol. 42, no. 7, pp. 1912–1916, 2011.

[58] G. Zahnd, K. Kapellas, M. Van Hattem, and A. Van Dijk, "A fully-automatic method to segment the carotid artery layers in ultrasound imaging: application to quantify the compression-decompression pattern of the intima-," *Ultrasound Med. Biol.*, vol. 43, no. 1, pp. 239–257, 2017.

[59] N. Ikeda, N. Dey, A. Sharma, *et al.*, "Automated segmental-IMT measurement in thin/thick plaque with bulb presence in carotid ultrasound from multiple scanners: stroke risk assessment," *Comput. Methods Programs Biomed.*, vol. 141, pp. 73–81, Apr. 2017.

[60] L. Xiao, Q. Li, Y. Bai, L. Zhang, and J. Tang, "Automated measurement method of common carotid artery intima-media thickness in ultrasound image based on Markov random field models," *J. Med. Biol. Eng.*, vol. 35, no. 5, pp. 651–660, Oct. 2015.

[61] R.-M. Menchón-Lara, J.-L. Sancho-Gómez, and A. Bueno-Crespo, "Early-stage atherosclerosis detection using deep learning over carotid ultrasound images," *Appl. Soft Comput.*, vol. 49, pp. 616–628, 2016.

Chapter 20
Ultrasound carotid plaque video segmentation

Christos P. Loizou[1] *and Constantinos S. Pattichis*[2]

Border identification of the atherosclerotic carotid plaque, the common carotid artery (CCA), degree of stenosis, as well as the characteristics of the arterial wall (plaque size, composition and elasticity), may add additional clinical information for the assessment of future cardiovascular events. We propose and evaluate in this chapter an integrated system for the segmentation of atherosclerotic carotid plaque in ultrasound videos of the CCA. The system is based on video frame normalization, speckle reduction filtering, M-mode-state-based identification, parametric active contours and snake's segmentation. The cardiac cycle in each video is first identified and the video M-mode is generated, thus identifying systolic and diastolic states. The video is segmented for a time period of at least one full cardiac cycle by initializing the algorithm in the first video frame. Human manual assistance may be provided if needed. The atherosclerotic plaque borders are tracked and segmented in the subsequent frames. We also propose an initialization method for positioning the snake as close as possible to the plaque borders, based on morphology operators, where initial contours are estimated every 20 video frames. The performance of the algorithm is evaluated on 43 real CCA digitized videos from B-mode longitudinal ultrasound segments and is compared to the manual segmentations of an expert, available every 20 frames in a time span of 3–5 s, covering in general two cardiac cycles. The segmentation results were very promising, according to the expert objective evaluation, with a true-negative fraction (TNF) specificity of 83.7% ± 7.6%, a true-positive fraction (TPF) sensitivity of 85.42% ± 8.1%, between the ground truth and the proposed segmentation method, a kappa index (KI) of 84.6% and an overlap index (OI) of 74.7%. We also computed the cardiac state identification for the CCA. It is shown that the integrated system presented in this chapter can be used for the video segmentation of the CCA plaque in ultrasound videos.

20.1 Introduction

It was documented that the size and composition of carotid atherosclerotic plaque are independent predictors of future cardiovascular events [1]. It was also shown

[1]Department of Electrical Engineering, Computer Engineering and Informatics, Cyprus University of Technology, Cyprus
[2]Department of Computer Science, University of Cyprus, Cyprus

that vulnerable plaques are usually found as containing a large lipid core, a thin fibrous cap [2]. The accurate segmentation of the atherosclerotic carotid plaque in ultrasound B-mode video (see also Figure 20.1(a)) will allow the extraction of important anatomical properties of the artery wall and plaque. These are useful to the physicians, and they may be used to evaluate plaque development, the

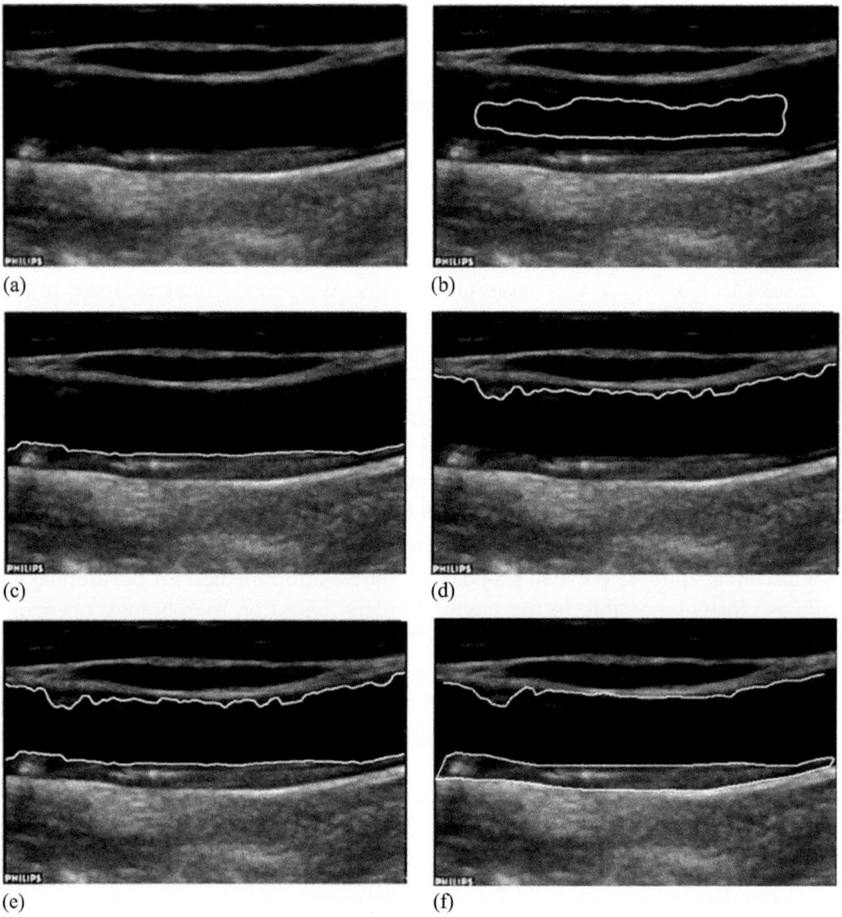

Figure 20.1 *(a) First video frame (after normalized and despeckle filtering), (b) initialization contour using the Chan–Vese model produced by thresholding and morphological closing, (c) initialization at the far wall of the CCA using the Chan–Vese model segmentation, (d) initialization at the near wall of the CCA using the Chan– Vese model segmentation, (e) Chan–Vese model final segmentation result (additional morphological processing has been applied to the Chan–Vese result) and (f) final snakes segmentation of plaque at the far wall of the CCA and lumen at the near wall of the CCA*

process of atherosclerosis as well as in modeling and evaluating the risks for future cardiovascular events. Ultrasound, elastography and other imaging methods such as spectroscopic photoacoustic imaging can also be integrated to advance the characterization of the plaques and corresponding vulnerability [3] as the variation in the mechanical properties of the different tissue types is huge [4]. There have been different quantitative methods proposed and developed in the past few years for the CCA segmentation [5,6] as well as plaque heterogeneity and plaque echogenicity characterization [2–5].

It is accepted that the experts are little confident that there is adequate evidence to determine which interventions to use for different patient populations [3] and, therefore, the availability and evaluation of different characteristics of carotid plaque is of outmost importance. However, the manual segmentation of the plaque in the CCA in ultrasound video is a tedious, time-consuming task and suffers from large inter- and intraobserver variability [5–26]. It is therefore difficult to trace boundaries for each time frame of the cardiac cycle and for large volume of data sets [6,7]. It was shown in [8] that manual delineation of the CCA intima and adventitia borders, which is made by experts, produced errors that were different for the intima and the adventitia borders. When manual delineation of plaques is performed, then errors are further amplified. Therefore, still the need exists for the development of new semiautomated tools and techniques for the assessment of the risk of stroke from ultrasound videos of the CCA incorporating plaque segmentation.

Currently, the ability to predict and identify which patients will have a stroke is poor, and the current practice of assessing the risk of stroke relies on measuring the thickness of the CCA wall (intima-media thickness, IMT) [9,10] or the artery lumen stenosis by identifying the plaque borders in the carotid artery [6]. It was shown that the IMT as well as the degree of artery stenosis can reliably be delineated in still B-mode ultrasound images [1,6,9,10]. The identification of the moving borders of the atherosclerotic carotid plaque and the extraction of the systolic and diastolic video states [7] may also provide additional information of an individual's stroke risk, and treatment of asymptomatic patients may be improved [11].

We present in this chapter an integrated system for the video segmentation of the CCA based on our previous work [6,10,24] for facilitating the quantitative assessment of the atherosclerosis disease. The snake contour was repositioned using the level set formulation of Chan and Vese [13] (see also [10] and [24] for additional details), using random initialization. There are only few studies published in the literature so far for the segmentation of atherosclerotic carotid plaque in ultrasound CCA videos [7,24,25], where a significant number of cases (N) was used for their evaluation, as also shown in Table 20.1. Destrempes *et al.* [7] proposed and evaluated a Bayesian-based video segmentation method on 33 videos, which required manual corrections. In [24], the authors used a Bayesian-based segmentation model and evaluated the method on 33 video sequences. Loizou *et al.* [24] proposed a video carotid plaque segmentation method based on active contours, which was evaluated on 43 videos of the CCA. Gastounioti *et al.* [25] presented a graph-based motion-driven method which was evaluated on 120 image

Table 20.1 Atherosclerotic carotid plaque segmentation techniques. © 2014, reprinted with the permission from [4]

Study	Segmentation method	AIC	*N*
Ultrasound Imaging 2-D			
Mao [16]	Discrete dynamic contour	No	7
Loizou [6]	Active contour model	Yes	80
Delsanto [21]	Gradient-based snake with fuzzy *k*-means	Yes	56
Bonanno [23]	Edge based	Yes	44
Ultrasound video			
Destrempes [7]	Bayesian model	No	33
Loizou [24]	Active contour model	Yes	43
Gastounioti [25]	Graph-based motion driven	No	120
Ultrasound imaging 3-D			
Cheng [26]	3-D-Set evolution	Yes	10
Ukwatta [28]	Level sets	No	21

AIC, automatic initial contour; *N*, number of cases investigated.

sequences of the CCA. Still, several other studies investigated the segmentation of atherosclerotic carotid plaque in ultrasound images. An overview of these techniques is given in Table 20.1. Mao *et al.* [16] proposed a discrete dynamic contour model for extracting the carotid artery lumen in 2-D transversal ultrasound images. Loizou *et al.* [6] proposed a plaque segmentation method, which was based on the Williams and Shah snake [20], for the extraction of the CCA using an automated contour estimation and applied on 80 ultrasound images of the CCA. The atherosclerotic carotid plaque in [21] was segmented in 56 2-D longitudinal ultrasound images using a gradient-based snake segmentation method and fuzzy *K*-means algorithm with an initialization based on pixel intensity. In [28], a three-dimensional (3-D) semiautomated segmentation method using sparse field level sets, where the users choose anchor points on each boundary, was proposed for the segmentation of 3-D CCA images. More recently, Bonanno *et al.* [23] proposed a direct 3-D segmentation method based on a 3-D level-set evolution approach to refine the initial plaque borders which was evaluated on 44 images of the CCA. All the above methods, with the exception of [7] (where ultrasound video segmentation of the plaque in the CCA was proposed), have investigated and proposed different solutions for the segmentation of the atherosclerotic carotid plaque in ultrasound images of the CCA.

Additionally, a number of other techniques not shown in Table 20.1 have been investigated for the atherosclerotic carotid plaque segmentation, where a significantly smaller subset of images was used for algorithm evaluation. More specifically, Hamou *et al.* [14] proposed a method based on the Canny edge detector to detect the plaque in longitudinal CCA ultrasound images. A morphology-based approach for the carotid contour extraction was proposed in [15] for longitudinal ultrasound images of the CCA, incorporating speckle reduction filtering, contour quantization, morphological contour detection and a contour enhancement stage. Abolmaesumi *et al.* [17] introduced a method based on the star algorithm improved by Kalman filtering, for the plaque segmentation in transversal carotid ultrasound images. A semi-automatic method for plaque segmentation in 3-D images of the CCA using the balloon model introduced in [18] was proposed by Gill *et al.* [19]. In [22], the Hough transform was applied to perform segmentation of plaque in four 2-D cross-sectional ultrasound images of the CCA. Finally, in [27], an automated segmentation method for 3-D ultrasound carotid plaque based on a geometrically deformable model, taking advantage of both the local and regional detectors, was proposed.

It is shown from the above that different methods were investigated for the segmentation of the atherosclerotic carotid plaque in ultrasound images and videos. Although a number of studies have been proposed for the segmentation of the CCA plaque from ultrasound images, yet these studies were evaluated on a relatively limited number of subjects. Also, a very limited number of studies have been proposed for the video segmentation of the CCA plaque. Therefore, the need still exists for the development, implementation, and evaluation, of an integrated system enabling the automated segmentation of ultrasound video carotid plaque.

20.2 Methodology and materials used

20.2.1 Acquisition of ultrasound videos and manual delineation of atherosclerotic plaque

We acquired a total of 43 B-mode longitudinal ultrasound videos (from 38 asymptomatic subjects, aged 56 ± 12 and 5 symptomatic, aged 53 ± 16 subjects, 17 female and 26 male) of the CCA bifurcation of subjects. The videos representing different types of atherosclerotic plaque formation with irregular geometry typically found in this blood vessel. Almost all subjects demonstrated a left or a right CCA stenosis of 30% or larger. The videos were acquired by the ATL HDI-5000 ultrasound scanner (Advanced Technology Laboratories, Seattle, USA) and were recorded digitally on a magneto-optical drive, with a size of 576 × 768 pixels with 256 gray levels, a pixel size of 59 μm (17 pixels per mm) and having a frame rate of 100 frames per second. The ATL HDI-5000 ultrasound scanner is equipped with a 256-element fine pitch high-resolution 50-mm linear array, a multielement ultrasound scan head with an extended operating frequency range of 5–12 MHz, and it offers real spatial compound imaging. The video segmentations were performed for 3–5 s intervals, covering in general 2–3 cardiac cycles.

An expert neurologist with more than 20 years of clinical experience manually delineated the plaque borders, between plaque and artery wall, and the borders between plaque and blood, after image normalization and speckle reduction filtering (see Section 20.2.3), using MATLAB® software developed by our group [24,32]. The manual segmentations traced in the first frame could be transferred in the second frame and then could be readjusted by the expert accordingly. The procedure used for carrying out the manual delineation was the one established and documented in the asymptomatic carotid stenosis and risk of stroke project protocol [29] for still images of the CCA. In cases where several plaques were located in the

CCA, comprising multiple components, each plaque was segmented independently so that each contour initialization represents a different plaque.

20.2.2 *Video normalization and speckle reduction filtering of ultrasound videos*

Brightness adjustments of ultrasound videos were carried out based on the method introduced in [30]. This improves image compatibility by reducing the variability introduced by different gain settings, different operators, different equipment and facilitates ultrasound tissue comparability [30]. Algebraic (linear) scaling of the first video frame was manually performed by linearly adjusting the image so that the median gray-level value of the blood was 0–5, and the median gray level of the adventitia (artery wall) was 180–190 [24,30]. The intensity of the gray-level values on the video frames ranged from 0 to 255. Thus, the brightness of all pixels in the video frame was readjusted according to the linear scale defined by selecting the two reference regions [24]. The subsequent frames of the video were then normalized based on the selection of the first frame.

For speckle reduction, the filter DsFlsmv, introduced in [31], was applied to each consecutive frame prior the plaque segmentation. The filters of this type utilize first-order statistics such as the variance and the mean of a pixel neighborhood and may be described with a multiplicative noise model [31,32]. The moving window size for the despeckle filter DsFlsmv was 5×5 and the number of iterations applied to each video frame was two, where a complete description of the filter and its parameters can be found in [31–34].

20.2.3 *Plaque contour initialization and snakes segmentation*

Before running the video plaque snake's segmentation algorithm, an initialization procedure, based on the Chan and Vese active contour, for positioning the initial snake contour in the first frame of the video, as close to the area of interest (plaque borders), was applied [10].

The Williams and Shah snake segmentation method [20] was used to deform the snake and segment the plaque borders in each video frame. The snake contour, $v(s)$, adapts itself by a dynamic process that minimizes an energy function (E_{snake} (v, s) defined as [20]:

$$E_{\text{snake}}(v(s)) = E_{\text{int}}(v(s)) + E_{\text{image}}(v(s)) + E_{\text{external}}(v(s))$$
$$= \int_s \left(\alpha_s E_{\text{cont}}(v(s)) + \beta_s E_{\text{curv}}(v(s)) + \gamma_s E_{\text{image}}(v(s)) + E_{\text{external}}(v(s))\right) ds. \tag{20.1}$$

where $E_{\text{int}}(v(s))$, $E_{\text{image}}(v(s))$, $E_{\text{external}}(v(s))$, $E_{\text{cont}}(v(s))$, $E_{\text{curv}}(v(s))$ are the internal, image, external, continuity and curvature energies of the snake, and $\alpha(s)$, $\beta(s)$ and $\gamma(s)$ the strength, tension and stiffness parameters, respectively. For the Williams and Shah snake, the strength, tension and stiffness parameters were equal to

$\alpha_s = 0.6$, $\beta_s = 0.4$ and $\gamma_s = 2$, respectively. The sampled contour points resulting from the previous step were used for the active contour initialization. The first and the last points on the contour resulting from the initialization procedure presented in the previous section are connected to form a closed initial snake contour. The final plaque contour resulting from the snake deformation is mapped from the first video frame to the second and is sampled to provide the initialization for the snake deformation. The segmentation is carried out for a full cardiac cycle, which is identified using the procedure in Section 20.2.5. In every 20 video frames, the entire initialization procedure is repeated in order to detect the plaque borders again, reposition the snake and reassure that the snake contour will not converge away from the area of interest. If there were multiple plaques in the CCA video, then the entire methodology is repeated for each plaque. Two more examples of video plaque segmentation are shown in Figure 20.2.

20.2.4 M-mode image generation, boundary extraction, state identification and manual delineation

The M-mode image (see Figure 20.3(d)) can be generated in such a way that it crosses all plaque borders having maximum motion in opposite directions [35]. The procedure of the M-mode generation is illustrated in Figure 20.3 and also described in [36].

Figure 20.3(a) presents the first video frame of the cardiac cycle from a B-mode ultrasound video of the left CCA, after normalization and despeckle filtering acquired from a male symptomatic subject at the age of 64 (having a stent on the right CCA and a stenosis of 40%–50%). Figure 20.3(b) presents the automated snakes segmentations of the plaque boundaries at the far wall of the CCA and the lumen segmentation at the near wall. The segmented atherosclerotic plaque is shown in Figure 20.3(c), whereas Figure 20.3(d) presents the despeckled M-mode image generated from the CCA video for the first 1,200 frames (12 s).

Perpendicular lines that cross the major axis of the plaque (from Figure 20.3(c) were placed automatically at the major axis quintiles (20%, 40%, 60% and 80%). By scanning the intensity values along the straight perpendicular line selected by the user, the M-mode image is generated, by taking this line as the *Y*-axis, and each frame of the video as the *X*-axis (see Figure 20.3(d)). Four M-mode images were generated for each of the corresponding four perpendicular lines. The manual delineations, as well as all other measurements, were performed using a system implemented in MATLAB from our group [6,24]. The M-mode images were converted to binary images, and morphological operators were applied to smooth the edges. Then, edge detection was applied on each M-mode image in order to derive the initial near and far wall boundaries, and the rate of change [36]. The snake segmentation system [6] was also used to refine the derived snakes contours (see Figure 20.3(e)) found on the M-mode image. From the derived contours at the far and near wall boundaries of the M-mode image, the diastolic and systolic diameters (plaque–lumen) of the carotid artery were calculated. This was done by finding corresponding maxima and minima (and vice versa) at the near and far

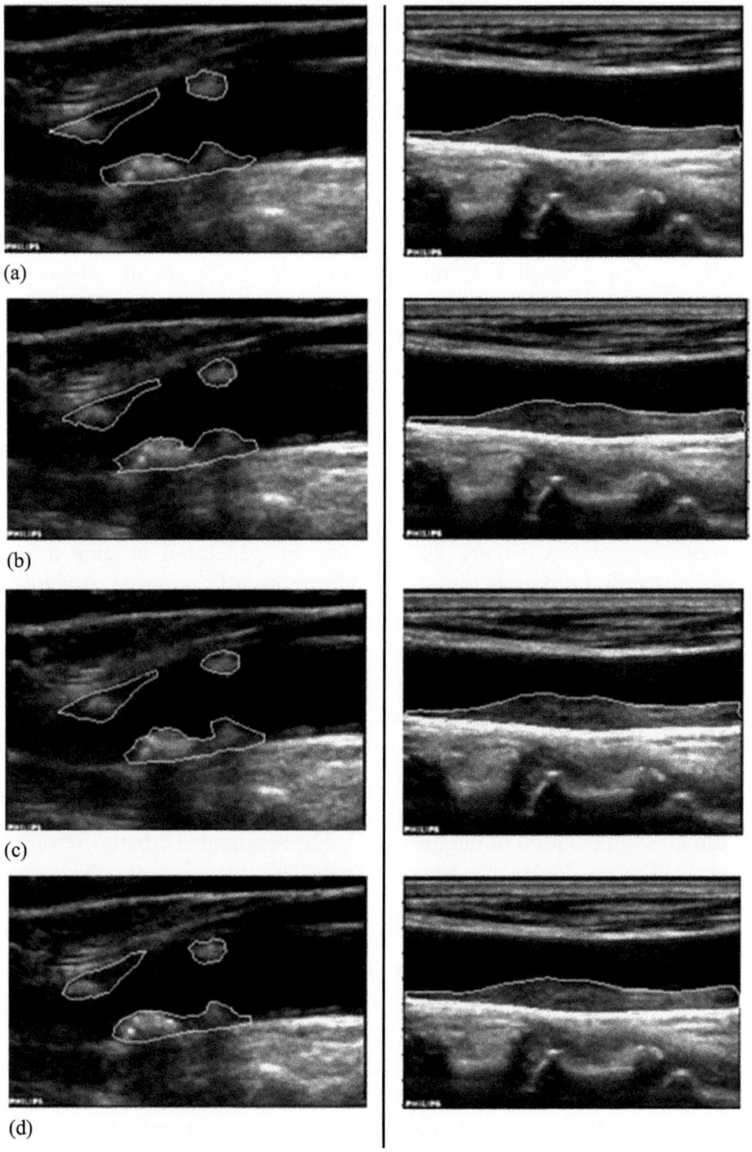

Figure 20.2 Examples of plaque segmentation of atherosclerotic carotid plaques appearing at the CCA at the (a) 50th, (b) 60th, (c) 70th and (d) 150th video frames of the videos. Left column: a female asymptomatic subject with three different plaques at the near and far wall of the CCA, at the age of 61 with a left CCA stenosis of 35%–40%. Right column: male symptomatic subject at the age of 64, a stent on the right CCA and with a stenosis of 40%–50%

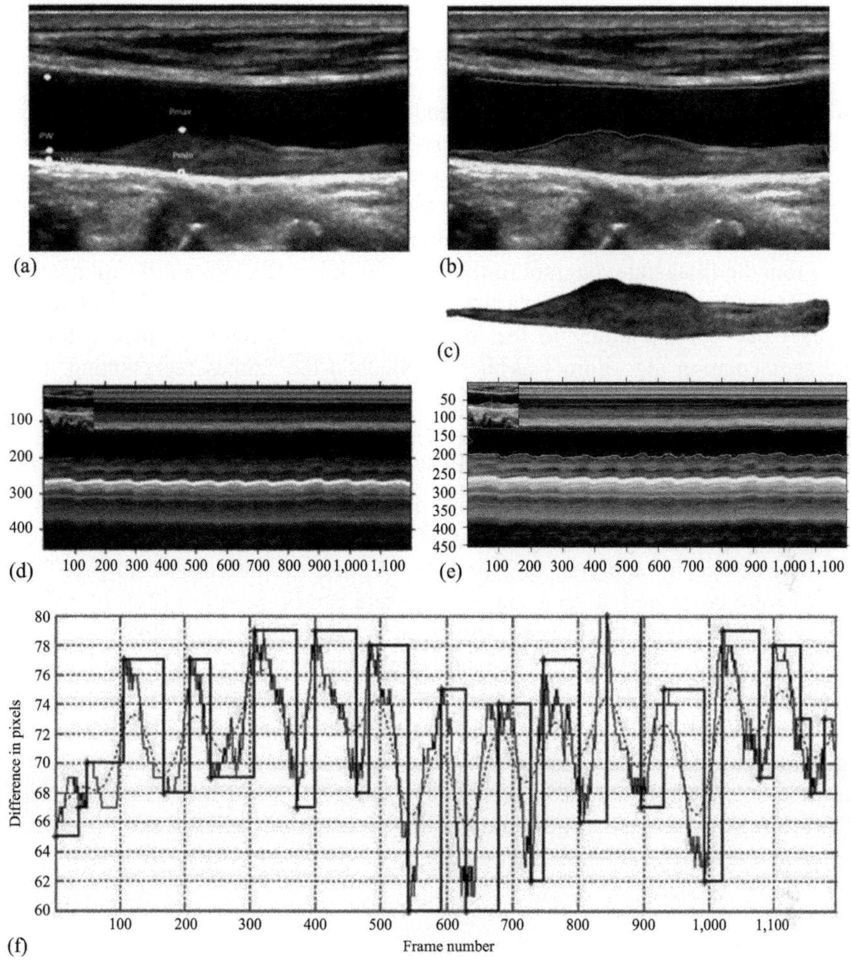

Figure 20.3 M-mode generation (see Section 20.2.4), (a) first normalized despeckled (with DsFlsmv) frame of a B-mode ultrasound video of the CCA, (b) segmentation of the plaque boundaries and the near wall of the CCA using snakes [5], (c) extracted atherosclerotic carotid plaque, (d) M-mode image generated from the CCA video for a selected B-mode line (after despeckling), (e) M-mode states superimposed on the original M-mode image at the far and near walls, respectively, (f) diameter change (averaged across the major plaque axis quintiles, with step diagram and systolic and diastolic frames of the video with maximum carotid diameter during distension (*) and maximum carotid diameter during contraction) (see also (a)). For the points adventitia wall (AW), plaque wall (PW), media-adventitia wall (MAW), plaque at maximum point (P_{max}) and plaque at minimum point (P_{min}) (see also [24] for definition). Diastolic and systolic frames (from 0 to 1,200) (100 frames per second = 12 s). Contraction frames: 1, 36, 168, 240, 372, 464, 543, 629, 728, 803, 896 and 993. Distension Frames: 49, 106, 208, 306, 400, 483, 592, 680, 747, 844 and 931. Minimum carotid diameter: 2 mm at frame 543. Maximum carotid diameter: 2.67 mm at frame 844

wall boundaries of the M-mode image and then estimating their difference, which is the diameter rate of change (see Figure 20.3(f)). The extracted contours for the rate of change were averaged to form the final state diagram of the video (see Figure 20.3(f) showing final states of the video), where diastolic and systolic frames were estimated at the maxima and minima of the curve.

From the final state diagram of the video in Figure 20.3(f), a full cardiac cycle was selected by identifying the starting and ending frames of the cycle. The frames of the video corresponding to the identified cardiac cycle were then extracted. The segmentation algorithm was then applied on the frames representing a full cardiac cycle.

20.2.5 Evaluation of the segmentation method and state diagram

The video segmentation methods were evaluated using the *TPF* and the TNF corresponding to sensitivity and specificity [37]. Ratios of overlapping areas can also be assessed by applying the similarity *KI* and the OI as used in [6]. These indices were computed at each video frame and can be found in [24]. In order to further evaluate the state-based identification algorithm, the following metrics between the automated and the manual state diagram timings were computed for each subject (video). The metrics were used to assess the agreement between the manual (M) and the automated (A) segmentation methods [24,32,33]: the root-mean-square error (RMSE), the normalized mean-square error (NMSE), the mean absolute error (MAE), the mean average absolute error, the carotid diameter during contraction (CDC), the carotid diameter during distension (CDD) and the percentage of the carotid wall distension [24].

20.3 Results

Figure 20.2 presents two different examples of video plaque segmentation with atherosclerotic plaques appearing at the CCA in the left and right column, respectively. The segmentations were performed for the first and second cardiac cycle, for the 50th, 60th, 70th and 150th video frames of the video, respectively. It is observed that the proposed segmentation algorithm is able to follow the plaque borders consistently as a result of the initialization procedures followed.

Table 20.2 tabulates the quantitative results of the statistical analysis based on TNF, TPF, KI and OI for the proposed video segmentation method performed for 1–2 cardiac cycles, on 43 ultrasound videos of the CCA. The results of the automated segmentation method are compared with the manual tracings of the expert which are considered to be the ground truth. The results show that the proposed method using the proposed initialization method agrees with the expert by correctly detecting no plaque (TNF) in (83.7% $\pm$ 7.6%) of the cases, by correctly detecting a plaque (TPF) in (85.42% $\pm$ 8.1%) of the cases. The similarity KI and the OI, for the proposed video snakes segmentation method, were equal to 84.6% and 74.7% using the two different initialization techniques, respectively. There was no

Table 20.2 Performance evaluation metrics for the plaque video segmentation method. Sensitivity (TPF), specificity (TNF), KI and overlap index (OI) for the video segmentation methods performed on $N = 43$ ultrasound videos of the CCA.

Segmentation method	N	TPF (%)	TNF (%)	KI (%)	OI (%)
Loizou [6]	Images ($N = 80$)	83 ± 7	81 ± 7	81	69
Loizou [24]	Videos ($N = 43$)	85 ± 8	84 ± 8	84.6	75
Destrempes [7]	Videos ($N = 33$)	84 ± 8	94 ± 4	85	80
Golemati [22]	Images ($N = 4$)	98 ± 1	96 ± 10	–	–

N, number of images or videos; TNF, true-negative fraction; TPF, true-positive fraction; KI, kappa index; OI, overlap index.

significant difference between the two methods for all metrics investigated using a pair t-test at $p < 0.05$. However, a small improvement was observed in almost all evaluation metrics when the segmentations were performed with the second initialization method. It should further be noted that the snake contour may be attracted occasionally to local minima and converge to a wrong location. This occurred in less than 10% of the cases (i.e., in four videos).

Figure 20.3(e) presents the M-mode image of the video, where the video states are superimposed at the far and near wall, respectively. The insert on the left upper side of the images in Figure 20.3(d) and (e), indicates the straight perpendicular line that can also be selected by the user of the proposed system in order to generate the M-mode image. Finally, in Figure 20.3(f), the diameter change is presented with the help of a step diagram showing systolic (1, 36, 168, 240, 372, 464, 543, 629, 728, 803, 896, 993) and diastolic frames (49, 106, 208, 306, 400, 483, 592, 680, 747, 844, 931) of the video. The maximum CDD (2 mm at frame 543 indicated with an *) and maximum CDC (2.67 mm at frame 844 indicated with an *) are also shown.

Table 20.3 presents the results of the evaluation metrics between the manual and the automated state diagrams (mean ± std) in microseconds for the asymptomatic and the symptomatic subjects, respectively. The RMSE, NRMSE, MAE and the mean absolute relative error (MARE) were for all videos 125.41 ± 11.77, 121.16 ± 10.38, 119.06 ± 11.96 and 5.43 ± 0.95 μs, respectively. The t-test gave statistically significant differences between the asymptomatic and symptomatic cases for all evaluation metrics tabulated in Table 20.3.

Table 20.4 illustrates the results of the CDC, CDD and the % of carotid wall distension (%CWD) for the asymptomatic and the symptomatic subjects (mean ± std). The CDC, CDD and the %CWD were for the asymptomatic/the symptomatic group $5.13 \pm 0.34/5.48 \pm 0.29$ mm, $5.89 \pm 0.31/6.27 \pm 0.35$ mm and $10.2\% \pm 1.03\%/16.09\% \pm 0.83\%$, respectively. The t-test, shown in the last row of Table 20.4, performed between the values obtained for the asymptomatic and symptomatic cases, at $p < 0.05$, gave no statistically significant differences between them.

Table 20.3 Evaluation metrics between manual and automatic states in μs (mean±std)

Videos	RMSE	NRMSE	MAE	MARE
AS ($N=38$)	191±13	213±12	183±20	7±1
SY ($N=5$)	60±10	44±8	55.50±4.20	3.8±0.9
t-Test between AS and SY[1]	S ($p=0.04$)	S ($p=0.002$)	S ($p=0.03$)	S ($p=0.03$)

N, number of videos; AS, asymptomatic; SY, symptomatic; RMSE, relative mean square error; NRMSE, normalized mean square error; MAE, mean absolute error; MARE, mean absolute relative error; S, significantly different.
[1]Test carried out at $p < 0.05$.

Table 20.4 Carotid diameter during contraction (CDC), carotid diameter during distension (CDD) and % of carotid wall distension (%CWD) for the automated segmentations (mean ± std)

Videos	CDC (mm)	CDD (mm)	%CWD
AS ($N=38$)	5 ± 0.4	5.9 ± 0.3	10±1
SY ($N=5$)	5.5 ± 0.3	6.3 ± 0.4	16.1 ± 0.8
t-Test between AS and SY[1]	NS ($p=0.6$)	NS ($p=0.1$)	NS ($p=0.4$)

NS, nonsignificantly different.
[1]Test carried out at $p < 0.05$.

20.4 Discussion

The results of the proposed integrated video segmentation method can be favorably compared with the results of the segmentation of the carotid plaque in ultrasound images presented in [6], and also with the results presented in [7,22] (see also Table 20.1). Comparing the proposed video segmentation method with the one presented in [6], one may observe that the TNF, TPF, KI and OI are larger in this study. This may be attributed to the fact that the videos used here were of better quality when compared to the images used in [6]. The results reported in [22] are better than the ones reported in [6] as well as in this study, but it should also be taken into consideration that the number of images used in [22] was very small (only four ultrasound images of the CCA) when compared to the study in [6,7], where 80 and 33 videos were used, respectively. Furthermore, in [7], where video segmentation of atherosclerotic carotid plaque in 33 video sequences was proposed, similar results were obtained for the KI and OI (see also Table 20.2). Also, the specificity was 94.1% ± 4.2% in [7] versus 84.3% ± 7.5% here. It should also be noted that the standard deviations obtained for the presented work are larger when compared to the ones obtained in [7].

The results of Table 20.3 show that all error measurements (RMSE, NRMSE, MAE and MARE), calculated in this study, are much smaller with much smaller standard deviations than the ones obtained in recent studies [25,36], where M-mode-state-based identification in ten CCA videos was investigated. The smaller deviations obtained in this study could be attributed to the fact that a heterogeneous group of videos was investigated in [36].

The results of Table 20.4 are also consistent with [25,36] (CDC = 5.26 ± 0.52 mm, CDD = 5.81 ± 0.59 mm, %CWD = 10.32% ± 4.71%) where M-mode-state-based identification in ten ultrasound videos of the CCA was performed.

In [21,22], where image segmentation of the atherosclerotic carotid plaque was performed, images were neither normalized nor despeckled, nor was an automatic contour estimation used as in this study. The video normalization method presented in this study ensures that the segmentation method and the results are not dependent on the equipment used. This is not the case for the video segmentation method proposed in [7], where the region-based segmentation was established using the statistical distribution of the gray level of the frames whilst speckle noise was not taken into consideration. Furthermore, the results of this study showed that the proposed video segmentation method performs very closely to the method for atherosclerotic plaque segmentation presented in [6]. The presented work can also be favorably compared with the recent video segmentation study in [7], performed on 33 subjects (see also Table 20.2).

In [21,22], the initialization of the segmentation algorithm was performed automatically based on the echogenicity of the lumen and the plaque, or the Hough transform, respectively. These methods were tested on image sequences but were processed individually. In the presented methodology, it was assumed that if the method performed satisfactorily for an individual image, it might also perform well for a whole sequence of images, each one processed individually. However, a more sophisticated tracking procedure, taking into consideration the interrelations between neighboring frames by utilization motion estimation, could be taken into consideration in future work. Such a method could achieve automated video segmentation with even less manual intervention.

Initial contour estimation for segmenting ultrasound images was also proposed in [38], derived from the polar image by combining information extracted from the probability function of the contour position, and more specifically from the function maximum location and the first zero crossing of its derivative. Then, starting from the initial contour, a region of interest was automatically selected and the process iterated until the snake contour evolution could be ignored. In [39], a cost function was calculated and used as an input to the image plaque segmentation algorithm. In [19], a dynamic balloon model [18] represented by a triangular mesh was applied for detecting the plaque borders on two 3-D ultrasound carotid images where the initial contour was placed manually. In all of these studies as well as in the present study, the significance of the initial contour placement was not exhaustively investigated in order to estimate how this influences the final segmentation result.

By identifying the states of the CCA, the normal and abnormal plaque motion can be investigated. It was shown in [7,35], as well as in the present study, that M-mode-state-based modeling derived from B-mode videos can be used successfully to derive the carotid states and assess the corresponding wall changes. This work also shows that state-based video modeling can be used to identify video segments dynamic behavior in ultrasound videos of the CCA. However, further work is needed for validating the proposed method and for differentiation between normal and abnormal state-based plaque motion analysis.

In [40], it was shown that M-mode ultrasound analysis can be a sensitive tool for measurements of strain decrease with increasing age and male sex and strain increase with smoking and obesity when evaluated on the right CCA. Therefore, it might be used for screening of "unsuccessful vascular aging" and still potentially reversible subclinical carotid atherosclerosis thereby lowering the cutoff value of vascular damage towards the values of unaffected population. It provides opportunities for introduction of different therapeutic or lifestyle change strategies for reduction or retardation of overt clinical manifestation of cerebrovascular disease.

In [35], the states of echocardiogram videos were identified based on a state classifier detector, which first detects the view boundaries using histogram-based comparison and edge change ratio. The accuracy of the classifier was 97.19% which was higher than two existing approaches [41,42]. Misclassification error of state detection was less than 13% which is reasonably low.

Future research perspectives may be orientated towards the development of new M-mode identification algorithms, and motion field of the arterial wall. Further, the separation between healthy and diseased arterial wall remains to be studied in detail.

20.4.1 Limitations of the video segmentation method

There are some limitations in the proposed methodology that are summarized below. Cases of plaque type I and type V [6,29,30] were not considered for segmentation. If the plaque is of type I, borders are not visible well. Plaques of type V produce acoustic shadowing and the plaque is also not visible well [29]. However, there are also inherent difficulties for segmentation of the carotid videos and the corresponding plaques that arise not only from the use of different protocols but also due to differences in anatomy as well as the extent of the atherosclerosis and plaque presence. The presence of extensive and severe carotid stenosis may cause the initialization to completely fail as there will be difficulty in establishing the lumen. In addition, the presence of extensive plaques in the near wall may cause inaccurate segmentation of the far wall adventitia. It should be noted that the parameters for each processing step (e.g., the size of the moving pixel window, the number of iterations and the number of frames for which the contour was reinitialized) were selected for maximum performance.

In everyday clinical practice, the ultrasonographer manipulates the transducer and mentally transforms the 2-D images into anatomical volume, or structure, or lesion, in order to make a diagnosis. The 3-D ultrasound attempts to provide the ultrasonographer with a more realistic reconstruction and visualization of the 3-D structure under investigation thus overcoming the limitations of 2-D imaging, reducing the variability of assessment aiding in improved diagnosis. The additional information may also enable evaluation of changes in the volume but also in the surface morphology providing additional information for stroke risk analysis [27]. The use of 3-D techniques has primarily focused on measuring volume changes through time to monitor disease progression [43–45]. Landry *et al.* [43] demonstrated that plaque volume change can be reliably measured using 3-D ultrasound. They showed that a 20%–35% change can be measured with 95% confidence for plaques of volume <100 mm^3. For larger plaques (volume >100 mm^3), with 95% confidence, they showed that we can measure finer changes of the order of 10%–20%, respectively. Chiu *et al.* [44] developed a 3-D segmentation method for measuring the combined thickness of the plaque, the intima and media (vessel wall plus plaque thickness or VWT). The authors proposed the use of 3-D VWT and VWT-change maps for identifying disease progression in relation to disturbances of flow. The authors extended their work in [45], where they measured VWT volume changes for assessing and monitoring carotid artery disease.

20.5 Concluding remarks

We presented in this chapter a method which proposes an integrated system, which may be used for the segmentation of atherosclerotic carotid plaque in longitudinal ultrasound videos or image sequences. The proposed method is based on different preprocessing steps, which includes video frames normalization and despeckling and active contours segmentation. We anticipate that the proposed system will be incorporating in the future medical practice and will be able to reduce the time which is required for the video analysis. Another anticipation is to reduce the subjectivity that accompanies manual delineations and measurements. Future work will focus on improving the segmentation procedure, such that it can process satisfactorily special plaque cases and difficult to segment videos, taking for example into consideration a statistical approach to initialize and teach the snake about the blood flow and plaque area [40] as was also investigated in [6]. The system will also be further used to investigate longitudinal and radial strain movement of the wall and plaque in ultrasound videos of the CCA. The extracted strain parameters may offer additional clinical information on the severity of the atherosclerosis disease.

References

[1] W. E. Hellings, W. Peeters, F. L. Moll, *et al.*, “Composition of carotid atherosclerotic plaque is associated with cardiovascular outcome: A prognostic study,” Circulation, vol. 121, no. 17, pp. 1941–1950, May 2010.

[2] C. Schmitt, G. Soulez, R. L. Maurice, M.-F. Giroux, and G. Cloutier, “Noninvasive vascular elastography: Toward a complementary characterization tool of atherosclerosis in carotid arteries,” Ultrasound Med. Biol., vol. 33, no. 12, pp. 1841–1858, 2007.

[3] I. M. Graf, J. Su, D. Yeager, J. Amirian, R. Smalling, and S. Emelianov, “Methodical study on plaque characterization using integrated vascular

ultrasound, strain and spectroscopic photoacoustic imaging," in Proc. SPIE 7899, 2011, vol. 789902, pages 4.

[4] H. Ribbers, R. G. P. Lopata, S. Holewijn, *et al.*, "Noninvasive two-dimensional strain imaging of arteries: Validation in phantoms and preliminary experience in carotid arteries in vivo," Ultrasound Med. Biol., vol. 33, no. 4, pp. 530–540, 2007.

[5] H. Shi, C. C. Mitchell, M. McCormick, M. A. Kliewer, R. J. Dempsey, and T. Varghese, "Preliminary in vivo atherosclerotic carotid plaque characterization using the accumulated axial strain and relative lateral shift strain indices," Phys. Med. Biol., vol. 53, pp. 6377–6394, 2008.

[6] C. P. Loizou, C. S. Pattichis, M. Pantziaris, and A. N. Nicolaides, "An integrated system for the segmentation of atherosclerotic carotid plaque," IEEE Trans. Inf. Technol. Biomed., vol. 11, no. 6, pp. 661–667, Nov. 2007.

[7] F. Destrempes, J. Meunier, M.-F. Giroux, G. Soulez, and G. Cloutier, "Segmentation of plaques in sequences of ultrasonic B-mode images of carotid based on motion estimation and a Bayesian model," IEEE Trans. Biomed. Eng., vol. 58, no. 8, pp. 2202–2211, 2011.

[8] J. F. Polak, M. J. Pencina, D. H. O'Leary, and R. B. D'Agostino, "Common-carotid artery intima-media thickness progression as a predictor of stroke in multi-ethnic study of atherosclerosis," Stroke, vol. 42, pp. 3017–3021, 2011.

[9] Q. Liang, I. Wendelhag, J. Wikstrand, and T. Gustavsson, "A multiscale dynamic programming procedure for boundary detection in ultrasonic artery images," IEEE Trans. Med. Imaging, vol. 19, no. 2, pp. 127–142, Feb. 2000.

[10] S. Petroudi, C. P. Loizou, M. Pantziaris, and C. S. Pattichis, "Segmentation of the common carotid intima-media complex in ultrasound images using active contours," IEEE Trans. Biomed. Eng., vol. 59, no. 11, pp. 3060–3069, Nov. 2012.

[11] D. Kashiwazaki, T. Yoshimoto, T. Mikami, *et al.*, "Identification of high-risk carotid artery stenosis: Motion of intraplaque contents detected using B-mode ultrasonography," J. Neurosurg., vol. 117, no. 3, pp. 574–578, 2012.

[12] C. P. Loizou, C. S. Pattichis, S. Petroudi, M. Pantziaris, T. Kasparis, and A. N. Nicolaides, "Segmentation of atherosclerotic carotid plaque in ultrasound video," in 34th Ann. Int. Conf. IEEE Eng. Med. Biol., EMBC, San Diego, USA, 2012, Aug. 28–Sep. 1, pages 4, Paper WeA03.2.

[13] T. Chan and L. Vese, "Active contours without edges," IEEE Trans. Image Process., vol. 10, pp. 266–277, 2001.

[14] A. Hamou and M. El.-Sakka, "A novel segmentation technique for carotid ultrasound images," in Int. Conf. on Acoustic Speech and Signal Process., ICASSP, 2004, pp. III-521–III-524.

[15] A. R. Abdel-Dayen and M. R. El.-Sakka, "A novel morphological-based carotid artery contour extraction," Can. Conf. Electr. Comput. Eng., vol. 4, pp. 1873–1876, 2–5 May 2004.

[16] F. Mao, J. Gill, D. Downey, and A. Fenster, "Segmentation of carotid artery in ultrasound images: Method development and evaluation technique," Med. Phys., vol. 27, no. 8, pp. 1–10, Aug. 2000.

[17] P. Abolmaesumi, M. R. Sirouspour, and S. E. Salcudean, "Real-time extraction of carotid artery contours from ultrasound images," in Proc. IEEE Int. Conf. Computer Based Medical Systems, 2000, pp. 181–186.
[18] L. D. Cohen, "On active contour models and balloons," Comput. Vision Graphics Image Process.: Image Understanding (CVGIP:IU), vol. 53, no. 2, pp. 211–218, 1991.
[19] J. D. Gill, H. M. Ladak, D. A. Steinman, and A. Fenster, "Segmentation of ulcerated plaque: A semi-automatic method for tracking the progression of carotid atherosclerosis," in Proc of 22nd Annual Intern. Confer. of the IEEE, Engineering in Medicine & Biology Society, Chicago, IL, 23–28 July 2000, pp. 1–4.
[20] D. Williams and M. Shah, "A fast algorithm for active contour and curvature estimation," GVCIP: Image Understanding, vol. 55, no. 1, pp. 14–26, 1992.
[21] S. Delsanto, F. Molinari, P. Giustetto, W. Liboni, S. Badalamenti, and J. S. Suri, "Characterization of completely user-independent algorithm for carotid artery segmentation in 2D ultrasound images," IEEE Trans. Instrum. Meas., vol. 56, no. 4, pp. 1265–1274, 2007.
[22] S. Golemati, J. Stoitsis, E. G. Sifakis, T. Balkisas, and K. S. Nikita, "Using the Hough transform to segment ultrasound images of longitudinal and transverse sections of the carotid artery," Ultrasound Med. Biol., vol. 33, no. 12, pp. 1918–1932, 2007.
[23] L. Bonanno, F. Sottile, R. Ciurleo, *et al.*, "Automatic algorithm for the segmentation of atherosclerotic carotid plaque," J. Stroke Cardiovasc. Dis., vol. 26, no. 2, pp. 411–416, 2017.
[24] C. P. Loizou, S. Petroudi, C. S. Pattichis, M. Pantziaris, A. N. Nicolaides, "An integrated system for the segmentation of atherosclerotic carotid plaque in ultrasound video," IEEE Trans. Ultrason. Ferroelectr. Freq. Control, vol. 61, no. 1, pp. 86–101, 2014.
[25] A. Gastounioti, A. Sotiras, K. S. Nikita, N. Paragios, "Graph-based motion-driven segmentation of the carotid atherosclerotique plaque in 2D Ultrasound sequences," in Medical Image Computing & Computer-Assisted Intervention, MICCAI 2015, Part III, LNCS 9351, pp. 551–559, Munich, Germany, Oct. 2015.
[26] J. Cheng, Y. Yu, and B. Chiu, "Direct 3D segmentation of carotid plaque for 3D ultrasound images," in IEEE Biomd. Circuits & Systems Conf. (BioCAS), Shanghai, China, 17–19 Oct. 2016, pp. 123–126.
[27] A. Zahalka and A. Fenster, "An automated segmentation method for three-dimensional carotid ultrasound images," Phys. Med. Biol., vol. 46, no. 4, pp. 1321–1342, 2001.
[28] E. Ukwatta, J. Yuan, D. Buchanan, *et al.*, "Three-dimensional segmentation of three-dimensional ultrasound carotid atherosclerosis using sparse field level sets," Med. Phys., vol. 40, no. 5, 17 pages, 2013.
[29] A. N. Nicolaides, M. Sabetai, S. K. Kakkos, S. Dhanjil, T. Tegos, and J. M. Stevens, "The asymptomatic carotid stenosis and risk of stroke study," Int. Angiol., vol. 22, no. 3, pp. 263–272, 2003.

[30] T. Elatrozy, A. Nicolaides, T. Tegos, A. Zarka, M. Griffin, and M. Sabetai, "The effect of B-mode ultrasonic image standardization of the echodensity of symptomatic and asymptomatic carotid bifurcation plaque," Int. Angiol., vol. 17, no. 3, pp. 179–186, 1998.

[31] J. S. Lee, "Digital image enhancement and noise filtering by using local statistics," IEEE Trans. Pattern Anal. Mach. Intell., vol. PAMI-2, no. 2, pp. 165–168, 1980.

[32] C. P. Loizou, C. S. Pattichis, C. I. Christodoulou, R. S. H. Istepanian, M. Pantziaris, and A. Nicoliades, "Despeckle filtering in ultrasound imaging of the carotid artery," IEEE Trans. Ultrason. Ferroelectr. Freq. Control, vol. 52, no. 2, pp. 1653–1669, 2005.

[33] C. P. Loizou, T. Kasparis, P. Christodoulides, *et al.*, "Despeckle filtering in ultrasound video of the common carotid artery," in Proc. 12th Int. Conf. Bioinf. & Bioeng. (BIBE), Larnaca, Cyprus, Nov. 11–13, 2012, pages 4.

[34] C. P. Loizou, T. Kasparis, P. Papakyriakou, L. Christodoulou, M. Pantziaris, and C. S. Pattichis, "Video segmentation of the common carotid artery intima-media complex," in Proc. 12th Int. Conf. Bioinf. & Bioeng. Proc. (BIBE), Larnaca, Cyprus, Nov. 11–13, 2012, pages 4.

[35] A. Roy, S. Sural, J. Mukherjee, and A. K. Majunmdar, "State based modeling and object extraction from echocardiogram video," IEEE Trans. Inf. Technol. Biomed., vol. 12, no. 3, pp. 366–376, 2008.

[36] C. P. Loizou, M. Pantziaris, C. S. Pattichis, and E. Kyriakou, "M-mode state-based identification in ultrasound videos of the common carotid artery," in Proc. 4th Int. Symp. on Commun. Contr. and Sign. Process., ISCCSP 2010, Limassol, Cyprus, Mar. 3–5, 2010, pages 6.

[37] C. Metz, "Basic principles of ROC analysis," Semin. Nucl. Med., vol. 8, pp. 283–298, 1978.

[38] E. Brusseau, C. L. De Korte, F. Mastick, J. Schaar, and A. F. W. Van der Steen, "Fully automatic luminal contour segmentation in intracoronary ultrasound imaging-A statistical approach," IEEE Trans. Med. Imaging, vol. 23, no. 5, pp. 554–566, 2004.

[39] M. E. Olszewski, A. Wahle, S. C. Vigmostad, and M. Sonka, "Multidimensional segmentation of coronary intravascular ultrasound images using knowledge-based methods," in Proc SPIE, Med. Image: Image Processing, 2005, vol. 5747, pp. 496–504.

[40] M.-J. Jurasic, A. Lovrencic-Huzjan, M. R. Bedekovic, and V. Demarin, "How to monitor vascular aging with an ultrasound," J. Neurol. Sci., vol. 257, pp. 139–142, 2007.

[41] S. Ebadollahi, S. F. Chang, and H. Wu, "Automatic view recognition in echocardiogram videos using parts-based representation," in Proc. IEEE Comp. Soc. Conf. on Comp. Vision and Pattern Recog., Jun. 2004, vol. 2, pp. 2–9.

[42] S. Kevin, J. H. Park, B. Georgescu, C. Simopoulos, J. Otsuki, and D. Comaniciu, "Image-based multiclass boosting and echocardiographic

view classification," in Proc. IEEE Comp. Soc. Conf. on Comp. Vision and Pattern Recog., Jun. 2006, vol. 2, pp. 1559–1565.

[43] A. Landry, J. D. Spence, and A. Fenster, "Measurement of carotid plaque volume by 3-dimensional ultrasound," Stroke, vol. 35, no. 4, pp. 864–869, 2004.

[44] B. Chiu, M. Egger, J. D. Spence, G. Parraga, and A. Fenster, "Quantification of carotid vessel wall and plaque thickness change using 3D ultrasound images," Med. Phys., vol. 35, no. 8, pp. 3691–3710, Aug. 2008.

[45] B. Chiu, M. Egger, J. D. Spence, G. Parraga, and A. Fenster, "Development of 3D ultrasound techniques for carotid artery disease assessment and monitoring," Int. J. CARS, vol. 3, pp. 1–10, 2008.

Chapter 21

Ultrasound asymptomatic carotid plaque image analysis for the prediction of the risk of stroke

Efthyvoulos Kyriacou[1] *and Andrew Nicolaides*[2]

21.1 Introduction

High-resolution vascular B-mode and Doppler ultrasound provide information not only on the degree of carotid artery stenosis but also on the characteristics of the arterial wall including the size and consistency of atherosclerotic plaques [1]. Carotid stenosis alone has limitations in predicting risk and does not show plaque vulnerability and instability, thus other ultrasonographic plaque morphologic characteristics have been studied for better prediction of the risk stroke. Plaque echogenicity as assessed by B-mode ultrasound has been found to reliably predict the content of soft tissue and the amount of calcification in carotid plaques. Additionally, it has been reported that subjects with echolucent atherosclerotic plaques have increased the risk of ischemic cerebrovascular events [2]. More recent studies by Nicolaides *et al.* [3], Topakian *et al.* [4] and Kyriacou *et al.* [5] showed that plaque echolucency and plaque morphology can be used to predict stroke. Other studies have reported that plaques that are more echolucent and heterogeneous are often associated with higher cerebrovascular risk and the development of ipsilateral neurological symptoms [3,6–10]. In contrast, homogeneous hypoechoic and hyperechoic plaques without evidence of ulceration usually remain asymptomatic.

Prediction of risk is important as it will aid clinicians in the selection of asymptomatic cases at higher risk. Equally important is the establishment of a method that will allow for objective and quantitative evaluation of high risk cases, that are the ones that would most benefit from endarterectomy.

Atherosclerosis of the internal carotid artery (ICA) is known to be an important risk factor for stroke. Using the North American Symptomatic Carotid Endarter. Trial (NASCET) [11] method for the determination of stenosis, the risk of stroke has been shown to range between 0.1% and 1.6% per year for asymptomatic individuals with ICA stenosis <75%–80%. The risk rises to 2%–3% per year

[1]Department of Computer Science and Engineering, Frederick University, Cyprus
[2]Cyprus Cardiovascular Disease Educational Research Trust (CDERT), Cyprus

for individuals with higher grades of stenosis. In the past two decades, carotid endarterectomy was extensively used for the reduction of stroke risk. This is because two randomized controlled trials, almost a decade apart, the ACAS in 1995 [12] and the ACST in 2004 [13] reported that in patients with asymptomatic ICA stenosis >60%–70% (using the NASCET method) carotid endarterectomy reduced the risk of stroke from 2% to 1% per year. However, in these trials, carotid endarterectomy was associated with a 2%–3% perioperative rate of stroke or death making it marginally effective for asymptomatic patients.

This chapter presents methods that can be used for evaluation of high cerebrovascular risk using the texture and morphological appearance of plaques in combination with a number of clinical factors for the estimation of the stroke risk. Images and results presented are based on the analysis of images that were collected through a multicenter cohort study of patients with asymptomatic ICA called Asymptomatic Carotid Stenosis and Risk of Stroke (ACSRS) [3].

21.2 Collected data

The data (ultrasound scans and clinical data) were collected from patients based on a predefined protocol as follows: Patients were assessed as asymptomatic and included in the monitored group based on the following criteria/characteristics. Newly referred (<3 months) patients with 50%–99% ICA stenosis in relation to the carotid bulb diameter (ECST method) without previous ipsilateral cerebral or retinal ischemic (CORI) symptoms and without neurological abnormalities were recruited to the study after written informed consent. Patients who had contralateral cerebral hemispheric/retinal or vertebrobasilar symptoms or signs of stroke/transient ischemic attack (TIA) were included if asymptomatic for at least 6 months prior to recruitment. For patients with bilateral carotid atherosclerosis, the side with the more severe stenosis was considered ipsilateral (the study artery) [3].

At baseline, when all patients were asymptomatic; clinical and duplex ultrasound scanning data were collected. This procedure was repeated at 6 months intervals until a primary endpoint or the end of the study was reached. Exit points (i.e., when follow-up was stopped) were any of the above endpoints, death from any cause, carotid endarterectomy, stenting or loss to follow-up. Thus, patients that died, had carotid endarterectomy or had an ipsilateral ischemic event (often followed by a carotid endarterectomy) have been followed up to the event only. Apart from the ipsilateral fatal strokes, there was no overlap between these events. Clinical data included parameters like total cholesterol, LDL cholesterol, HDL cholesterol, Kreatinine, Triglycerides, etc. as published in [3]. Duplex ultrasound scanning data were performed using a protocol and standard procedure specified during the study. These included artery stenosis and plaque characteristics based on image analysis algorithms as described in the following paragraphs and published in [3,5].

Table 21.1 Number of asymptomatic and stroke (including TIAs) cases, separated into subgroups according to ECST stenosis and NASCET stenosis. Follow-up 6 months to 8 years (mean, 48 months) [3]. Groups of years of event are for ≤3 years group1 and >3 years group2

ECST st (%)	NASCET st (%)	No.	Asymp.	Stroke	Group 1/2
All		1,121	991 (88.4%)	108 (9.6%)	65–27
50–69	<50	198	182 (92%)	12 (6.1%)	13–5
70–89	50–82	598	533 (89.1%)	56 (9.4%)	28–11
90–99	83–99	325	276 (84.9%)	40 (12.3%)	24–11

TIAs, transient ischemic attacks; ECST, European Carotid Surgery Trial; NASCET, North American Symptomatic Carotid Endarter. Trial.

The total number of patients collected through the study was 1,121 out of which 108 strokes or TIAs were recorded. The data characteristics of the different groups are shown in Table 21.1. Stroke and TIA subjects are used in this chapter. These can be further divided into group1 short-term period (event happened in ≤3 years from baseline) and group2—long-term period (event happened in >3 years from baseline) in case we want to further divide the risk groups.

21.3 Imaging feature sets

Several image analysis features can been used in the statistical analysis and automated classification models as described in [5,9,14,15]. These features presented in this chapter were also presented in previous published studies and can be computed using the "Plaque Texture Analysis software" by LifeQ medical (http://www.lifeqmedical.com/). The standardization of images was done using an image normalization protocol as documented in [3]. The image analysis algorithms used for this chapter are described in the following subsections.

21.3.1 Statistical features

The statistical features (SF) features are based of first order statistical analysis and they are resolution independent [5,16]. The following SF features were computed:

1. *Mean value*

   The mean of the gray level values $I_1, \ldots, I_N$ of the pixels of the segmented plaque.

$$\bar{I} = \frac{1}{N}\sum_{j=1}^{N} I_j \tag{21.1}$$

2. *Median value*

   The median I_{med} of the distribution of the gray level values $I_1, \ldots, I_N$ is the value of the middle item of the distribution.

3. *Standard deviation*

$$\sigma = \sqrt{\frac{1}{N-1}\sum_{j=1}^{N}(I_j - \bar{I})^2} \tag{21.2}$$

4. *Skewness*

$$\text{Skew} = \frac{1}{N}\sum_{j=1}^{N}\left[\frac{I_j - \bar{I}}{\sigma}\right]^3 \tag{21.3}$$

The skewness characterizes the degree of asymmetry of a distribution around its mean.

5. *Kurtosis*

$$\text{Kurt} = \left\{\frac{1}{N}\sum_{j=1}^{N}\left[\frac{I_j - \bar{I}}{\sigma}\right]^4\right\} - 3 \tag{21.4}$$

Kurtosis measures the peakedness or flatness of a distribution in relation to a normal distribution.

21.3.2 Spatial gray level dependence matrices

The spatial gray level dependence matrices (SGLDM) [16,17] are based on the estimation of the second-order joint conditional probability density functions (pdfs), $f(i, j, d, \theta)$. The $f(i, j, d, \theta)$ is the probability that two pixels (k,l) and (m,n) with distance d in direction specified by the angle θ, have intensities of gray level i and gray level j. The estimated values for these pdfs will be denoted by $P(i, j, d, \theta)$. In a $N_x \times N_y$ image, let $L_x = \{1, 2, \ldots, N_x\}$ be the horizontal spatial domain, $L_y = \{1, 2, \ldots, N_y\}$ be the vertical spatial domain and $I(x,y)$ be the image intensity at pixel (x,y). Formally, for angles quantized at 45° intervals, the unnormalized pdfs are defined by

$$P(i,j,d,0^\circ) = \#\ \{((k,l),(m,n)) \in (L_y \times L_x) \times (L_y \times L_x) : k - m = 0, |l - n| = d, I(k,l) = i, I(m,n) = j\} \tag{21.5}$$

$$P(i,j,d,45^\circ) = \#\{((k,l),(m,n)) \in (L_y \times L_x) \times (L_y \times L_x) : (k - m = d, |l - n| = d) \text{ or } (k - m = -d, l - n = d), I(k,l) = i, I(m,n) = j\} \tag{21.6}$$

$$P(i,j,d,90^\circ) = \{((k,l),(m,n)) \in (L_y \times L_x) \times (L_y \times L_x) : |k - m| = d, l - n = 0, I(k,l) = i, I(m,n) = j\} \tag{21.7}$$

$$P(i,j,d,135^\circ) = \#\ \{((k,l),(m,n)) \in (L_y \times L_x) \times (L_y \times L_x) : (k - m = d, l - n = d) \text{ or } (k - m = -d, l - n = -d), I(k,l) = i, I(m,n) = j\} \tag{21.8}$$

where # denotes the number of elements in the set.

Haralick *et al.* [17] proposed the following texture measures which can be extracted from the SGLDM:

Notation:

$p(i,j)$ is the (i,j)th entry in the normalized spatial gray level dependence matrix,

$$p(i,j) = p(i,j)/R,$$

where R is a normalizing constant.

$p_x(i)$ is the ith entry in the marginal probability matrix obtained by summing the rows of $p(i,j)$

$$p_x(i) = \sum_{j=1}^{N_g} p(i,j) \tag{21.9}$$

N_g is the number of distinct gray levels in the quantized image.

$$\sum_i \text{ means } \sum_{i=1}^{N_g}, \text{ and } \sum_j \text{ means } \sum_{j=1}^{N_g}.$$

$$p_y(i) = \sum_{i=1}^{N_g} p(i,j) \tag{21.10}$$

$$p_{x+y}(k) = \sum_{\substack{i=1 \\ i+j=k}}^{N_g} \sum_{j=1}^{N_g} p(i,j), \quad k = 2, 3, \ldots, 2N_g \tag{21.11}$$

$$p_{x-y}(k) = \sum_{\substack{i=1 \\ |i-j|=k}}^{N_g} \sum_{j=1}^{N_g} p(i,j), \quad k = 0,\ 1, \ldots, N_g - 1 \tag{21.12}$$

Texture measures:

1. *Angular second moment*

$$f_1 = \sum_i \sum_j \{p(i,j)\}^2 \tag{21.13}$$

The angular second moment is a measure for homogeneity of the image.

2. *Contrast*

$$f_2 = \sum_{i=1}^{N_g-1} n^2 \left\{ \sum_{\substack{i=1 \\ |i-j|=n}}^{N_g} \sum_{j=1}^{N_g} p(i,j) \right\} \tag{21.14}$$

The contrast is a measure of the amount of local variations present in the image.

3. *Correlation*

$$f_3 = \frac{\sum_i \sum_j (i,j)p(i,j) - \mu_x\mu_y}{\sigma_x\sigma_y} \tag{21.15}$$

where μ_x, μ_y and σ_x, σ_y are the mean and standard deviation values of p_x and p_y, respectively. Correlation is a measure of gray tone linear dependencies.

4. *Sum of squares: variance*

$$f_4 = \sum_i \sum_j (i-\mu)^2 p(i,j) \tag{21.16}$$

5. *Inverse difference moment*

$$f_5 = \sum_i \sum_j \frac{1}{1+(i-j)^2} p(i,j) \tag{21.17}$$

6. *Sum average*

$$f_6 = \sum_{i=2}^{2N_g} i p_{x+y}(i) \tag{21.18}$$

7. *Sum variance*

$$f_7 = \sum_{i=2}^{2N_g} (i-f_6)^2 p_{x+y}(i) \tag{21.19}$$

8. *Sum entropy*

$$f_8 = \sum_{i=2}^{2N_g} p_{x+y}(i)\log\{p_{x+y}(i)\} \tag{21.20}$$

9. *Entropy*

$$f_9 = \sum_i \sum_j p(i,j)\log(p(i,j)) \tag{21.21}$$

10. *Difference variance*

$$f_{10} = \text{variance of } p_{x-y} \tag{21.22}$$

11. *Difference entropy*

$$f_{11} = \sum_{i=0}^{N_g-1} p_{x-y}(i)\log\{p_{x-y}(i)\} \tag{21.23}$$

12. *Information measures of correlation*

$$f_{12} = \frac{HXY - HXY1}{\max\{HX, HY\}} \tag{21.24}$$

$$f_{13} = (1 - \exp[-2.0(HXY2 - HXY)])^{1/2} \tag{21.25}$$

$$HXY = -\sum_i \sum_j p(i,j)\ \log(p(i,j)) \tag{21.26}$$

where HX and HY are entropies of p_x and p_y, and

$$HXY1 = -\sum_i \sum_j p(i,j)\log\{p_x(i)p_y(j)\} \tag{21.27}$$

$$HXY2 = -\sum_i \sum_j p_x(i)p_y(j)\log\{p_x(i)p_y(j)\} \tag{21.28}$$

For a chosen distance d (in this work $d = 1$ was used), we have four angular gray level dependence matrices, i.e., we obtain four values for each of the above 13 texture measures. The mean and the range of the four values of each of the 13 texture measures comprise a set of 26 texture features which can be used for classification. Some of the 26 features are strongly correlated with each other, and a feature selection procedure may be applied in order to select a subset or linear combinations of them. In this work, the mean values and the range of values were computed for each feature for $d = 1$ and they were used as two different feature sets.

21.3.3 Morphological analysis

Morphological features associated with plaque composition as described in [15] were also considered. This leads to the consideration of morphological features that come from: (i) dark regions associated with lipid, thrombus, blood or hemorrhage (ii) bright regions associated with collagen and calcified components and (iii) medium-brightness regions that fall between them. As discussed in [15], the most promising results were given by morphological analysis of the dark image components. Following image normalization, the binary L images are generated using

$$L = \{(i,j):\ \text{such that } I(i,j) < 25\} \tag{21.29}$$

where I denotes the normalized image. A multiscale morphological decomposition of each binary image is generated using the difference images.

$$\begin{aligned} d_0(L;B) &= L - L \circ B, \\ d_1(L;B) &= L \circ B - L \circ 2B \\ &\vdots \\ d_{n-1}(L;B) &= L \circ (n-1)B - L \circ nB, \end{aligned} \tag{21.30}$$

where B denotes the '+' structural element, $\circ$ denotes the morphological open operation and d_n denotes the binary difference image. The binary difference images are then used to generate the morphological pdf using

$$\mathrm{pdf}_K(n,B) = A(d_n(L;B))/A(L). \tag{21.31}$$

where $A(L)$ represents the number of pixels in the image and n was allowed to vary from 1 to 70. The cumulative distribution function (cdf) was defined in terms of the probability density function (pdf) using

$$\mathrm{cdf}_L(n,B) = \begin{cases} 0, & n = 0, \\ \sum_{r=0}^{n-1} \mathrm{pdf}_L(r,B), & n > 0. \end{cases} \tag{21.32}$$

images that gave significant differences in the classification of symptomatic vs asymptomatic cases which were used as texture features. This led to the use of

$$\mathrm{pdf}_L(r,B), \mathrm{cdf}(p,B),\ r,p = 1,\ldots,5. \tag{21.33}$$

as explained in [15].

21.4 Risk modeling

21.4.1 Classifiers

Risk modeling was carried out using the Support Vector Machine (SVM) (and the LibSVM [18] library for MATLAB®) and the Probabilistic Neural Networks (PNNs) classifiers. The classifier was trained to classify the feature sets investigated into two classes: (i) asymptomatic plaques or (ii) stroke (including TIAs) (or symptomatic) plaques, i.e., unstable plaques.

The SVM method [18] is initially based on a nonlinear mapping of the initial data set using a function $\varphi(.)$ and then the identification of a hyperplane which is able to achieve the separation of two categories of data. The vectors defining the hyperplanes can be chosen to be linear combinations with parameters α_i of images of feature vectors that occur in the database. With this choice of a hyperplane, the points x in the feature space that are mapped into the hyperplane are defined by the relation

$$\sum \alpha_i K(x_i, x) = \text{constant}\ () \tag{21.34}$$

If $K(x,y)$ becomes small as y grows further from x, each element in the sum measures the degree of closeness of the test point x to the corresponding database point x_i. In this way, the sum of kernels above can be used to measure the relative nearness of each test point to the data points originating in one or the other of the sets to be discriminated.

Details about the implementation of the SVM algorithm used can be found in [18]. The SVM network was investigated using Gaussian Radial Basis Function (RBF) kernels; this was decided as the rest of the kernel functions could not achieve satisfactory results. The SVM with RBF kernel was investigated using 10-fold cross-validation in order to identify the best possible parameters.

The PNN [19] classifier was used for developing classification models for the problem under study. The PNN falls within the category of nearest-neighbor classifiers. For a given vector $\mathbf{w}$ to be classified, an activation α_i is computed for each of the two classes of plaques ($i = 1,\ldots,2$). The activation α_i is defined to be the total distance of $\mathbf{w}$ from each of the M_i prototype feature vectors $\mathbf{x}_j^{(i)}$ that belong to the i th class:

$$\alpha_i = \sum_{j=1}^{M_i} \exp\left[-\beta\left(\mathbf{w} - \mathbf{x}_j^{(i)}\right)^T\left(\mathbf{w} - \mathbf{x}_j^{(i)}\right)\right], \quad (21.35)$$

where β is a smoothing factor. This classifier was investigated for several spread radii in order to identify the best radius for the current problem.

21.4.2 Evaluation

The performances of the classifier systems were measured using the following parameters: (i) true positives when the system correctly classifies plaques as symptomatic, (ii) false positives where the system wrongly classifies plaques symptomatic while they are asymptomatic, (iii) false negatives when the system wrongly classifies plaques as asymptomatic while they are symptomatic and (iv) true negatives when the system correctly classifies plaques as asymptomatic. To evaluate the ability of the classifiers to predict high risk cases, the Sensitivity, which is the likelihood that a symptomatic plaque will be detected given that it is symptomatic, and Specificity which is the likelihood that a plaque will be classified as asymptomatic given that it is asymptomatic, were also evaluated.

For the overall performance, the correct classification (CC) rate, which gives the percentage of correctly classified plaques, is also provided [20] (see Table 21.3).

21.5 Results

A total of 1,121 patients between 39 and 89 years (mean age $\pm$ SD—70.0 $\pm$ 7.7, 61% male) were recruited during 1998–2002 with a follow-up of 6–96 months (mean 48 months) in the context of the ACSRS study (see Table 21.2). A total of 130 first ipsilateral CORI events occurred (59 strokes of which 12 were fatal, 49 TIAs and 22 amaurosis fugax). There were 49 first contralateral CORI events (18 ischemic strokes

Table 21.2 List of risk factors—feature sets investigated for the data sets given in Table 21.2 for the asymptomatic and stroke (including TIAs) plaques. For the continuous variables, mean ± standard deviation, and for categorical variables the frequency of yes/no are tabulated. Univariate analysis (t-test) was carried out for the continuous parameters and the P value is given, and chi-square test for the categorical parameters. Features that are significantly different at P<0.001 were used for the risk modeling as given in the last column

	Asymptomatic ($N = 991$)	Stroke (inc. TIAs) ($N = 108$)	*P* value	Used in clasif.
FS 1: ACSRS Clinical and plaque features [3]				
Stenosis (%ECST)	77.64 ± 12.830	81.52 ± 11.673	0.002	Yes
Log(GSM + 40)	4.301 ± 0.313	4.058 ± 0.250	0.000	Yes
(Plaque Area)1/3	3.40 ± 0.676	3.987 ± 0.794	0.000	Yes
DWAs (# of Yes cases) [3]	614	88	0.000	Yes
History of contr. TIAs and/or Stroke (# of Yes cases)	139	34	0.000	Yes
FS 2: Texture Features—SGLDM [14]				
SGLDM_ASM_mean	4.42 ± 0.738	3.92 ± 0.838	0.000	Yes
SGLDM_con_mean	0.026 ± 0.0802	0.0676 ± 0.1150	0.000	Yes
ln(SGLDM_con_mean)	−5.813 ± 1.8080	−4.018 ± 1.7830	0.000	Yes
SGLDM_SAV_range	0.306 ± 0.1341	0.412 ± 0.1482	0.000	Yes
SGLDM_SVAR_mean	94.692 ± 49.2841	61.211 ± 33.3339	0.000	Yes
SGLDM_ent_mean	5.018 ± 0.8032	4.512 ± 0.9301	0.000	Yes
ln(SGLDM_ent_mean)	2.245 ± 0.1992	2.114 ± 0.2382	0.000	Yes
SGLDM_diffvar_m ean	7.0951 ± 1.2341	6.220 ± 1.3939	0.000	Yes
FS 3: Texture Features—Morphology [15]				
L Image cdf for $n = 1$	0.0438 ± 0.0451	0.019 ± 0.0218	0.000	Yes
L Image cdf for $n = 2$	0.120 ± 0.1063	0.057 ± 0.0611	0.000	Yes
L Image cdf for $n = 3$	0.208 ± 0.1641	0.103 ± 0.1054	0.000	Yes
L Image cdf for $n = 4$	0.294 ± 0.2110	0.148 ± 0.1358	0.000	Yes
L Image cdf for $n = 5$	0.374 ± 0.2491	0.193 ± 0.1628	0.000	Yes
L Image pdf for $n = 1$	0.0438 ± 0.0451	0.019 ± 0.0218	0.000	Yes
L Image pdf for $n = 2$	0.076 ± 0.0646	0.037 ± 0.0100	0.000	Yes
L Image pdf for $n = 3$	0.088 ± 0.0662	0.047 ± 0.0475	0.000	Yes
L Image pdf for $n = 4$	0.086 ± 0.0609	0.044 ± 0.0330	0.000	Yes
L Image pdf for $n = 5$	0.080 ± 0.0563	0.045 ± 0.0331	0.000	Yes

TIAs, transient ischemic attacks; ECST, European Carotid Surgery Trial; GSM, Gray Scale Median; DWA, Discrete White Areas (Present or Absent) [3]; SGLDM, Spatial Gray Level Dependence Matrices; ASM, Angular Second Moment; CON, Contrast; SAV, Sum Average; SVAR, Sum Variance; ENT, Entropy; Diffvar, Difference Variance.

of which 7 were fatal, 22 TIAs and 9 amaurosis fugax). There were two vertebrobasilar strokes. Amaurosis Fugax (AF) cases were excluded from the study thus having 1,099 cases.

Features with significant difference at $P<0.001$ were used in the prediction models. Figure 21.1 shows examples of normalized gray scale and color contoured images of segmented plaques with selected plaque features for both asymptomatic and symptomatic plaques.

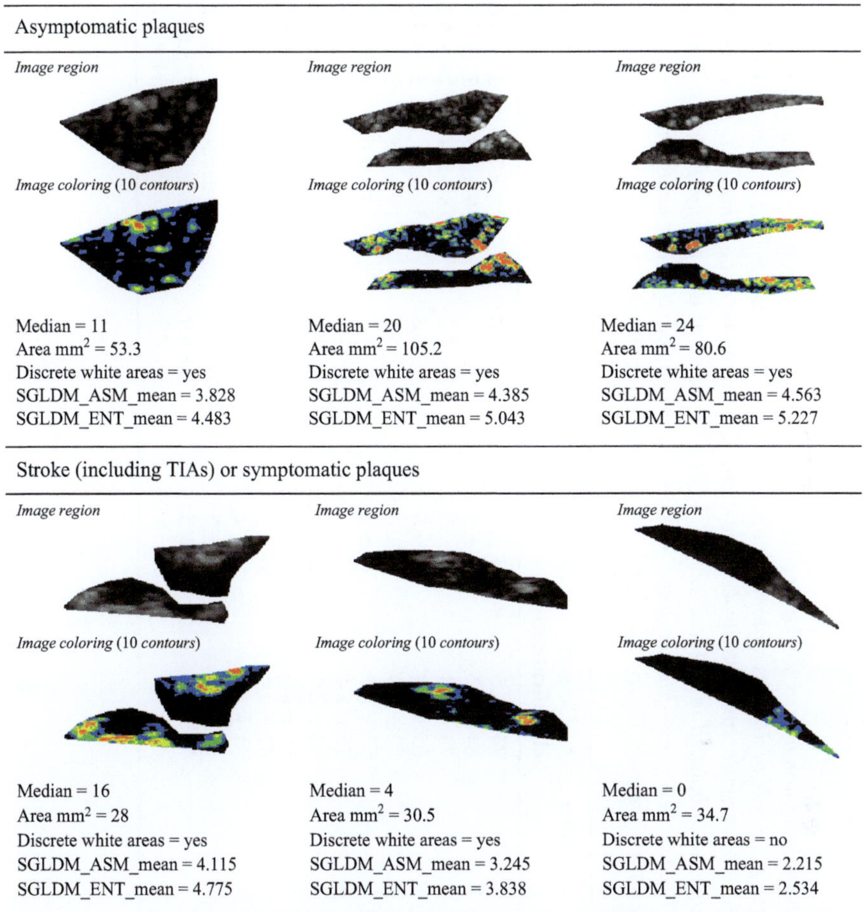

Figure 21.1 Examples of normalized gray scale and color contoured images of segmented plaques with selected plaque features: (a) asymptomatic and (b) stroke (including TIAs) or symptomatic (see Table 21.2 for feature description)

It is noted that as documented in the ACSRS study [3], comorbid conditions such as LDL, diabetes, etc. were not associated with the development of stroke in this population because they were high or present in the majority of patients. Also, the population of patients is with >50% carotid stenosis and are all high risk arteriopaths. Compared to the clinical features, it is interesting to note that the mean values for the different texture features give relatively large differences between asymptomatic and stroke cases. Unfortunately, texture features also exhibit higher variations than clinical features.

Table 21.3 tabulates the results from several runs using the SVM and PNN classifiers. The best CC in combination with high sensitivity and high specificity

Table 21.3 High risk modeling prediction results of asymptomatic vs stroke (including TIAs), measures (mean ± standard deviation) are given for 2,000 runs (10 bootstrapping sets of 100 asymptomatic and 100 stroke (including TIAs) cases drawn at random from the corresponding 991 asymptomatic, and 108 stroke cases; and the leave one out method was then run on each of the 200 set). Features sets used as tabulated in Table 21.2: FS 1: ACSRS Clinical and plaque features; FS 2: Texture Features—SGLDM; FS 3: Texture Features—Morphology. Risk modeling was carried out using the Probabilistic Neural Networks (P) and the Support Vector Machines (S) classification models

FS 1: ACSRS	FS 2: SGLDM	FS 3: Morphology	Classifier	% Correct classifications	% Sensitivity	% Specificity	% False negatives	% False positives
+			S	74 ± 2.5	78 ± 3.8	71 ± 4.0	23 ± 3.8	30 ± 4.0
+			P	64 ± 4.2	64 ± 3.3	65 ± 5.3	36 ± 3.3	35 ± 5.3
	+		S	**77 ± 1.8**	82 ± 3.4	72 ± 1.2	**18 ± 3.4**	**28 ± 1.2**
	+		P	65 ± 4.8	65 ± 6	65 ± 4.6	35 ± 6	35 ± 4.6
		+	S	72 ± 1.8	82 ± 4.3	63 ± 3.2	18 ± 4.3	37 ± 3.2
		+	P	63 ± 2.2	70 ± 3.6	56 ± 4.6	30 ± 3.6	44 ± 4.6
+	+		S	**76 ± 2.4**	79 ± 3.5	72 ± 3.0	**21 ± 3.5**	**28 ± 3.0**
+	+		P	64 ± 2.9	63 ± 4.9	66 ± 3.2	37 ± 4.9	34 ± 3.2
+		+	S	**76 ± 2.6**	80 ± 5	71 ± 6.3	**20 ± 5**	**29 ± 6.3**
+		+	P	67 ± 2.9	69 ± 3.9	64 ± 3.2	31 ± 3.9	36 ± 3.2
	+	+	S	74 ± 3.5	78 ± 4.7	70 ± 9.7	22 ± 4.7	30 ± 9.7
	+	+	P	65 ± 3.9	65 ± 5.9	65 ± 3.2	35 ± 5.9	35 ± 3.2
+	+	+	S	75 ± 4.2	78 ± 5.0	73 ± 6.9	22 ± 5.0	27±6.9
+	+	+	P	64 ± 3.5	63 ±4.2	66 ± 4.2	37 ± 4.2	34 ± 4.2

Bold values indicate the best results.

Table 21.4 Confusion matrices for the best SVM prediction model and of the corresponding PNN model based on FS2 Texture—SGLDM features. Sym. represents high risk cases that ended up having a stroke (including TIAs), whereas Asym. represents asymptomatic cases. AF cases were excluded from the study

	Prediction			
Observed	**a**	**SVM**	**b**	**PNN**
	Sym.	**Asym.**	**Sym.**	**Asym.**
Sym. 108	89 (82%)	19 (18%)	71 (65%)	37 (35%)
Asym. 991	277 (28%)	714 (72%)	346 (35%)	645 (65%)
Total 1099	366	733	417	682

Positive Predictive Value, PPV = 24% (SVM), 17% (PNN); Negative Predictive value, NPV = 97% (SVM), 94.5% (PNN); Correct Classifications = 73% (SVM), 65% (PNN).

was achieved using the SVM classifier and the SGLDM features. High-risk modeling using the prediction results of asymptomatic vs stroke (including TIAs) is given in Table 21.3 based on the feature sets tabulated in Table 21.3: FS 1: ACSRS Clinical and plaque features; FS 2: Texture Features— SGLDM; FS 3: Texture Features—Morphology. Risk modeling was carried out using the PNNs (P) and the SVM s (S) classification models. The results are the average of 2,000 runs, where 10 bootstrapping sets of 100 asymptomatic and 100 stroke (including TIAs) cases were drawn at random from the corresponding 991 asymptomatic and 108 stroke cases.

Table 21.4 tabulates the results of the best risk prediction model based on SVM using the SGLDM plaque texture features. It can be seen that for this model, for the 1,099 cases from the ACSRS dataset, the SVM model could correctly predict at baseline 89 out of the 108 cases that were symptomatic.

21.6 Conclusions

This chapter demonstrates how image texture and morphology analysis algorithms are used in order to classify ultrasound images of carotid plaques. Until now, the results using different classifiers are very promising and have the potential for computer assisted identification of patients with asymptomatic carotid stenosis at increased risk of stroke. The results using image texture analysis algorithms presented in this chapter [5] are comparable with previous work carried out with different datasets [15,16]. The Haralick SGLDM texture features gave best results in all studies whereas the SF gray scale median proved again a good and simple descriptor for plaque instability.

Morphological features help us understand the inter-relations among different intensity regions. We have examined morphological results from dark, mid-range and high intensity regions. We have found that there was significant overlap between the pattern spectra coming from symptomatic and asymptomatic plaques.

Furthermore, as we expected, *pdf* estimates were visually verified to be noisier than cumulative distribution function estimates. For larger morphological components, the *pdf* started to decrease, and the variance in the estimates increased significantly. Thus, most of the discriminating power was concentrated in the smaller components for lower scales.

The application of these techniques in combination with analysis of videos and motion of plaques is something that is still under research investigation and looks that is going to give some more promising results.

References

[1] M. Reiter, R. Horvat, S. Puchner, *et al.*, "Plaque imaging of the internal carotid artery – correlation of B-flow imaging with histopathology", *American Journal of Neuroradiology*, vol. 28, pp.122–126, 2007.

[2] E. Mathiesen, K. Bonan, O. Joakimsen, "Echolucent plaques are associated with high risk of ischemic cerebrovascular events in carotid stenosis: the Tromso Study", *Circulation,* vol. 103, pp.2171–2175, 2001.

[3] A. Nicolaides, S. Kakkos, E. Kyriacou, *et al.*, "Asymptomatic internal carotid artery stenosis and cerebrovascular risk stratification," *Journal of Vascular Surgery*, vol. 52, no. 4, pp.1486–1496, Dec. 2010.

[4] R. Topakian, A. King, S. Kwon, A. Schaafsma, M. Shipley, H. Markus, "Ultrasonic plaque echolucency and emboli signals predict stroke in asymptomatic carotid stenosis", *Neurology*, vol.77, pp.751–758, 2011.

[5] E.C. Kyriacou, S. Petroudi, C.S. Pattichis, *et al.*, "Prediction of high risk asymptomatic carotid plaques based on ultrasonic image features," *IEEE Transactions on Information Technology in Biomedicine*, vol.16, no.5, pp.966–973, 2012.

[6] A. AbuRahma, J. Wulu, B. Crotty, "Carotid plaque ultrasonic heterogeneity and severity of stenosis", *Stroke*, vol.33, pp.1772–1775, 2002.

[7] A.L. Leahy, P.T. McCollum, T.M. Feeley, *et al.*, "Duplex ultrasonography and selection of patients for carotid endarterectomy: plaque morphology or luminal narrowing?", *Journal of Vascular Surgery*, vol.8, pp.558–562, 1998.

[8] M. Langsfeld, A.C. Gray-Weale, R.J. Lusby, "The role of plaque morphology and diameter reduction in the development of new symptoms in asymptomatic carotid arteries," *Journal of Vascular Surgery*, vol.9, pp.548–557, 1989.

[9] S.K. Kakkos, J.M. Stevens, A.N. Nicolaides, *et al.*, "Texture analysis of ultrasonic images of symptomatic carotid plaques can identify those plaques associated with ipsilateral embolic brain infarction," *European Journal of Vascular and Endovascular Surgery*, vol.33, no.4, pp.422–429, 2007.

[10] A.C. Gray-Weale, J.C. Graham, J.R. Burnett, *et al.*, "Carotid artery atheroma: comparison of preoperative B-mode ultrasound appearance with carotid endarterectomy specimen pathology," *Journal of Cardiovascular Surgery*, vol.29, pp. 676–681, 1988.

[11] A. Fox, "How to measure carotid stenosis", *Radiology*, vol.186, pp.316–318, 1993.

[12] Executive Committee for the Asympt. Carotid Atheroscl. Study, "Endarterectomy for asymptomatic carotid artery stenosis," *Journal of the American Medical Association*, vol.273, pp.1421–1428, 1995.

[13] MRC Asymptomatic Carotid Surgery Trial (ACST) Collaborative Group, "Prevention of disabling and fatal strokes by successful carotid endarterectomy in patients without recent neurological symptoms: randomized controlled trial," *Lancet*, vol.363, pp.1491–1502, 2004.

[14] C.I. Christodoulou, C.S. Pattichis, M. Pantziaris, A. Nicolaides, "Texture based classification of atherosclerotic carotid plaques," *IEEE Transactions on Medical Imaging,* vol.22, no.7, pp.902–912, 2003.

[15] E. Kyriacou, M. Pattichis, C.S. Pattichis, *et al.*, "Classification of atherosclerotic carotid plaques using morphological analysis on ultrasound images," *Journal of Applied Intelligence*, vol.30, no.1, pp.3–23, 2009.

[16] E. Kyriacou, M. Pattichis, C. Christodoulou, *et al.*, Ultrasound imaging in the analysis of carotid plaque morphology for the assessment of stroke, in Plaque Imaging: Pixel To Molecular Level, editors are: Suri, Yuan, Wilson and Laxminarayan. Studies in Health Technology and Informatics, Vol.113, pp.241–275, IOS Press, 2005, ISBN: 1–58603–516- 9.

[17] R.M. Haralick, K. Shanmugam, I. Dinstein, "Texture features for image classification", *IEEE Transactions on Systems, Man, and Cybernetics*, vol.SMC-3, pp.610–621, 1973 Nov.

[18] C.C. Chang, C.J. Lin. "LIBSVM: a library for support vector machines", *ACM Transactions on Intelligent Systems and Technology*, vol.2, no.3, 2011. (Software available at: http://www.csie.ntu.edu.tw/~cjlin/libsvm).

[19] S.M. Ross, *Introduction to probability and statistics for engineers and scientists.* 3rd ed. Amsterdam: Elsevier/Academic Press, 2014.

[20] H. Ma, A.I. Bandos, H.E. Rockette, D. Gur, "On use of partial area under the ROC curve for evaluation of diagnostic performance," *Statistics in Medicine,* vol.32, no.20, pp.3449–3458, 2013.

Chapter 22

3D segmentation and texture analysis of the carotid arteries

Aaron Fenster[1], Bernard Chiu[2], and Eranga Ukwatta[3]

22.1 Introduction

Stroke is the second leading cause of mortality and morbidity worldwide, and its incidence is expected to grow in the developing world. Stroke can occur as a result of a blockage of a cerebral artery by a thrombotic embolus, with about 87% of strokes resulting in regional brain ischemia. Generation of thrombosis and subsequent cerebral emboli is a result of disruption of atherosclerotic plaques at and near the carotid bifurcation (BF). Patients who have been identified to have carotid plaques may have an elevated risk for stroke and may either change their diet and lifestyle habits, or be treated with medical interventions for their carotid atherosclerosis. Thus, identification of patients with carotid plaques who may be at risk for stroke as well as accurate and precise methods to monitor carotid plaque changes are critical in the management of patients at risk for stroke. Since patients may need to be imaged serially to monitor changes, noninvasive, imaging-based methods are needed to provide a direct measurement of carotid plaques for quantification of the disease burden and for monitoring carotid plaque changes in response to nonsurgical management of carotid atherosclerosis.

Carotid atherosclerosis is typically quantified using duplex 2D ultrasound (2D US). This approach is used as a clinical standard for assessing the severity of the disease at the carotid BF and is an important factor of the patient's eligibility for endarterectomy. Measurements of intima-media thickness (IMT) at the common carotid artery (CCA) using 2D US imaging has been shown to be associated with the risk of stroke. However, more recent studies suggest that three-dimensional (3D)-based measurements of carotid atherosclerosis, expressed in terms of total wall volume and total plaque volume (TPV), is more sensitive than lumen stenosis or IMT.

[1]Imaging Research Laboratories, Robarts Research Institute, Western University, Canada
[2]Department of Electronic Engineering, City University of Hong Kong, Hong Kong
[3]Department of Systems and Computer Engineering, Carlton University, Canada

The noninvasiveness of magnetic resonance (MR) imaging, which provides excellent soft-tissue contrast, makes it ideally suited for quantification and monitoring of carotid plaques and obtaining morphological measurements for the monitoring of carotid atherosclerosis. Numerous publications have reported on methods to segment the carotid arteries and plaques in MR images. These include morphological measurements such as vessel wall volume (VWV), vessel wall thickness (VWT), plaque composition, and inflammation.

Although MR imaging of the carotid arteries provide excellent information, its cost and availability in some countries makes it difficult to use in response to the large number of patients who need monitoring of changes of the disease in response to therapy. 3D ultrasound (3D US) imaging is the best alternative for providing 3D information on the carotid arteries and its use has been explored in clinical trials. Over the last decade, techniques have been developed to use 3D US images to obtain volumetric, morphological, and textural measurements rapidly and noninvasively. Research laboratories have developed 3D US imaging techniques for a variety of applications, including the carotid arteries, and many ultrasound imaging vendors have included this capability in their systems. These advances have allowed investigators to use 3D US for imaging the carotid arteries and explore quantification methods of carotid atherosclerosis. Since 3D US can provide 3D views of the carotid arteries, it overcomes the variability of the use of conventional 2D US as the user will not need to mentally integrate multiple 2D images to produce a 3D impression of the disease in the carotid arteries. Since carotid plaques change in three dimensions, 3D US imaging has the potential to provide sensitive and reproducible biomarkers of carotid atherosclerosis.

Quantification of carotid atherosclerosis requires delineation (segmentation) of the carotid media-adventitia (MAB) and lumen-intima (LIB) boundaries. These boundaries have been segmented using manual methods, which are tedious and prone to errors and variability. Over the past few years, investigators have developed various semiautomated and automated methods for fast and robust 3D segmentation of the carotid MAB and LIB from the 3D US images. These methods have the potential to assist the analysis of carotid atherosclerosis and use for monitoring patients at risk for stroke.

While segmentation of MAB and LIB provides accurate and robust metrics of the morphology of the carotid arteries and plaques within them, ultrasound images contain more information about the tissues being imaged. Specifically, image textural information can also provide information about the plaques' echogenicity, which is related to the composition of the plaque. Since lipid cores and intraplaque hemorrhage are believed to destabilize plaque, quantification of these plaque components adds to the information needed to assess plaque vulnerability to disruption and potentially causing stroke. Thus, investigators have explored carotid plaque texture in MR and 3D US images with intent to provide information on the composition of carotid plaques and their vulnerability to disruption.

In this chapter, we review 3D US-based methods for segmentation of carotid plaques and their use in quantifying plaque composition using image texture metrics. Specifically, we review algorithms used to segment the MAB and LIB of

CCA, internal carotid artery (ICA), and external carotid artery (ECA). We also review methods, which have used these segmented boundaries to provide information on plaque composition using image texture metrics.

22.2 3D carotid ultrasound imaging

22.2.1 Advantages of 3D US

2D US imaging is used globally to diagnose carotid atherosclerosis. Generation of 2D US images requires the user to manipulate the hand-held US transducers over the neck while real-time 2D images are generated using B-mode and Doppler techniques. Although this approach is used extensively, it suffers from the following limitations for use in diagnosis of vulnerable plaques and monitoring of progression and regression of carotid atherosclerosis:

- Users of conventional 2D US imaging must mentally integrate many 2D US images to form an impression of 3D carotid arterial pathology. Many users can perform the procedure effectively; however, this approach does not permit volumetric analysis of the carotid plaques and monitoring changes in the vessels.
- The same view of the carotid arteries must be imaged over long time periods to provide accurate and informative quantitative metrics of progression and regression of carotid plaques in response to nonsurgical therapy. Since monitoring may last for a few years, it is very difficult to reproduce the same view using conventional 2D US.

3D US systems are now available on most commercial US systems and researchers have developed specialized approaches for a variety of applications to generate 3D US images [1–5]. Some systems used in cardiology can produce 3D US information in real time. Researchers can now take advantage of low cost computers to reconstruct 3D US images as the 2D US images are acquired (i.e., in real time) limited only by the acquisition time. Thus, efficient and cost effective 3D US systems and techniques are now available to researchers for further development of quantitative carotid plaque metrics. The developers of 3D US systems in commercial companies and research laboratories are now challenged to develop efficient, accurate, and reproducible software tools for extracting additional meaningful information from these 3D US images. Specifically, for carotid arterial image analysis, the challenge is to extract quantitative information of plaque volume to be used in monitoring of progression and regression of carotid atherosclerosis and plaque composition analysis to identify vulnerable plaques.

Although 3D US transducers with matrix arrays of piezoelectric elements are now available on some ultrasound machines, we briefly review two carotid US imaging techniques developed by researchers for generating these images. Details about the technical aspects of these methods can be found in recent review articles and books on the subject [6–13].

Analysis of carotid disease requires imaging of the CCA and its two branches. Thus, imaging of these vessels requires at least a 4-cm scan length along the vessel. To accomplish this, researchers have developed methods to acquire images of the carotid arteries using conventional 2D transducers using either a mechanical or free-hand methods to track the transducer as it is moved along the vessel. The mechanical approach makes use of a motorize assembly to translate the transducer along the neck, allowing acquisition of 2D US images at regular intervals, which are reconstructed into a 3D US image. The free-hand method makes use of an external tracking method to track the position and orientation of the transducer as it is moved freely.

22.2.2 Mechanical systems for 3D imaging of the carotid arteries

These systems use a motorized mechanism to translate linearly a conventional 2D US transducer over the carotid arteries (Figure 22.1). As the transducer is translated, conventional B-mode 2D images of the carotid arteries are acquired at regular spatial intervals, such as 0.25 or 0.5 mm, depending on the 2D US image update frame rate. This approach results in a series of 2D US images with a known predefined spacing, which are parallel to each other, making 3D reconstruction possible in real time (see Figure 22.2 e.g., 3D US image). Furthermore, the length of the scan can be variable as the mechanical mechanisms can be built of different lengths. Typically, this type of approach can allow scans as long as 6 cm. If the 2D US images are acquired every 0.25 mm and the 2D US frame rate is 30 frames per second, a 4 cm length will require 160 2D US images, which will be acquired into the computer via a digital frame grabber in 5.3 s.

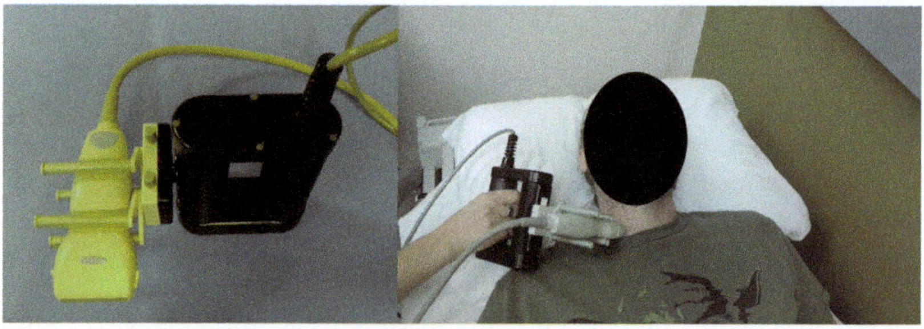

(a) (b)

Figure 22.1 (a) Photograph of a mechanical linear scanning mechanism used in our laboratory to acquire 3D US images of the carotid arteries. The scanning mechanism is hand-held so that the transducer is oriented transverse to the vessel and is translated along it while 2D US images from the US machine are acquired into a computer via a digital frame grabber and reconstructed into a 3D US image as the images are acquired. (b) Photograph showing the hand-held device with the transducer ready to be scanned

The resolution in the 3D US images will not be isotropic since this approach uses a series of equally spaced 2D US images. Thus, the spatial resolution of the image perpendicular to the scanning direction (i.e., transverse to the vessel axis) will depend on the resolution in-plane of the acquired 2D US images. The spatial resolution in the direction of the scanning motion (i.e., along the artery) will depend on the elevational resolution of the US transducer and the spacing between the acquired images. Since the acquired images are collected with spacing typically less than half of the US beam width, the spacing of the acquired images should not affect the elevational resolution of the 3D US image. However, the spacing between acquired images can be optimized through experimentation and quantification of the resolution. As Figure 22.2 shows, the 3D US image has poorer resolution in the direction along the vessel than in-pane in the transverse plane. Clearly, a transducer with good elevational resolution would produce optimal results [6].

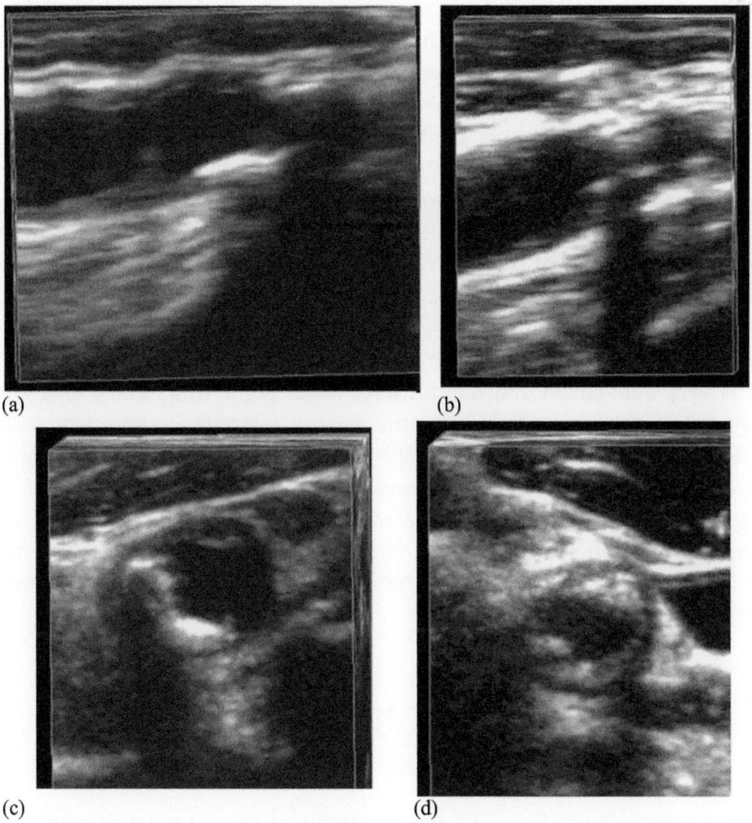

Figure 22.2 3D US views of the carotid arteries of two different patients with complex and ulcerated carotid plaques. For each patient, a transverse (a) and (c) and longitudinal (b) and (d) views are shown side by side

22.2.3 Free-hand 3D US imaging

Mechanical 3D US scanning devices using external fixtures are bulkier than 2D US transducers and can be awkward at times. Thus, researchers have developed free-hand scanning approaches that avoid any external motorized fixture. The free-hand approaches require a method to track the transducer as it is moved over the arteries. Over the past two decades, various methods have been used to track the transducer allowing the user to freely move the conventional US transducer. Optical, mechanical, acoustic, and electro-magnetic approaches have been investigated and used to track the transducer to generate 3D images and for image-guided intervention [14]. Because the US transducer is moved freely over the anatomy, the image location, orientation, and spacing of the images are not pre-defined and are under control by the user. Thus, the user must be trained to move the transducer at a velocity that is appropriate for the US image refresh rate so that images are acquired with the proper spacing with no gaps between them. Several approaches for tracking of US transducers have been developed, but the most common approach makes use of magnetic field sensing technology: Ascension—Bird sensor [15]; Polhemus—Fastrack sensor [16]; and Northern Digital—Aurora sensor [17].

The magnetic field sensor method uses a time-varying 3D magnetic field transmitter placed near the patient's neck. To sense the magnetic field strength, a small receiver containing three orthogonal coils (providing 6 degrees-of-freedom) is mounted on the transducer. The transducer's position and orientation are calculated using the strength of the three components of the local magnetic field. The tracking of the transducer is sufficiently rapid to allow use of this information to reconstruct the 3D US image.

Although the free-hand 3D US scanning approach using a magnetic field sensor is very convenient and unobtrusive, it has some limitations. Uncontrolled environment, such as significant electromagnetic interference and nearby ferrous (or highly conductive) metals, can compromise the accuracy of the tracking. These effects can result in geometric distortions in the 3D US image especially if ferrous (or highly conductive) metals are located nearby. Current magnetic field sensors have improved significantly; however, to minimize these potential sources of error, the position of the sensor relative to the transmitter must be calibrated accurately and precisely [18–26].

22.3 Quantitative analysis of 3D carotid US images

22.3.1 Texture analysis

Volume measurements of carotid plaque and its changes have been shown to be important metrics of carotid atherosclerosis. These metrics include TPV [27–29] and total VWV [30,31]. However, despite the sensitivity and specificity of these metrics, 3D carotid images have not been fully exploited to provide information about the composition of the arterial wall or plaque. Compositional analysis may provide information on plaque vulnerability and insights into the mechanisms related to plaque regression and progression. Thus, 3D US-based texture features may offer the required information on carotid plaque and vessel wall on plaque composition and its changes.

Image texture analysis of 2D carotid ultrasound images have been used to successfully differentiate between symptomatic and asymptomatic subjects [32,33]. These image texture-based methods have been extended to 3D US images [34,35].

22.3.1.1 Texture feature calculation

Awad *et al.* [34] investigated carotid vessel wall/plaque texture features using texture analysis to detect changes in the carotid wall and plaque in response to atorvastatin therapy. The images were obtained in a study in which 21 patients were in the placebo group and 17 subjects were in the atorvastatin group. All subjects were imaged at baseline and three at month following [29].

In this method, the 3D US carotid images were first normalized using two reference points: the gray-scale median of the blood and adventitia and the plaques segmented manually. The texture features used were: first order statistics, spatial gray-level dependence matrix, gray-level run length statistics, gray-level difference statistics, neighborhood gray tone difference matrix, laws texture energy measures, and Fourier power spectrum. These texture features were applied to each slice of the 3D carotid US images and 135 texture features were calculated. The change of each texture feature for each slice was then calculated by subtracting the baseline value from the value at 3 months. The average (AV_i) and the standard deviation (SD_i) values of each feature change (Δf) were then calculated for all the 3D carotid image slices, generating 270 texture features. Analysis of the correlation (COR) between left and right carotid arteries, resulted in a low COR for texture (COR = 0.27) and VWV percentage change (COR = 0.03). Thus, the dataset used in this study consisted of 70 objects [35 subjects × 2 carotid arteries (left and right)], and 270 texture features [135 $AV_i(\Delta f)$ + 135 $SD_i(\Delta f)$].

22.3.1.2 Feature selection

The best texture features selection was based on a comparison to the percentage volume change of the vessel wall. Three goodness measures were used: the distance between the two classes, the *p*-value of the Wilcoxon rank sum, and accuracy of the classifiers.

The distance measure between the two classes was computed thus:

$$\text{dis} = \frac{|m_1 - m_2|}{\sqrt{\sigma_1^2 + \sigma_2^2}} \tag{22.1}$$

where m_1 and m_2 are the mean values and σ_1 and σ_2 are the standard deviations of the atorvastatin and placebo groups for each feature. Thus, the features with the largest distance between the two classes would be best. The Wilcoxon measure evaluates a two-sided rank sum test of the null hypothesis that feature values of the two classes have equal medians. The best features for this measure are the ones with the smallest *p*-value.

Using an accuracy metric, which measures the percentage of the correctly classified carotid arteries, six classifiers were used to rank the individual features according: (1) Linear discriminant (LDC), (2) Quadratic discriminant (QDC), (3) Parzen (PARZENC), (4) Logistic linear (LOGLC), (5) Nearest mean (NMC), and (6) Naive Bayes (NAIVEBC). The features that produce the highest classification accuracy were considered to be best.

22.3.1.3 Classification

To estimate the accuracy of each classifier/multiclassifier for each feature set, the average accuracy (and SD) was computed over 1,000 trials with 80% of the randomly selected images used for training and the other 20% for evaluation. All the features were normalized by subtracting the mean and dividing by the standard deviation. The performance evaluated using Receiver operating characteristic (ROC) curves was also used to evaluate performance of the texture features.

22.3.1.4 Results

In Awad *et al.,* [34] selection of the best features that would classify the placebo and atorvastatin groups correctly and comparing them with the VWV percentage change (ΔV%), which is the VWV change divided by the value at baseline. Results of the ranking of the features based on distance between the atorvastatin and placebo groups (22.1) are shown in Table 22.1. The ranks of the features according to the *p*-value of Wilcoxon rank sum test are shown in Table 22.2. Ranking the features according to the median value of the average accuracies of the classifiers are shown in Table 22.3. These tables show that many of the selected top features are common for the three metrics.

The average ($\pm$SD) of AUC over 1,000 trials for ΔV% are 0.617 ($\pm$0.15), using the LDC classifier, which is the best classifier for the VWV feature.

Table 22.1 The top features based on distance measure [34]

Rank	Features	Distances
1	SD_i_FPS_[16,32)&[67.5,112.5)	0.519925
2	AV_i_GLRLS _Run nonuniformity_AV_s	0.504522
3	AV_i_FPS_[2,4)&[112.5,157.5)	0.4703
4	AV_i_FPS_[−22.5,22.5)	0.460846
5	AV_i_FPS_[8,16)&[22.5,67.5)	0.44193
6	AV_i_FPS_[64,128)&[−22.5,22.5)	0.433214
7	AV_i_FPS_[4,8)&[−22.5,22.5)	0.428599
8	AV_i_FPS_[64,128)	0.421249
9	AV_i_FPS_[2,4)	0.420104
10	AV_i_FPS_[32,64)&[22.5,67.5)	0.414708
11	AV_i_FPS_LAP	0.410841
12	AV_i_LAWS_L7W7	0.409942
21	Volume_Change Percentage	0.379832

Figure 22.3(a) shows the ROC curve for ΔV% using LDC classifier, and Figure 22.3(b) shows the ROC curve for AV_i_LAWS_L7R7 texture feature, using the NAIVEBC classifier, the best classifier for this texture feature, with an average and standard deviation of AUC over 1,000 trials of 0.721 (±0.13), respectively, which represents a significant improvement in performance.

22.3.2 Semiautomated segmentation algorithms of 3D US carotid images

Although, manual delineation is still widely used for the carotid MAB and LIB segmentation, semiautomated segmentation algorithms are preferred over the manual delineation because manual techniques are tedious, time-consuming and may be subject to high operator variability. Manual segmentation also demands more training and expertise from the operators. Therefore, developing semi-automated techniques for segmentation and analysis is important for translating the use of 3D carotid US phenotypes to clinical research and ultimately to clinical care. However, due to the low image contrast of the vessel boundaries and less distinguishable intensity histograms, it is challenging for algorithms to segment 3D carotid US images robustly.

As shown in Table 22.4, the algorithms developed for the segmentation of the carotid artery MAB and LIB can be broadly categorized into two groups, which is based on the measurement of interest: methods that segment only the carotid artery LIB and ones that segment both the MAB and LIB. In this chapter, we briefly review all such algorithms, but focus more on the segmentation methods that are specifically designed for segmenting both boundaries for the purpose of generating volumetric phenotypes of plaque burden.

Most recent segmentation tasks are performed using optimization-based approaches, such as, active contours [44], level sets [45], sparse field level sets [46]. Except for graph cuts, rest of the approaches are formulated in the continuous

Table 22.2 The top features based on Wilcoxon measure [34]

Rank	Features	*p*-Values
1	AV_i_GLRLS _Run nonuniformity_AV_s	0.002132
2	SD_i_FPS_[16,32)&[67.5,112.5)	0.002802
3	AV_i_LAWS_L7W7	0.007848
4	AV_i_FPS_[2,4)&[112.5,157.5)	0.009659
5	SD_i_FPS_[32,64)&[67.5,112.5)	0.020524
6	AV_i_FPS_[64,128)	0.021175
7	SD_i_FPS_[128,256)&[67.5,112.5)	0.021175
8	AV_i_FPS_[−22.5,22.5)	0.023965
9	AV_i_FPS_[4,8)&[−22.5,22.5)	0.026262
10	AV_i_FPS_[2,4)	0.026262
11	AV_i_FPS_LAP	0.026262
12	AV_i_FPS_[112.5,157.5)	0.027069
35	Volume_Change Percentage	0.076

Table 22.3 Top features based on the median accuracy measure (mean ± sd) [34]

Rank	Feature	LDC	QDC	LOGLC	NMC	NAIVEBC	PARZENC	Median
1	SD_i_FPS_[128,256)&[67.5,112.5)	65.12 ± 11.98	62.82 ± 11.88	54.92 ± 12.03	65.12 ± 11.98	54.75 ± 11.69	62.23 ± 11.96	63.87
2	AV_i_LAWS_L7R7	63.55 ± 11.98	59.51 ± 12.31	53.70 ± 11.90	63.55 ± 11.98	74.42 ± 13.43	67.96 ± 10.96	63.63
3	SD_i_FPS_[16,32)&[67.5,112.5)	65.08 ± 11.96	59.28 ± 11.08	55.65 ± 11.69	65.08 ± 11.96	57.41 ± 10.73	61.90 ± 11.54	63.49
4	AV_i_LAWS_L7W7	63.25 ± 11.77	64.24 ± 12.72	53.55 ± 11.66	63.25 ± 11.77	63.39 ± 11.63	62.02 ± 11.88	63.32
5	AV_i_FPS_[4,8)&[−22.5,22.5)	64.75 ± 12.22	59.05 ± 12.39	55.19 ± 12.05	64.75 ± 12.22	52.85 ± 12.79	60.38 ± 12.20	62.57
6	AV_i_FPS_[112.5,157.5)	62.50 ± 12.01	61.25 ± 11.87	52.45 ± 12.13	62.50 ± 12.01	55.07 ± 12.12	60.68 ± 11.97	61.85
7	AV_i_FPS_[2,4)&[112.5,157.5)	62.86 ± 11.86	59.64 ± 12.62	63.00 ± 11.76	62.86 ± 11.86	60.22 ± 12.98	56.58 ± 11.38	61.54
8	SD_i_FPS_[32,64)&[67.5,112.5)	63.03 ± 12.14	59.95 ± 11.39	62.82 ± 12.17	63.03 ± 12.14	59.91 ± 11.14	59.28 ± 11.84	61.39
9	AV_i_FPS_[256,512)	61.97 ± 12.60	58.96 ± 12.74	62.02 ± 12.60	61.97 ± 12.60	60.52 ± 12.59	58.79 ± 11.55	61.24
10	AV_i_FPS_[4,8)&[112.5,157.5)	61.01 ± 12.11	60.56 ± 10.91	60.96 ± 12.14	61.01 ± 12.11	59.99 ± 11.81	61.58 ± 11.56	60.98
11	AV_i_GLRLS_Run nonuniformity_SDs	61.27 ± 11.88	59.45 ± 11.04	61.30 ± 11.88	61.27 ± 11.88	49.99 ± 11.93	60.28 ± 9.89	60.78
12	AV_i_GLRLS_Run nonuniformity_AVs	60.70 ± 12.83	60.46 ± 12.46	60.75 ± 12.83	60.70 ± 12.83	56.49 ± 13.42	59.94 ± 12.64	60.58
89	Volume Change Percentage	57.22 ± 12.11	51.82 ± 11.48	57.18 ± 12.18	57.22 ± 12.11	46.28 ± 12.08	49.73 ± 10.18	54.50

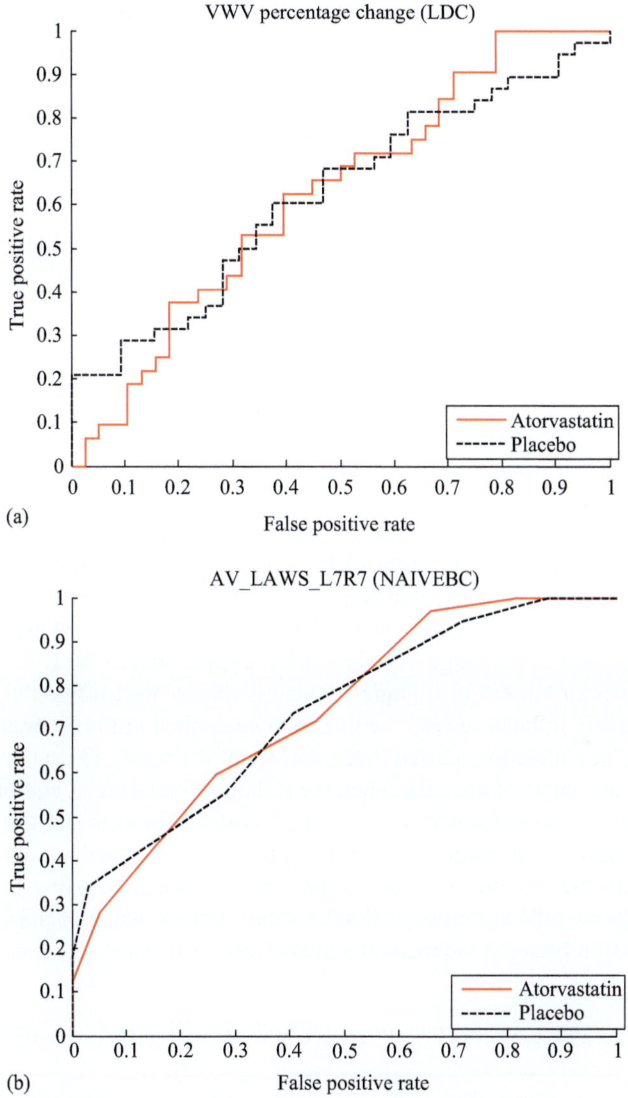

Figure 22.3 ROC curve for (a) LDC classifier using the percentage volume change feature (AUC = 0.6242), (b) NAIVEBC classifier using laws texture energy measure (L7R7) (AUC = 0.741) [34]

domain. In graph cuts, segmentation is formulated as a discrete graph problem, where a min-cut/max-flow model is solved to differentiate the object from background. In the continuous-domain approaches, an objective function is defined to guide the segmentation, which incorporates a measure of goodness of the desired segmentation boundary/surface. The objective function is then iteratively minimized to locate the desired boundary. The objective functions typically contain two types of energy terms: external energy term, derived from the (preprocessed) image data, and internal energy terms, derived from high-level knowledge about the expected shape of the boundaries. In some texts, external energy term is also referred to as the data term, as it is created using image boundary data and/or regional data. Relative importance of each term is determined during the parameter tuning phase of the algorithm and is heavily dependant on the quality of image data. Depending on the strength of the data term, this parameter(s) is tuned for the segmentation task at hand. For a segmentation problem of images with high signal-to-noise ratio and clearly defined image boundaries, data term is usually assigned relatively higher weight to drive the segmentation.

22.3.3 2D and 3D methods for segmenting LIB from 3D US images

As shown in Table 22.4, some methods have been developed to delineate only the carotid artery LIB for the purpose of computing lumen stenosis [41–43,47]. All of the methods are formulated as an energy minimization problem with slightly different external and internal energy terms.

Gill *et al.* [41] described one of the first attempts at developing a semi-automated method for carotid artery LIB segmentation from 3D US images. The algorithm consisted of three main steps: (1) manual placement of the initial seed mesh within the lumen, (2) automated inflation of the mesh toward the LIB, and (3) iteratively refined using image edge-based forces proximal to the LIB. The balloon model consists of a mesh of triangles, which is then placed inside the artery. The model is quickly inflated toward the LIB with an applied uniform force on vertices of the mesh, in a direction normal to the surface of the mesh. The model represents the appropriate shape of the LIB, when the inflation forces are at equilibrium. This mesh is then further deformed using image-based forces to locate the LIB. However, edge-based segmentation alone is not adequate to stop leaking at low-contrast boundaries in 3D US images. This algorithm was validated using only a single 3D US image and the algorithm yielded a submillimeter value of 0.35 mm for the mean separation between the manual and algorithm LIB surface. Since the method

Table 22.4 Summary of segmentation methods for 3D carotid US images

Paper	Year	Dim.	LIB	MAB	Time (min)	Number of images
Ukwatta *et al.* [36]	2011	2D	Level set	Level set	2.8 ± 0.4	21
Ukwatta *et al.* [37]	2013	3D	Level set	Level set	1.72	21
Hossain *et al.* [38]	2015	2D	Level set	Level set		10
Ukwatta *et al.* [39]	2011	2D	Coupled level sets	Coupled level sets	3.7	21
Yang *et al.* [40]	2011	2D	Active shape	Active shape	4.4 ± 0.6	68
Gill *et al.* [41]	2000	3D	Dynamic balloon model	–	30 s	1
Zahalka *et al.* [42]	2001	2D	Active contours	–	25 s/slice	2
Lorza *et al.* [43]	2013	3D	Graph cuts	–	3	12

requires manual initialization of a seed, there is inherent variability in the segmentation. The variability analysis studies have shown that this semiautomated algorithm has been less variable than the intraobserver variability for manual segmentation. However, the algorithm needed to be validated using multiple images to adequately evaluate its robustness and usefulness in practice.

Zahalka *et al.* [42] proposed a method similar to the one described by Gill *et al.* [41] for segmenting the carotid artery LIB. The method uses a geometrically deformable model (GDM) with an external energy based on the image gradient and internal energy based on curvature of the contour. In GDMs, the contour/surface is defined as a set of vertices, which are connected by edges and the internal and external energies are calculated independently at each vertex. One of the major drawbacks of this work is that the method has been validating using only 3D US images of phantoms. However, 3D US images of patients usually tend to have more image artifacts, such as shadowing and motion and low image quality, making the image segmentation task much more challenging.

Lorza *et al.* [43] described a semiautomated method for segmentation of the carotid artery LIB from 3D US images using a graph cuts approach. The method requires initialization of seed points in the internal, external, and common carotid arteries. Afterwards, the centerline between these points was constructed, which is used as an initialization to the graph cuts algorithms. The optimal LIB surface was found around the centerline using graph cuts. Finally, a 3D segmentation is obtained by solving the graph cut optimization problem. The method was tested on 12 3D US images from six subjects including three patients with a moderate carotid artery stenosis. Several segmentation evaluation metrics were used in the evaluation, including the Dice coefficient (DC), which measures the regional overlap of algorithm and manual segmentations. In comparison to manual segmentation, the method yielded an average DC of 84% for healthy volunteers and 66.7% for patient data.

22.3.4 2D methods that segment both the LIB and MAB from 3D US images

In this section, our focus is on the segmentation methods that are designed specifically for segmenting both the carotid artery MAB and LIB for the purpose of generating volumetric phenotypes of plaque burden. Ukwatta *et al.* [36] proposed a combined 2D segmentation method to segment the MAB and LIB from 3D US images using a modified sparse field level set method [48]. Their method was the first technique that was proposed for segmenting both boundaries from 3D US images for the purpose of computing volumetric measurements of plaque burden. This method works on a slice-by-slice basis on transverse slices extracted from 3D US images. Ukwatta *et al.* [39] extended the previous method by using a coupled level set approach to simultaneously segment the MAB and LIB. For both techniques, the areas from individual segmentations are summed together to generate the VWV measurement. Since each slice is segmented independently at an inter-slice distance (ISD) of 1 mm, the methods require user interaction on every slice. Although the slice thickness of the 3D US images is approximately 0.15 mm, the methods make an assumption of no considerable change in the vessel morphology within an ISD of 1 mm.

Yang *et al.* [49] used active shape models (ASM) to segment the carotid artery MAB and LIB slice-wise, which involved a large number of training images to generate models. The shape of an object is usually represented by a set of points in ASM. The ASM algorithm matches the set of model points to an image, controlled by the statistical model of shape, which locates the valid range of shape variation from the training set of labeled images. However, the shape of the LIB could be different between subjects, which is also affected by the degree of stenosis. Their method yielded a DC of 92.8 ± 3.3 and 94.4 ± 3.2 for the MAB and LIB, respectively.

Hossain *et al.* [38] described a method similar to one proposed by Ukwatta *et al.* [36] for segmenting the MAB and LIB from 3D US images. Their method used distance regularized level set method with smoothness energy, region-based energy, edge-based energy and a stopping criterion to segment the MAB and LIB. The algorithm was initialized by seed points on the MAB and LIB in 2D cross-sectional slices in 3D US image. To further smooth the MAB and to stop any leaking, an ellipse fitting and a stopping boundary-based energy are used. Their method yielded an DC of 88.78% and 94.81% for the MAB and LIB, respectively.

Here, we have chosen to describe the method proposed by Ukwatta *et al.* [36] in more detail. The segmentation pipeline of their method is shown in Figure 22.4. Their method initializes the boundary close to the actual boundary by choosing four or more anchor points on each boundary on each transverse slice to be segmented. After initialization, two level set segmentations with different energies were used to segment the MAB and LIB. The MAB was segmented initially, where the

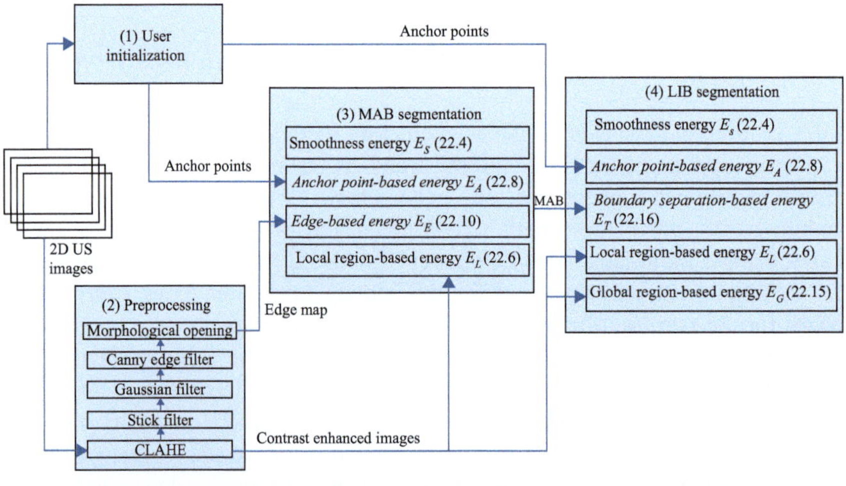

Figure 22.4 Block diagram of the segmentation pipeline [36]

segmented MAB contour was used to constrain the LIB segmentation from leaking in regions with low image contrast.

22.3.4.1 MAB segmentation

Since the carotid artery MAB has neither a strong edge nor consistent regional features for segmentation, a combination of various criteria were used for the MAB segmentation. For example, the MAB has high image contrast at parallel locations to the US beam direction, whereas the orthogonal locations of the boundary would generally have low image contrast and the image intensities of the interior and exterior of the outer wall are heterogeneous. Therefore, an objective function combining local region-based, edge-based energies, and user interaction are used for the outer wall segmentation. Edge-based forces drive the segmentation successfully in the presence of strong image gradients, whereas the local region-based forces localize the boundary in the local neighborhood. The local region-based energy, which was originally proposed by Lankton *et al.* [46] assumes that at each point on the object boundary, the local interior and exterior neighborhoods can be modeled by their mean intensities within the localized circular region. The anchor-point energy encourages the contour to pass through each anchor point, placed by the observer, when segmentation is within a user-defined distance to an anchor point. When the contour points are away from the anchor point by more than a user-defined distance there is no influence by this energy term.

22.3.4.2 LIB segmentation

Similar to the MAB segmentation, a combination of numerous criteria is used for the lumen segmentation to utilize its characteristics. For instance, the LIB boundary has an irregular shape due to the presence of plaque and does not typically contain sharp, high contrast edges. In addition, the intensity distribution of the interior of the LIB is fairly homogeneous. Therefore, a combination of local region-based and global region-based forces is employed to segment the LIB. To stop the leaking at the low-contrast boundaries, the previously segmented MAB is used to constrain the current LIB segmentation.

This algorithm was evaluated with 231 2D carotid US slices extracted from 21 3D US images. The algorithm segmentations were compared to the manual segmentations on a slice-by-slice basis. The algorithm yielded high DC s (>92%), submillimeter errors for the mean absolute distance (MAD) and maximum absolute distance (MAXD) and a comparable coefficient of variation (COV) (5.1% vs. 3.9%) to manual segmentations for the MAB and LIB, respectively (see Table 22.5 for more details). The minimum detectable difference of the algorithm in computing the VWV was comparable (64.2 vs. 50.3 mm^3) to manual segmentations. Using this method, the total segmentation time is reduced by 5.5 min in comparison to the manual segmentation (2.8 vs. 8.3 min). Out of the mean time of 2.8 min, 1.2 min is required for the computation and the 1.6 min for the initialization by the observer. The authors also reported on a coupled level set segmentation method to segment both boundaries simultaneously [39] for a more robust segmentation.

Table 22.5 Overall CCA segmentation results for the segmentation algorithm [36] for 231 2D US images extracted from 21 3DUS images. MAD is the MAD error and MAXD is the MAXD error

Metric	MAB segmentation	LIB segmentation
Volume error (%)	2.4 ± 1.9	5.8 ± 2.7
Dice coefficient (%)	95.6 ± 1.5	92.8 ± 3.1
MAD (mm)	0.2 ± 0.1	0.3 ± 0.1
MAXD (mm)	0.6 ± 0.3	0.6 ± 0.4

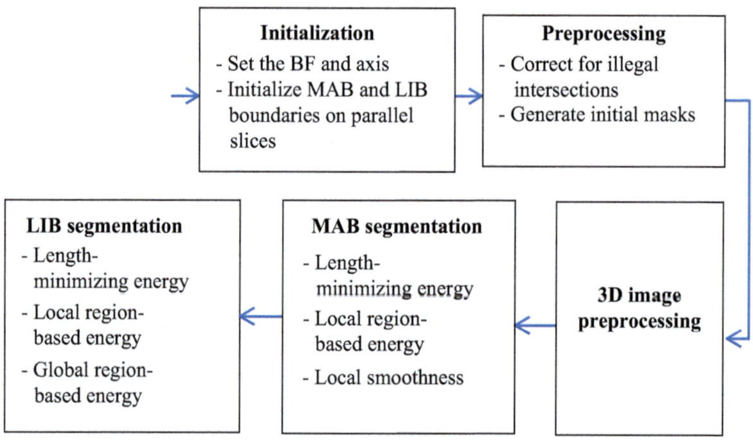

Figure 22.5 Steps involved in 3D segmentation algorithm pipeline [37], which is similar to the previous 2D segmentation method proposed by Ukwatta et al. [36]

This study was validated using the global metrics such as DC, MAD, MAXD and volume errors, which is sufficient for generating 3D US VWV. However, when the algorithm is required to be used for generating VWT maps, the algorithm must be validated using localized techniques. Chiu *et al.* [50] conducted a study, which evaluated the algorithm using standardized carotid maps for the population.

22.3.4.3 3D methods that segment both LIB and MAB from 3D US images

One of the main drawbacks of the previous method proposed by Ukwatta *et al.* [36] is that it still requires a considerable amount of user interaction on each slice to obtain a good segmentation. For some reason, if the user decides to segment each and every slice of the 3D image, a 2D segmentation technique would take a long time.

Ukwatta *et al.* [37] described a direct 3D segmentation algorithm to delineate the outer wall and lumen of the carotid CCA from 3D US images. The segmentation pipeline of the algorithm is shown in Figure 22.5. The algorithm uses a similar initialization approach used previously for the 2D segmentation, but requires initialization only on a smaller subset of transverse slices than used in the 2D method [36]. A direct 3D segmentation method has the potential for reducing user interaction over a 2D method, while increasing the robustness of the segmentation by integrating out-of-plane image information. The 3D method used very similar energy functions to the 2D approach and an extension to the 2D sparse field level set method.

Some example segmentation results of the 3D algorithm are shown in Figure 22.6. The algorithm-generated accuracy and intraobserver variability results are comparable to the previous methods, but with fewer user interactions. For example, for the ISD of 3 mm, the algorithm yielded an average DC of 94.4% ± 2.2% and 90.6% ± 5.0% for the MAB and LIB and the COV of 6.8% for computing the VWV of the CCA, while requiring only 1.72 min (vs. 8.3 min for manual segmentation) for a 3D US image.

22.3.5 Segmentation algorithms of carotid plaque from 3D US images

The segmentation of plaque boundaries is an even more challenging task than the lumen and outer wall segmentations due to the fuzzy boundaries of the plaque. Unlike the measurement of 3D US TPV, which requires observers to distinguish plaque-lumen and plaque-outer vessel wall boundaries, the measurement of 3D US VWV requires an observer to manually outline the LIB/plaque and MAB boundaries—similarly to the measurement of IMT. These boundaries are more straightforward to interpret than plaque-lumen and plaque-wall boundaries in 3D US images. Furthermore, the measurement of TPV from 3D US images requires trained observers who are experts in 3D US image interpretation and in distinguishing vessel wall from plaque in 3D US images.

22.3.5.1 Manual segmentation of plaque from 3D US images

Currently, TPV measurements are obtained by manual segmentation of the plaque [27,28,51–53]. Initially, the observer defines the medial axis of the artery in longitudinal view. After familiarizing with the orientation and geometry of the plaque using a multiplaner reformatting software, the observer outlines the plaque boundary on transverse slices with ISD of 1 mm. After outlining the complete plaque, the software generate a 3D surface from there contours. Limitations of this approach include image interpretation and measurement differences within and between observers, long training times for observers, and long durations to perform manual segmentations.

22.3.5.2 Semiautomated segmentation of plaque from 3D US images

Although, there are several methods that have been developed for the 2D segmentation of the plaque from 2D US images, there are only few studies [54,55] that

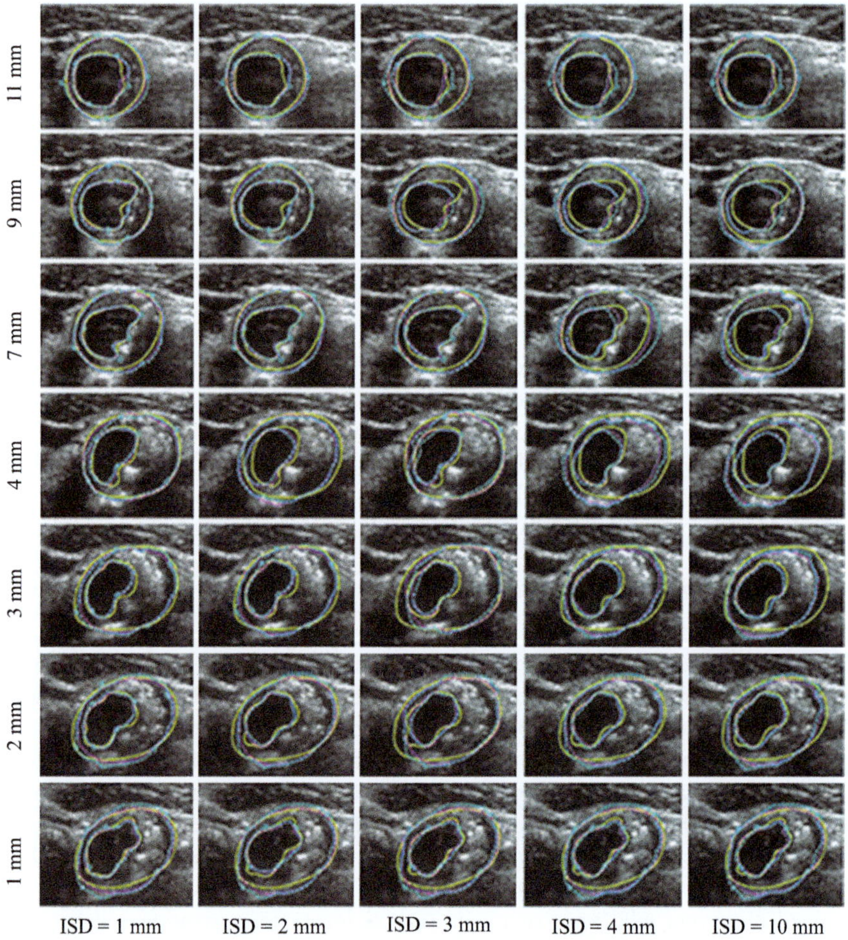

Figure 22.6 2D slice-by-slice comparisons of algorithm segmentations to manual segmentations for a subject with a moderate stenosis (stenosis is between 30% and 70%). Results for ISD from 1 to 4 and 10 mm are shown. The accuracy dropped at 4 and 10 mm. The contours are as follows: Continuous yellow contour—mean manual MAB and LIB, dashed purple contour—mean algorithm MAB and LIB, and cyan dashed contour—one round of algorithm MAB and LIB. Each row corresponds to the distance from the BF and each column corresponds to the ISD used for initialization [37]

describe a semiautomated tool to generate the TPV measurement from 3D US images. The summary of these studies is shown in Table 22.6. Buchanan *et al.* [55] reported on a semiautomated plaque estimated method to outline the plaque boundaries from 3D US images thereby computing TPVs. The workflow of their

Table 22.6 Summary of segmentation methods of carotid plaque from 3D US images

Paper	Year	Dim.	Plaque	Time (min)	No. of images
Buchanan *et al.*	2011	2D	Level set	2.8 ± 0.4	21
Cheng *et al.*	2013	2D	Level set	4.9 s/slice	26

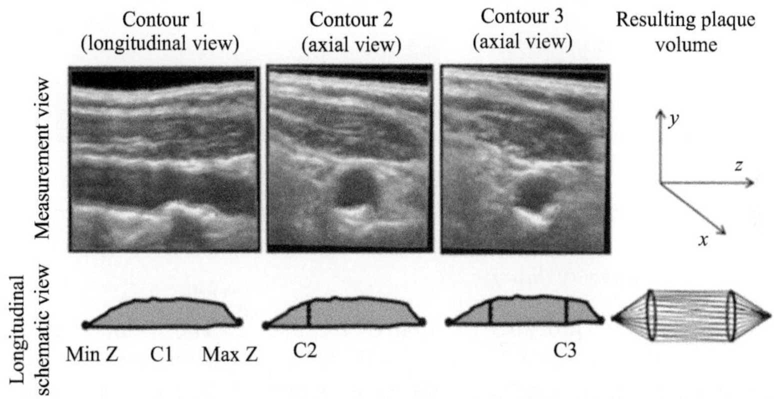

Figure 22.7 User input for semiautomated TPV measurement. In the longitudinal view (and with assistance from the axial view, not shown) the user identifies the maximum and minimum z-values representing the end points of the plaque (Min Z and Max Z). The user identifies the mid-point of the plaque (C1) and finally C2 and C3 are identified and generated in the axial view. Uniform plaque geometry between C2 and C3 is assumed and a final volume is generated [55]

method is shown in Figure 22.7. For the initialization, the observer defines the beginning and end points of the plaque in the long axis view, followed by two contours in the transverse view to identify the regions of greatest change in shape. The algorithm was evaluated with 22 plaque from 10 3D US images. An example comparison of the manually- and algorithm-generated plaque surfaces are shown in Figure 22.8. The algorithm-generated plaque volume and the manual one were significantly correlated ($r = 0.99$, $p < 0.001$) while maintaining a mean COV of $\approx$12.0%. One of the main drawbacks of this method is that it currently does not use any image information by the algorithm. After the algorithm segmentation is obtained, the ability to adjust the segmented boundary by the user is highly desirable.

Cheng *et al.* [54] proposed a semiautomated segmentation of the carotid plaques from 3D US images using the level set method. In comparison to the method by Buchanan *et al.* [55], this method utilizes image information in the segmentation. The objective function of the level set method incorporated smoothness energy, a global region-based energy, a local region-based energy, and prior

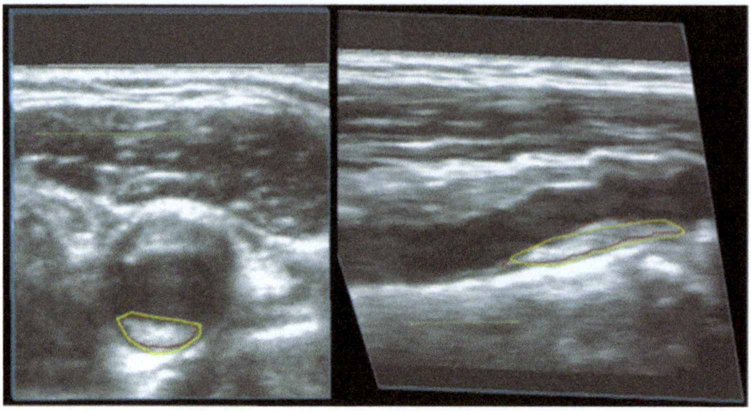

(a) (b)

Figure 22.8 Representative manual and semiautomated segmentation boundaries. (a) axial view, (b) longitudinal view. Manual (red) algorithm contours (yellow)

knowledge about the probable location of the plaque. The method utilizes the presegmented boundaries of MAB and LIB as region of interest for the plaque segmentation. Example results of algorithm-generated plaque segmentation are shown in Figure 22.9, where they closely resemble manual segmentations. The algorithm yielded difference in TPV of -5.3 ± 12.7 and -8.5 ± 13.8 mm^3 and absolute difference in TPV of 9.9 ± 9.5 and 11.8 ± 11.1 mm^3.

22.4 Local quantification of carotid atherosclerosis based on 3D US images

22.4.1 3D vessel-wall-plus-plaque thickness (VWT) map

Although TPV and VWV measured from 3D US images provide direct and reproducible measurements for stroke risk stratification and serial monitoring of disease progression, we hypothesized that quantification of spatiotemporal distribution of vessel wall and plaque burden will improve the sensitivity for treatment evaluation and the accuracy in risk stratification. Chiu *et al.* proposed the first technique to extract the change of vessel-wall-plus-plaque thickness (VWT-Change) on a point-by-point basis, to display the VWT-Change distribution as a 3D map and to evaluate whether the point-wise VWT-Change was statistically significant after segmentation variability had been taken into account [56].

The algorithm consists of four major steps as illustrated in Figure 22.10. The lumen and the outer wall boundaries were segmented from a 3D US image as shown in Figure 22.10(a). The segmentation can be performed either manually [56] or semiautomatically [37]. To evaluate the detected VWT-Change in relation of segmentation variability, five repeated segmentations were performed for both the lumen and outer wall boundaries as shown in Figure 22.11. If the segmentation

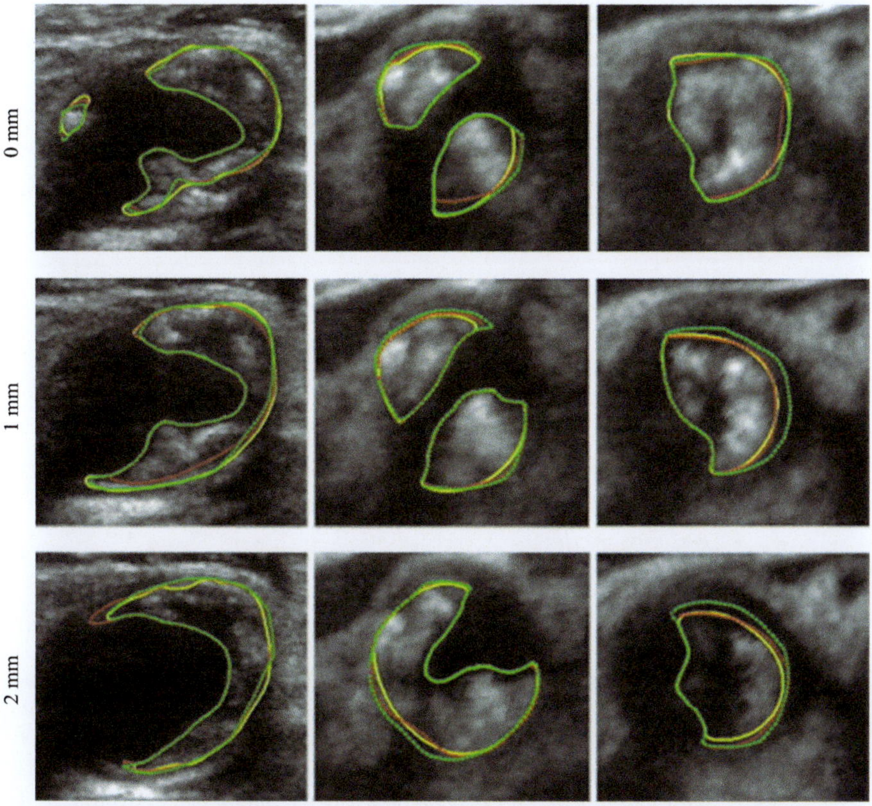

Figure 22.9 Example results of algorithm and manual segmentations for three patients (one subject in each column). The panels in the rows were obtained at distances of 0, 1, and 2 mm from the carotid bifurcation. Yellow solid contours = algorithm results, red dashed contours = results of operator 1, green dashed contours = results of operator 2 [54]

was performed on each transverse slice of a 3D US image as shown in Figure 22.10(a), a stack of contours would be generated for each of the lumen and outer wall boundaries, and subsequently reconstructed into surfaces as shown in Figure 22.10(b). This surface reconstruction step would not be required if a direct 3D segmentation algorithm was applied [37]. Mean lumen and outer wall surfaces were computed by first establishing corresponding points between the five repeated segmentations by the symmetric correspondence algorithm, followed by taking the mean of each set of five correspondence points as shown in Figure 22.11. Then, the symmetric correspondence technique was applied to match the mean lumen and the outer wall surfaces on a point-by-point basis, establishing a pair of correspondence points, denoted by p_W and p_L in Figure 22.11, thereby providing the mean measurement for the point-wise VWT, $\overline{T} = \|p_W - p_L\|$, which were color-coded and

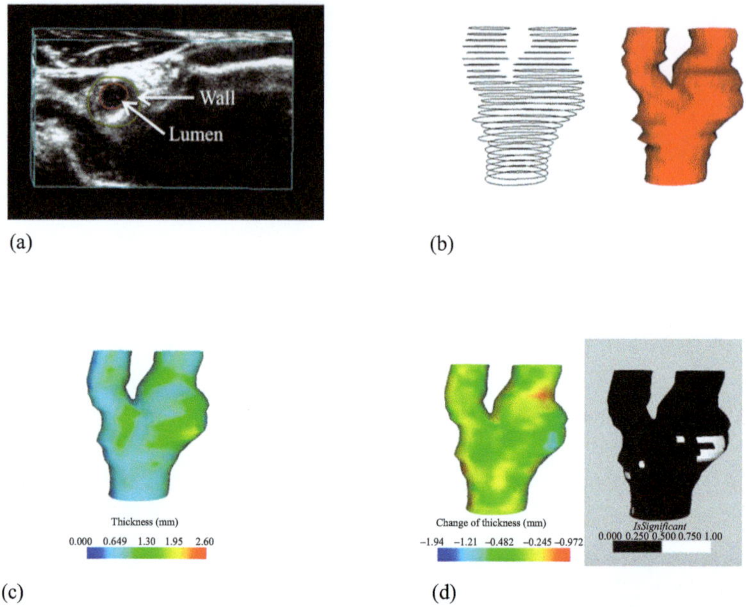

Figure 22.10 Schematic for the construction of 3D VWT-Change map [56]: (a) segment arterial wall and lumen from 3D US images, (b) reconstruct arterial wall and lumen surfaces, (c) compute the mean and standard deviation of the vessel-wall-plus-plague thickness (VWT) based on multiple segmentations of the arterial wall and lumen, and (d) compute VWT-Change from baseline to the second scanning session and determine whether the point-wise VWT-Change is statistically significant

superimposed on the outer wall surface for visualization and assessment as shown in Figure 22.10(c). This thickness distribution map is referred to as *3D VWT map* for later reference.

To account for the standard error (SE) of $\overline{T}$ for later statistical analysis, intersections were obtained between the line joining the correspondence points on the mean boundaries and the repeated segmentations of the lumen and outer wall boundaries as shown in Figure 22.11. The standard deviation of outer wall segmentation, s_W was obtained by taking the standard deviation of the five intersections on the repeatedly segmented outer wall boundaries. The standard deviation of lumen segmentation, s_L, was obtained in a similar manner. With s_W and s_L thus defined and the number of repeated outer wall and lumen segmentations denoted by η_w and η_L, respectively, (equal to 5 in our previous publications [53,56], the SE of $\overline{T}$ can be expressed as

$$\mathrm{SE}_{\overline{T}} = \sqrt{\frac{s_W^2}{\eta_W} + \frac{s_L^2}{\eta_L}} \tag{22.2}$$

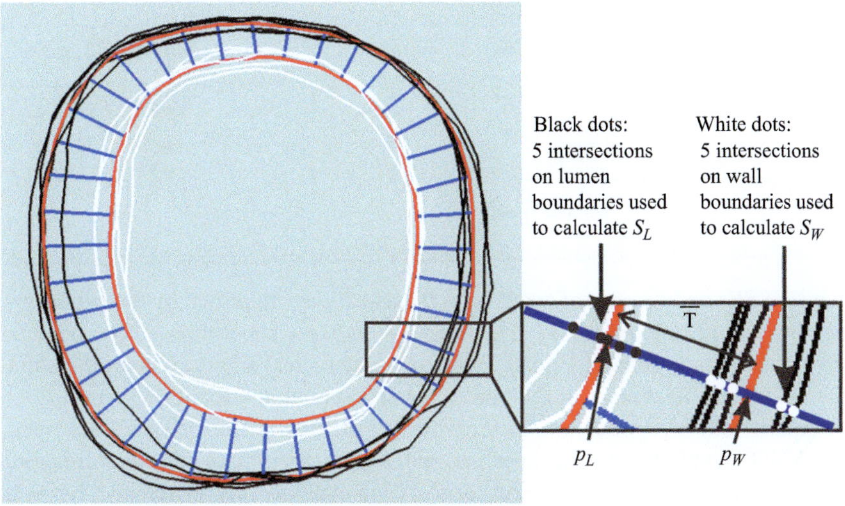

Figure 22.11 *The technique for determining point-wise mean and standard deviation of VWT. The black and white boundaries represent repeated segmentations for the wall and lumen boundaries, respectively. The red curves represent the mean wall and lumen boundaries. The line joining the two correspondence points p_L and p_w intersects the five wall and lumen boundaries. The local standard deviations of the wall and lumen boundaries, S_L and S_w, respectively, can be computed from these intersections. The standard deviation of the local VWT can be computed based on s_L and s_W according to (22.2) [50]*

with a degree of freedom [57]

$$v_{\overline{T}} = \frac{\left(s_W^2/\eta_W + s_L^2/\eta_L\right)^2}{\frac{\left(s_W^2/\eta_W\right)^2}{\eta_W - 1} + \frac{\left(s_L^2/\eta_L\right)^2}{\eta_L - 1}} \tag{22.3}$$

For serial monitoring of therapeutic treatment effect, such as in assessment of the effect of atorvastatin [30,56,58], 3D VWT maps were generated at baseline and the follow-up imaging session, and registered using the modified iterative closest point technique introduced in Chiu *et al.* [59] Then, the 3D VWT maps were matched on a point-by-point basis, and the point-wise *VWT-Change,* ΔVWT, were obtained by $\overline{T}_2 - \overline{T}_1$, where $\overline{T}_1$ and $\overline{T}_2$ denote the point-wise mean VWT on the baseline and the follow-up maps, respectively. Figure 22.10(di) shows an example *3D VWT-Change* map, constructed by superimposing the point-wise ΔVWT measurements on the outer wall surface. To evaluate whether each point-wise ΔVWT measurement is statistically different from 0, a *t*-test was performed by evaluating the statistics $\Delta VWT/SE_{\Delta VWT}$, with the SE and degrees of freedom of ΔVWT given by the following equations:

$$\mathrm{SE}_{\Delta\mathrm{VWT}} = \sqrt{\mathrm{SE}^2_{\overline{T}_1} + \mathrm{SE}^2_{\overline{T}_2}} \tag{22.4}$$

$$v_{\Delta\mathrm{VWT}} = \frac{\left(\mathrm{SE}^2_{\overline{T}_1} + \mathrm{SE}^2_{\overline{T}_2}\right)^2}{\frac{\left(\mathrm{SE}^2_{\overline{T}_1}\right)^2}{v_{\overline{T}_1}} + \frac{\left(\mathrm{SE}^2_{\overline{T}_2}\right)^2}{v_{\overline{T}_2}}} \tag{22.5}$$

where the SEs and degrees of freedom of $\overline{T}_1$ and $\overline{T}_2$ are identified by the subscripts, and given by (22.2) and (22.3). The *t*-test results were superimposed on the outer wall as shown in Figure 22.10(dii), showing the statistical significance of the point-wise ΔVWT measurement in relation to the segmentation variability.

Apart from its application on identifying statistical difference between point-wise VWTs exhibited in the baseline and follow-up images, the quantification method described above has been applied to evaluate the difference between manual and algorithm segmentations from the 3D US images of carotid arteries [50,52] and neonatal lateral ventricles [60]. Unlike in assessing VWT-Change, no registration was required as both the manual and algorithm segmentations were generated in the same image.

22.4.2 2D Carotid template

Although the 3D VWT-Change map provides rich information on the distribution, the geometry of the map is highly subject-specific, thereby hindering quantitative comparisons of different subjects in a study cohort and even of the same subject imaged by different imaging modalities or at different time points. For this reason, clinical investigations involving the VWT-Change maps [61,62] were limited to qualitative visual matching. To address this issue, Chiu *et al.* developed a technique to map 3D carotid maps onto a carotid template [63].

22.4.2.1 Arc-length scaling (AL) approach

Chiu *et al.* introduced the arc-length scaling (AL) approach for carotid template construction [63], which we refer to as the AL approach hereafter for easy reference. The first step of this algorithm involves transforming the 3D carotid surface to a standard coordinate system with BF located at origin and longitudinal direction of CCA aligned with *z*-axis. Centroids denoted by C_{ECAup} and C_{ICAup} in Figure 22.12(a) were obtained from the external and internal carotid contours that were closest to the BF (BF), and the line from C_{ECAup} and C_{ICAup} was aligned with the *x*-axis.

Then, the ICA and CCA of the 3D carotid surface were cut by two planes, labeled as P_{ICA} and P_{CCA} in Figure 22.12(a), respectively, and unfolded into two connected 2D rectangular domains as shown in Figure 22.12(b). Figure 22.12(a) shows two example contours on the CCA and ICA surfaces, labeled as Contours 1 and 2, respectively, which were mapped to two straight lines shown in Figure 22.12(b).

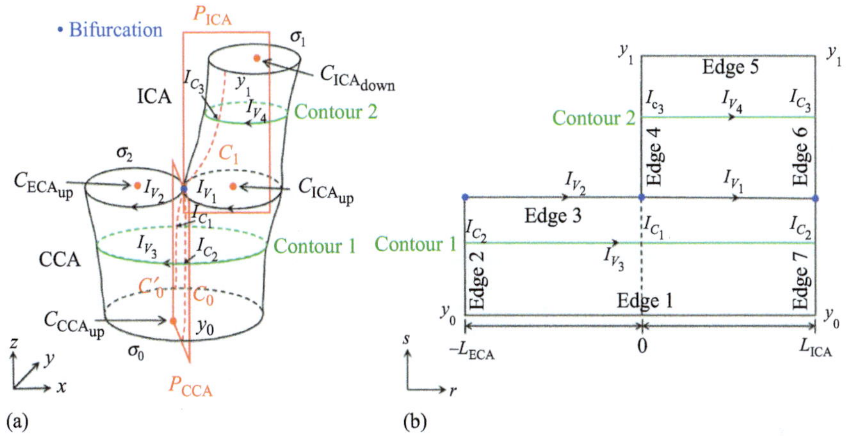

Figure 22.12 Construction of the 2D carotid template using the arc-length scaling (AL) approach. (a) Two planes P_{ICA} and P_{CCA} cut the internal and external carotid (ICA and ECA) surfaces, respectively. (b) The 2D map generated by the AL approach [64]

The width of the 2D map was specified by L_{ECA} and L_{ICA}, which were obtained in a standard way related to the average surface area of the entire set of carotid arteries under investigation as described in Chiu *et al.* [63].

22.5 Optimization of correspondence by minimizing the description length

Although the carotid template constructed by the AL approach adjusted for the anatomic variability of the carotid arteries exhibited in a subject population, the quality of the surface correspondence was not optimized in any sense. Mismatches of point correspondence may lead to higher variability in the point-wise VWT-Change. For this reason, Chen and Chiu developed a method to optimize the correspondence quality [64] based on minimizing the description length (DL), which is referred to as the minimum DL (MDL) approach hereafter to facilitate later discussion. It was shown that the MDL approach played an important role in improving interscan reproducibility of VWT measurements. Figure 22.13 shows the flowchart of the algorithm. Each step is described in detail below.

After the initial map was generated by the AL approach, it was sampled in a 0.3-mm interval horizontally and vertically, resulting in a set of N landmarks with one-to-one mapping with the corresponding 3D map. Generalized Procrustes alignment was applied to rescale and align all carotid arteries based on these landmarks. To facilitate later discussion, we denote the set of N landmarks associated with the jth subject by a $3N$-dimensional vector $L_j = [x_{1j} \dots x_{Nj} y_{1j} \dots y_{Nj} z_{1j} \dots z_{Nj}]^T$, where the 3D coordinates of the ith landmark was denoted by (x_{ij}, y_{ij}, z_{ij}).

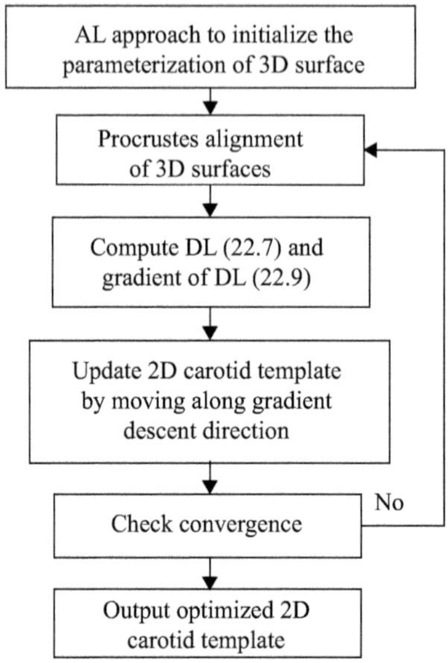

Figure 22.13 The flowchart of the minimum description length (MDL) approach for correspondence optimization [64]

After the Procrustes alignment, the vectors containing the landmarks of all carotid arteries were concatenated to form the landmark configuration matrix **L**:

$$\mathbf{L} = [L_1 L_2 \ldots L_S] \tag{22.6}$$

where S is the total number of arteries. A statistical shape model can be constructed based on the established landmarks:

$$\overline{L} + \sum_m b_m p_m \tag{22.7}$$

where $\overline{L} = \frac{1}{S}\sum_{i=1}^{S} L_i$ and b_m is a constant specifying the weight of each principal components p_m, which is an eigenvector of the covariance matrix of **L**. Singular value decomposition (SVD) of the centered and unbiased matrix $\mathbf{A} = \frac{1}{\sqrt{S-1}}(\mathbf{L} - \overline{\mathbf{L}})$, where $\overline{\mathbf{L}} = [\underbrace{\overline{L}\,\overline{L} \ldots \overline{L}}_{S}]$, can be performed to obtain eigenvalues (λ_m) and eigenvectors (p_m) of the covariance matrix associated with **L** [65].

The DL, denoted by F, is defined as

$$F = \sum_m \varsigma_m \tag{22.8}$$

where

$$\varsigma_m = \begin{cases} 1 + \log(\lambda_m/\lambda_{\text{cut}}), & \lambda_m > \lambda_{\text{cut}} \\ \lambda_m/\lambda_{\text{cut}}, & \lambda_m \leq \lambda_{\text{cut}} \end{cases} \tag{22.9}$$

and λ_{cut} is a cut-off constant that accounts for noise in the training surfaces. We adopt the same cut λ_{cut} value of 0.0032 as in the DL calculation [65–67].

The gradient of F with respect to horizontal and vertical reparameterizations at each landmark l_{ij}, whose 3D coordinates are $(a_{ij}, a_{i+N,j}, a_{i+2N,j})$ in the matrix **A**, can be written as follows:

$$\begin{aligned}\frac{\partial F}{\partial \Delta r} &= \sum_k \frac{\partial F}{\partial a_{kj}} \frac{\partial a_{kj}}{\partial \Delta r} \quad k \in \{i, i+N, i+2N\} \\ \frac{\partial F}{\partial \Delta s} &= \sum_k \frac{\partial F}{\partial a_{kj}} \frac{\partial a_{kj}}{\partial \Delta s} \quad k \in \{i, i+N, i+2N\}\end{aligned} \tag{22.10}$$

$\partial F/\partial a_{ij}$ can be obtained based on the SVD result for **A** [66], $\partial a_{ij}/\partial \Delta r$ and $\partial a_{ij}/\partial \Delta s$ could be computed as the surface gradient as established mathematically [64]. With $(\partial F/\partial \Delta r, \partial F/\partial \Delta s)$ obtained using (22.10), each landmark was moved along the gradient descent direction $(-\partial F/\partial \Delta r, -\partial F/\partial \Delta s)$ to minimize F in each iteration. One iteration of the DL minimization algorithm concluded when 2D maps for all arteries investigated were deformed and resampled. Procrustes alignment was performed again based on the new set of landmarks and a new iteration of DL minimization followed. The algorithm terminated if the number of iterations exceeded 200 and the reduction of DL in an iteration was lower than 10^{-3}.

22.5.1 Role of DL minimization to improve reproducibility of 3D US VWT measurements

Ten subjects were involved in a previous study focusing on the evaluation of the interscan reproducibility in 3D US-based VWV and TPV measurements [61]. 3D carotid ultrasound images were acquired for these subjects at baseline and 2 weeks later. No physiological changes were expected for these patients with stable atherosclerosis within 2 weeks. For each image, the arterial lumen and outer wall were each repeatedly segmented five times. These patient images were evaluated [59] to demonstrate the improvement in the reproducibility of 3D US-based VWT measurements by the introduction of the correspondence optimization strategy described in the previous section. A total of 20 3D VWT and SE maps were generated (10 subjects × 2 images/subject), which were subsequently transformed onto the carotid template using the AL and the MDL approaches. As the VWT maps obtained at the two different time points for each subject were mapped to the carotid template, point-wise ΔVWT for individual subjects could be computed, which were averaged to obtain the group-average ΔVWT at each point p_i on the carotid template, denoted by $\overline{\Delta\mathrm{VWT}}(p_i)$. As described in [64], a t-test can be performed to evaluate whether $\overline{\Delta\mathrm{VWT}}(p_i)$ is significantly different from 0, and the interscan reproducibility of VWT for the entire group of ten subjects can be assessed by the percentage of points on the carotid map with $\overline{\Delta\mathrm{VWT}}$ significantly different from 0. The results showed that the percentage of points with $\overline{\Delta\mathrm{VWT}}$ significantly different from 0 was 18% for the AL approach, which was reduced to

11% after DL minimization were performed. Although no physiological changes were expected for this population of subjects, a degree of interscan variability was expected due to sonographer change, patient positioning, and different neck orientations. We showed the MDL approach was effective in minimizing interscan variability.

22.5.2 Novel biomarker based on 2D carotid template

Although the 2D VWT-Change map provides rich information on the change in VWT distribution and allows for quantitative comparison among patients, clinical conclusions are difficult to be drawn based on the complex VWT-Change distribution represented by thousands of VWT-Change data points per patient. To address this issue, Chiu *et al.* developed a biomarker to provide simple and sensitive assessment of therapeutic effect on atherosclerosis [63]. The biomarker was developed based on a feature selection algorithm, which was applied to identify regions of interest (ROI) where the VWT-Change measurements are most correlated with treatment group identity. Figure 22.14 demonstrates the application of the feature selection technique for identifying ROI where the differences in VWT-Change measurements between subjects receiving atorvastatin and placebo were largest. It was established that this subject-based mean VWT-Change computed over the ROI was more sensitive than the mean VWT-Change computed over the entire 2D map for each patient as well as existing biomarkers, including the IMT, total plaque area (TPA), and VWV. *The sample size required to detect treatment effect in a 6-month therapy with 90% power at a 5% significance level is 35 per group using our new biomarker, compared to 17,465, 2,260, 133 and 97 per group required by IMT, TPA, VWV and the mean VWT computed over the entire 2D map, respectively.* These results provide strong evidence to show that the new biomarker was much more sensitive to effect of the therapy.

The introduction of this sensitive quantification technique for carotid atherosclerosis allows many proof-of-principle longitudinal studies to be performed before a more costly study involving a larger population is held to validate the results. Moreover, this technique can also be applied to cross-sectional studies aiming at assessing the contributions by potential risk factors to the development of atherosclerosis. One such example is our previously described clinical study that involved only 61 patients, but was able to show that the VWT burden in smokers was greater than ex-smokers in a statistically significant manner [68]. This population did not fulfill the diagnostic criteria for chronic obstructive pulmonary disease (COPD), but was associated with mild functional pulmonary abnormalities detectable by 3He MR perfusion imaging. This finding supports the existence of a relationship between carotid atherosclerosis and COPD even in their very early stages, and suggests an opportunity for early detection of carotid atherosclerosis by inclusion of 3D US in the clinical workflow in the management of COPD patients, which is important because cardiovascular events are leading causes of death for these patients.

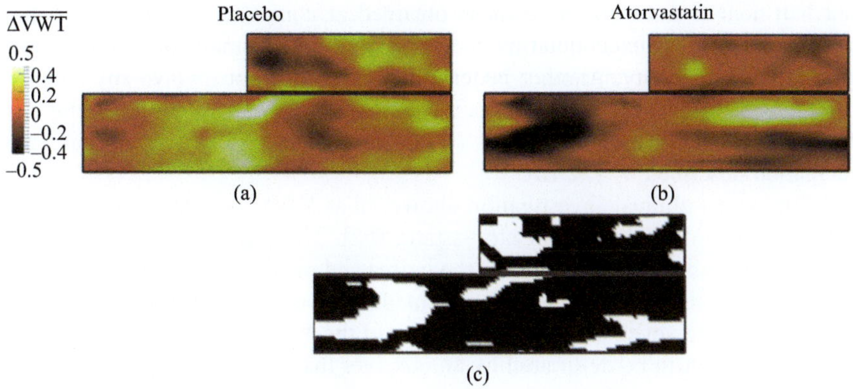

Figure 22.14 The average 2D ΔVWT maps for (a) 10 placebo and (b) 10 atorvastatin subjects involved in the study described in [29]. (c) ROI in white were selected, which exhibits larger difference in ΔVWT between placebo and atorvastatin subjects [50]

22.6 Future perspectives

3D US has been demonstrated to be capable of providing reproducible plaque and VWV measurements. These global measurements are shown to be sensitive to treatment effect [58] and valuable in predicting strokes [69]. Although these global parameters provide rich information for treatment effect evaluation and risk stratification, the localized nature of carotid atherosclerosis suggested that more sensitive biomarkers can be developed if the spatial distribution of vessel wall and plaque burden is taken into consideration. In this chapter, we reviewed techniques developed for local vessel wall and plaque burden monitoring and clinical study results that showed the elevated sensitivity of the local VWT-Change biomarker as compared to VWV. Although substantial progress has been made in the development of sensitive quantification tools required for monitoring carotid atherosclerosis, further technical development and validation studies are required before the proposed quantification framework can be used as a routine clinical tool for atherosclerosis assessment.

An important requirement for VWT-Change quantification is the registration of the baseline and follow-up 3D US images. Rigid registration introduced previously [59] was applied in Sections 22.1 and 22.3 without considering the potential nonlinear misalignment in the carotid images due to different head positioning and orientations [70]. Although optimization of correspondence described in Section 22.5 is expected to handle the misalignment and lead to yet more sensitive biomarkers by reducing the variability in VWT-Change measurements, these hypotheses are required to be validated in our ongoing clinical investigations. Moreover, the correspondence optimization method currently requires 4 h to converge, and must be significantly accelerated in order to be used in clinical analyses. As reported in Chen and Chiu [64], the correspondence quality provided after the first half-hour is comparable to those obtained at convergence. Thus, an option would be to limit the execution time to 30 min and make a small compromise in the correspondence quality. Another better option that does not involve any compromise in the correspondence quality is to capitalize on the parallel processing capability of graphical processing unit (GPU) to accelerate the gradient direction calculation described by (22.10).

A previous clinical investigation showed that VWV was less sensitive than TPV in evaluating the effect of atorvastatin [62]. The lower sensitivity of VWV may be attributable to its inclusion of the intima and media layers, the thickening of which is more related to hyperintensive medial hypertrophy than carotid atherosclerosis [71]. However, a major shortcoming of the TPV phenotype is that plaques are more difficult to be delineated by an observer than vessel wall and lumen. For this reason, measuring TPV is more time-consuming and prone to observer variability. We are currently developing a 3D plaque segmentation technique and will incorporate plaque measurements in our analysis framework.

References

[1] S. Natarajan, L. S. Marks, D. J. Margolis, *et al.*, "Clinical application of a 3D ultrasound-guided prostate biopsy system," Urologic Oncology 29, 334–342 (2011).

[2] G. Treece, R. Prager, A. Gee and L. Berman, "3D ultrasound measurement of large organ volume," Medical Image Analysis 5, 41–54 (2001).

[3] A. Fenster and D. B. Downey, "3-dimensional ultrasound imaging: A review," IEEE Engineering in Medicine and Biology 15, 41–51 (1996).

[4] T. R. Nelson and D. H. Pretorius, "Three-dimensional ultrasound of fetal surface features," Ultrasound in Obstetrics & Gynecology 2, 166–174 (1992).

[5] R. N. Rankin, A. Fenster, D. B. Downey, P. L. Munk, M. F. Levin and A. D. Vellet, "Three-dimensional sonographic reconstruction: techniques and diagnostic applications.," AJR American Journal of Roentgenology 161, 695–702 (1993).

[6] A. Fenster, D. B. Downey and H. N. Cardinal, "Three-dimensional ultrasound imaging," Physics in Medicine and Biology 46, R67-R99 (2001).

[7] T. R. Nelson, D. B. Downey, D. H. Pretorius and A. Fenster, Three-Dimensional Ultrasound. (Lippincott-Raven, Philadelphia, PA, 1999).

[8] T. R. Nelson and D. H. Pretorius, "Three-dimensional ultrasound imaging," Ultrasound in Medicine & Biology 24, 1243–1270 (1998).

[9] K. Baba and D. Jurkovic, Three-Dimensional Ultrasound in Obstetrics and Gynecology, 1 ed. (The Parthenon Publishing Group, New York, 1997).

[10] D. B. Downey and A. Fenster, "Three-dimensional ultrasound: A maturing technology," Ultrasound Quarterly 14, 25–40 (1998).

[11] A. Fenster and D. Downey, "Three-dimensional ultrasound imaging," in Handbook of Medical Imaging, Volume 1, Physics and Psychophysics,

Vol. 1, edited by J. Beutel, H. Kundel and R. Van Metter (SPIE Press, Bellingham, WA, 2000), pp. 433–509.

[12] A. Fenster and D. B. Downey, "Three-dimensional ultrasound imaging," Annual Review of Biomedical Engineering 02, 457–475 (2000).

[13] A. Fenster and D. Downey, "Basic principles and applications of 3-D ultrasound imaging," in An Advanced Signal Processing Handbook, edited by S. Stergiopoulos (CRC Press, Boca Raton, 2001), pp. 14-11–14-34.

[14] N. Pagoulatos, D. R. Haynor and Y. Kim, "A fast calibration method for 3-D tracking of ultrasound images using a spatial localizer," Ultrasound in Medicine and Biology 27, 1219–1229 (2001).

[15] E. M. Boctor, M. A. Choti, E. C. Burdette and R. J. Webster Iii, "Three-dimensional ultrasound-guided robotic needle placement: an experimental evaluation," The International Journal of Medical Robotics 4, 180–191 (2008).

[16] G. Treece, R. Prager, A. Gee and L. Berman, "3D ultrasound measurement of large organ volume," Medical Image Analysis 5, 41–54 (2001).

[17] J. Hummel, M. Figl, M. Bax, H. Bergmann and W. Birkfellner, "2D/3D registration of endoscopic ultrasound to CT volume data," Physics in Medicine and Biology 53, 4303–4316 (2008).

[18] L. Mercier, T. Lango, F. Lindseth and D. L. Collins, "A review of calibration techniques for freehand 3-D ultrasound systems," Ultrasound in Medicine & Biology 31, 449–471 (2005).

[19] F. Lindseth, G. A. Tangen, T. Lango and J. Bang, "Probe calibration for freehand 3-D ultrasound," Ultrasound in Medicine & Biology 29, 1607–1623 (2003).

[20] F. Rousseau, P. Hellier and C. Barillot, "Confhusius: a robust and fully automatic calibration method for 3D freehand ultrasound," Medical Image Analysis 9, 25–38 (2005).

[21] D. F. Leotta, "An efficient calibration method for freehand 3-D ultrasound imaging systems," Ultrasound in Medicine & Biology 30, 999–1008 (2004).

[22] M. J. Gooding, S. H. Kennedy and J. A. Noble, "Temporal calibration of freehand three-dimensional ultrasound using image alignment," Ultrasound in Medicine & Biology 31, 919–927 (2005).

[23] S. Dandekar, Y. Li, J. Molloy and J. Hossack, "A phantom with reduced complexity for spatial 3-D ultrasound calibration," Ultrasound in Medicine & Biology 31, 1083–1093 (2005).

[24] T. C. Poon and R. N. Rohling, "Comparison of calibration methods for spatial tracking of a 3-D ultrasound probe," Ultrasound in Medicine & Biology 31, 1095–1108 (2005).

[25] A. H. Gee, N. E. Houghton, G. M. Treece and R. W. Prager, "A mechanical instrument for 3D ultrasound probe calibration," Ultrasound in Medicine & Biology 31, 505–518 (2005).

[26] K.-L. Chien, T.-C. Su, J.-S. Jeng, *et al.*, "Carotid artery intima-media thickness, carotid plaque and coronary heart disease and stroke in Chinese," PLoS ONE 3, e3435 %U http://www.google.ca/q=maximum+diameter+of

+carotid+artery&hl=en&ei=tLY3439TJ_AJs3437wngfLq_HdDg&start=3440&sa=N&fp=e4100ea3438dfe2176d (2008).

[27] A. Landry, J. D. Spence and A. Fenster, "Measurement of carotid plaque volume by 3-dimensional ultrasound," Stroke 35, 864–869 (2004).

[28] A. Landry, J. D. Spence and A. Fenster, "Quantification of carotid plaque volume measurements using 3D ultrasound imaging," Ultrasound in Medicine & Biology 31, 751–762 (2005).

[29] C. D. Ainsworth, C. C. Blake, A. Tamayo, V. Beletsky, A. Fenster and J. D. Spence, "3D ultrasound measurement of change in carotid plaque volume: a tool for rapid evaluation of new therapies," Stroke 36, 1904–1909 (2005).

[30] M. Egger, J. D. Spence, A. Fenster and G. Parraga, "Validation of 3D ultrasound vessel wall volume: an imaging phenotype of carotid atherosclerosis," Ultrasound in Medicine & Biology 33, 905–914 (2007).

[31] M. Egger, A. Krasinski, B. K. Rutt, A. Fenster and G. Parraga, "Comparison of B-mode ultrasound, 3-dimensional ultrasound, and magnetic resonance imaging measurements of carotid atherosclerosis," Journal of Ultrasound in Medicine: Official Journal of the American Institute of Ultrasound in Medicine 27, 1321–1334 %U http://www.jultrasoundmed.org/cgi/content/abstract/1327/1329/1321 (2008).

[32] C. I. Christodoulou, C. S. Pattichis, M. Pantziaris and A. Nicolaides, "Texture-based classification of atherosclerotic carotid plaques," IEEE Transactions on Medical Imaging 22, 902–912 (2003).

[33] E. C. Kyriacou, S. Petroudi, C. S. Pattichis, *et al.*, "Prediction of high-risk asymptomatic carotid plaques based on ultrasonic image features," IEEE Transactions on Information Technology in Biomedicine: A Publication of the IEEE Engineering in Medicine and Biology Society 16, 966–973 (2012).

[34] J. Awad, A. Krasinski, G. Parraga and A. Fenster, "Texture analysis of carotid artery atherosclerosis from three-dimensional ultrasound images," Medical Physics 37, 1382–1391 (2010).

[35] A. van Engelen, T. Wannarong, G. Parraga, *et al.*, "Three-dimensional carotid ultrasound plaque texture predicts vascular events," Stroke 45, 2695–2701 (2014).

[36] E. Ukwatta, J. Awad, A. D. Ward, *et al.*, "Three-dimensional ultrasound of carotid atherosclerosis: Semiautomated segmentation using a level set-based method," Medical Physics 38, 2479 (2011).

[37] E. Ukwatta, J. Yuan, D. Buchanan, *et al.*, "Three-dimensional segmentation of three-dimensional ultrasound carotid atherosclerosis using sparse field level sets," Medical Physics 40, 052903 (2013).

[38] M. M. Hossain, K. AlMuhanna, L. Zhao, B. K. Lal and S. Sikdar, "Semi-automatic segmentation of atherosclerotic carotid artery wall volume using 3D ultrasound imaging," Medical Physics 42, 2029–2043 (2015).

[39] E. Ukwatta, J. Awad, A. D. Ward, D. Buchanan, G. Parraga and A. Fenster, "Coupled level set approach to segment carotid arteries from 3D ultrasound

images," in Biomedical Imaging: From Nano to Macro, 2011 IEEE International Symposium on, (2011), pp. 37–40.
[40] X. Yang, M. Ding, L. Lou, M. Yuchi, W. Qiu and Y. Sun, "Common carotid artery lumen segmentation in B-mode ultrasound transverse view images," International Journal of Image, Graphics and Signal Processing (IJIGSP) 3, 15 (2011).
[41] J. D. Gill, H. M. Ladak, D. A. Steinman and A. Fenster, "Accuracy and variability assessment of a semiautomatic technique for segmentation of the carotid arteries from three-dimensional ultrasound images," Medical Physics 27, 1333–1342 (2000).
[42] A. Zahalka and A. Fenster, "An automated segmentation method for three-dimensional carotid ultrasound images," Physics in Medicine and Biology 46, 1321–1342 (2001).
[43] A. M. Lorza, D. D. Carvalho, J. Petersen, *et al.*, "Carotid artery lumen segmentation in 3D free-hand ultrasound images using surface graph cuts," Medical Image Computing and Computer-Assisted Intervention: MICCAI ... International Conference on Medical Image Computing and Computer-Assisted Intervention 16, 542–549 (2013).
[44] M. Kass, A. Witkin and D. Terzopoulos, "Snakes: Active contour models," International Journal of Computer Vision 1, 321–331 (1988).
[45] S. Osher and J. A. Sethian, "Fronts propagating with curvature dependent speed: algorithms based on Hamilton-Jacobi formulations," (1988).
[46] S. Lankton and A. Tannenbaum, "Localizing region-based active contours," IEEE Transactions on Image Processing 17, 2029–2039 %U http://2066.2102.2021.2104/scholar?hl=en&lr=&q=cache:NvAgJ2024nThCMJ:www.shawnlankton.com/wp-content/uploads/articles/lankton-lrbac-TIP-2008.pdf+related:NvAgJ2024nThCMJ:scholar.google.com/ (2008).
[47] Z. Wei, G. Wan, L. Gardi, G. Mills, D. Downey and A. Fenster, "Robot-assisted 3D-TRUS guided prostate brachytherapy: system integration and validation," Medical Physics 31, 539–548 (2004).
[48] R. T. Whitaker, "A level-set approach to 3D reconstruction from range data," International Journal of Computer Vision 29, 203–231 %U http://dx.doi.org/210.1023/A:1008036829907 (1998).
[49] X. Yang, J. Jin, M. Xu, *et al.*, "Ultrasound common carotid artery segmentation based on active shape model," Computational and Mathematical Methods in Medicine 2013, 345968 (2013).
[50] B. Chiu, E. Ukwatta, S. Shavakh and A. Fenster, "Quantification and visualization of carotid segmentation accuracy and precision using a 2D standardized carotid map," Physics in Medicine and Biology 58, 3671–3703 (2013).
[51] A. Fenster, C. Blake, I. Gyacskov, A. Landry and J. D. Spence, "3D ultrasound analysis of carotid plaque volume and surface morphology," Ultrasonics 44, e153–e157 (2006).
[52] A. Landry, C. Ainsworth, C. Blake, J. D. Spence and A. Fenster, "Manual planimetric measurement of carotid plaque volume using three-dimensional ultrasound imaging," Medical Physics 34, 1496–1505 (2007).

[53] J. D. Spence, C. Blake, A. Landry and A. Fenster, "Measurement of carotid plaque and effect of vitamin therapy for total homocysteine," Clinical Chemistry and Laboratory Medicine. 41, 1498–1504 (2003).

[54] J. Cheng, H. Li, F. Xiao, *et al.*, "Fully automatic plaque segmentation in 3-D carotid ultrasound images," Ultrasound in Medicine & Biology 39, 2431–2446 (2013).

[55] D. Buchanan, I. Gyacskov, E. Ukwatta, T. Lindenmaiera, A. Fenster and G. Parraga, "Semi-automated Segmentation of Carotid Artery Total Plaque Volume from Three Dimensional Ultrasound Carotid Imaging," in SPIE Medical Imaging, (San Diego, 2011).

[56] B. Chiu, M. Egger, J. D. Spence, G. Parraga and A. Fenster, "Quantification of carotid vessel wall and plaque thickness change using 3D ultrasound images," Medical Physics 35, 3691–3710 (2008).

[57] F. E. Satterthwaite, "An approximate distribution of estimates of variance components," Biometrics 2, 110–114 (1946).

[58] A. Krasinski, B. Chiu, J. D. Spence, A. Fenster and G. Parraga, "Three-dimensional ultrasound quantification of intensive statin treatment of carotid atherosclerosis," Ultrasound in Medicine & Biology 352009 #2721, 1763–1772 (2009).

[59] B. Chiu, V. Shamdasani, R. Entrekin, C. Yuan and W. S. Kerwin, "Characterization of carotid plaques on 3-dimensional ultrasound imaging by registration with multicontrast magnetic resonance imaging," Journal of Ultrasound in Medicine: Official Journal of the American Institute of Ultrasound in Medicine 31, 1567–1580 (2012).

[60] Y. Chen, W. Qiu, J. Kishimoto, *et al.*, "A framework for quantification and visualization of segmentation accuracy and variability in 3D lateral ventricle ultrasound images of preterm neonates," Medical Physics 42, 6387–6405 (2015).

[61] M. Egger, B. Chiu, J. Spence, A. Fenster and G. Parraga, "Mapping spatial and temporal changes in carotid atherosclerosis from three-dimensional ultrasound images," Ultrasound in Medicine & Biology 34, 64–72 (2008).

[62] A. Krasinski, B. Chiu, A. Fenster and G. Parraga, "Magnetic resonance imaging and three-dimensional ultrasound of carotid atherosclerosis: Mapping regional differences," Journal of Magnetic Resonance Imaging 29, 901–908 %U http://dx.doi.org/910.1002/jmri.21709 (2009).

[63] B. Chiu, B. Li and T. W. Chow, "Novel 3D ultrasound image-based biomarkers based on a feature selection from a 2D standardized vessel wall thickness map: a tool for sensitive assessment of therapies for carotid atherosclerosis," Physics in Medicine and Biology 58, 5959–5982 (2013).

[64] Y. Chen and B. Chiu, "Correspondence optimization in 2D standardized carotid wall thickness map by description length minimization: A tool for increasing reproducibility of 3D ultrasound-based measurements," Medical Physics 43, 6474 (2016).

[65] T. Heimann, I. Wolf, T. Williams, H.P. Meinzer, "3D active shape models using gradient descent optimization of description length," Information Processing in Medical Imaging, 19, 566–577 (2005).
[66] A. Ericsson, K. Astrom, "Minimizing the description length using steepest descent," Proc. British Machine Vision Conference, Norwich, United Kingdom, 2, 93–102, (2003).
[67] H.H. Thodberg, "Minimum Description Length shape and appearance models," Information Processing in Medical Imaging, 18, 51–62 (2003).
[68] J. Cheng, D. Pike, T. W. Chow, M. Kirby, G. Parraga and B. Chiu, "Three-dimensional ultrasound measurements of carotid vessel wall and plaque thickness and their relationship with pulmonary abnormalities in ex-smokers without airflow limitation," The International Journal of Cardiovascular Imaging 32, 1391–1402 (2016).
[69] T. Wannarong, G. Parraga, D. Buchanan, *et al.*, "Progression of carotid plaque volume predicts cardiovascular events," Stroke 44, 1859–1865 (2013).
[70] N. D. Nanayakkara, B. Chiu, A. Samani, J. D. Spence, J. Samarabandu and A. Fenster, "A "twisting and bending" model-based nonrigid image registration technique for 3-D ultrasound carotid images," IEEE Transactions on Medical Imaging 27, 1378–1388 (2008).
[71] J. D. Spence and R. A. Hegele, "Noninvasive phenotypes of atherosclerosis: similar windows but different views," Stroke 35, 649–653 (2004).

Chapter 23

Carotid artery mechanics assessed by ultrasound

R.G.P. Lopata[1]*, M.C.M. Rutten*[1]
and M.R.H.M. van Sambeek[2]

23.1 Introduction

23.1.1 Anatomy

The carotid artery is an important blood vessel, supplying the brain with oxygen and nutrients. Two carotid arteries are found, one on either side of the neck, see Figure 23.1. It bifurcates into the external carotid artery, that is mainly responsible for supplying the facial muscles with blood, and the internal carotid artery that ensures blood flow to the brain. It connects (together with the vertebral arteries) to the circle of Willis, from which the entire brain is supplied with blood. The circle of Willis introduces redundancy of supplying vessels, thus ensuring that occlusion of one carotid artery does not result in cerebral ischemia.

23.1.2 Tissue composition

Figure 23.1 shows the anatomy of a healthy (*center panel*) and stenosed case (*right panel*). The healthy carotid has a diameter of $d = 6-8$ mm with a wall thickness h of 500−700 μm. The wall thickness increases with age (arterial aging), but the diameter remains more or less constant due to remodeling (Reneman *et al.*, 1986). The wall consists of three layers: the intima, the media and the adventitia. The intima is a 5−10-μm layer of endothelial cells, backed with an elastic lamina called the internal elastic lamina. A healthy intima appears as a thin white line delineating the transition from lumen to vessel wall, in a B-mode ultrasound (US) image of the carotid artery (see Figure 23.2). The media (300−400 μm) consists of layers of smooth muscle cells intertwined with sheets of collagen and elastic fibers (elastin) and appears as a black hypoechoic line next to the intima in a B-mode image of the carotid. The thickness of the intima and media combined can be assessed with US and is known as the IMT (intima-media thickness) measurement. The IMT is a

[1]Cardiovascular Biomechanics, Department of Biomedical Engineering, Eindhoven University of Technology, The Netherlands
[2]Department of Vascular Surgery, Catharina Ziekenhuis Eindhoven, The Netherlands

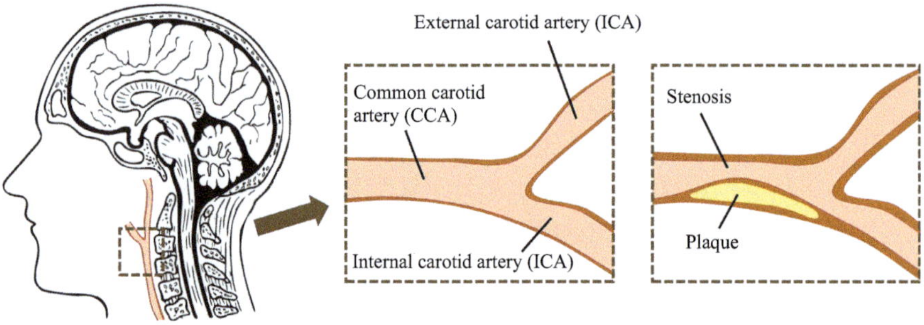

Figure 23.1 Anatomy of the neck with the carotid artery (left panel). The dashed box indicates the region, that is, typically examined with US imaging. A close-up of the common carotid artery and bifurcation into the internal and external carotid artery is found in the center panel, whereas an illustration of a stenosed carotid artery with elevated wall thickness is shown in the right panel

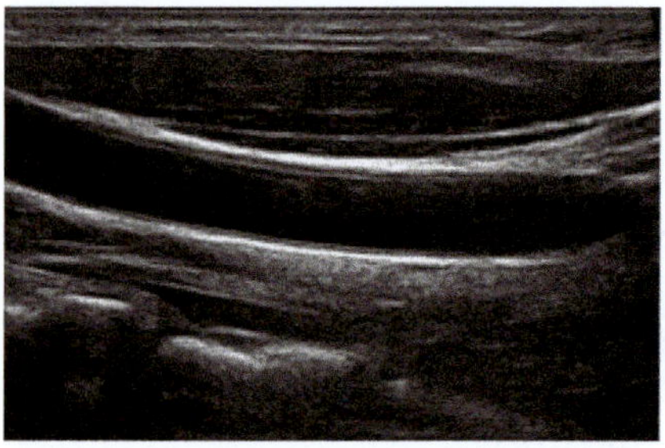

Figure 23.2 Longitudinal B-mode image of a healthy common carotid artery. The thin clear line at the lumen, together with the darker line next to it, makes up the intima-media thickness of the vessel

measure for vascular age and health. The smooth muscle cells in the media are responsible for vasoconstriction and vasodilation, primarily to regulate the vessel diameter with respect to flow. The contraction is mediated due to endothelial activity in the intima. Finally, the adventitial layer, that comprises 25% to 30% of the wall, is a layer of fibers, vasa vasorum and connective tissue (collagen).

23.1.3 Atherosclerosis

Carotid stenosis is the result of atherosclerosis, which is a process that develops over time. The vessel wall increases in thickness and its morphology changes. Fatty streaks are formed in the vessel wall (disposition of lipid), see also Figure 23.3. In response to the fatty streak formation, inflammation occurs and macrophages

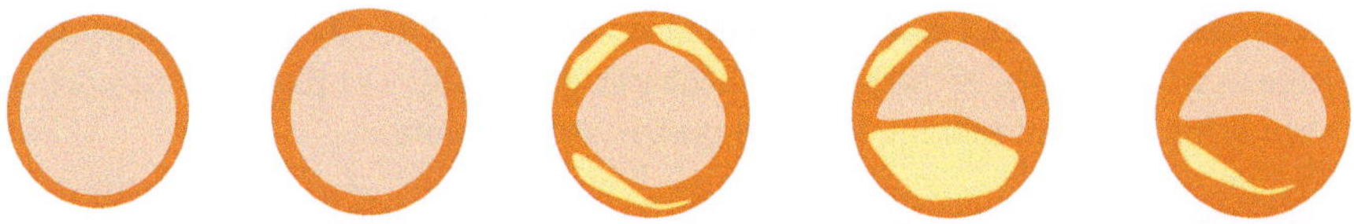

Figure 23.3 From left to right: healthy (young) carotid artery; carotid artery with increased wall thickness due to arterial aging; formation of fatty streaks; stenosed artery with an atherosclerotic, vulnerable plaque; stenosed, fibrotic stenosis

infiltrate the wall. At first, the arterial walls remodel by dilating and thereby preserving the original lumen surface area. Once this mechanism fails, growth is more predominant at the inside of the wall, resulting in stenosis formation. At later stages, micro- or larger calcifications may occur (Redgrave *et al.*, 2010; Finn *et al.*, 2010).

Carotid stenoses can have different morphologies. The so-called **plaque** can consist of mostly fibrotic tissue, which is known as a *stable plaque* (Figure 23.3). The plaque can have small regions of fatty streaks, often paired with calcifications, throughout the plaque. However, the plaque can also consist of a large lipid pool, separated from the blood flow by a thin fibrous cap, and often neovascularization of the plaque (Redgrave *et al.*, 2006; van Gils *et al.*, 2013). These stenoses form the class of **vulnerable plaques** (Virmani *et al.*, 2006). Once ruptured, the interior of the plaque flows into the bloodstream inducing a thrombotic response that results in a large blood clot. This blood clot can lead to local ischemia further downstream in the affected tissue. In case of the brain, and depending on the severity of the ischemia, a transient ischemic accident, cerebrovascular accident or stroke occurs. Around 15%–20% of all strokes is caused by carotid plaque rupture (Chaturvedi *et al.*, 2005; Howard *et al.*, 2015).

23.1.4 Treatment of stenotic arteries

Patients that are diagnosed with a stenotic carotid artery are examined using duplex US. Surgery is decided upon when the grade of stenosis (decrease in normal luminal surface area) is 70%–99%. The current standard in treatment of carotid stenosis is endarterectomy. In this procedure, the intima and part of the media at the stenotic site are surgically removed and the resulting arteriotomy is patched. However, postoperative analysis of plaque geometry and morphology revealed that only one out of six excised plaques was vulnerable (Rothwell and Warlow, 1999). More recent clinical studies have shown a number to treat (NTT) of nine symptomatic patients to prevent one stroke. In asymptomatic patients, this number is even higher (NTT = 21) (NOA, 1995, 1998). Hence, a better predictor for plaque vulnerability is required to not only prevent strokes but also reduce overtreatment and the unnecessary risks and costs involved. One way to do that may be the assessment of plaque vulnerability by measuring mechanical properties of plaque constituents *in vivo* using US, and relating those to plaque vulnerability.

23.2 Mechanical behavior of carotid arteries

The mechanical behavior of carotid arteries is mainly determined by the fibers in the vessel wall. Elastin and collagen fibers are found, both with different orientation and acting in different pressure ranges, resulting in nonlinear mechanical behavior. In general, the deformation of an artery is the result or response of its loading and its mechanical properties. Blood pressure here is the input signal, whereas strain in all directions (Figure 23.4) is the response (= output) depending on the mechanical behavior. We will first explore loading and deformation, after which typical parameters and relations between loading and deformation will be introduced.

23.2.1 Loading of arteries

The carotid artery is constantly loaded or pressurized by the fluctuating arterial blood pressure. During the cardiac cycle, the blood pressure p typically varies between 80 and 120 mmHg, similar to the brachial blood pressure. In SI units, this corresponds to a pressure of 10.7–16.0 kPa. The blood pressure induces a stress in the wall. A frequently used linear approach to approximate the average circumferential **wall stress** is the law of Laplace:

$$\begin{aligned} \sigma_{\theta\theta} &= \frac{pd}{2h} = \frac{pr}{h} \\ \sigma_{rr} &\approx 0 \end{aligned} \tag{23.1}$$

with r the radius of the artery $\left(= \frac{1}{2}d\right)$. Here, it is assumed that the pressure in the lumen is $p_i = p$, whereas the outside pressure is $p_o = 0$. The Laplace approximation is valid for thin-walled tubes, typically when $h < \frac{1}{10}r$. Considering its thickness to radius ratio, a carotid artery should be regarded as a thick-walled tube. An expression

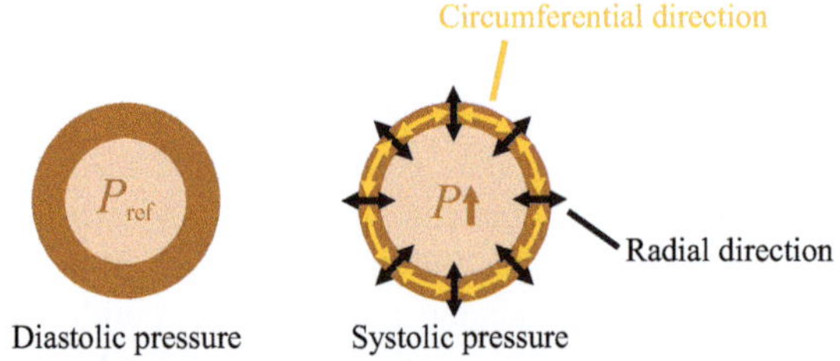

Figure 23.4 Transverse cross section of the carotid in end-diastolic (left) and end-systolic phase (right). Increasing pressure during systole results in thinning of the wall in the radial direction (black) and circumferential elongation (yellow)

for the circumferential and radial stress can be derived by solving the Lamé equations:

$$\begin{aligned} \sigma_{\theta\theta}(r) &= \frac{pr_i^2}{r_o^2 - r_i^2}\left(1 + \frac{r_0^2}{r^2}\right) \\ \sigma_{rr}(r) &= \frac{pr_i^2}{r_o^2 - r_i^2}\left(1 + \frac{r_0^2}{r^2}\right) \end{aligned} \tag{23.2}$$

with r_i and r_o the inner and outer radius, and $r_i \leq r \leq r_o$ (Mascarenhas *et al.*, 2016).

23.2.2 Deformation of arteries

In healthy carotid arteries, the pressure induces a deformation of the artery: the circumference increases while its wall thickness decreases. This deformation is known as **strain** and is often represented with the Greek letter ε, see also Chapter 14. Mathematically, strain in three dimensions is a linear transformation from an undeformed body into a deformed body, describing the relative changes in shape of that body. Three-dimensional strain is represented by a 3×3 matrix or tensor. Deformation in arteries is often expressed in cylindrical coordinates. The strain tensor for cylindrical coordinates is

$$\varepsilon = \begin{bmatrix} \varepsilon_{rr} & \varepsilon_{r\theta} & \varepsilon_{rz} \\ \varepsilon_{\theta r} & \varepsilon_{\theta\theta} & \varepsilon_{\theta z} \\ \varepsilon_{zr} & \varepsilon_{z\theta} & \varepsilon_{zz} \end{bmatrix} \tag{23.3}$$

with the principal components on the diagonal, ε_{rr} is the radial strain, i.e., wall thinning or thickening; $\varepsilon_{\theta\theta}$ is circumferential strain, i.e., elongation or shortening of the circumference of the artery, and finally, ε_{zz} is the longitudinal strain that resembles shortening or lengthening of the vessel axis/length. The other components are so-called **shear strains.** Especially in healthy young volunteers, a considerable shear strain in the $r - z$ direction has been measured.

For a normal blood pressure of 80–120 mmHg, the circumferential strain is roughly 7%–11%. This corresponds to a diameter increase in the range of roughly 400–900 μm. The radial strain will be roughly in the same range but with opposite sign (= compressional strain). Longitudinal strain ε_{zz} is low: 0%–2%. This is the result of the presence of *in vivo* axial prestretch, which reduces cyclic lengthening and shortening of arteries to a minimum. This prestretch is typically 20%–50% in healthy arteries.

23.2.3 Pressure–diameter relation

A traditional way in assessing and visualizing the mechanical behavior of the artery is a so-called **pressure–diameter curve**. This is more or less an equivalent of the pressure–volume loops that are measured in the heart, although the underlying mechanics are of course different. An example is shown in Figure 23.5.

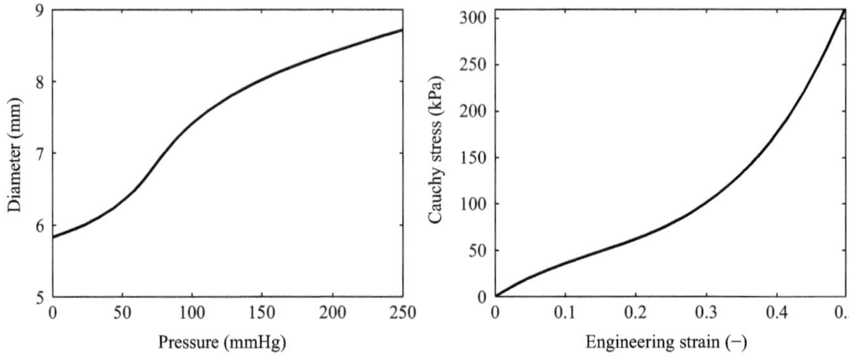

Figure 23.5 Pressure–diameter curve for a carotid artery (left) and the corresponding stress–strain curve with Cauchy stress and engineering strain (right)

The relation is typically **nonlinear**, i.e., an incremental or stepwise increase in pressure will not always result in a proportional increase in diameter (Holzapfel *et al.*, 2000). In the case that the systolic and diastolic mechanical responses are not identical, i.e., the unloading behavior differs from the loading behavior, the vessel may be viscoelastic (see also Section 23.2.6). Especially, in larger arteries, at physiological deformation levels, the effect of viscoelasticity is fairly low.

One could linearize the mechanical behavior of the carotid artery by only considering the systolic phase of the cardiac cycle and linearize the pressure–diameter curve within the working range. The benefit of such a simplification is the fact that the entire behavior can be described with one parameter, e.g., using the compliance or distensibility (Hoeks *et al.*, 1990).

23.2.3.1 Compliance and distensibility

We can convert the pressure–diameter into a pressure–volume curve, see Figure 23.6, by considering a certain segment with length l. The slope of this curve is a well-known measure for its elasticity, i.e., the **compliance** of the artery. The volume–compliance is defined as

$$C_V = \frac{\Delta V}{\Delta p} = \frac{V_{\text{sys}} - V_{\text{dia}}}{p_{\text{sys}} - p_{\text{dia}}} \tag{23.4}$$

with ΔV the increase in volume from end-diastolic volume V_{dia} to end-systolic volume (V_{sys}), and Δp the corresponding increase in pressure. The non-SI unit of compliance is [ml/mmHg], whereas the SI unit is (m^3/Pa). For example, let's consider a carotid of 20 cm in length, with a radius of 7 mm. The initial volume of this segment is $V_{\text{dia}} = 7.7 \cdot 10^{-6}$ m^3, or 7.7 ml. When the pressure increases from 80 to 120 mmHg, $\Delta p = 120{-}80 = 40$ mmHg $= 5.3$ kPa. Let's assume a circumferential strain of 10% as a result for Δp. The increase in volume is then $\Delta V = 1.6$ ml ($= 1.6 \cdot 10^{-6}$ m^3), resulting in a compliance of

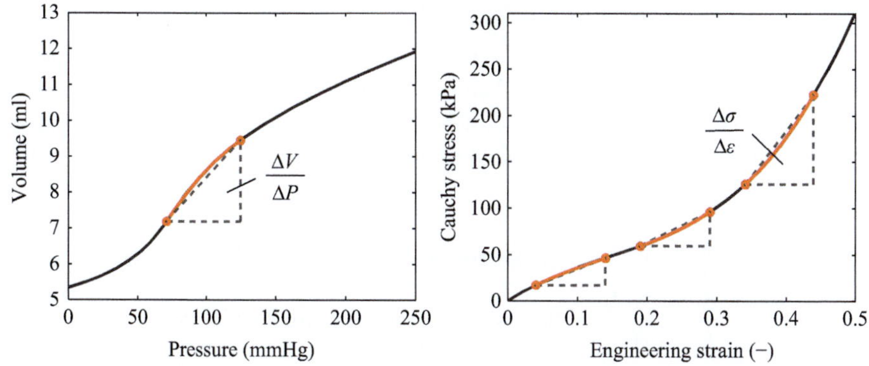

Figure 23.6 Pressure–volume curve vs. compliance (local derivative) (left) and the corresponding stress–strain curve with three different approximations of the Young's modulus (right)

$$\begin{aligned} C_V &= \frac{\Delta V}{\Delta p} = \frac{1.6}{40} \approx 0.04\text{ml/mmHg} \\ &= \frac{1.6 \cdot 10^{-6}}{5.3 \cdot 10^{3}} \approx 3 \cdot 10^{-10}\text{m}^3/\text{Pa} \end{aligned} \tag{23.5}$$

In the previous example, the volume–compliance is estimated. However, in case of 2-D data, one can measure the surface–area compliance:

$$C_A = \frac{\Delta A}{\Delta p} \tag{23.6}$$

with ΔA the change in surface area in m^2, and C_A in m^2/Pa.

Unfortunately, the volume–compliance C_V is highly dependent on the total length l that is considered. The compliance of an artery of 10 cm is half the value reported in the previous example. To partially circumvent these problems, one can either normalize the volume compliance for length (C_V/l) or calculate the **distensibility**.

The distensibility is defined as the compliance per end-diastolic volume:

$$D_V = \frac{C_V}{\Delta V_0} = \frac{\Delta V}{V_0 \Delta p} \tag{23.7}$$

or

$$D_A = \frac{C_A}{\Delta A_0} = \frac{\Delta A}{A_0 \Delta p} \tag{23.8}$$

both in Pa^{-1}. For the previous example, the carotid distensibility was $D_V = 3.93 \cdot 10^{-5}\ Pa^{-1} \approx 39\ MPa^{-1}$. Hence, a high value for distensibility implies that the common carotid artery (CCA) is highly elastic.

23.2.4 Stress–strain behavior

In biomechanical literature, tissue mechanics are analyzed using stress–strain relationships rather than pressure–diameter relationships. In fact, most constitutive material models describe the relation between stress and strain, independent of tissue geometry (hence, strain and not diameter). Here, the choice of stress and strain measures normally:

$$
\begin{aligned}
\sigma &= \frac{F}{A} && \text{Cauchy stress} \\
\varepsilon &= \frac{\Delta l}{l_0} = \frac{l - l_0}{l_0} && \text{Engineering strain, for small deformation}
\end{aligned}
\tag{23.9}
$$

with F, A and l the instantaneous force, surface and length, respectively (and l_0 the original length). For large deformations, geometrically nonlinear strain measures are used, i.e., strain that is, a nonlinear function of the stretch λ, ($\lambda = \frac{l}{l_0}$).

The pressure–diameter curve of a carotid artery can be converted into a stress–strain curve, see (Figure 23.5). It can easily be derived that the stress–strain behavior is also nonlinear. This is caused by the collagen fiber structure and orientation (Holzapfel *et al.*, 2004, 2015). At low pressures, the elastin fibers stretch and determine the mechanical behavior. The collagen fibers are known for their wavy structure and entangled orientation at low pressure. Once the pressure increases, they disentangle and the load is borne by the collagen fibers. These fibers are much stiffer, hence the increasing slope in the stress–strain curve. Degradation of elastin or collagen, other processes such as collagen disposition, or the presence of calcifications, will alter the stress–strain behavior significantly.

23.2.4.1 Elasticity moduli and stiffness

The relation between stress and strain is called the material law or constitutive law. For a simple linear elastic material, subjected to small deformations, the constitutive equation is

$$\sigma = E\varepsilon \tag{23.10}$$

with E the Young's modulus. Due to tissue nonlinearity, depending on the strain range, the total Young's modulus will differ in the carotid artery, see Figures 23.5 and 23.6. In such a case, one can calculate what is called the incremental Young's modulus, for a certain stress or strain range:

$$E_{\text{inc}} = \frac{\Delta\sigma}{\Delta\varepsilon} = \frac{\sigma_2 - \sigma_1}{\varepsilon_2 - \varepsilon_1} \tag{23.11}$$

resulting in E_{inc} as a function of blood pressure. For example, in a healthy CCA, a pressure of 120/80 mmHg results in a strain of 7%. The incremental modulus is then $E_{\text{inc}} \approx 500$ kPa. In a hypertensive patient, the mean arterial pressure is higher, say a systolic/diastolic pressure of 160/110 mmHg. In this example, the incremental modulus increases from $E_{\text{inc}} = 500–700$ kPa. The total modulus (for the entire pressure range from 0 to 120 mmHg) results in a total strain of 32%, and a modulus of $E = 350$ kPa

For large deformations, the neo-Hookean model can be used. This model is given by

$$\sigma = -p\mathbf{I} + G(\mathbf{B} - \mathbf{I}) \tag{23.12}$$

with G the shear modulus, **B** the left Cauchy–Green or Finger deformation tensor and **I** the identity matrix. For small deformations, $G \approx \frac{1}{3}E$. It can be shown that for a carotid artery, the circumferential stress is given by

$$\sigma_{\theta\theta} = G\left(\lambda_{\theta\theta}^2 - 1/\lambda_{\theta\theta}^2\right)/\lambda_{zz} + \sigma_{rr} \tag{23.13}$$

with $\sigma_{\theta\theta}$ and θ_{rr}, the circumferential and radial stress, respectively. For thin-walled tubes, θ_{rr} may be omitted.

You can appreciate the nonlinearity in the strain measures (quadratic and hyperbolic terms), although the parameter between stress and the nonlinear strain measure is still a single parameter and therefore a linear one (G).

23.2.4.2 Pulse wave velocity

The blood pressure propagates through the arterial system as a wave, see Figure 23.7. The phase velocity c_0, or **pulse wave velocity**, depends on the vessel geometry and material properties. A relationship was derived by Moens and Korteweg in 1878 (Westerhof *et al.*, 2010):

$$c_0 = \sqrt{\frac{E_{\text{inc}} h_0}{\rho d_0}} \tag{23.14}$$

with ρ the mass density in kg/m^3. Hence, one can measure the incremental Young's modulus (or shear modulus) by measuring the diameter, wall thickness and the pulse wave velocity. Typical values for healthy arteries are 5–7 m/s. Let us choose $c_0 = 6.5$ m/s and use the geometric properties of the carotid artery of the previous example. Plugging this into the equation, assuming $\rho = 1{,}050$ kg/m^3,

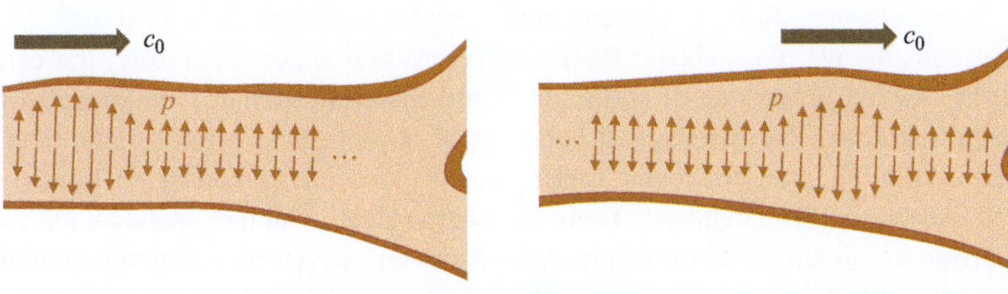

Figure 23.7 The pulse wave of the blood pressure p traveling through the carotid artery with speed c_0 causes the vessel to dilate

we find $E_{\text{inc}} \approx 517$ kPa, which is in the same range as obtained from the stress–strain data.

23.2.4.3 Stiffness vs. elasticity

The material properties described in the previous section should not be confused with stiffness. Stiffness is a property that holds information of material properties in combination with geometric properties of a structure. For a vessel, the circumferential stiffness S is defined as

$$S = Eh \tag{23.15}$$

in Pa m. In other words, arteries with the same (incremental) modulus but different wall thickness will show differences in stiffness and thus different distension and strain. Hence, in the aging population, an increase in IMT indicates an increase in stiffness, but not necessarily in modulus (although the latter increases as well due to elastin degradation or atherosclerosis).

23.2.5 Nonlinearity

Several nonlinear models have been proposed that describe the nonlinear behavior of biological tissue, such as the carotid wall, more accurately. Most widely used are the models by Delfino *et al.* (1997), Fung (1993), Raghavan *et al.* (1996), Holzapfel *et al.* (2000). These models focus on isotropic nonlinearity or split the material behavior into an isotropic and anisotropic part. However, these models require extensive tensile or inflation experiments and data regarding the unloaded geometry. Considering the limited pressure and strain ranges *in vivo*, application of these models, or estimation of all material properties, is cumbersome, if possible at all.

23.2.6 Anisotropy and viscoelasticity

Carotid arteries are **anisotropic** due to the fibrous nature of the tissue, especially in the media and adventitia. To predict the correct stresses, one needs to take into account the fiber structure in the constitutive model, which is beyond the scope of this book. Extensive discussion on this topic can be found in Holzapfel *et al.* (2004) and Sommer and Holzapfel (2012).

Some **viscoelasticity** is present in the carotid wall, which is a mixture of different constituents, viscoelastic fibers (collagen) and water. Therefore, the carotid wall has mixed properties of solid and liquid material, formally making it a poroelastic material. The mechanical behavior of poroelastic materials is beyond the scope of this chapter; however, under load, a poroelastic material behaves very much like viscoelastic material. There is a creep effect, which expresses itself in the hysteresis in the stress–strain or pressure–diameter curves. This is why sometimes vascular tissue is described as being viscoelastic. In the long term, viscoelasticity is not of interest for mechanical characterization of materials (Garca *et al.*, 2012; Holzapfel *et al.*, 2004).

23.3 US-based assessment of carotid mechanics

US can be used to visualize the plaque. Figure 23.8 shows examples of conventional focused US for A-mode, M-mode (motion mode) and B-mode (2-D brightness mode). B-mode is normally used for carotid imaging, often combined with Color Flow to improve contrast with the lumen (Figure 23.9). The role of US in mechanical characterization of carotids is 2-fold:

- Geometry assessment: measurement of the IMT, diameter, etc.
- Motion estimation: for the assessment of volume changes, distensibility, strain imaging, elastography, etc.

US geometry assessment, specifically segmentation of carotid echography, has been dealt with in the previous chapter. So here, we will discuss this briefly from a diagnostic perspective and focus primarily on the latter, i.e., motion tracking. A third source of information would be flow assessment to estimate or measure pressure (drop), wall shear stress and stenosis grade. This is beyond the scope of this chapter.

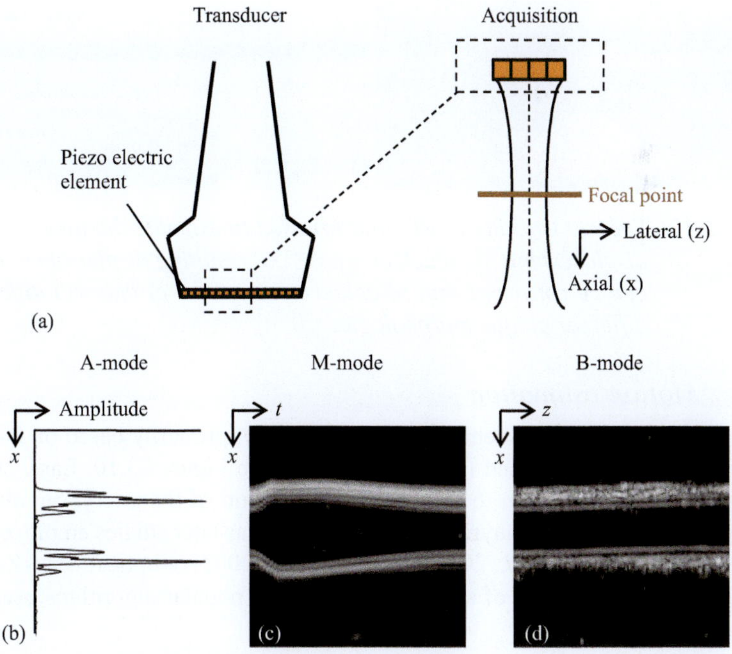

Figure 23.8 A linear array transducer (left) that performs conventional 2-D line-by-line scanning (a) of a carotid artery. Conventional modes include A-mode (b), M-mode (c) and B-mode (d), obtained in an excised porcine carotid artery mounted in a water tank

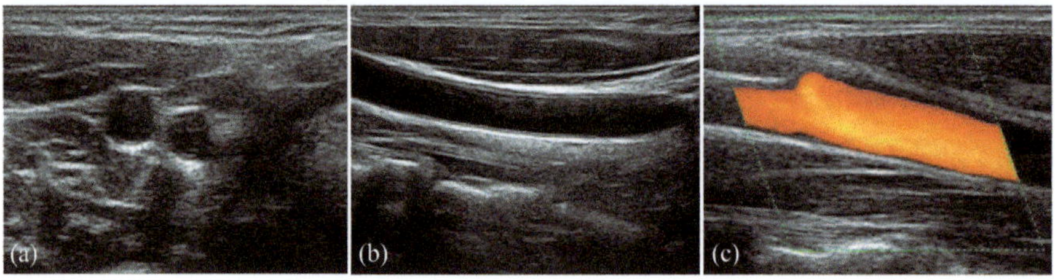

Figure 23.9 Cross-sectional (a), longitudinal (b) and color flow mode (c) images of a healthy carotid artery

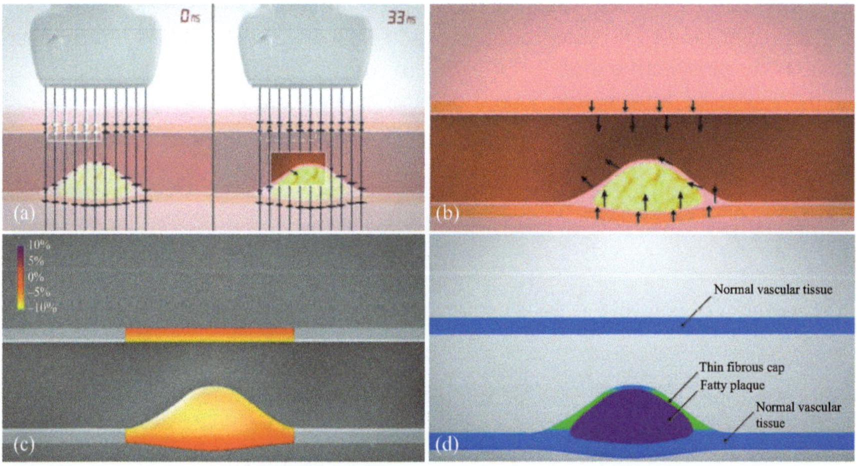

Figure 23.10 Speckle tracking of RF data (a) used to estimate the local displacements (b, black arrows). The resulting displacement data can be converted into so-called strain maps (c) that will differ for different plaque morphologies (d)

23.3.1 Motion estimation

Motion estimation has been demonstrated extensively, primarily based on B-mode or radio frequency (RF)-based (speckle) tracking, see Figure 23.10. Early studies have used motion estimation to measure the distension of the artery, but also the velocity of distension (Boutouyrie *et al.*, 1992), whereas later studies employed 2-D speckle tracking (Zahnd *et al.*, 2011; Golemati *et al.*, 2003) or optical flow (Zakaria *et al.*, 2010). For the basics of speckle tracking, and popular algorithms used, see Chapter 14, etc.

23.3.1.1 Compliance and distensibility estimation

Compliance: By measuring the transverse or longitudinal area as a function of time, using the aforementioned motion analysis, the compliance can be estimated (Marlatt *et al.*, 2013; Pascaner *et al.*, 2015; Van Merode *et al.*, 1988; Gamble *et al.*,

1994; Hansen *et al.*, 1995). Typically, the brachial arm pressure is assessed with a pressure cuff and assumed to be equal to the carotid pressure. Using (23.6), the average area compliance is then calculated (diastole to systole). In the case of the longitudinal cross section, one could assume rotational symmetry to convert the diameter–length information to a volume $V(t) = \frac{\pi}{4}d(t)^2\Delta l$ and estimate the volume compliance using (23.4). In the transverse cross section, this could be performed by multiplying the area with a slice thickness Δl.

Compliance measurements are highly susceptible to out-of-plane motion. A huge bias can be caused when geometrical changes are mistaken for distension. The same holds for transverse cross-sections in case of tapered vessels. Motion along the axis will result in a change in area.

Finally, 3-D US can be used to estimate the true volume over time, although current scanners do not have sufficient resolution and contrast, let alone frame rate, to give an accurate estimate.

Distensibility: The aforementioned methods to estimate compliance can be simply adapted to measure distensibility (Hoeks *et al.*, 1990). The change in area or volume is divided by the diastolic area or volume estimate [see (23.7) and (23.8)]. See Kawasaki *et al.* (2009) and Gamble *et al.* (1994) for examples and Engelen *et al.* (2015) for a large-scale study on reference values.

23.3.2 Elastometry

Data on diameter and wall thickness over time can also be used to estimate the Young's modulus or the shear modulus, depending on the modeling assumptions used. One can use Laplace's law to estimate circumferential stress (23.1), diameter to estimate circumferential stretch or strain:strain:

$$\begin{aligned}\lambda_{\theta\theta} &= \frac{d(t)}{d(0)} \\ \varepsilon_{\theta\theta} &= \lambda_{\theta\theta} - 1\end{aligned} \tag{23.16}$$

and estimate either E or G. In this case, a single number is found for the entire wall, which is known as elastometry (Boekhoven *et al.*, 2016; Riley *et al.*, 1992; Nakagawa *et al.*, 2004). Other numbers include the so-called carotid β-index (Weisz *et al.*, 2014).

23.3.3 Pulse wave velocity imaging

A second option for estimating the Young's modulus is pulse wave velocity measurements or imaging. In this case, one measures or assumes a certain wall thickness h_0, measures the initial diameter d_0, uses a literature value for the density ρ_0 and then estimates the pulse wave velocity c_0, leaving E as the only variable. The pulse wave speed is estimated by tracking the diameter in 2-D in the longitudinal cross section. By determining the time of peak distension for each RF line, c_0 can be estimated (Figure 23.11).

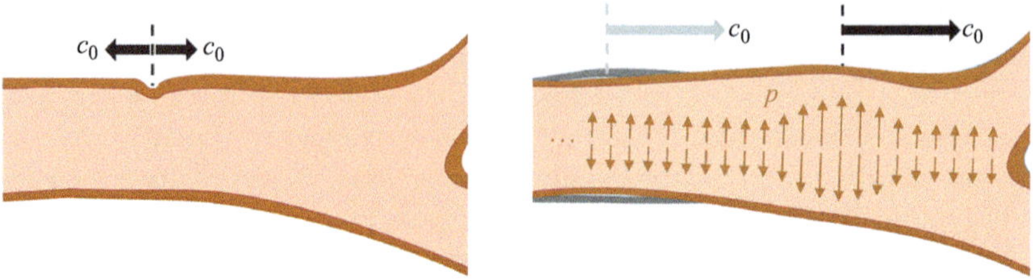

Figure 23.11 Shear wave elastography (left) vs. pulse wave velocity imaging (right). In shear wave imaging, a "push" is given and its wave propagation measured using tracking, whereas in pulse wave velocity imaging, the natural deformation caused by the systolic blood pressure is tracked

In conventional beamformed RF, the frame rate is limited. Therefore, a single estimate of c_0 for the entire image is feasible (so "elastometry"). Current advances in ultrafast imaging enable acquisition in the kHz range, yielding a detailed dataset with the propagation of the wavefront as a function of time for all lines. As a result, one can determine the pulse wave velocity for each RF line, providing an elastogram with a value for E for each line. This spatial information can be used to distinguish local differences in material properties (Luo *et al.*, 2012; Li *et al.*, 2017).

23.3.4 Shear wave elastography

Rather than measuring the modulus using pulse wave velocity, one can also apply a local perturbation of the tissue (using an external device or focused US) and track its propagation in either the circumferential or longitudinal direction, depending on the image view (Figure 23.11). The speed of the shear waves depends on the shear modulus (and for small deformation thus on the Young's modulus):

$$\begin{aligned} c_{0,s} &= \sqrt{\frac{G}{\rho_0}} \\ \text{or}: & \\ E &= 3G = 3c_{0,s}^2\rho_0 \end{aligned} \tag{23.17}$$

This is known as **shear wave elastography** or **pulse wave elastography**. Measuring the shear wave is again executed by plane wave (ultrafast) imaging and determining the local shear wave velocity and has been performed in carotid arteries (Garrard *et al.*, 2015; Balahonova *et al.*, 2013). In transverse cross sections, the circumferential propagation is tracked, which is considerably less trivial due to the change in angle with respect to the US propagation direction and shear wave reflections.

23.3.5 Strain imaging

As stated earlier, strain is the response of a mechanical system (= material properties and geometry) to its loading (here: blood pressure). Hence, the assessment of

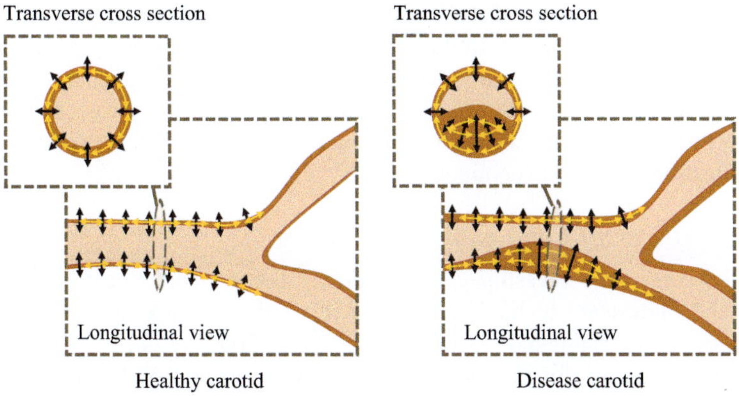

Figure 23.12 Strains found in the transverse (insert) and longitudinal cross sections. In the healthy case (left), strains are found in the radial (black) and circumferential (yellow) directions in the transverse cross section, whereas radial (black) and longitudinal strains (yellow) are present in the longitudinal cross section. In the diseased case, the principal strains obey local coordinates (right) and are not exactly positioned in the radial (black) or circumferential/longitudinal (yellow) directions

strain is a way to visualize the mechanical behavior without estimating the actual material properties. Here, strain is a surrogate for elasticity. It was shown in atherosclerotic plaques in both coronaries and carotid arteries that high strain regions in the shoulders of the plaques are present and may be linked to the risk of rupture (De Korte *et al.*, 2000; Schmitt *et al.*, 2007; Paini *et al.*, 2007).

Strain imaging at the level of resolution needed for vascular applications is typically done using RF data, see Figure 23.10 (Ribbers *et al.*, 2007), although B-mode speckle tracking has also been demonstrated (Carvalho *et al.*, 2015; Saito *et al.*, 2012). For an extensive description of block-matching techniques using B-mode and RF data, see Chapter 14. In a nutshell, strain is estimated from high-precision, high-resolution, 1-D or 2-D displacement fields, acquired by cross-correlation of the US data, or performing image registration or optical flow techniques (Chapters 13 and 15).

Radial strains are often encountered in the longitudinal cross sections, see Figure 23.12, and in the case of intravascular ultrasound (IVUS) also in the transverse cross section. Longitudinal strains are low and are estimated in the lateral direction. The lack of phase information renders these measurements to be quite noisy (Ribbers *et al.*, 2007), although shear strain has been successfully estimated using RF data (Idzenga *et al.*, 2011).

In transverse cross sections, estimation of radial and circumferential strains is possible, but it depends on the region in the artery whether you can estimate these strains with high accuracy or not. If radial/circumferential strain aligns with the US axial direction, the highest resolution is obtained (Figure 23.12). In case these strains align with the lateral direction, the lack of phase and resolution is a problem. Recent developments using strain compounding or plane wave coherent compounding have shown to tackle these issues (Hansen *et al.*, 2009). In the case of stenotic arteries, local coordinates are required, depending on the geometry of the plaque. Principal component analysis often is used to estimate these strains in a straightforward manner (Zervantonakis *et al.*, 2007).

23.3.6 (Inverse) finite element modeling

Several studies have investigated the coupling between functional US measurements and finite element models. Using a forward or inverse approach, material properties can be estimated (Masson *et al.*, 2011; Sousa *et al.*, 2016), which has also been applied to, for instance, aortic aneurysms using 3-D US data (van Disseldorp *et al.*, 2016; Wittek *et al.*, 2013).

References

NOA. Endarterectomy for asymptomatic carotid artery stenosis. Executive Committee for the Asymptomatic Carotid Atherosclerosis Study. *Journal of the American Medical Association*, 273(18): 1421–1428, May 1995. ISSN 0098-7484.

NOA. Randomised trial of endarterectomy for recently symptomatic carotid stenosis: final results of the MRC European Carotid Surgery Trial (ECST). *Lancet*, 351(9113): 1379–1387, May 1998. ISSN 0140-6736.

T. Balahonova, L. Hamchieva, O. Pogorelova, M. Tripoten, and A. Rogoza. Shear wave elastography of the common carotid artery: the first experience of application. *Ultrasound in Medicine & Biology*, 39(5): S63–S63, 2013.

R. W. Boekhoven, M. F. Peters, M. C. Rutten, M. R. van Sambeek, F. N. van de Vosse, and R. G. Lopata. Inflation and bi-axial tensile testing of healthy porcine carotid arteries. *Ultrasound in Medicine & Biology*, 42(2): 574–585, Feb. 2016. ISSN 03015629. doi: 10.1016/j. ultrasmedbio.2015.09.019. URL http://linkinghub.elsevier.com/retrieve/pii/S0301562915005803.

P. Boutouyrie, S. Laurent, A. Benetos, X. J. Girerd, A. P. Hoeks, and M. E. Safar. Opposing effects of ageing on distal and proximal large arteries in hypertensives. *Journal of Hypertension. Supplement: Official Journal of the International Society of Hypertension*, 10(6): S87–S91, Aug. 1992. ISSN 0952-1178.

D. D. B. Carvalho, Z. Akkus, S. C. H. van den Oord, *et al.* Lumen segmentation and motion estimation in b-mode and contrast-enhanced ultrasound images of the carotid artery in patients with atherosclerotic plaque. *IEEE Transactions on Medical Imaging*, 34(4): 983–993, Apr. 2015. ISSN 0278-0062, 1558-254X. doi: 10.1109/TMI.2014.2372784. URL http://ieeexplore.ieee.org/document/6964810/.

S. Chaturvedi, A. Bruno, T. Feasby, *et al.* and Therapeutics and Technology Assessment Subcommittee of the American Academy of Neurology. Carotid endarterectomy—an evidence-based review: report of the Therapeutics and Technology Assessment Subcommittee of the American Academy of Neurology. *Neurology*, 65(6): 794–801, Sep. 2005. ISSN 1526-632X. doi: 10.1212/01.wnl.0000176036.07558.82.

C. L. De Korte, A. F. Van Der Steen, E. I. Cspedes, *et al.* Characterization of plaque components and vulnerability with intravascular ultrasound elastography. *Physics in Medicine and Biology*, 45(6): 1465, 2000. URL http://iopscience.iop.org/0031-9155/45/6/305.

A. Delfino, N. Stergiopulos, J. E. Moore, and J. J. Meister. Residual strain effects on the stress field in a thick wall finite element model of the human carotid bifurcation. *Journal of Biomechanics*, 30(8): 777–786, Aug. 1997. ISSN 0021-9290.

L. Engelen, J. Bossuyt, I. Ferreira, *et al.* Reference values for local arterial stiffness. Part A: Carotid artery. *Journal of Hypertension*, 33(10): 1981–1996, Oct. 2015. ISSN 0263-6352. doi: 10.1097/HJH.0000000000000654.

A. V. Finn, M. Nakano, J. Narula, F. D. Kolodgie, and R. Virmani. Concept of vulnerable/unstable plaque. *Arteriosclerosis, Thrombosis, and Vascular Biology*, 30(7): 1282–1292, Jul. 2010. ISSN 1524-4636. doi: 10.1161/ATVBAHA.108.179739.

Y.-C. Fung. *Biomechanics Mechanical Properties of Living Tissues*. Springer New York, New York, NY, 1993. ISBN 978-1-4757-2257-4 1-4757-2257-5. URL http://dx.doi.org/10.1007/978-1-4757-2257-4.

G. Gamble, J. Zorn, G. Sanders, S. MacMahon, and N. Sharpe. Estimation of arterial stiffness, compliance, and distensibility from M-mode ultrasound measurements of the common carotid artery. *Stroke*, 25(1): 11–16, 1994. URL http://stroke.ahajournals.org/content/25/1/11.short.

A. Garca, M. A. Martnez, and E. Pea. Viscoelastic properties of the passive mechanical behavior of the porcine carotid artery: influence of proximal and distal positions. *Biorheology*, 49(4): 271–288, 2012. ISSN 1878-5034. doi: 10.3233/BIR-2012-0606.

J. Garrard, P. Ummur, S. Nduwayo, *et al.* Shear wave elastography may be superior to greyscale median for the identification of carotid plaque vulnerability: a comparison with histology. *Ultraschall in der Medizin – European Journal of Ultrasound*, 36(04): 386–390, Jun. 2015. ISSN 0172-4614, 1438-8782. doi: 10.1055/s-0034-1399676. URL http://www.thieme-connect.de/DOI/DOI?10.1055/s-0034-1399676.

S. Golemati, A. Sassano, M. J. Lever, A. A. Bharath, S. Dhanjil, and A. N. Nicolaides. Carotid artery wall motion estimated from B-mode ultrasound using region tracking and block matching. *Ultrasound in Medicine & Biology*, 29(3): 387–399, 2003. URL http://www.sciencedirect.com/science/article/pii/S0301562902007603.

F. Hansen, P. Mangell, B. Sonesson, and T. Lnne. Diameter and compliance in the human common carotid artery—variations with age and sex. *Ultrasound in Medicine & Biology*, 21(1): 1–9, 1995. ISSN 0301-5629.

H. Hansen, R. Lopata, and C. L. De Korte. Noninvasive carotid strain imaging using angular compounding at large beam steered angles: validation in vessel phantoms. *IEEE Transactions on Medical Imaging*, 28(6): 872–880, 2009.

A. Hoeks, P. Brands, F. Smeets, and R. Reneman. Assessment of the distensibility of superficial arteries. *Ultrasound in Medicine & Biology*, 16(2): 121–128, 1990. URL http://www.sciencedirect.com/science/article/pii/0301562990901394.

G. A. Holzapfel, J. A. Niestrawska, R. W. Ogden, A. J. Reinisch, and A. J. Schriefl. Modelling non-symmetric collagen fibre dispersion in arterial walls. Journal of the Royal Society Interface, 12(106), pii: 20150188, 2015. doi: 10.1098/rsif.2015.0188. PMID: 25878125. 2015.

G. A. Holzapfel, T. C. Gasser, and R. W. Ogden. A new constitutive framework for arterial wall mechanics and a comparative study of material models. *Journal of Elasticity and the Physical Science of Solids*, 61(1–3): 1–48, 2000. URL http://link.springer.com/article/10.1023/A:1010835316564.

G. A. Holzapfel, G. Sommer, P. Regitnig, *et al.* Anisotropic mechanical properties of tissue components in human atherosclerotic plaques. *Transactions of the ASME-K – Journal of Biomechanical Engineering*, 126(5): 657–665, 2004.

D. P. J. Howard, G. W. van Lammeren, P.M. Rothwell, *et al.* Symptomatic carotid atherosclerotic disease: correlations between plaque composition and ipsilateral stroke risk. *Stroke: A Journal of Cerebral Circulation*, 46(1): 182–189, Jan. 2015. ISSN 1524-4628. doi: 10.1161/STROKEAHA.114.007221.

T. Idzenga, H. Hansen, R. Lopata, and C. De Korte. Estimation of longitudinal shear strain in the carotid arterial wall using ultrasound radiofrequency data. *Ultraschall in der Medizin – European Journal of Ultrasound*, 33(7): E275-82, 2012. doi: 10.1055/s-0029-1245936. Epub 2011 Jan 11. PMID: 21225566.

J. Luo, R. X. Li, and E. E. Konofagou. Pulse wave imaging of the human carotid artery: an in vivo feasibility study. *IEEE Transactions on Ultrasonics, Ferroelectrics and Frequency Control*, 59(1): 174–181, Jan. 2012. ISSN 0885-3010. doi: 10.1109/TUFFC.2012.2170. URL http://ieeexplore.ieee.org/document/6138741/.

T. Kawasaki, S. Fukuda, K. Shimada, *et al.* Direct measurement of wall stiffness for carotid arteries by ultrasound strain imaging. *Journal of the American Society of Echocardiography*, 22(12): 1389–1395, Dec. 2009. ISSN 08947317. doi: 10.1016/j. echo.2009.09.011. URL http://linkinghub.elsevier.com/retrieve/pii/S0894731709008542.

X. Li, J. Jiang, H. Zhang, *et al.* Measurement of carotid pulse wave velocity using ultrafast ultrasound imaging in hypertensive patients. *Journal of Medical Ultrasonics*, 44(2): 183–190, Apr. 2017. ISSN 1346-4523, 1613-2254. doi: 10.1007/s10396-016-0755-4. URL http://link.springer.com/10.1007/s10396-016-0755-4.

K. L. Marlatt, A. S. Kelly, J. Steinberger, and D. R. Dengel. The influence of gender on carotid artery compliance and distensibility in children and adults: carotid artery elasticity in youth and adults. *Journal of Clinical Ultrasound*, 41(6): 340–346, Jul. 2013. ISSN 00912751. doi: 10.1002/jcu.22015. URL http://doi.wiley.com/10.1002/jcu.22015.

E. J. Mascarenhas, M. F. Peters, J. Nijs, M. C. Rutten, F. N. van de Vosse, and R. G. Lopata. Assessment of mechanical properties of porcine aortas under physiological loading conditions using vascular elastography. *Journal of the Mechanical Behavior of Biomedical Materials*, 59:185–196, Jun. 2016. ISSN 17516161. doi: 10.1016/j. jmbbm.2015.12.009. URL http://linkinghub.elsevier.com/retrieve/pii/S175161611500483X.

I. Masson, H. Beaussier, P. Boutouyrie, S. Laurent, J. D. Humphrey, and M. Zidi. Carotid artery mechanical properties and stresses quantified using in vivo data from normotensive and hypertensive humans. *Biomechanics and Modeling in Mechanobiology*, 10(6): 867–882, Dec. 2011. ISSN 1617-7940. doi: 10.1007/s10237-010-0279-6.

N. Nakagawa, H. Hasegawa, and H. Kanai. Cross-sectional elasticity imaging of carotid arterial wall in short-axis plane by transcutaneous ultrasound. *Japanese Journal of Applied Physics*, 43(5B):3220–3226, 2004.

A. Paini, P. Boutouyrie, D. Calvet, M. Zidi, E. Agabiti-Rosei, and S. Laurent. Multiaxial mechanical characteristics of carotid plaque: analysis by multi-array echotracking system. *Stroke: A Journal of Cerebral Circulation*, 38(1): 117–123, Jan. 2007. ISSN 1524-4628. doi: 10.1161/01.STR.0000251796.38954.b2.

A. F. Pascaner, D. Craiem, M. E. Casciaro, R. Danielo, S. Graf, and E. Guevara. Continuous assessment of carotid intima–media thickness applied to estimate a volumetric compliance using B-mode ultrasound sequences. *Physiological Measurement*, 36(3): 397–407, Mar. 2015. ISSN 0967-3334, 1361-6579. doi: 10.1088/0967-3334/36/3/397. URL http://stacks.iop.org/0967-3334/36/i=3/a=397? key=crossref.fc89e38bf87ea28bc93d3410ee0b961b.

M. L. Raghavan, M. W. Webster, and D. A. Vorp. Ex vivo biomechanical behavior of abdominal aortic aneurysm: assessment using a new mathematical model. *Annals of Biomedical Engineering*, 24(5): 573–582, Oct. 1996. ISSN 0090-6964.

J. N. E. Redgrave, J. K. Lovett, P. J. Gallagher, and P. M. Rothwell. Histological assessment of 526 symptomatic carotid plaques in relation to the nature and timing of ischemic symptoms: the Oxford plaque study. *Circulation*, 113(19): 2320–2328, May 2006. ISSN 1524-4539. doi: 10.1161/CIRCULATION AHA.105.589044.

J. N. E. Redgrave, J. K. Lovett, and P. M. Rothwell. Histological features of symptomatic carotid plaques in relation to age and smoking: the oxford plaque study. *Stroke: A Journal of Cerebral Circulation*, 41(10): 2288–2294, Oct. 2010. ISSN 1524-4628. doi: 10.1161/STROKEAHA.110.587006.

R. S. Reneman, T. Van Merode, P. Hick, A. M. Muytjens, and A. P. Hoeks. Age-related changes in carotid artery wall properties in men. *Ultrasound in Medicine & Biology*, 12(6): 465–471, 1986. URL http://www.sciencedirect.com/science/article/pii/0301562986902188.

H. Ribbers, R. G. Lopata, S. Holewijn, G. Pasterkamp, J. D. Blankensteijn, and C. L. De Korte. Noninvasive two-dimensional strain imaging of arteries: validation in phantoms and preliminary experience in carotid arteries in vivo.

Ultrasound in Medicine & Biology, 33(4): 530–540, 2007. URL http://www.sciencedirect.com/science/article/pii/S0301562906018618.

W. A. Riley, R. W. Barnes, G. W. Evans, and G. L. Burke. Ultrasonic measurement of the elastic modulus of the common carotid artery. The Atherosclerosis Risk in Communities (ARIC) Study. *Stroke*, 23(7): 952–956, 1992. URL http://stroke.ahajournals.org/content/23/7/952.short.

P. M. Rothwell and C. P. Warlow. Prediction of benefit from carotid endarterectomy in individual patients: a risk-modelling study. European Carotid Surgery Trialists' Collaborative Group. *Lancet*, 353(9170): 2105–2110, Jun. 1999. ISSN 0140-6736.

M. Saito, H. Okayama, K. Inoue, *et al.* Carotid arterial circumferential strain by two-dimensional speckle tracking: a novel parameter of arterial elasticity. *Hypertension Research*, 35(9): 897–902, 2012. URL http://www.nature.com/hr/journal/v35/n9/abs/hr201239a. html.

C. Schmitt, G. Soulez, R. L. Maurice, M.-F. Giroux, and G. Cloutier. Noninvasive vascular elastography: toward a complementary characterization tool of atherosclerosis in carotid arteries. *Ultrasound in Medicine & Biology*, 33(12): 1841–1858, 2007. URL http://www.sciencedirect.com/science/article/pii/S0301562907002694.

G. Sommer and G. A. Holzapfel. 3D constitutive modeling of the biaxial mechanical response of intact and layer-dissected human carotid arteries. *Journal of the Mechanical Behavior of Biomedical Materials*, 5(1): 116–128, Jan. 2012. ISSN 1878-0180. doi: 10.1016/j. jmbbm.2011.08.013.

L. C. Sousa, C. F. Castro, C. C. Antnio, *et al.* Computational simulation of carotid stenosis and flow dynamics based on patient ultrasound data—a new tool for risk assessment and surgical planning. *Advances in Medical Sciences*, 61(1): 32–39, Mar. 2016. ISSN 1898-4002. doi: 10.1016/j. advms.2015.07.009.

E. M. van Disseldorp, N. J. Petterson, M. C. Rutten, F. N. van de Vosse, M. R. van Sambeek, and R. G. Lopata. Patient specific wall stress analysis and mechanical characterization of abdominal aortic aneurysms using 4D ultrasound. *European Journal of Vascular and Endovascular Surgery*, 52(5): 635–642, 2016. doi: 10.1016/j.ejvs.2016.07.088. Epub 27 Sept. 2016. PMID: 27665991.

M. J. van Gils, M. C. Bodde, L. G. M. Cremers, D. W. J. Dippel, and A. van der Lugt. Determinants of calcification growth in atherosclerotic carotid arteries; a serial multi-detector CT angiography study. *Atherosclerosis*, 227(1): 95–99, Mar. 2013. ISSN 1879-1484. doi: 10.1016/j. atherosclerosis.2012.12.017.

T. Van Merode, P. J. Hick, A. P. Hoeks, K. H. Rahn, and R. S. Reneman. Carotid artery wall properties in normotensive and borderline hypertensive subjects of various ages. *Ultrasound in Medicine & Biology*, 14(7): 563–569, 1988. URL http://www.sciencedirect.com/science/article/pii/0301562988901226.

R. Virmani, A. P. Burke, A. Farb, H. K. Gold, A. V. Finn, and F. D. Kolodgie. Plaque Rupture. In R. Virmani, J. Narula, M. B. Leon, and J. T. Willerson, editors, *The Vulnerable Atherosclerotic Plaque*, pages 37–59. Blackwell Publishing, Oxford, UK, Oct. 2006. ISBN 978-0-470-98757-5 978-1-4051-5859-6. URL http://doi.wiley.com/10.1002/9780470987575.ch3.

S. H. Weisz, J. Magne, R. Dulgheru, P. Caso, L. A. Pirard, and P. Lancellotti. Carotid artery and aortic stiffness evaluation in aortic stenosis. *Journal of the American Society of Echocardiography*, 27(4): 385–392, Apr. 2014. ISSN 08947317. doi: 10.1016/j. echo.2013.12.014. URL http://linkinghub.elsevier.com/retrieve/pii/S0894731713009887.

N. Westerhof, N. Stergiopulos, and M. I. M. Noble. *Snapshots of Hemodynamics: An Aid for Clinical Research and Graduate Education*. Springer Verlag, New York, 2nd edition, 2010. ISBN 978-1-4419-6362-8. OCLC: ocn648920959.

A. Wittek, K. Karatolios, P. Bihari, *et al.* In vivo determination of elastic properties of the human aorta based on 4D ultrasound data. *Journal of the Mechanical Behavior of Biomedical Materials*, 27: 167–183, 2013. doi: 10.1016/j. jmbbm.2013.03.014. Epub 15 Apr. 2013. PMID: 23668998.

G. Zahnd, L. Boussel, A. Marion, *et al.* Measurement of two-dimensional movement parameters of the carotid artery wall for early detection of arteriosclerosis: a preliminary clinical study. *Ultrasound in Medicine & Biology*, 37(9): 1421–1429, 2011. URL http://www.sciencedirect.com/science/article/pii/S0301562911011057.

T. Zakaria, Z. Qin, and R. L. Maurice. Optical-flow-based b-mode elastography: application in the hypertensive rat carotid. *IEEE Transactions on Medical Imaging*, 29(2): 570–578, 2010.

I. K. Zervantonakis, S. D. Fung-Kee-Fung, W.-N. Lee, and E. E. Konofagou. A novel, view-independent method for strain mapping in myocardial elastography: eliminating angle and centroid dependence. *Physics in Medicine and Biology*, 52(14): 4063–4080, Jul. 2007. ISSN 0031-9155. doi: 10.1088/0031-9155/52/14/004.

Chapter 24

Carotid artery wall motion and strain analysis using tracking

Spyretta Golemati[1] *and Konstantina S. Nikita*[2]

Abstract

In this chapter, a number of speckle-tracking-based methodologies are outlined, suitable for the estimation of motion and strain of the carotid artery from ultrasound images. Various versions of intensity- and phase-based techniques have been suggested and validated mostly in phantoms, in *in silico* and *in vitro* data. Waveforms showing displacements, velocities and accelerations can be obtained from these methods, and a number of indices can then be calculated. Spatial mapping (imaging) of tissue strains can be achieved with elastography, a major application of motion analysis. Through their application in real data, these methods are promising for revealing valuable quantitative *in vivo* information about arterial mechanics. Compared to other ultrasound-based indices, a major advantage of motion-derived indices is that they provide functional, rather than mere anatomical, information, which is more sensitive to early wall changes. Their full potential in predicting, diagnosing and monitoring carotid-related disorders, such as cerebrovascular events, as well as in characterising the burden of other diseases, remains to be confirmed in large clinical trials, towards an integrated personalised approach for disease management and increased patient safety.

24.1 Introduction

The carotid artery is the artery that brings blood to the brain. There are two carotid arteries in the arterial tree, one in the left and one in the right side of the neck, originating from the aortic arch in the thorax and the right subclavian artery in the neck, respectively. Anatomically, each carotid artery starts as a common branch and then divides into the internal carotid, which takes blood to the brain, and the external carotid, which takes blood to the organs of the face. Average diameter values of the common carotids in adult males and females have been reported to be

[1]Medical School, National and Kapodistrian University of Athens, Greece
[2]School of Electrical and Computer Engineering, National Technical University of Athens, Greece

6.5 and 6.1 mm, respectively, and of the internal carotids 5.1 and 4.7 mm, respectively [1]. Anatomical differences between the left and right sides have been reported, in terms of lengths and diameters, with the left carotid being longer and with smaller diameter than the right [2].

As is the case with all arteries, the wall of the carotid is composed of three distinct layers, namely the tunica intima, the tunica media and the tunica adventitia. The main components of these layers are elastin, collagen and smooth muscle cells, and it is the relative proportion, geometric configuration and arrangement of these components that determine the stability, resilience and mechanical behaviour of the arterial wall.

The arterial wall *in vivo* is in constant movement, following the periodic movement of the heart during each cardiac cycle. Mechanical forces due to blood pressure and flow, as well as those originating from surrounding tissue, induce deformations of the arterial tissue [3]. Stresses and strains can be calculated from the forces and deformations, respectively. Stress is defined as the force per unit surface area over which the force is exerted. Strain relates the tissue dimensions before and after deformation. Arterial deformations consist of rapid distension following ventricular systole, whereby 50% or more of the stroke volume is transiently accommodated, and of retraction during diastole. Arterial stresses and strains occur in all spatial directions, i.e. circumferential, longitudinal and radial directions. Stresses and strains in the circumferential and longitudinal directions are tensile because the vessel tends to distend in these directions with pressurisation. Strains and stresses in the radial direction are compressive as the wall tends to be narrowed with pressurisation.

The largest motion and derived strains have been reported in the direction of vessel diameter changes, and the lowest in the direction corresponding to wall thickness changes. Specifically, most conduit arteries undergo 8%–10% oscillation in external diameter or about 15% oscillation in internal diameter. Motion and strains in the direction of diameter change have been intensely investigated in a number of studies and correlated with various pathological conditions. Motion and strains in the longitudinal direction, i.e. along the arterial centreline, have not been studied as much as those in the circumferential direction, because they had been assumed to be negligible compared to the latter [4]. Recent ultrasound scanners, in combination with sophisticated motion estimation algorithms, have allowed the calculation of the longitudinal component of common carotid artery movement, indicating in addition that its amplitude was comparable to the diameter change [5–7].

In the course of its lifetime, the carotid artery wall undergoes changes in its anatomical, morphological and mechanical properties. Ageing is responsible for reduced elastin and smooth muscle cell content within the arterial wall, in favour of collagen, and this is in turn reflected in decreased wall mobility and elasticity [8]. The latter are also related to anatomical alterations, consisting in increased diameters. Changes in carotid diameters in males and females between 15 and 70 years of age have been reported using a phase-locked echo-tracking system. The mean carotid diameter increased more rapidly in males and was larger than in females from 25 years of age [9]. Reduced wall elasticity, i.e. increased stiffness, reduces the reservoir function of the conduit arteries near the heart and increases pulse wave velocity, thus increasing systolic and pulse pressures. As these two pressures determine the peak loads on the cardiovascular system, their increase has an unfavourable effect on the strength of the system [8]. The presence of a number of diseases, including not only cardiovascular disorders, like hypertension, but also other diseases, like periodontal and neurological diseases, amplify age-related carotid artery wall alterations. In addition to these diffuse diseases, atheromatous plaque, consisting in the build-up of fatty material in the inner arterial wall, which is the focal lesion specific to the arterial wall, alters the local geometry and the properties of the arterial wall.

Ultrasound imaging is the modality of choice for diagnosis and monitoring of carotid artery disease, due to a number of relative benefits, including non-invasive assessment of disease severity and tissue morphology [13]. Modern ultrasound systems allow real-time imaging of moving structures as well as storage of temporal image sequences, or cine loops, for further processing. Tissue motion can be quantitatively estimated from these sequences provided they are acquired at sufficiently high frame rates. Tissue motion can be estimated in one dimension (1D), namely along the direction of the ultrasound beam, using M(otion)-mode or Tissue Doppler Imaging (TDI). Radio frequency (RF) and B(brightness)-mode are the appropriate modalities for studying tissue motion in two or in three dimensions.

The estimation of carotid artery wall motion from ultrasound images is a task of considerable importance but has remained particularly challenging in clinical practice and prone to significant variability [13]. Objective quantification of normal motion patterns is important for the study of local mechanical phenomena involved in arterial function under normal conditions, as well as with ageing, due to disease, injury and following treatment. However, ultrasound imaging presents many challenges for interpretation. Arterial tissue motion is particularly complex, including thickness changes, translation, rotation and shear. In addition to this, unlike other imaging modalities, ultrasound images are characterised by the so-called speckle, which tends to reduce the image contrast and image details, as well as by an inherent trade-off between spatial resolution and penetration depth, which both degrade image quality. Furthermore, anatomical borders lack continuity, further limiting the applicability of common image analysis techniques.

This chapter provides a comprehensive overview of methodologies for estimating motion and strain of the carotid artery using speckle tracking from ultrasound images. In this context, the basic principles of ultrasound-based motion and strain analysis are described, and the major findings are highlighted, derived from applications in real human data, along with their pathophysiological and clinical implications.

24.2 Methods for motion and strain analysis

Carotid artery wall motion regards the complex, three-dimensional (3-D) dynamic pattern of deformations experienced by the tissue as a result of exerted stresses.

In general, tissue motion can be described by displacements as well as by displacement-derived indices, namely velocities (first derivatives of displacements) and accelerations (second derivatives of displacements). Strains (relative displacements with respect to an initial position) and strain rates (first derivatives of strains) can also be used to describe motion patterns. Tissue stiffness, which characterises the overall mechanical behaviour of the underlying material, can be estimated by combining strain and stress (pressure-based) measurements.

A large number of methods have been suggested for measuring ultrasound-image-based motion and strain of the carotid artery wall, towards quantifying and interpreting local mechanical phenomena. M-mode and TDI can be used to estimate tissue motion in a single dimension, namely the radial one. M-mode has been applied to study movement of arterial walls along a single ultrasound beam. As the organ boundaries that produce reflections move relative to the probe, this can be used to determine the velocity of specific organ structures [14]. TDI, which measures velocity of tissue motion based on the Doppler principle, was one of the early attempts in this direction. In TDI, the frequency shift of ultrasound signals reflected from moving objects is used to quantify the high-amplitude, low-velocity signals of tissue motion [15].

More recently, speckle tracking and image registration have been commonly applied to estimate arterial wall motion in two-dimensional (2-D) and 3-D ultrasound image sequences [16]. Figure 24.1 shows examples of 2-D B-mode ultrasound images of a longitudinal and a transverse section of a normal carotid artery, along with the motion directions that can be interrogated. Radial and longitudinal motion can be estimated in longitudinal section images, whereas different directions of radial motion can be estimated in transverse section images. Speckle is the characteristic pattern of ultrasound images, derived by interfering echoes of a transmitted waveform that originate from tissue heterogeneities [17] (see also Chapter 2). Specifically, speckle is caused by waves scattering off small particles in the tissue being scanned and alternately reinforcing and then cancelling each other. Although speckle may be related to image noise, it carries useful information about the underlying tissue activity. Speckle-tracking methods analyse motion by tracking the intensity or the interference patterns produced by speckle over time.

A number of practical issues need to be taken into account in carotid artery motion analysis protocols. (i) Arterial wall physiology affects subject and probe setup, as the constantly moving artery may not be easily imaged during a sufficient time window (e.g. a few seconds). Also, the common carotid artery is usually easier to image than its internal branch, which may not be easily accessible in many subjects. (ii) Physical principles of ultrasound imaging affect appropriate selection of scanner setting values. These should be carefully selected, so as to ensure reliable acquisition of the interrogated motion phenomena. Quantitative estimation of tissue displacement is achieved with the application of the selected speckle-tracking algorithm to the recorded image sequence.

Various speckle-tracking methods, including block matching (BM) and differential methods, have been applied in the study of carotid artery wall motion. Despite their popularity in similar applications, these algorithms are limited by

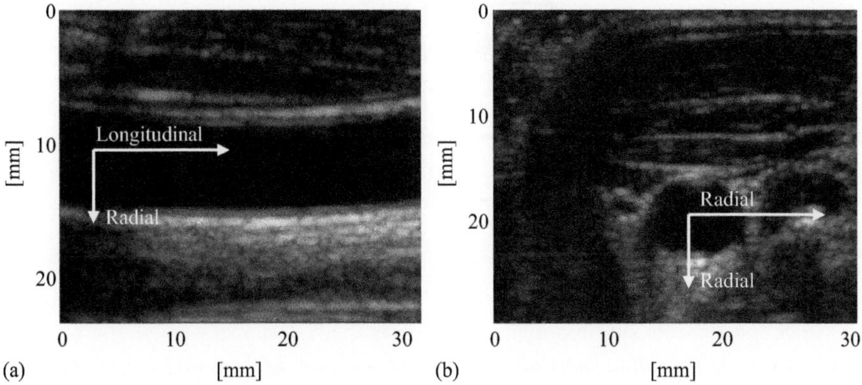

Figure 24.1 Examples of B-mode ultrasound images of a longitudinal (a) and a transverse (b) section of a normal carotid artery. Radial and longitudinal directions for motion analysis are indicated

tissue-deformation-induced decorrelation, and, in 2-D image recordings, out-of-plane motions [17], which may significantly alter image patterns over time and limit the ability of speckle-tracking methods to correlate consecutive frames.

BM holds a prominent position in carotid artery wall tracking due to its simplicity and robustness to noise (see Chapter 14). Conventional BM consists in finding a region in an image that best matches a region selected in the first, or, in one of the previous images in a sequence, termed the 'reference image' (Figure 24.2). This definition relies on the assumption that the reference block remains constant over time and motion, which is valid if the frame rate is sufficiently high. The method relies on a good measure of similarity, which yields large values when the selected and the interrogated image regions coincide in intensity patterns and small values otherwise. A number of similarity measures have been suggested, including the correlation coefficient, the normalised correlation coefficient, the sum of absolute differences and the sum of squared differences. The search for the best matched block is typically constrained to a search window, the size of which has to be appropriately chosen. A large search window allows accurate tracking of rapid movements that could be lost with a smaller window but increases the possibility for mismatch and the algorithm's computational complexity. Yli-Ollila *et al.* suggested an enhanced version of the conventional BM through the use of luminance optimisation [18]. Specifically, the algorithm optimises the contrast of each following frame by detecting the luminance of the selected region of interest (ROI) in the current frame and forcing the following frame to match the luminance and dynamic range of that ROI. This facilitates selection of optimal ROI in the next frame. An alternative approach to BM was suggested by Albinsson *et al.* based on the expansion of the conventional technique with an additional reference block [19]. The two reference blocks originate from two consecutive frames. The evaluation of the method in *in silico*, phantom and

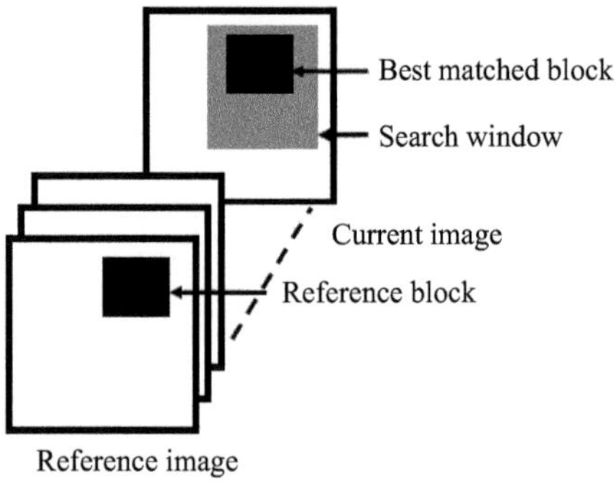

Figure 24.2 Schematic representation of BM strategy. Motion of a block of pixels is estimated by searching for the most similar block of pixels in a search window at subsequent frames

in vivo data showed improved accuracy and the possibility to reduce the size of the reference blocks while maintaining the performance.

Adaptive BM (ABM) is an extension of the conventional BM, which updates the reference block considering one or more of the previous frames, in an attempt to improve the performance of BM, through the incorporation of the temporal dimension into the motion estimation pipeline. Proposed update strategies include single-frame, multiframe and finite impulse response filtering [7]. Kalman filtering has also been suggested for ABM [10], and compared to the previous ABM strategies, it was shown to be the most robust one, which minimised the mean tracking error, on the grounds of a benchmarking procedure based on *in silico* data [7].

Optical flow (OF) is the term used to describe the velocity field generated by the relative motion between an object and the camera in a sequence of frames. To estimate OF, a constraint regarding the smoothness of the velocity field needs to be determined. The smoothness constraint requires that the energy of the image derivatives is minimal. A common way to constrain velocity is to use gradient constraints from neighbouring pixels, assuming they share the same 2-D velocity. In reality, there may be no single velocity value that simultaneously satisfies all regional pixels, so the velocity that minimises the constraint errors is found instead. This is a modification with respect to the conventional Lucas–Kanade method, which does not use a weighted function in the least squares estimator. In addition to BM, differential methods have also been applied to investigate motion in the carotid artery. Golemati *et al.* compared the performances of BM- and OF-based methods, in terms of *in silico* data, and suggested OF using weighted least squares as the optimal method [11]. OF was also used to produce elastograms, from B-mode, rather than from the usual RF, images of the carotid artery [12].

Image registration methods estimate motion by frame-to-frame or groupwise registering successive ultrasound frames with a deformable shape-tracking approach (see also Chapter 15). The deformation field is parameterised using smooth basis functions, such as B-splines. To regularise the motion, the energy

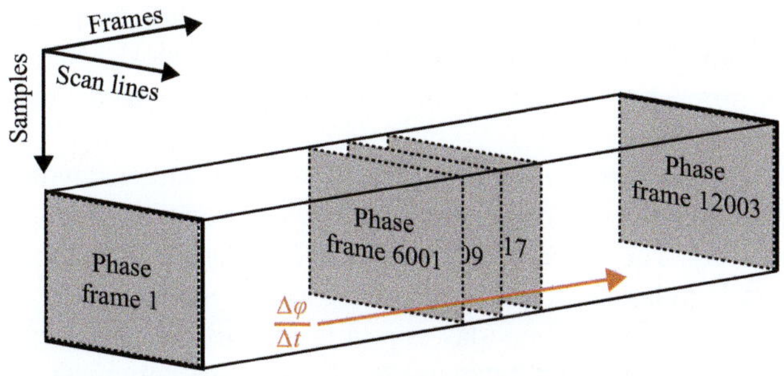

Figure 24.3 Schematic representation of the 3-D phase-difference matrix. 2014. Reprinted from [22], with permission from Elsevier

function is optimised, by adding extra cost terms. The B-spline free-form deformation model, which registers pairs of images at systole and diastole, was used to extract the 2-D displacement field from contrast-enhanced ultrasound images of the carotid artery [20]. A nonrigid feature-based registration algorithm has been proposed for elastic alignment of dynamic-3-D ultrasound images [21]. The algorithm relied on image intensity and gradient information to perform feature-based matching in image sequences, using prior information from both the fixed and previous moving images.

Motion estimation methodologies generate vectors, which can be processed so as to extract quantitative indices. Motion vectors corresponding to displacements of individual image areas over the total duration of the recording can be quantified in terms of amplitude, frequency or, in the case of pairs of areas, the synchronisation. Standard indices include radial strain (RS), longitudinal strain (LS), circumferential strain (CS) and shear strain (SS) indices, as well as distensibility or compliance indices, when pressure measurements are available.

Compared to the previously presented intensity-based methods, phase-based approaches consist in processing the information carried by the phase of the images, namely in the frequency domain. A phase difference method has been recently suggested, based on plane wave imaging, which allows high-definition motion analysis of carotid tissue [22]. The method consists of RF signal beamforming in the Fourier domain, and calculation of individual pixel velocities from the time differences of signal phases (Figure 24.3). Tissue distension and acceleration can also be estimated by integrating and differentiating, respectively, pixel velocities. A phase-based OF method was used by Zahnd *et al.* to improve tracking of longitudinal tissue motion of the intima-media complex [23]. The method relies on introducing a pattern of periodic longitudinal oscillations in the RF signals and tracking the motion from the derived analytic signals [24].

Motion-based indices, e.g. strains, can be used to estimate arterial stiffness, if a measure of stress is available. The stress–strain relationship has been identified in the carotid artery *in vivo*, using diameter-derived strain estimates along with applanation-tonometry-based stress measures [25]. With the use of different assumptions, relying on the linear elastic two-parallel spring model and the 2-D, nonlinear, hyperelastic model, a number of Young's moduli can be calculated from such relationship. These moduli characterise the mechanical behaviour of elastin and collagen fibres, both separately and combined, as well as the behaviour of the different arterial layers.

Spatial mapping (imaging) of tissue strains can be achieved with elastography, a major application of motion analysis, which was introduced in the early 1990s by Ophir *et al.* [26]. The technique consists of calculating 2-D local tissue strain through cross-correlation of RF segments for the estimation of the time shift resulting from inherent deformations. Strain represents the displacements of tissue particles with respect to a reference position and is the parameter that is mapped with conventional elastography. The more recently suggested shear wave elastography maps elastic moduli, i.e. the ratio of stress and strain, where stress is induced by the shear wave of the device [27].

The Lagrangian speckle model estimator (LSME) was proposed by Maurice and Bertrand to describe speckle motion by following local characteristics of the speckle field. The method involves an analytical description of the decorrelation that enables the derivation of an appropriate inverse filter for speckle restoration [28]. The full 2-D strain tensor derived by this method was then used to produce elastograms of the carotid artery, with the additional use of von Mises coefficients to address mechanical artefacts due to different directions between tissue motion and ultrasound beam propagation [29]. Along the same line, a LSME-based compensative model, allowing the computation of the scanning angle, was suggested by Mercure *et al.*, to compensate for the angle dependence of motion estimates and reduce the bias in strain estimates, namely, when investigating longitudinal vessel segments [30]. It was demonstrated that the model allows the estimation of scanning angle with less than 3- and 4-degree errors, according to experiments in vessel-mimicking phantoms and in *in vivo* human carotid arteries, respectively, and with low variability. Recently, a non-invasive vascular elastography approach was suggested, based on the LSME, which relied on local angle compensation using kinematics constraints, and on the application of a filtering process on the time-varying strain curve to reduce as much as possible the impact of motion artefacts [31].

Validation of methods is a crucial part of the motion estimation procedure and has mostly relied on the use of specially devised phantoms, which simulate the acoustic properties of biological tissue, as well as of *in silico* data. Comparison with manual tracings has also been reported in one study [32], but this is generally a very challenging and time-consuming task. Cinthio *et al.* [33] used a cylindrical agar phantom attached to and moved by an *X–Y* system, the movement of which was measured by two high-resolution triangulation lasers. Bang *et al.* [34] made free-hand scans of a rubber–foam phantom at rest by sideways translation of the probe. A vessel wall phantom was described for use in ultrasound studies of wall motion, consisting of a vessel made of polyvinyl alcohol and a gear pump to affect motion [35]. Larsson *et al.* suggested the use of sonomicrometry to validate RS, LS and CS of the carotid artery in phantoms [36]. Recently, a novel phantom design protocol was suggested, allowing fabrication of walled carotid bifurcation phantoms with high acoustic compatibility, artery-like vessel elasticity and stenotic narrowing feature, useful for assessing wall motion and flow dynamics [37]. A phantom was designed and fabricated by Sjostrand *et al.* using a 3-D printer, which incorporates relative longitudinal motion of adjacent wall layers, thus allowing validation of longitudinal arterial movements [38].

The use of tissue-mimicking phantoms is useful for validation experiments but requires specialised equipment which may not be readily available. *In silico* models allow simulation of ultrasound images, for evaluating transducers and focusing schemes as well as motion analysis methods. FIELD II is an ultrasound simulation package, which provides a useful framework to simulate ultrasound fields by incorporating realistic transducer features [39]. A comprehensive *in silico* framework was recently developed by Gastounioti *et al.*, for benchmarking different carotid artery motion estimators [7]. The framework consists of real ultrasound images of normal and diseased subjects, which can be displaced using mathematical models of displacement in the radial and longitudinal directions, and then corrupted with noise of different types and levels.

24.3 Estimation of motion and strain of the carotid artery in health and disease

Motion and strain of the carotid arterial tissue has been estimated in different clinical scenarios using the previously presented methods, in an attempt to demonstrate their usefulness towards better understanding the mechanical phenomena taking place in the arterial wall and their changes with ageing and in the presence of disease. Components of these kinematic properties in different spatial directions have been measured at different locations along the normal and diseased (plaque-laden) carotid artery, namely along the common and internal branches. Of particular interest are motion patterns adjacent to plaque and those of normal, nonatheromatous, carotid tissue in the presence of a diffuse disease.

Some of the early attempts to measure 1-D carotid artery wall motion included the application of M-mode and TDI. M-mode was used to estimate minimal and maximal diameters and calculate stiffness and distensibility indices; moderate repeatability was reported for these indices [40]. Tissue velocities were measured with TDI, showing different patterns between the anterior and posterior walls [41]. Both studies observed increased stiffness and reduced distensibility with age.

Motion estimation in 2D using speckle tracking allows a more complete description of local phenomena as well as the study of anisotropy, i.e. the different mechanical behaviour of tissue in different directions. More importantly, it has allowed the study of the longitudinal component of tissue motion, namely along the axis of the vessel, which has not been investigated as commonly as the radial component. The estimation of the longitudinal component of motion, either on its own or in combination with the radial one, has revealed valuable information about arterial tissue biomechanics. One of the first studies in this area demonstrated that RS, i.e. change of arterial diameter normalised by the diastolic diameter, was significantly higher than LS, i.e. the change of distance along the arterial wall normalised by the distance at diastole (10.2 $\pm$ 4.5% vs. 2.5 $\pm$ 0.89%) [42], which is indicative of the anisotropic behaviour of arterial tissue. That study also showed that radial and longitudinal displacements decreased as a function of the distance from the near and far walls, with the steepest decrease taking place between 0 and 2 mm from the wall–lumen interface. A later study reported a distinct multiphasic longitudinal pattern of motion during the cardiac cycle that is of the same magnitude as the diameter change in the common carotid artery of healthy humans [5]. The same study also showed that the intima-media complex exhibited larger longitudinal movement than the adventitia, indicating the presence of SS within the wall. Attenuation of longitudinal movement across the arterial wall and tissue was also found here.

Using vector velocity imaging (VVI) to analyse offline B-mode images of young healthy volunteers, Svedlund and Gan demonstrated that most longitudinal kinematic parameters, including displacements, velocities, strains and strain rates, were similar in the right and left common carotids, which is suggestive of bilateral symmetry [43]. Similarity was also reported for these parameters in the near and far walls of the right common carotid. Zahnd *et al.* found that the amplitude of longitudinal movement was progressively attenuated along the length of the artery, being larger in regions located closer to the heart and smaller in regions located towards the head (Figure 24.4) [44]. This phenomenon might be explained by the tissue viscoelastic properties in combination with tethering forces acting on the wall. Principal component analysis was used to characterise the longitudinal displacement waveform, beyond amplitude-based features [45]. The estimation of two principal components could account for more than 92% of motion variation in the waveforms obtained. Specifically, the first principal component was significantly correlated to pulse pressure, indicating that the main dominant base waveform of the longitudinal motion was related to blood pressure. The second principal component exhibited significant correlations to known stiffness indices, indicating that the stronger biphasic structure of the motion curve, was associated with higher distensibility and compliance, as well as reduced carotid artery stiffness. The same group used a transfer function in an attempt to derive how the energy from the blood pressure moves the innermost arterial wall longitudinally and how the kinetic energy is then transferred to the outermost arterial layer [46]. The power spectra showed that the main kinetic energy of the longitudinal motion lies in the band 0–3 Hz with a peak at 1.1 Hz. Energy transfer from blood pressure to longitudinal wall motion exhibited high variability among subjects, whereas energy loss across wall layers was characterised by an average 17% of amplitude and a visible 18.9 ms delay at 1 Hz.

A relationship was recently reported between patterns of carotid artery longitudinal motion and left ventricular rotational mechanics in young healthy individuals [47]. Specifically, longitudinal displacements were associated with local blood velocity and with rotation of the left ventricular base, but not with longitudinal septal displacements. These observations suggest a complex relationship between the influences of local blood velocity and left ventricular rotation within the context of a

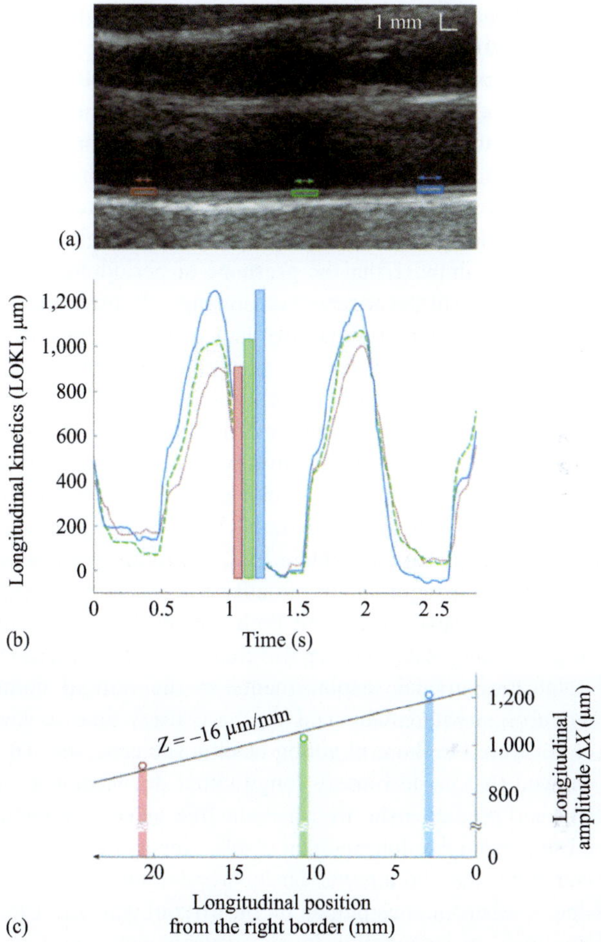

Figure 24.4 Example of amplitude ΔX of longitudinal kinetics (b) in three locations along the arterial wall (a) of a healthy subject. Vertical bars correspond to peak-to-peak amplitudes ΔX of each tracked point. (c) Attenuation coefficient Z of the corresponding cine loop, determined by linear regression (solid line) of the three tracked points (circles). For each tracked point, the x- and y-coordinates correspond to the abscissa X of the region of interest in (a) and the estimated motion amplitude ΔX in (b), respectively. 2015. Reprinted from [44], with permission from Elsevier

structural ventricular–vascular coupling theory. The application of high-frame-rate plane-wave imaging has allowed the estimation of tissue dynamics, including displacements, velocities and accelerations, at the sub-micrometre and sub-millisecond scales, which is promising for interrogating unexplored tissue phenomena, such as imaging of the pulse wave [22]. Stiffness of the carotid artery wall, in terms of the

Young's moduli estimated from the stress–strain relationship, is higher in collagen fibres compared to elastin [25] and seems to increase with age [48].

The presence of a pathological condition, either related to the cardiovascular system or not, may alter the motion pattern of the carotid artery wall, yielding important implications about the overall burden of the condition. In elderly diabetic subjects, the amplitudes of diameter change and of longitudinal displacements of the near and far arterial walls of the left common carotid were significantly lower compared to those of healthy volunteers [49]. Carotid longitudinal motion was additionally found to be impaired in the presence of periodontal disease, and the strongest correlates of such displacement were ageing, adiposity and blood pressure [50]. Accordingly, carotid longitudinal displacement may provide information about the vascular abnormalities related to cardiovascular risk factors, complementing information obtained from current non-invasive techniques. Tat *et al.* estimated longitudinal wall displacements and intramural SS in the common carotid artery of seven individuals with spinal cord injury (SCI), considered at high cardiovascular risk, and in seven able-bodied participants. Bidirectional motion patterns, including motion retrograde to blood flow during systole, followed by antegrade motion during diastole, characterised longitudinal movement. The retrograde intramural SS was significantly smaller by 60.2% in subjects with SCI, exhibiting smaller peak displacements in both the intima–media and adventitia, while in the antegrade direction, no group differences were observed [51]. Systolic, diastolic and total longitudinal displacements in the normal common carotid artery of elderly subjects with established coronary artery disease were found significantly lower compared to those in young healthy subjects [43]. The same group subsequently showed that carotid artery longitudinal displacements reflected cardiovascular status and predicted short-term event-free survival in medium- to high-risk patients and suggested that longitudinal displacements per se or in combination with IMT measurement may be a novel cardiovascular surrogate biomarker [52].

The presence of atheromatous plaque on the arterial wall alters local geometry and morphology and, consequently, local displacement and motion patterns. Mokhtari-Dizajl *et al.* used OF to estimate systolic and diastolic diameters of the right common carotid artery, proximal to plaque, from sequences of B-mode and colour Doppler ultrasound images [53]. They subsequently calculated standard arterial stiffness indices, which were found to be significantly different in subjects with severe, i.e. greater than 40%, stenosis compared to subjects with mild or no stenosis. Axial and lateral plaque strains were shown to differentiate calcified from noncalcified plaque [54]. Non-calcified hypoechoic plaque exhibited more than 20% accumulated axial strain over a cardiac cycle, indicating easier deformation due to the periodic pulsation and blood flow, whereas calcified plaque exhibited moderate accumulated axial strain (~5%). Soft plaque demonstrated significantly larger relative lateral shift values (2–3 mm) than calcified plaque (less than 1 mm), indicating easier stretch, compression and lateral movement during the cardiac cycle. Calcified plaque generally remained in their location and did not stretch as much as soft plaque. With VVI, Svedlund and Gan showed that low total longitudinal displacement of the common carotid was associated with increased atherosclerotic plaque burden, determined by increased values of bifurcation IMT and plaque area, in both mice and humans [55]. Soleimani *et al.* generated longitudinal motion waveforms of healthy subjects and of patients with carotid artery stenoses lower and greater than 50%, and they reported a strong and graded association between axial stress and severity of carotid stenosis [56]. The non-invasive elastography approach was used to quantify the strain behaviour of near and far walls in longitudinal images of normal and atherosclerotic, i.e. with greater than 50% stenosis, internal carotid arteries [31]. Maximal and minimal strain values of the far walls were significantly higher in the healthy group. The mean systolic, diastolic and cumulated axial strains could distinguish the two groups after normalisation by the pressure gradient between acquired images, implying that these measures may help to diagnose vulnerable plaques.

In a group of subjects with symptomatic and asymptomatic atheromatous plaque, symptomatic ones showed decreased amplitude of radial and longitudinal motion of the wall, higher motion amplitude of the plaque top surface and higher relative movement between the plaque top and bottom surfaces [7] (Figure 24.5). The application of these methodologies to patients with carotid atherosclerosis revealed the discriminatory capacity of kinematic and strain features of carotid tissue between symptomatic and asymptomatic cases, showing also that the deformation of both the atherosclerotic lesion and the normal wall adjacent to the lesion should be considered [57]. Using speckle-tracking ultrasound, common carotid artery wall motion was estimated in 12 patients with carotid plaque causing either moderate (less than 80%) or severe (greater than 80%) stenosis, and in 23 healthy participants [58]. Although healthy individuals were found to have a retrograde wall motion pattern, a distinct anterograde pattern was noted with plaque presence. Importantly, patients with severe plaque stenosis had greater anterograde motion (0.53 ± 0.36 mm) than those with moderate stenosis (0.17 ± 0.15 mm), likely owing to high wall shear stresses associated with greater peak systolic velocities at the site of stenosis (severe: 342.0 ± 99.4 cm/s, moderate: 177.5 ± 31.2 cm/s). Recently, an association was demonstrated between carotid plaque strain and cognitive function [59]. Specifically, subjects with higher axial, lateral and SS (Figure 24.6) performed poorly on cognitive assessment compared to other subjects. This behaviour might be due to the presence of micro-emboli, which may lead to cognitive impairment, possibly as a result of the rupture of vulnerable plaque associated with increased strain, because higher strain is indicative of larger deformation and increased probability of plaque rupture. Using contrast-enhanced ultrasound, Zhang *et al.* associated registration-based elasticity and intraplaque neovascularisation, demonstrating that softer plaque is related to increased neovascularisation [20].

24.4 Discussion and future perspectives

In this chapter, a number of speckle-tracking-based methodologies were outlined, suitable for the estimation of motion and strain of the carotid artery from ultrasound

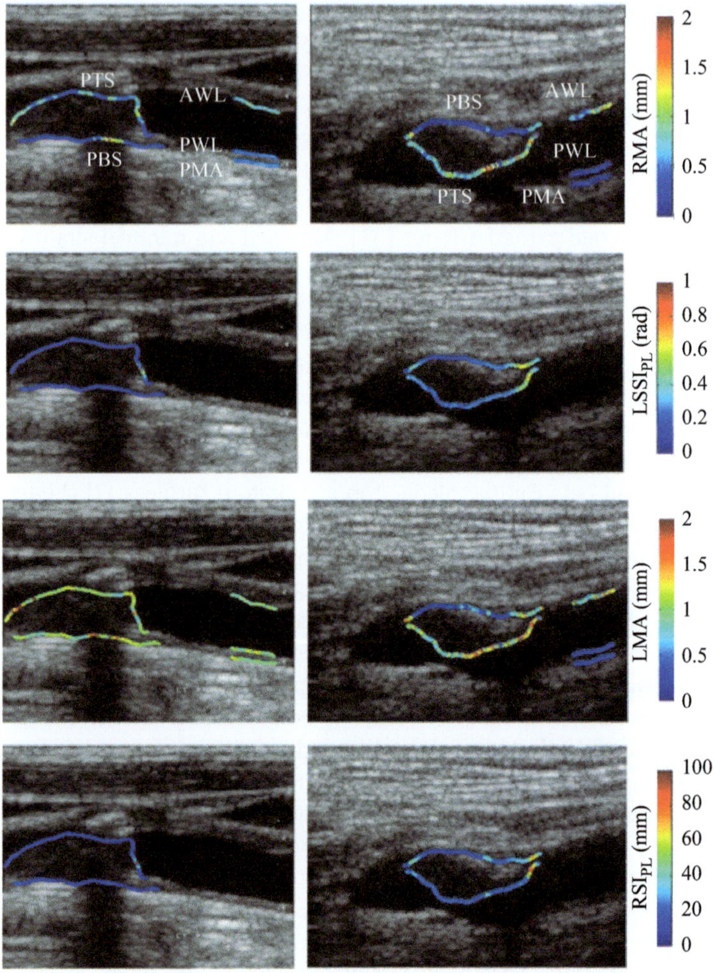

Figure 24.5 Examples of colour-coded distributions of various motion-derived indices for an asymptomatic (left column) and a symptomatic (right column) patient with an atherosclerotic plaque on the posterior and the anterior wall, respectively. White labels indicate the selected ROIs for each case. RMA/LMA: radial/longitudinal motion amplitude; $LSSI_{PL}$: longitudinal strain index at plaque; RSI_{PL}: radial strain index at plaque. 2013. Reprinted from [7], with permission from IOP Publishing

images. Various versions of BM and other techniques have been suggested and validated in phantoms, in *in silico* and *in vitro* data, as well as through comparisons with visual estimations. Waveforms showing displacements, velocities and accelerations can be obtained from these methods, and a number of indices can then be calculated. Spatial mapping (imaging) of tissue strains can be achieved with

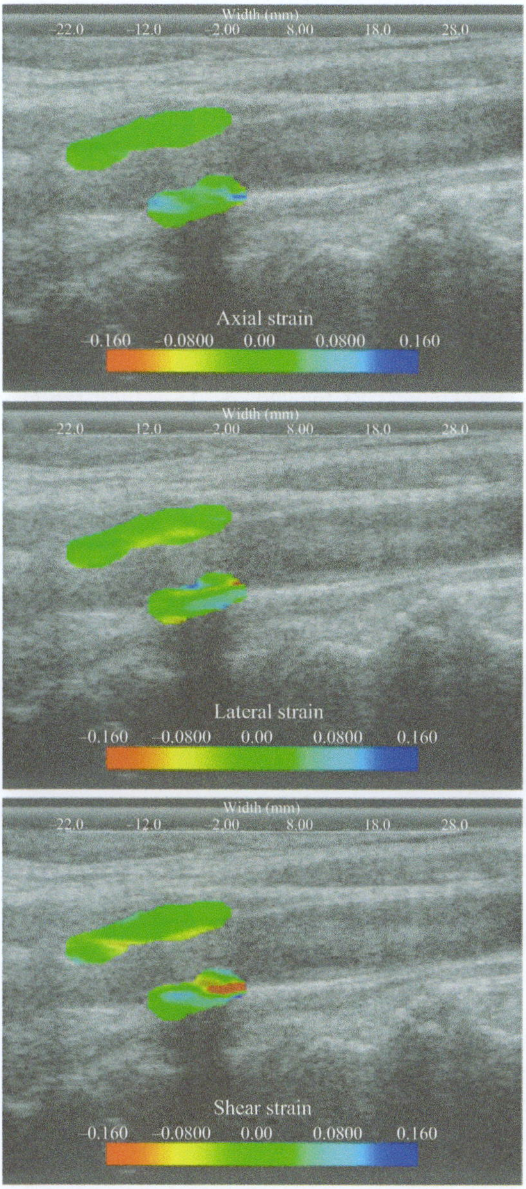

(a)

(b)

(c)

Figure 24.6 Axial (a), lateral (b) and shear (c) strain images in the segmented region overlaid on the B-mode image. 2016. Reprinted from [59], with permission from Elsevier

elastography, a major application of motion analysis. The methods have been used in real data, addressing different physiological and pathophysiological phenomena, and revealed valuable quantitative *in vivo* information about arterial mechanics (see also Chapter 22). Compared to other ultrasound-based indices, a major advantage of motion-derived indices is that they provide functional, rather than mere anatomical information, which is more sensitive to early wall changes.

Ultrasound-based motion and strain estimation allows the investigation of a number of local mechanical phenomena in the arterial wall. One of the first achievements of speckle-tracking methods was the estimation of the longitudinal component of motion, which had not been as interrogated as the radial one. Furthermore, local tissue motion analysis allows the study of SS, anisotropy, bilateral asymmetry and movement variability along the arterial wall. The use of image phase information, rather than amplitude, has allowed the estimation of additional mechanical phenomena, including pulse wave imaging, using ultra-fast technologies.

The clinical usefulness of the indices describing the above-mentioned phenomena lies in their potential ability to reflect tissue changes as a result of ageing, drug or other treatment, and due to the presence of a disease, including the carotid-specific atheromatous plaque. It is interesting to note that carotid artery motion and strain are altered in the presence of a number of diseases, not necessarily cardiovascular-related; these include diabetes, periodontal disease and neurological disorders. In these, as well as in a number of other pathologies, associations have been reported between disease burden and ultrasound-derived indices, such as the IMT. This suggests that many diseases have an overall burden, some aspects of which can be picked up by carotid ultrasound. It is also indicative of the fact that new valuable information can be collected about a given disease by this simple imaging method, which points towards a novel direction in this line of research, namely ultrasound-based mechanical changes of the carotid artery tissue in the presence of a given disorder.

The presence of an atheromatous plaque on the arterial wall alters the local motion patterns, and their estimation is more challenging because of the increased complexity of the local kinematic phenomena. Different motion patterns have been reported for different plaque types, namely calcified vs. non-calcified plaque, as well as symptomatic vs. asymptomatic ones. Plaque has been shown to affect the motion of the adjacent wall and to induce relative movement within itself, which may be responsible for plaque rupture resulting in cerebrovascular events. The association between plaque movement and the risk for stroke is one of the major clinical applications of motion analysis, holding promise for improved prevention of stroke. Changes of plaque motion as a result of treatment may also provide valuable information for disease monitoring.

To confirm the clinical usefulness of carotid artery ultrasound-based motion patterns, application of the previously mentioned methodologies in large clinical trials is required, including different types of subjects and a variety of additional indices. Such prospective trials, with long-term follow-ups, will identify the most robust motion-derived indices for disease diagnosis, prevention and monitoring. The investigation of potential associations between motion-derived indices and (i) other ultrasound-image-based indices, including, for example, IMT and texture indices and (ii) disease biomarkers, such as biochemical indices, will allow a more integrated and in-depth approach to arterial biomechanics. In addition to this, given that ultrasound is a low-cost imaging modality, it allows a cost-efficient use in clinical practice.

In conclusion, carotid artery wall motion and strain analysis using tracking has shown promise in describing a variety of local kinematic and mechanical properties. Its full potential in predicting, diagnosing and monitoring of carotid-related disorders, such as cerebrovascular events, as well as in characterising the burden of other diseases remains to be confirmed in large clinical trials, towards an integrated personalised approach for disease management and increased patient safety.

References

[1] Krejza J., Arkusjewski M., Kasner S. E., *et al.* 'Carotid artery diameter in men and women and the relation to body and neck size'. *Stroke* 2006, vol. 37(3), pp. 1103–1105.

[2] Manbachi A., Hoi Y., Wasserman B. A., Lakatta E. G., Steinman D. A. 'On the shape of the common carotid artery with implications for blood velocity profiles'. *Physiol. Meas.* 2011, vol. 32(12), pp. 1885–1897.

[3] Wagenseil J. E., Mecham R. P. 'Vascular extracellular matrix and arterial mechanics'. *Physiol. Rev.* 2009, vol. 89, pp. 957–989.

[4] Nichols W. W., O'Rourke M. *F. McDonald's Blood Flow in Arteries*. London: Arnold, 1998.

[5] Cinthio M., Ahlgren Å. R., Bergkvist J., Jansson T., Persson H. W., Lindström K. 'Longitudinal movements and resulting shear strain of the arterial wall'. *Am. J. Physiol. Heart Circ. Physiol.* 2006, vol. 291(1), pp. H394–H402.

[6] Larsson M., Kremer F., Claus P., Kuznetsova T., Brodin L. A., D'hooge J. 'Ultrasound-based radial and longitudinal strain estimation of the carotid artery: a feasibility study'. *IEEE Trans. Ultrason. Ferroelectr. Freq. Control* 2011, vol. 58(10), pp. 2244–2251.

[7] Gastounioti A., Golemati S., Stoitsis J. S., Nikita K. S. 'Adaptive block matching methods for carotid artery wall motion estimation from B-mode ultrasound: in silico evaluation & in vivo application'. *Phys. Med. Biol.* 2013, vol. 58(24), pp. 8647–8661.

[8] Greenwald S. E. 'Ageing of the conduit arteries'. *J. Pathol.* 2007, vol. 211(2), pp. 157–172.

[9] Hansen F., Mangell P., Sonesson B., Länne T. 'Diameter and compliance in the human carotid artery – variations with age and sex'. *Ultrasound Med. Biol.* 1995, vol. 21(1), pp. 1–9.

[10] Gastounioti A., Golemati S., Stoitsis J., Nikita, K. S. 'Comparison of Kalman-filter-based approaches for block matching in arterial wall motion analysis from B-mode ultrasound'. *Meas. Sci. Technol.* 2011, vol. 22, p. 9.

[11] Golemati S., Stoitsis J. S., Gastounioti A., Dimopoulos A. C., Koropouli, V., Nikita K. S. 'Comparison of block matching and differential methods for

motion analysis of the carotid artery wall from ultrasound images'. *IEEE Trans. Inf. Technol. Biomed.* 2012, vol. 16(5), pp. 852–858.

[12] Zakaria T., Qin Z., Maurice R. L. 'Optical-flow-based B-mode elastography: application in the hypertensive rat carotid'. *IEEE Trans. Med. Imaging* 2010, vol. 29(2), pp. 570–578.

[13] Nikita K. S. 'Atherosclerosis: the evolving role of vascular image analysis'. *Comput. Med. Imaging Graph.* 2013, vol. 37(1), pp. 1–3.

[14] Cobbold R. S. *Foundations of Biomedical Ultrasound*. Oxford University Press Inc.: New York, NY, USA, 2007.

[15] Ho C. Y., Solomon C. D. 'A clinician's guide to tissue Doppler imaging'. *Circulation* 2006, vol. 113, pp. e396–e398.

[16] Golemati S., Gastounioti A., Nikita K. S. 'Ultrasound-image-based cardiovascular tissue motion estimation'. *IEEE Rev. Biomed. Eng.* 2016, vol. 9, pp. 208–218.

[17] Wells P. N. T., Halliwell M. 'Speckle in ultrasonic imaging'. *Ultrasonics* 1981, vol. 19, pp. 225–229.

[18] Yli-Ollila H., Laitinen T., Weckström M., Laitinen T. M. 'Axial and radial waveforms in common carotid artery: an advanced method for studying arterial elastic properties in ultrasound imaging'. *Ultrasound Med. Biol.* 2013, vol. 39(7), pp. 1168–1177.

[19] Albinsson J., Brorsson S., Ahlgren Å. R., Cinthio M. 'Improved tracking performance of Lagrangian block-matching methodologies using block expansion in the time domain: in silico, phantom and in vivo evaluations'. *Ultrasound Med. Biol.* 2014, vol. 40(10), pp. 2508–2520.

[20] Zhang Q., Li C., Zhou M., *et al.* 'Quantification of carotid plaque elasticity and intraplaque neovascularization using contrast-enhanced ultrasound and image registration-based elastography'. *Ultrasound Med. Biol.* 2015, vol. 62, pp. 253–262.

[21] Khallaghi S., Leung C. G., Hastudi-Zaad K., Foroughi P., Nguan C., Abolmaesumi P. 'Experimental validation of an intrasubject elastic registration algorithm for dynamic 3D ultrasound images'. *Med. Phys.* 2012, vol. 39(9), pp. 5488–5497.

[22] Kruizinga P., Mastik F., van den Oord S. C. H., *et al.* 'High-definition imaging of carotid artery wall dynamics'. *Ultrasound Med. Biol.* 2014, vol. 40(10), pp. 2392–2404.

[23] Zahnd G., Salles S., Liebgott H., Vray D., Sérusclat A., Mouli P. 'Real-time ultrasound-tagging to track the 2D motion of the common carotid artery in vivo'. *Med. Phys.* 2015, vol. 42(2), pp. 820–830.

[24] Salles S., Chee A. J., Garcia D., Yu A. C., Vray D., Liebgott H. '2-D arterial wall motion imaging using ultrafast ultrasound and transverse oscillations'. *IEEE Trans. Ultrason. Ferroelectr. Freq. Control* 2015, vol. 62(6), pp. 1047–1058.

[25] Khamdaeng T., Luo J., Vappou J., Terdtoon P., Konofagou E. E. 'Arterial stiffness identification of the human carotid artery using the stress–strain relationship in vivo'. *Ultrasonics* 2012, vol. 52, pp. 402–411.

[26] Ophir J., Céspedes E. I., Ponnekanti H., Yazdi Y., Li X. 'Elastography: a quantitative method for imaging the elasticity in biological tissues'. *Ultrason. Imaging* 1991, vol. 13(2), pp. 111–134.

[27] Couade M., Pernot M., Prada C., *et al.* 'Quantitative assessment of arterial wall biomechanical properties using shear wave imaging'. *Ultrasound Med. Biol.* 2010, vol. 36(10), pp. 1662–1676.

[28] Maurice R. L., Bertrand M. 'Lagrangian speckle model and tissue-motion estimation – theory'. *IEEE Trans. Med. Imaging* 1999, vol. 18(7), pp. 593–603.

[29] Maurice R. L., Ohayon J., Frétigny Y., Bertrand M., Soulez G., Cloutier G. 'Noninvasive vascular elastography: theoretical framework'. *IEEE Trans. Med. Imaging* 2004, vol. 23(2), pp. 164–180.

[30] Mercure E., Deprez J. F., Fromageau J., *et al.* 'A compensative model for the angle-dependence of motion estimates in noninvasive vascular elastography'. *Med. Phys.* 2011, vol. 38(2), pp. 727–735.

[31] Mercure E., Destrempes F., Roy Cardinal M. H., *et al.* 'A local angle compensation method based on kinematics constraints for non-invasive vascular axial strain computations on human carotid arteries'. *Comput. Med. Imaging Graph.* 2014, vol. 38(2), pp. 123–136.

[32] Zahnd G., Orkisz M., Sérusclat A., Moulin P., Vray, D. 'Evaluation of a Kalman-based block matching method to assess the bi-dimensional motion of the carotid artery wall in B-mode ultrasound sequences'. *Med. Image Anal.* 2013, vol. 17(5), pp. 573–585.

[33] Cinthio M., Ahlgren Å. R., Jansson J. T., Eriksson A., Persson H. W., Lindström K. 'Evaluation of an ultrasonic echo-tracking method for measurements of arterial wall movements in two dimensions'. *IEEE Trans. Ultrason. Ferroelect. Freq. Control* 2005, vol. 52(8), pp. 1300–1311.

[34] Bang J., Dahl T., Bruinsma A., Kaspersen J. H., Hernes T. A. N., Myhre H. O. 'A new method for analysis of motion of carotid plaques from RF ultrasound images'. *Ultrasound Med. Biol.* 2003, vol. 29, pp. 967–976.

[35] Dineley J., Meagher S., Poepping T. L., McDicken W. N., Hoskins P. R. 'Design and characterisation of a wall motion phantom'. *Ultrasound Med. Biol.* 2006, vol. 32, pp. 1349–1357.

[36] Larsson M., Heyde B., Kremer F., Brodin L. A., D'hooge J. 'Ultrasound speckle tracking for radial, longitudinal and circumferential strain estimation of the carotid artery – an in vitro validation via sonomicrometry using clinical and high-frequency ultrasound'. *Ultrasonics* 2015, vol. 56, pp. 399–408.

[37] Chee A. J. Y., Ho C. K., Yiu B. Y. S., Yu, A. C. H. 'Walled carotid bifurcation phantoms for imaging investigations of vessel wall motions and blood flow dynamics'. *IEEE Trans. Ultrason. Ferroelect. Freq. Control* 2016, vol. 63(11), pp. 1852–1864.

[38] Sjostrand S., Widerstrom A., Ahlgren A., Cinthio M. 'Design and fabrication of a conceptual arterial ultrasound phantom capable of exhibiting

longitudinal wall movement'. *IEEE Trans. Ultrason. Ferroelectr. Freq. Control* 2016, vol. 64(1), pp. 11–18.

[39] Jensen J. 'Field: a program for simulating ultrasound systems'. *Med. Biol. Eng. Comput.* 1996, vol. 34, pp. 546–556.

[40] Gamble G., Zorn, J., Sanders G., MacMahon S., Sharpe N. 'Estimation of arterial stiffness, compliance and distensibility from M-mode ultrasound measurements of the common carotid artery'. *Stroke* 1994, vol. 25(1): pp. 11–16.

[41] Schmidt-Trucksäss A., Grathwohl D., Schmid A., *et al.* 'Assessment of carotid wall motion and stiffness with tissue Doppler imaging'. *Ultrasound Med. Biol.* 1998, vol. 24(5), pp. 639–646.

[42] Golemati S., Sassano A., Lever M. J., Bharath A. A., Dhanjil S., Nicolaides A. N. 'Motion analysis of carotid atherosclerotic plaque from B-mode ultrasound'. *Ultrasound Med. Biol.* 2003, vol. 29(3), pp. 387–399.

[43] Svedlund S., Gan L. M. 'Longitudinal wall motion of the common carotid artery can be assessed by velocity vector imaging'. *Clin. Physiol. Funct. Imaging* 2011, vol. 31(1), pp. 32–38.

[44] Zahnd G., Balocco S., Sérusclat A., Moulin P., Orkisz M., Vray D. 'Progressive attenuation of the longitudinal kinetics in the common carotid artery: preliminary in vivo assessment'. *Ultrasound Med. Biol.* 2015, vol. 41, (1), pp. 339–345.

[45] Yli-Ollila H., Tarvainen M. P., Laitinen T. P., Laitinen T. M. 'Principal component analysis of the longitudinal carotid wall motion in association with vascular stiffness: a pilot study'. *Ultrasound Med. Biol.* 2016, vol. 42(12), pp. 2873–2886.

[46] Yli-Ollila H., Tarvainen M. P., Laitinen T. P., Laitinen T. M. 'Transfer function analysis of the longitudinal movement of the common carotid artery wall'. *Front Physiol.* 2016, vol. 7(651), 10pp.

[47] Au J. S., Ditor D. S., McDonald M. J., Stöhr E. J. 'Carotid artery longitudinal wall motion is associated with local blood velocity and left ventricular rotational, but not longitudinal, mechanics'. *Physiol. Rep.* 2016, vol. 4(14), pii. e12872.

[48] Golemati S., Tzortzi M., Li R. X., Russo C., Konofagou E. E. 'Noninvasive assessment of age-related arterial changes using the carotid stress-strain relationship in vivo: a pilot study'. *Proceedings of the 2015 IEEE International Ultrasonics Symposium*; Taipei, Taiwan, Oct 2015.

[49] Zahnd G., Boussel L., Marion A., *et al.* 'Measurement of two-dimensional movement parameters of the carotid artery wall for early detection of arteriosclerosis: a preliminary clinical study'. *Ultrasound Med. Biol.* 2011, vol. 37 (9), pp. 1421–1429.

[50] Zahnd G., Vray D., Sérusclat A., *et al.* 'Longitudinal displacement of the carotid wall and cardiovascular risk factors: associations with aging, adiposity, blood pressure and periodontal disease independent of cross-sectional distensibility and intima-media thickness'. *Ultrasound Med. Biol.* 2012, vol. 38(10), pp. 1705–1715.

[51] Tat J., Au J. S., Keir P. J., MacDonald M. J. 'Reduced common carotid artery longitudinal wall motion and intramural shear strain in individuals with elevated cardiovascular disease risk using speckle tracking'. *Clin. Physiol. Funct. Imaging*, Jul 2015, doi: 10.1111/cpf.12270.

[52] Svedlund S., Eklund C., Robertsson P., Lomsky M., Gan L. M. 'Carotid artery longitudinal displacement predicts 1-year cardiovascular outcome in patients with suspected coronary artery disease'. *Arterioscler. Thromb. Vasc. Biol.* 2011, vol. 31(7), pp. 1668–1674.

[53] Mokhtari-Dizajl M., Montazeri M., Saberi H. 'Differentiation of mild and severe stenosis with motion estimation in ultrasound images'. *Ultrasound Med. Biol.* 2006, vol. 32(10), pp. 1493–1498.

[54] Shi H., Mitchell C. C., McCormick M., *et al.* 'Preliminary in vivo atherosclerotic carotid plaque characterization using the accumulated axial strain and relative lateral shift strain indices'. *Phys. Med. Biol.* 2008, vol. 53(22), pp. 6377–6394.

[55] Svedlund S., Gan L. M. 'Longitudinal common carotid artery wall motion is associated with plaque burden in man and mouse'. *Atherosclerosis* 2011, vol. 217(1), pp. 120–124.

[56] Soleimani E., Mokhtari-Dizaji M., Saberi H. 'A novel non-invasive ultrasonic method to assess total axial stress of the common carotid artery wall in healthy and atherosclerotic men'. *J. Biomech.* 2015, vol. 48(10), pp. 1860–1867.

[57] Gastounioti A., Makrodimitris S., Golemati S., Kadoglou N. P. E., Liapis C. D., Nikita K. S., 'A novel computerized tool to stratify risk in carotid atherosclerosis using kinematic features of the arterial wall'. *IEEE J. Biomed. Health Inform.* May 2015, vol. 19(3), pp. 1137–1145.

[58] Tat J., Psaromiligkos I. N., Daskalopoulou S. S. 'Carotid atherosclerotic plaque alters the direction of longitudinal motion in the artery wall'. *Ultrasound Med. Biol.* 2016, vol. 42(9), pp. 2114–2122.

[59] Wang X., Jackson D.C., Mitchell C. C., *et al.* 'Classification of symptomatic and asymptomatic patients with and without cognitive decline using non-invasive carotid plaque strain indices as biomarkers'. *Ultrasound Med. Biol.* 2016, vol. 42(4), pp. 909–918.

Chapter 25

IVUS tracking: advantages and disadvantages of intravascular ultrasound in the detection of artery geometrical features and plaque type morphology

V. Kigka[1,2], T. Exarchos[1,2], G. Rigas[1,2], A. Sakellarios[1,2], P. Siogkas[1,2], L.K. Michalis[3,4] and D.I. Fotiadis[1,2,3]

Abstract

Intravascular ultrasound (IVUS) is an invasive coronary imaging modality which provides insights in the diagnosis and therapy of coronary artery disease. The main advantage of IVUS compared to other coronary imaging techniques such as traditional invasive angiography, is that it allows the tomographic assessment of: the lumen area, the external elastic membrane area, the plaque size, the distribution and the composition of the plaque. It can safely detect and characterize the following types of plaques: necrotic core, fibrous plaque and calcified plaque. One other aspect worth mentioning is that it also provides accurate measurement of the luminal dimensions of the artery of interest. With IVUS, lipid-laden lesions appear hypoechoic, fibromuscular lesions generate low-intensity echoes and fibrous or calcified tissues are echogenic. However, IVUS suffers from a few drawbacks directly connected to its innate image quality. For example, calcium obscures the underlying wall, a phenomenon called acoustic shadowing. One other major image quality issue that emerges from the use of IVUS is the so-called speckle noise, which is the main reason for the grainy texture of IVUS images. This results to poor quality images, which makes their interpretation and processing nontrivial for computed-based diagnostic systems.

[1]Unit of Medical Technology and Intelligent Information Systems, University of Ioannina, Greece
[2]Department of Biomedical Research, Institute of Molecular Biology and Biotechnology, FORTH, Greece
[3]Michailideion Cardiology Center, Greece
[4]Department of Cardiology, Medical School, University of Ioannina, Greece

25.1 Introduction

The coronary artery disease (CAD), the most common form of heart disease, is according to the American Heart Association one of the main causes of death worldwide. CAD is characterized by atherosclerosis, which is the buildup of cholesterol and fatty deposits, known as atherosclerotic plaques, in the arterial wall. The development of atherosclerotic plaques obstructs the blood flow to the heart muscle and as a result, the heart lacks of oxygen and vital nutrients in order to work properly. This may lead to complications, such as angina (chest pain) and heart attack [1].

Due to the awareness of the mortality rate of CAD, different vascular imaging modalities have been developed over the last years to provide accurate diagnosis and support patient's treatment [2]. Coronary angiography is a predominant method for the detection of cardiovascular disease. However, despite the broad implementation of this technique, angiographic imaging portrays only 2D silhouette of the lumen and fails to depict the entire circumference of the vessel wall. On the contrary, the intravascular ultrasound (IVUS) modality overcomes this limitation and allows a reliable assessment of vessel morphology. IVUS is an invasive method using a specially designed catheter with a miniaturized ultrasound probe attached to the distal end of the catheter. It provides 2D cross-sectional high-resolution tomographic images of coronary arteries, which depict the luminal area, outer vessel wall, the composition of plaque and stent morphology [3].

IVUS is a widely used technique, not only in clinical applications, but also in research, especially in the study of plaque evolution, due to its ability to visualize the vessel wall with increased accuracy. Recent developments in IVUS image processing combined with the analysis of intravascular RF (IVUS-RF) backscatter signal allow the evaluation of the atherosclerotic plaque composition [4]. On the other hand, IVUS still has indigenous limitations, such as several artifacts and speckle noise, which affect the clinical interpretation of the IVUS image and the processing of medical images for computer-aided diagnosis, as well.

Thus, alternative invasive and noninvasive imaging modalities, which have their own strengths and weaknesses are nowadays available and able to detect atherosclerosis. More specifically, invasive [optical coherence tomography (OCT), angioscopy] and noninvasive techniques [computed tomographic coronary angiography (CTCA), magnetic resonance imaging] assess accurately the luminal pathology, provide quantification of plaque burden and characterize the type of atherosclerotic plaque [5].

However, IVUS is better in quantifying the percentage of the narrowing of stenosis and provides details for the nature of the plaque. Furthermore, IVUS is of particular use to determine the degree of stenosis in situations in which angiographic imaging is considered unreliable, such as for ostial lesions and when angiography cannot visualize the segment adequately [6].

The aim of this chapter is to present the IVUS imaging modality and its available image processing methodologies. The chapter is organized as follows: in the first section, the physical principles for IVUS acquisition are described and in the background section, several artifacts and difficulties, such as speckle noise are discussed. In the main body of the chapter, several artifact removal methodologies and the existing despeckling approaches are presented. Furthermore, automated and semiautomated border detection methodologies, atherosclerotic plaque characterization techniques and fusion approaches of coronary angiography and IVUS are extensively analyzed. The chapter is concluded with an overview of the IVUS imaging modality and future trends in IVUS imaging.

25.2 Background

25.2.1 Physical principles of IVUS imaging

Ultrasound is defined as the sound of frequency greater than 20,000 cycles per second (2 MHz), which is beyond the human hearing range. A special feature of ultrasound is its velocity in human soft tissues, which is around 1,540 m/s. The value of wave propagation velocity depends on the compressibility and the medium, where the wave is transmitted [7]. The production of ultrasound waves is based on transducers, devices that convert electrical energy to mechanical energy. These probes contain multiple piezoelectric crystals, which enable them to produce an ultrasound wave. Briefly, the electrical current passes through the piezoelectric (pressure-electric) crystalline material. Subsequently, the ultrasound wave propagates into the tissues and either is reflected or scattered. After reflection from tissue, part of ultrasound energy returns to the probe, where it distorts the shape of the transducer, according to the voltage passed through it. Thus, an electrical impulse is created that is converted into the image [8].

25.2.2 IVUS acquisition systems

The required equipment to perform IVUS imaging modality consists of a catheter, a transducer, a pullback device and a scanning console. IVUS catheter incorporates an ultrasound transducer combined usually with an inflatable balloon either with a stent, or without, in order to expand narrowed areas. Two different types of IVUS transducers are commercially available: the mechanical IVUS system and the solid-state IVUS system. The basic difference between these two types relies on the transmit and receive modes for monitoring ultrasound signals. The mechanical systems use a single-element mechanically rotating IVUS transducer, whereas the solid-state systems are based on a multielement phased-array transducer. Initially, the IVUS catheter is placed manually to the distal end of the coronary artery and then is pulled back, either manually or with automated pullback devices. The scanning console contains the electronics necessary for the storage of the IVUS data [9,10].

There are several advantages for the use of IVUS imaging in the evaluation of CAD. First of all, the full circumference of the vessel wall and not just two surfaces can be visualized, due to its tomographic orientation. Thus, a reliable assessment of vessels is provided, including cases, such as ostial or bifurcation stenoses, diffusely diseased segments, eccentric plaques, which are difficult to be assessed by angiography [6]. Moreover, IVUS has the potential to quantify the percentage of narrowing. Its penetrating nature provides remarkable images of the atherosclerotic plaque and provides insight into the nature of the plaque [11]. Finally, another important benefit by the use of IVUS is that it may reveal what in the past has been referred to as "re-stenosis," which may be a recurrence of the plaque buildup that may have previously been removed. Additionally, IVUS provides the physician the ability to identify buildup that may have been missed during angiogram or angioplasty [12].

25.2.3 IVUS disadvantages (artifacts-problems)

Despite the advantages that IVUS technique provides in the detection of region of interest (ROI) [lumen, media-adventitia (MA) borders and stent geometry], many artifacts are observed, impairing the quality of acquired images and must be taken into consideration. Some of them depend on the catheter design, while others are produced regardless of the type of the catheter [9,13]. In Figure 25.1, normal IVUS image without artifacts and typical IVUS images with artifacts are shown.

25.2.4 IVUS artifacts

25.2.4.1 Non-Uniform Rotational Distortion (NURD) and motion artifacts

Non-Uniform Rotational Distortion artifacts are observed when a mechanical catheter system is used. They are produced by an uneven drag of the drive cable of the mechanical catheter, which results to cyclic oscillations as a distortion of the image. Motion artifacts are caused by the nonstable catheter position, or the movement of the vessel before a complete creation of a circumferential image. Thus, a circular deformation of the image occurs.

25.2.4.2 Ring-down artifacts

Ring-down artifacts, a common phenomenon in medical ultrasound devices, occur for both types of catheters. They are observed as bright spots of variable thickness, which surround the IVUS catheter and are produced by acoustic oscillations of the transducer. These oscillations generate high-amplitude ultrasound signals that obscure the area surrounding the catheter.

25.2.4.3 Guide wire artifacts

Guide wire artifacts are usually observed in IVUS images and are presented as shadowing behind the guide wire. This type of artifact is delivered from the obstruction of the propagation of ultrasound signals, caused usually by the plastic sheath of the catheter.

25.2.4.4 Blood speckles

Due to the reflection of the signal by the red blood cells, IVUS images are characterized by blood speckles, which are spots moving with a characteristic pattern.

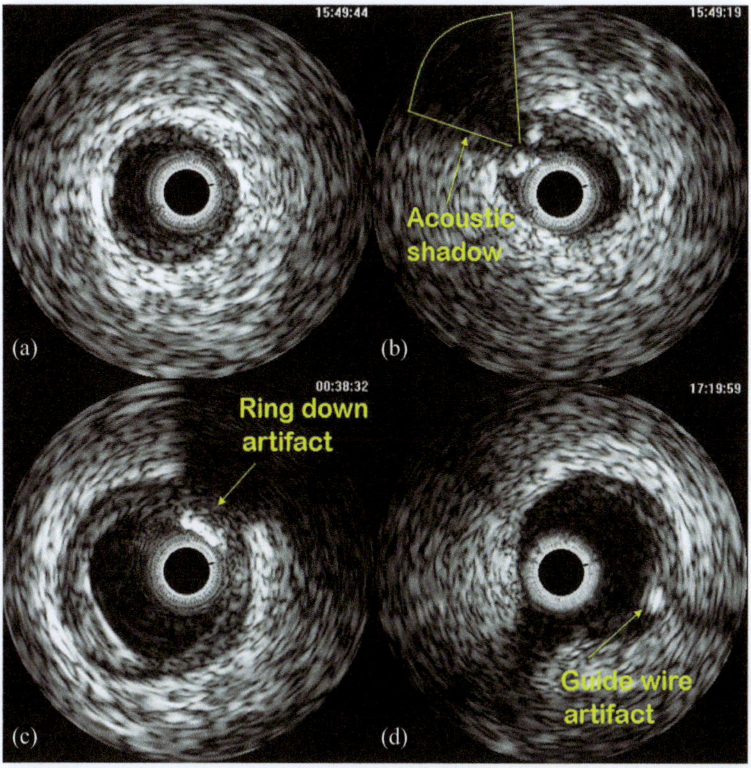

Figure 25.1 *(a) A normal IVUS image, (b) acoustic shadow artifact, (c) ring down artifact and (d) guide wire artifact*

25.2.4.5 Obliquity, eccentricity and vessel curvature problems

Vascular imaging methodologies assume that the vessel is circular and that the catheter is located in the center of the lumen, parallel to the long axis of the artery. Catheter obliquity and vessel curvature may lead to a false impression that the vessel is elliptical. Furthermore, the obliquity of the transducer, particularly in large vessels, may provide overestimation of vessel's dimensions and deterioration of image quality. The reduction of image quality is observed, because the amplitude of the echo signal reflected from an interface depends on the angle at which the beam strikes the interface. When the catheter is parallel to the vessel's long axis and the beam strikes the target at a 90° angle, then the strongest signals are obtained. Therefore, when the catheter is not located parallel to the vessel's long axis, the reflected signal is weak and the quality of the obtained images low.

25.2.4.6 Spatial orientation problem

Contemporary IVUS catheters lack constant orientation and there is no absolute anterior, posterior, left and right orientation in IVUS acquired images. On the other hand, there are some systems, in which images are rotated electronically to produce a constant orientation. However, these systems contribute only to images' interpretation and are not considered as a definitive standard. Actually, in everyday clinical practice, the use of perivascular landmarks, such as the pericardium, strands of muscle tissue and the venous system, can be considered as an important reference for the extraction of spatial orientation of the IVUS images.

25.3 Speckle noise in IVUS images

Apart from the various types of artifacts that are observed in the IVUS images, its inherent property of speckle noise consists also of an inhibiting factor as far as it concerns its wide use. Speckle noise affects not only medical doctors' interpretation of IVUS images, but also it prevents the medical image processing for computer-aided diagnoses. Speckle noise tends to reduce the quality of medical images, resolution and contrast, thereby limiting IVUS's diagnostic value and reliability [14].

Speckle noise affects all coherent medical systems, including medical ultrasound, in which images are produced by interfering echoes of a transmitted waveform. The superposition of acoustical echoes, characterized by random phases and amplitudes, produces noise that ranges from zero to a maximum, depending on whether the interference is destructive or constructive. The acquired image is thus corrupted by a random granular pattern that delays the interpretation of the image content and reduces detectability of the features of interest [15]. Speckle noise, in medical literature, is also known as "texture" and may provide useful and important diagnostic information [14].

A speckled image $V = \{V_1, V_2, V_3, ..., V_N\}$ is commonly modeled as $V_i = f_i\theta_i$ where $f = \{f_1, f_2, f_3, ..., f_N\}$ is noise-free ideal image and $\theta = \{\theta_1, \theta_2, \theta_3, ..., \theta_N\}$ is a unit mean random field [14].

25.3.1 *Model for speckle noise*

The model of speckle noise is given by

$$I(i,j) = R(i,j) \cdot u(i,j) + a(i,j), \tag{25.1}$$

where $I(i, j)$ is the noisy image, $R(i, j)$ denotes the intensity of the image without speckle, $u(t)$ and $a(t)$ are the multiplicative and additive components of the speckle noise, respectively. In the case of ultrasound images, only the multiplicative component u is considered. Thus, (25.1) can be simplified, by ignoring the additive component. This leads to the following model: $I(t) = R(\mathrm{t}) \cdot u(t)$, where $t\ (i, j)$ is the spatial coordinates of the current pixel.

25.3.2 *Need for denoising*

It is obvious that denoising of all types of ultrasound images is a predominant step in medical image processing. Loizou *et al.* [16] concluded that despeckling filtering improves the classification between asymptomatic and symptomatic ultrasound images of the carotid artery. Their study was focused on performing a comparative evaluation of ten different despeckling filters, based on texture analysis, image quality evaluation metrics and visual evaluation by medical experts.

Thus, it is essential to develop a number of alternative denoising methods that may result in despeckled images, without affecting important image features. As far as IVUS images are concerned, these methods aim to not only enhance human interpretation of ultrasound images, but also to facilitate image processing tasks, such as the detection of lumen and MA borders [17]. The desired grade of speckle smoothing depends on the expert's knowledge and on the clinical application. While numerous studies of 2D algorithms and commercially available software packages for denoising and analyzing ultrasound images have been proposed and described in detail, most of them are not employed in everyday clinical practice. Loizou *et al.* [18] introduced an integrated despeckling filtering toolbox for the ultrasound images of the common carotid artery. The basic aim of the proposed toolbox was to preprocess acquired images and to upgrade their quality. Thus, experts' image interpretation could be enhanced and tasks, such as segmentation or texture analysis, can be easier. This certain software can be characterized as a useful tool in the everyday clinical practice.

In the literature, there is a number of despeckling methods, performed in ultrasound images. However, in this section, only certain studies related to IVUS images despeckling are presented. As representative conventional noise reduction techniques, the median filter, the morphological analysis and the bilateral filters are widely used in the IVUS images. However, these filters have only the potential to reduce the speckle noise without preserving the edges of the atherosclerotic plaque successfully. On the contrary to this, anisotropic diffusion filter is known for its edge-preserving ability. When anisotropic diffusion filter is applied in IVUS images, an adaptive filtering depending on the local features of an edge is usually selected. Koga *et al.* [19] suggested a speckle noise reduction and edge-enhancement method in IVUS images by using an anisotropic diffusion filter, which is controlled by a weighted seperability of an IVUS image. This study is based on the Perona–Malik's Diffusion (PMD) [20] and its predominant goal is the edge-preserving smoothing of an image. The Perona–Malik's model is a diffusion-based algorithm, which involves simple, local and identical computations over the entire image lattice. The idea of this approach and the PMD is that the smoothed image $I(x, y, t)$ is considered as a convolution of the original image $I_0(x, y)$ with a Gaussian kernel $G(x, y, t)$

$$I(x,y,t) = I_0(x,y) * G(x,y,t), \tag{25.2}$$

The anisotropic diffusion equation is defined by:

$$I_t = \frac{\partial I}{\partial t} = \mathrm{div}(c(x,y,t)\nabla I) = c(x,y,t)\nabla I + \nabla c(x,y,t)\nabla I, \tag{25.3}$$

where $c(x, y, t) = g(\|\nabla I(x, y, t)\|)$ is the diffusion coefficient, ∇I represents the gradient of the image and $g(\cdot)$ is an edge stopping function.

Koga *et al.* [19] proposed that the diffusion strength of PMD is controlled locally and adaptively by the image seperability, which detects the elements of the inner (lower) and outer (upper) boundaries of the plaque. The weighted seperability of a pixel s is defined as

$$\eta_s^w = \eta_s \times \frac{(I_{\max} - \overline{I}_1)}{I_{\max}} \times \frac{\overline{I}_2}{I_{\max}}, \tag{25.4}$$

where $I_{\max}$ is the maximum intensity of whole image and $\overline{I}_1, \overline{I}_2$ are the means of intensity in the regions outside the luminal boundary and outside the adventitial boundary, respectively. In this approach, a weighted seperability controlled PMD (WSC-PMD) replaced the conventional one and an efficient edge-preserved speckle noise reduction is realized.

25.3.3 Wavelet transform denoising methods

Recently, several wavelet-thresholding approaches have been developed, which aim to remove the noise of the acquired image, retaining its characteristics. Wavelet-thresholding approaches are effective denoising techniques, due to their ability to capture the energy of a signal [21].

In general, the basic procedure for all wavelet-based techniques consists of the following steps:

1. Calculation of wavelet transform of the acquired image
2. Modification of noisy wavelet coefficients according to a rule
3. Computation of inverse transform by using the modified coefficients in order to get the denoised estimate [22]

The idea behind wavelet-based methods is wavelet thresholding either soft-thresholding or hard thresholding. In particular, coefficients which represent speckle noise must be removed, whereas coefficients which represent actual image edges must be retained.

Hard-Thresholding function cuts-off wavelet coefficients below a threshold and it is described as

$$W_\delta = \begin{cases} W, |W| \geq \delta \\ 0, |W| < \delta \end{cases}. \tag{25.5}$$

On the other hand, the Soft-Thresholding function threshold reduces all coefficients. The formula is

$$W_\delta = \begin{cases} \text{sign}(W)(|W| - \delta), |W| \geq \delta \\ 0, |W| < \delta \end{cases}, \tag{25.6}$$

where W is the wavelet coefficient, δ is a specific threshold and W_δ the wavelet coefficients. The threshold is defined as $\delta = \sigma\sqrt{2 \log N}$, where σ is the standard deviation of the noise and N is the size of the image.

The Wavelet Transform was deployed in many types of ultrasound images. Katouzian *et al.* [23] proposed a reliable denoising algorithm for IVUS images using exponential wavelet-like basis functions, known as Brushlets, to remove blood speckle noise. Brushlet functions belong to steerable wavelets and are explained in detail in [24]. In this approach, Katouzian concluded that this wavelet denoising approach is a reliable preprocessing step for accurate lumen border detection.

25.3.4 Curvelet transform denoising methods

Curvelet-transform attracts attention in ultrasound image denoising, due to its capability of recovering signals in different directions. Curvelet reconstructions exhibit higher quality than wavelet-based approaches, providing a higher quality recovery of edges. In order to reconstruct edge details in an image, curvelet technique uses a relatively small amount of coefficients. In [25,26], curvelet transforms are described in detail.

A comparative study between curvelet-based despeckling techniques and adaptive complex diffusion filters was proposed by Rizi and Setarehdan [27], who endeavored to reduce speckle noise, using curvelet transform and an adaptive complex diffusion filter and to compare their performances. They discovered that curvelet approach outperfoms and provided a better quality of a denoised IVUS image.

25.4 Segmentation techniques for border identification

The most important advantage of IVUS imaging modality is its ability to define in detail the lumen features, particularly luminal cross-sectional area, wall thickness and wall structure. In a typical IVUS image, three arterial regions can be distinguished: the lumen, the vessel wall, consisting of the intima and the media layers and the adventitia plus surroundings. These regions are separated by two borders: the lumen border, which is the boundary between lumen-wall interface and the MA border, which represents the boundary between the media and adventitia [28]. As is shown in Figure 25.2, IVUS can visualize both the inner (lumen border area) and the outer wall of the artery (media adventitia border area).

The fundamental goal of IVUS image segmentation is to detect in a reliable and fast manner the above-mentioned borders. Segmentation can be done either manually, which is an extremely time-consuming process, or via computer-aided techniques. To tackle the segmentation problem, researchers have developed several IVUS segmentation algorithms, which can detect the lumen and media adventitia boundaries. The efficiency of each algorithm is based not only on its ability to accurately define lumen and MA borders, but also on its automation. Generally, fully automated approaches attract more attention than those, requiring user intervention. However, in clinical applications, it is common to observe that automated segmentation techniques have achieved limited success, due to several extrinsic artifacts and parameters. Restrictions of IVUS image quality, such as lack

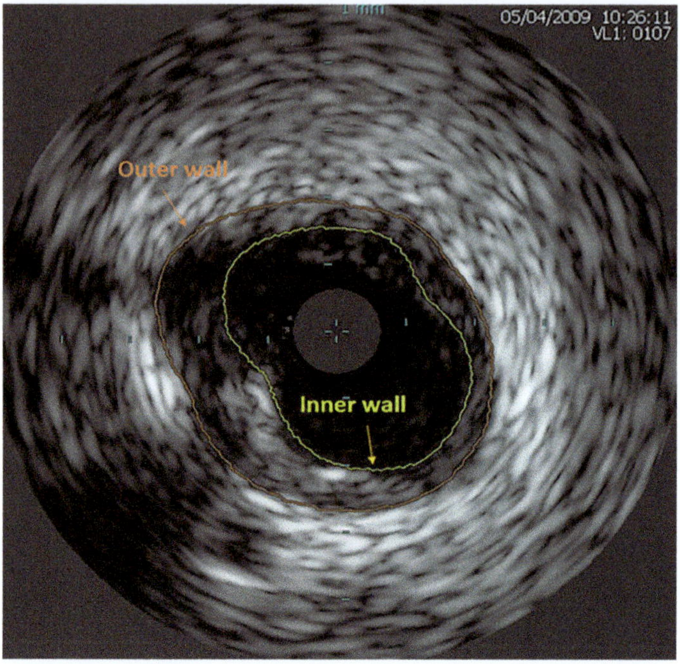

Figure 25.2 An IVUS image with annotated the inner wall and the outer wall of the artery

of homogeneity of ROI, high-intensity variation and shadowed regions, may result in automated segmentation of IVUS images.

This section presents existing techniques for IVUS image segmentation. The presented methods are divided into techniques, which are based on Edge-Tracking and Gradient, Active Contour, Statistics and Probabilities and Multiscale Expansion [10]. Table 25.1 summarizes the available IVUS segmentation techniques and provides the advantages, disadvantages and the results of each technique.

25.4.1 Edge-tracking and gradient-based techniques

The detection of lumen and MA boundaries usually relies on edge patterns of IVUS images and each boundary can be distinguished by the interactions of IVUS signal with either the blood-tissue interface or the smooth muscle cells. Thus, several hybrid algorithms and refinement techniques have been introduced, in order to incorporate edge features. This type of IVUS segmentation approaches usually requires precise initialization and is based on the energy minimization framework. The very first study on the detection of lumen and outer wall borders on IVUS images, based on such a principle, was proposed by Herrington *et al.* [29]. Sonka *et al.* [30] proposed a remarkable semiautomated method for IVUS image segmentation, by using global image information and heuristic graph searching. The key

Table 25.1 *Comparison of the developed IVUS segmentation methods*

Authors	Approach	Advantages	Disadvantages	Validation
Sonka *et al.* [30]	Edge-Tracking and Gradient based	Accurate border detection Fast	It is based on *a priori* knowledge which in some cases is not available	Linear Regression Analysis for luminal area: $y = 1.02x + 0.52\text{mm}^2$, $r = 0.96$, and for the plaque area: $y = 1.07x - 0.48\ \text{mm}^2$, $r = 0.95$
Birgelen *et al.* [32]	Edge-Tracking and Gradient based	Reproducible Interpolated contour tracing on the cross-sectional images	Deposits behind the calcium and the external vessel boundary cannot be traced	Mean differences were −0.65% to 3.86% for the luminal area
Kovalski *et al.* [37]	Active Contour based	Intrinsic parallel integration of axial and longitudinal factors Fully automated	Tuning of proper magnitudes to algorithm's parameters for adequate performance of algorithm is needed	Correlation plaque region: $y = 1.07x - 0.38\ \text{mm}^2$, $r = 0.98$
Shekhar *et al.* [39]	Active Contour based	Accurate Robust to artifacts	Requires further refinement of the weights of various forces, as in all deformable models	Mean error Luminal area error: 4.1% ($0.39\ \text{mm}^2$) Luminal perimeter error: 2.9% (0.38 mm) Media adventitial area error: 1.2% ($0.2\ \text{mm}^2$) Media adventitial area error: 1.3% (0.9 mm)
Plissiti *et al.* [41]	Active Contour based	Overcome IVUS images restrictions (artifacts, calcified regions, noise) Fast	The problem of side branches has not been overcome	Linear Regression Analysis for luminal area: $y = 0.97x + 6.13\ \text{mm}^2$, $r = 0.99$ and for the plaque area: $y = 1.01x - 5.47\ \text{mm}^2$, $r = 0.99$

(Continues)

Table 25.1 (*Continued*)

Authors	Approach	Advantages	Disadvantages	Validation
Gil *et al.* [42]	Statistical and probabilistic based	The model behaves well in low quality images	It detects only the inner wall	Mean error of the lumen: 0.15 ± 0.1
Taki *et al.* [43]	Statistical and probabilistic based	Automated	The sensitivity is reduced in small and discontinuous calcified regions of the images	Absolute difference for luminal area: Snake: 7.5367 ± 4.6274 Level set: 6.2653 ± 1.7284 Media adventitial area: Snake: 6.1232 ± 1.8332 Level set: 5.0179 ± 3.7915
Haas *et al.* [44]	Statistical and probabilistic based	Reliable results, independent of the catheter position and the total image brightness	It needs an extended histological evaluation	Expert A vs algorithm Difference of Inner contour: -0.025 ± 0.163 mm Difference of Outer contour: -0.064 ± 0.156 mm Expert B vs algorithm Difference of Inner contour: -0.030 ± 0.166 mm Difference of Outer contour: -0.027 ± 0.162 mm

(Continues)

Table 25.1 (Continued)

Authors	Approach	Advantages	Disadvantages	Validation
Brusseau *et al.* [45]	Statistical and probabilistic based	Fully automatic	Only luminal boundary is detected The cases of totally occlusive plaques, dissections and side-branches were not considered	Experts vs algorithm error 0.099 ± 0.032
Cardinal *et al.* [46]	Statistical and probabilistic based	Satisfactory overall performance	It requires to trace contours on more views during the initialization procedure for more complex lesions	Average distance between segmentation results and manually traced contours was 0.16 mm
Unal *et al.* [47]	Statistical and probabilistic based	Reliable	Slow	Mean difference $0.65 \pm 1.27\ mm^2$ for the luminal and $0.06 \pm 1.59\ mm^2$ for the media-adventitia area
Katouzian *et al.* [48]	Multiscale expansion based	Reliably classify simultaneously plaques and blood regardless of the transducer center frequency or spectrum	It detect only the luminal boundary	Linear Regression Analysis for luminal area: $y = 0.953x + 0.725$ $r = 0.9854$
Papadogiorgaki *et al.* [28]	Multiscale expansion based	Fully automated (does not require manual initialization) Fast	It is unreliable in calcified segments	Mean difference $0.13 \pm 1.21\ mm^2$ for the luminal and $0.06 \pm 1.59\ mm^2$ for the media-adventitia area

point of this method was the incorporation of an *a priori* knowledge of coronary artery anatomy and ultrasound image characteristics. The method was validated by 38 IVUS images and the computer-identified areas showed a high correlation with the observer-defined areas ($r = 0.96$, $y = 1.02x + 0.52\,\mathrm{mm}^2$ and $r = 0.95$, $y = 1.07 - 0.48\,\mathrm{mm}^2$ for the luminal and plaque area, respectively).

Two semiautomated segmentation techniques, in which the minimum-cost algorithm was applied, in order to find the optimal path within the vessel and detect both the lumen and MA borders, was implemented in [31,32]. The results were evaluated using both *in vivo* images and tubular phantom data. Birgelen *et al.* [32], based on the idea that edge points obtained from previously detected longitudinal contours may facilitate the contour detection in the cross-sectional images, concluded that the proposed analysis system provides accurate measurements of phantom dimensions and is useful for performing highly reproducible area and volume measurements in three-dimensional (3D) intracoronary ultrasound (ICUS) *in vivo*.

Later, Meier *et al.* [33] implemented a method, that allows a fully automated segmentation, without user's interaction, of the luminal and MA boundary. This approach consists of three phases: preproccessing (polar transform, local contrast enhancement, speckle noise reduction), segmentation process (including radial scanning, region growing, cost-function minimization techniques) and postprocessing (involving dropout filtering and outline smoothing) in order to refine the final segmentation. Two different datasets of 77 and 28 *in vivo* collected IVUS frames were used. The comparison with experts' annotation showed a good agreement (interclass and intraclass correlation coefficients ranged from 0.83 to 0.94). A modified optimization-based contour detection model was implemented by Zhongchi *et al.* [34]. More specifically, an alternative image cost function was used, as a combination of the gradient and the variance of image intensity in the radial direction. Subsequently, circular dynamic programing was performed, aiming to extract the minimal energy path, based on the optimal contour of the artery wall.

25.4.2 Active contour-based techniques

The active contour model [35], also known as snake or deformable model, is undoubtedly a useful tool in medical image segmentation. The active contour model is a parametrical curve and its energy functional is described by

$$E^*_{\mathrm{snake}} = \int_0^1 E_{\mathrm{snake}}(v(s))ds = \int_0^1 \left(E_{\mathrm{int}}(V(s)) + E_{\mathrm{image}}(v(s)) + E_{\mathrm{con}}(v(s))\right)ds, \tag{25.7}$$

where $v(s) = (x(s), y(s))$ represents the parametrical position of a snake, $\mathrm{E}_{\mathrm{int}}$ is the internal energy of the snake, E_{image} is the image energy and E_{con} is the energy caused by external constraint forces.

The basic idea behind active contour models is to place an approximate contour close to the desired features in an image and then to allow the contour to deform under the influence of external and internal forces in the energy function to snap to the desired features [35].

Active contour models have been incorporated in several border detection approaches of IVUS images. These models are called discrete dynamic contour (DDC) models, belonging to the general category of active contour ("snakes") methods and were firstly implemented by Lobregt and Viergever [36]. Few years later, Kovalski *et al.* [37] developed an automatic method for lumen and MA border extraction, based on active contour principles. The extraction of the features of interest was performed in three dimensions. They proposed a modification of the internal energy, by eliminating the elasticity term and they introduced a "balloon" force [38], that can assist the convergence process to overcome local energy minima caused by weak edges. The results of this approach demonstrated high correlation $r = 0.978$ and low variability $15.2 \pm 17.4\%$ and $6.5 \pm 7.6\%$ for lumen and MA borders, respectively, when comparing to manual tracing. Later, Shekhar *et al.* [39] presented an active surface segmentation algorithm for IVUS borders detection, which is an extension of the DDC models [36] and provides an accurate 3D reconstruction and visualization of coronary arteries and volumetric measurements. Briefly, in this 3D segmentation approach, an initial surface template is placed closed to the desired arterial wall borders. Then, this template is deformed to snap to it according to the external, internal and damping forces. In this method, the external force is the gradient of a 3D potential field, the internal force is based on the transverse and longitudinal curvature vectors in the local radial direction and the damping force is used to help the model to converge to its final shape. Despite this method was not fully automated and lumen and MA borders are detected in two distinct datasets, it attracted attention, since it demonstrated accurate and promising results (4.1% and 1.2% mean error for luminal and MA area, respectively). A year later, Klingensmith *et al.* [40] attempted to evaluate active surface segmentation techniques against a neighborhood-search technique.

Another interesting approach was proposed by Plissiti *et al.* [41], in which deformable models were used for lumen and MA borders detection. The segmentation procedure was applied in a sequence of IVUS frames and only for the first frame an initial user estimation of the borders was required. The use of a Hopfield neural network minimized the energy function of the deformable model and made the application computationally more efficient in the detection of MA borders, when calcified regions are present.

25.4.3 Statistical- and probabilistic-based techniques

Statistically based approaches for lumen boundaries detection rely usually on the assumption that the lumen and tissue appear in the image as gray-level pixels generated by two distinct normal distributions. Due to this idea, Gil *et al.* [42] introduced the very first region-based technique for luminal area detection. Its initial goal was to approximately compute an elliptical model, which is probably located close to the inner wall. The use of a fixed threshold allowed the extraction of an initial ellipse by means of a binarized image. A refinement algorithm was implemented, which by using an adaptive threshold, can discriminate different tissues. This algorithm was validated on 1,200 frames from eight different patients. Furthermore, Taki *et al.* [43] developed an automated method, for identifying intima and MA borders simultaneously, by using two different threshold values. It has been demonstrated that through an accurate discrimination between lumen and tissue regions, a reliable detection of vessel borders can be achieved by applying threshold techniques and classification algorithms. Haas *et al.* [44] proposed an automatic technique for IVUS image segmentation. The proposed model formulated an image generation model, based on Rayleigh distribution and proposed *a priori* knowledge about the contour. By employing a *maximum a posteriori* (MAP) estimator in an iterative process, final contours were found. This method was evaluated on 29 *in vivo* frames and its validation was realized by two expert observers. Although large variation was apparent between manual and automated defined boundaries ($0.01 \pm 5.99\%$ for lumen and $0.51 \pm 4.73\%$ for MA), this approach demonstrated satisfactory and promising results. In a similar manner [44], Brusseau *et al.* [45] introduced an algorithm, based on a contour, that evolved until it optimally separates regions with different statistical properties. This fully automated algorithm was dedicated to luminal contour segmentation of IVUS images. This study was based on statistical differences between blood and tissue scattering to deform the contour. A Rayleigh model for image brightness appearance was implemented and the final contour position was calculated by a MAP estimator and a constraint on the first zero crossing of image derivatives on the borders. Automatic contours were compared to those manually annotated by two experts, and the error was 0.099 ± 0.032.

Cardinal *et al.* [46] suggested a 3D IVUS segmentation model based on the combination of fast-marching methods and gray-level probability functions (PDFs) of vessel's structures. The model was validated both *in vivo* and realistic simulation of IVUS images. Despite the proposed method lacks automation and needs user intervention, a good overall performance was demonstrated, since the mean distance between the segmentation results and the manually identified contours was <0.16 mm.

Unal *et al.* [47] presented an automated shape-driven approach implemented in the polar domain to segment the arterial wall in IVUS images. Using intensity profiles from a training dataset, the probability distribution inside and outside the lumen was calculated and the luminal boundaries were delineated automatically. To identify MA borders, edge information was used. The approach seemed to perform reliably, since the extracted borders were in agreement with those estimated by the observers. ($0.65 \pm 1.27\ \text{mm}^2$ and $0.98 \pm 1.78\ \text{mm}^2$ were the difference error for luminal and outer vessel wall, respectively.)

25.4.4 Multiscale expansion-based techniques

Motivated by spectral analysis and spatial-frequency expansions, researchers developed multiscale expansion-based techniques for IVUS image segmentation.

Katouzian *et al.* [48] were the first, who proposed a multiscale expansion approach based on discrete wavelet packet frames for the automated detection of lumen borders in IVUS images. In a similar approach, Papadogiorgaki *et al.* [28] used both intensity information and the result of texture analysis, generated by a multilevel discrete wavelet frames decomposition to initialize desired contours.

25.5 Plaque characterization

The IVUS imaging modality, except of its ability to measure the luminal area dimensions and to detect the ROI, it is also considered as the gold standard in atherosclerotic plaque characterization. In the formation of atherosclerotic coronary lesions, a critical primary step is the accumulation and oxidation of low-density lipoprotein particles. These plaques consist of four main plaque types: calcium or dense calcium (DC), necrotic core (NC) or soft tissue, fibrous tissue (FT) and mixed or fibro-fatty tissue (FFT) [49].

Different studies have shown that plaque rupture may lead to the formation of thrombus and acute coronary syndrome (ACS). Thus, in order to detect and understand the process of ACS, researchers have developed a multitude of approaches regarding tissue characteristics evaluation of coronary plaque, since the histological composition plays an important role in the stability of the atherosclerotic plaque.

The methodologies of plaque characterization are divided into methodologies that use either gray-scale IVUS images or the backscatter IVUS signal. Table 25.2 summarizes these methods and provides their overall accuracy.

25.5.1 Methodologies developed for plaque characterization using gray-scale IVUS

Zhang *et al.* [50] proposed the first methodology for detecting and characterizing the atherosclerotic plaque. It was a novel automated texture-based method for plaque composition assessment, aiming to distinguish regions of soft (lipid rich) and hard plaque (fibrotic and calcified). In this approach, several texture descriptors, such as gray-level-based texture descriptors, co-occurrence matrices, run-length measures and fractal-based measures were used. Radial profile, long-run emphasis, fractal dimension were identified as the descriptors, which provided the best features for a correct plaque classification. Then, a classifier with a linear discrimination was employed for the classification of soft/hard regions. The method was evaluated, using expert-observers' annotations in 12 IVUS frames, which proved the validity of the obtained results (89.2% for hard plaque and 90.2% for soft plaque).

Similarly to the previous method, Brunenberg *et al.* [51], extracted different texture features combined with AdaBoost techniques for classification. The reliability of this method was tested against the annotations by medical experts in 30 IVUS images and the overall accuracy was 75.82%. Two years later, Santos Filho *et al.* [52] proposed an innovative application for automatic thresholding for the

Table 25.2 Comparison of the developed IVUS plaque characterization methods

Authors	Tissue classification	Validation dataset	Validation
Zhang *et al.* [50]	DC, NC, FT	12 IVUS images	Experts annotation Overall accuracy: 89.9%
Brunenberg *et al.* [51]	DC, NC, FT	30 IVUS images	Experts annotation Overall accuracy: 75.82%
Santos Filho *et al.* [52]	DC	43 plaque areas	Experts annotation Sensitivity: 84% Specificity: 72%
Zhang *et al.* [54]	DC	80 IVUS images	Experts annotation Sensitivity: 87.16% Specificity: 87.35%
Athanasiou *et al.* [55]	DC, NC, FT, FFT and the Media	300 VH-IVUS frames	VH-IVUS Accuracy DC: 84.87%, NC: 80.57%, FT: 77.4% and FFT: 64.47%
Athanasiou *et al.* [57]	DC, NC, FT	40 IVUS images	Experts annotation Overall accuracy: 86.17%
König *et al.* [56]	DC, NC, FT, FFT and the Media	889 histological cross-sections	Histology Accuracy DC: 96.7%, NC: 95.8%, FT: 93.5% and FFT: 94.1%
Kawasaki *et al.* [59]	FT, NC and FT-CA	724 histological cross-sections	Histology Accuracy DC: 93%, NC: 90%, FT-CA: 96%
Sathyanarayana *et al.* [61]	NC, FT-NC, FT and CA	1,200 histological cross-sections	Histology Accuracy NC: 97%, FT-NC: 98%, FT: 95% and CA: 98%

identification of calcified regions in gray-scale IVUS images. Adaptive thresholding and Otsu's method [53] were applied and the obtained sensitivity and specificity were 84% and 72%, respectively. Zhang *et al.* [54] introduced an approach, based on snakes and the Contourlet transform, limited only in the detection of calcified plaques. This methodology demonstrated a sensitivity of 87.16% and specificity of 87.35%. In contrast to the aforementioned approaches, Athanasiou *et al.* [55] suggested a three-step semiautomated method, in which atherosclerotic plaque was classified into four types of tissue: DC, NC, FT and FFT. In the first step, a well-validated previously mentioned approach [41] was used for the detection of ROI in an IVUS sequence. In the second step, a set of features for each pixel of ROI, such as the co-occurrence matrix, the local binary patterns, the mean value and the entropy, were extracted and in the third step, these pixels were classified using a random forest classifier. This technique produced promising results, with an overall accuracy of 85.65% when it was compared to 300 VH-IVUS frames [56]. Figure 25.3 depicts an example of color-coded characterized IVUS images. Apart from its high performance, another advantage of the suggested methodology is that it performs plaque characterization of the entire IVUS sequence and not only

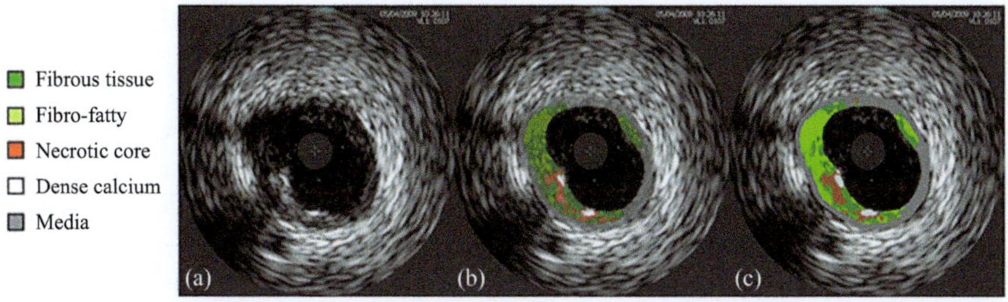

Figure 25.3 (a) Initial IVUS image, (b) virtual histology IVUS (VH-IVUS) image and (c) characterized IVUS image using the method described in [55]

of the end-diastolic IVUS frames. In addition to this, the standardized format of its estimations allowed recall, portability and data exchange.

A year later, Athanasiou *et al.* [57] proposed a hybrid approach, which provided complete atherosclerotic plaque characterization. Both classification methods and image filtering techniques were employed for correct classification of the IVUS image pixels. Using annotations of two medical experts in 40 IVUS frames, they validated their method, and produced an overall accuracy of 86.14%.

25.5.2 Methodologies developed for plaque characterization using the backscatter IVUS signal

Due to the fact that the visualization algorithms incorporated into the ultrasound consoles do not use all the information which might be present in radiofrequency (RF) signals, the assessment of the composition of coronary plaques using IVUS gray-scale images, is not fully functional. Thus, several methodologies based on the processing data from ultrasound backscattered RF signals have been developed. Nair *et al.* [58] confirmed that the use of IVUS RF data has the potential to predict coronary plaque composition. They indicated that autoregressive classification schemes outperformed over classic Fourier methods with accuracies of 90.4%, 92.8%, 90.9%, 89.5% for fibrous, fibrolipidic, calcified, calcified-necrotic regions, respectively.

Kawasaki *et al.* [59] introduced the integrated backscatter combined with conventional IVUS (IBIVUS), based on the implementation of the Fast Fourier Transform, as a new useful tool for evaluating the tissue structure of human coronary arterial plaques. The IB-IVUS system constructs color-coded tissue maps, providing a quantitative visual readout as four types of plaque composition: calcification, fibrosis, dense fibrosis and lipid pool. In a clinical study, Sano *et al.* [60] concluded that tissue characteristics of vulnerable plaque before ACS were different from those of stable angina plaques. Thus, the IB-IVUS predictive ability of ACS was demonstrated, by classifying plaque into vulnerable and stable angina.

iMap was introduced as another RF-based tissue characterization method, that is compatible with the latest 40 MHz mechanical IVUS imaging system. The iMap method, similar to other RF-based tissue characterization techniques, has the potential to classify the atherosclerotic plaque into four types: fibrotic, necrotic, lipidic and calcified. Sathyanarayana *et al.* [61] in an attempt to evaluate the iMap technique, performed an *ex-vivo* validation, using a swine animal model. The accuracy of their method was of the highest level of confidence: 97%, 98%, 95%, 98% for necrotic, lipidic, fibrotic and calcified tissues, respectively.

VH-IVUS analysis [56] is another promising technique for assessing atherosclerotic plaque, based on spectral analysis of the IVUS-RF data acquired with phased-array 20 MHz catheters. These are used to identify four different tissue types. This method identifies several features derived from the RF-signal, which were compared to the previously stored RF-pattern features of the four tissue types. VH-IVUS was able to identify four major plaque components (fibrous, fibrofatty, NC and dense calcified tissue) demonstrating an accuracy of 93.4%, 94.6%, 95.1%, 96.8% for each component, respectively, compared to histology.

Okubo *et al.* [62] attempted to compare directly IB-IVUS and VH IVUS for the same coronary arterial cross-section. This comparison demonstrated that the overall agreement between histological and IBIVUS diagnoses was higher ($\kappa = 0.81$, 95%, CI: 0.72–0.89) than between histological and VH-IVUS diagnoses ($\kappa = 0.66$, 95%, CI: 0.56–0.75).

25.6 IVUS-based hybrid imaging

25.6.1 Fusion of IVUS and coronary angiography

The assessment of coronary atherosclerosis requires an accurate representation of the vessel geometry and the plaque morphology. Several imaging modalities are available for the study of coronary anatomy. X-ray coronary angiography and IVUS are considered as the most popular techniques in interventional cardiology, in spite of each modality's limitations. For example, conventional contrast coronary angiography allows the estimation of the severity of a luminal stenosis, without providing any information about the plaque's composition and vulnerability. However, angiography combined with IVUS is able to overcome these limitations and deliver more information about vessel's geometry. Therefore, researchers proposed different fusion approaches of imaging modalities.

The first clinically applicable method was proposed by Wahle *et al.* [63]. In this approach, only two sets of angiographic images were required for the extraction of the IVUS catheter path. The first set was used to define the distal end of pull-back and the second one to define the other proximal end. Subsequently, 2D curves were defined, by the automatic IVUS catheter path extraction and corresponding points were identified in these curves, in order to define the 3D path of the IVUS catheter. A sequential triangulation algorithm, which is an approximation of the Frenet–Serret rules was applied to estimate the relative orientation of IVUS frames, after their assignments to their locations. Finally, an efficient methodology, which compared the projections of the path and final model onto the angiographic images and their silhouette in these, was applied for the definition of the absolute orientation.

Two years later, Slager *et al.* [64] proposed a true 3D reconstruction method of coronary arteries by fusing angiography and IVUS (ANGUS). In this method, the basic steps for true 3D reconstruction of an artery from IVUS and biplane angiography information were implemented. However, a quite different approach for catheter path extraction was applied, using a 3D circular segment as a first coreline approximation. Subsequently, the circular segment was stepwise adapted in 3D until its biplane projections ideally match with the actual drawings of the coreline.

Another approach for catheter path extraction was suggested by Bourantas *et al.* [65] employing a cubic-B spline. Initially, an efficient algorithm for the detection of ROI in IVUS images was used and then swept B-Spline surfaces were introduced in order to extract the catheter path. Bourantas *et al.* validated their method *in vivo* and *in vitro* and concluded that their method performed accurately and was able to depict the morphology of coronary arteries.

Furthermore, Wahle *et al.* [66] proposed an interactive virtual endoscopy system, in which fusion of biplane angiography and IVUS, combined with computational hemodynamics, morphologic analyses, and interactive 3D visualization provided information for diagnosis and evaluation of coronary interventions.

Bourantas *et al.* [5] developed an automated user-friendly system (ANGIOCARE), for rapid 3D coronary reconstruction, integrating angiographic and ICUS data. ANGIOCARE incorporates the method by Plissiti *et al.* [41] for border extraction. During the segmentation process, the user is able to check the borders in each frame in four longitudinal cut planes. In the case of failure of accurate detection of the borders, the process is interrupted, the corrections are made visually and the program was restarted from the corrected image. Apart from the detection of ROI, ANGIOCARE system incorporates the catheter path extraction from two end-diastolic X-ray images, in which the detected borders are placed perpendicularly.

25.6.2 Fusion of IVUS and coronary computed tomography

The previously presented fusion methodologies have the ability to provide only geometrically correct models of the coronary segments, without providing any information about the coronary bifurcations and the morphology of side branches. To address this limitation, van der Giessen *et al.* [67] suggested the fusion of IVUS and CTCA. They defined the centerline of the lumen by using CT (computer tomographic) images and then cross-sectional images were generated every 0.2 mm, perpendicularly to this centerline. These images are used to find a correspondence between IVUS and CT cross-sections.

25.7 Limitations of IVUS usability

Although IVUS consoles produced remarkably detailed view of vessel wall, IVUS imaging modality is accurate only in determining the thickness and echogenity of vessel wall structures and is not consistently able to provide actual histology of plaque. Thus, as far as IVUS clinical usability is concerned, there is lack of validated methods for objective or automated classification of atheromatic lesions [6].

However, the most significant limitations of IVUS usability are the artifacts that are generated by the contemporary devices. Artifacts of IVUS images, except for affecting adversely image quality, they reduce also the accuracy of quantitative measurements [68].

25.8 Future perspectives of IVUS

IVUS has been employed in clinical practice for more than two decades and its usefulness is widely known. However, there is still clinical future for IVUS, which might attract more attention, driven by clinical and technological developments [69]. Over the past few years, great efforts to overcome IVUS limitations have been observed, by developing new methodologies for improving the processing of acquired images and the visualization of plaque pathology. Furthermore, the current hybrid imaging approaches in combination with technological innovations and efficient algorithms have demonstrated promising results in the study of coronary atherosclerosis [70].

25.8.1 Future trends in 3D IVUS reconstruction

As previously mentioned, a geometrically correct 3D IVUS reconstruction model is able to eliminate IVUS's inherent technical limitations, as a tomographic technique. In the majority of studies, combination of IVUS data with biplane angiographic images allows the depiction of the true coronary anatomy. However, these studies were only experimentally validated and not incorporated in everyday clinical practice. Giannoglou *et al.* [71] argued that there is a lack of a widely accepted clinical 3D IVUS reconstruction tool, which would be valuable for interventional cardiologists. Thus, researchers should focus both on the further development of the existing software and on the advancing hardware capabilities in order to allow the implementation of a real-time 3D IVUS reconstruction.

Another future goal of IVUS imaging is to improve our understanding of complex lesions and improve our ability to deliver optimal interventional results. We should take into consideration that the existing artery imaging modalities should act synergistically. Therefore, the future in the imaging field is multimodality imaging. Synchronizing images acquired by two different resources is a difficult task, since there are many differences in each imaging method properties and positioning of the catheters in the coronary arteries. From a clinical point of view, such combined information would be very useful to guide percutaneous coronary interventions (PCIs).

An innovative clinically practical methodology for online co-registration of 3D quantitative coronary angiography and IVUS or OCT, proposed by Carlier *et al.* [72], aims to reach this target. The key idea of this approach is to combine the detailed information of intravascular imaging with the coronary tree overview as presented in angiography and to demonstrate which clinically relevant image at one position in one modality corresponds to the same position in the other modality. An ideal future co-registration system would require only time by the operators to observe the synchronized image data sets and the user's identification of landmarks to establish image synchronization.

25.8.2 Future technical development

The frequency of commonly used IVUS transducers ranges from 20 to 40 MHz. Increasing frequency from the currently available to 80 MHz might provide a much higher image resolution and could be valuable for the detection of vulnerable thin fibrous caps with lipid pools behind. However, this high level of frequencies is characterized by certain limitation factors, such as the difficulty of fabrication of miniature transducers of 80 MHz or higher and the strong tissue attenuation, as well. On the other hand, compared to the standard IVUS catheters, miniaturized 80 MHz transducers demonstrated superior imaging results in an *ex vivo* aortic specimen [73].

In general, new transducer technology could be characterized as a future technical development, since it would offer advancements in IVUS imaging such as increased image resolution, multifrequency devices, real-time volumetric ultrasound imaging capability [74] and software improvements to facilitate image interpretation.

25.9 Conclusions

This chapter focuses on the IVUS image processing methodologies, which aim to reduce inter-observer variability and facilitate IVUS processing. Due to its radial resolution, IVUS has become undoubtly an indispensable tool in research, since it allows an accurate evaluation of the plaque burden and estimation of atherosclerotic plaque evolution. However, although IVUS provides supplementary and valuable information for the management of complex PCI, many cardiologists are not familiar with this modality and its use in some cases is still limited.

References

[1] Fuster V, Badimon L, Badimon JJ, Chesebro JH. The pathogenesis of coronary artery disease and the acute coronary syndromes. New England Journal of Medicine. 1992;326(4): 242–50.
[2] Frangi AF, Amini A A, Bullitt E. Vascular imaging. IEEE Transactions on Medical Imaging. 2005;24(4): 433–5.
[3] Nissen SE, Yock P. Intravascular ultrasound. Novel Pathophysiological Insights and Current Clinical Applications. 2001; 103(4): 604–16.
[4] Mehta SK, McCrary JR, Frutkin AD, Dolla WJ, Marso SP. Intravascular ultrasound radiofrequency analysis of coronary atherosclerosis: an emerging technology for the assessment of vulnerable plaque. European Heart Journal. 2007;28(11): 1283–8.
[5] Bourantas CV, Kalatzis FG, Papafaklis MI, *et al.* ANGIOCARE: an automated system for fast three-dimensional coronary reconstruction by integrating angiographic and intracoronary ultrasound data. Catheterization and Cardiovascular Interventions: Official Journal of the Society for Cardiac Angiography & Interventions. 2008; 72(2): 166–75.
[6] Nissen SE, Yock P. Intravascular ultrasound novel pathophysiological insights and current clinical applications. Circulation. 2001; 103(4): 604–16.
[7] Kremkau FW. Physical principles of ultrasound. Seminars in Roentgenology. 1975; 10(4): 259–63.

[8] Katsarou O, Vavuranakis M. Basic Principles of Image Acquisition. Intravascular Imaging: Current Applications and Research Developments. IGI Global. 2011(1): 1–9.

[9] Mintz GS, Nissen SE, Anderson WD, *et al.* American College of Cardiology Clinical Expert Consensus Document on Standards for Acquisition, Measurement and Reporting of Intravascular Ultrasound Studies (IVUS). A report of the American College of Cardiology Task Force on Clinical Expert Consensus Documents. Journal of the American College of Cardiology. 2001;37(5): 1478–92.

[10] Katouzian A, Angelini ED, Carlier SG, Suri JS, Navab N, Laine AF. A state-of-the-art review on segmentation algorithms in intravascular ultrasound (IVUS) images. IEEE Transactions on Information Technology in Biomedicine: A Publication of the IEEE Engineering in Medicine and Biology Society. 2012; 16(5): 823–34.

[11] Tuzcu EM, Kapadia SR, Tutar E, *et al.* High prevalence of coronary atherosclerosis in asymptomatic teenagers and young adults. Evidence From Intravascular Ultrasound. 2001; 103(22): 2705–10.

[12] Aqel RA, Wells BJ, Hage FG, *et al.* Re-stenosis after drug-eluting stents in cardiac allograft vasculopathy. The Journal of Heart and Lung Transplantation. 2008;27(6): 610–5.

[13] Naka KK, Papamichael ND. Intravascular Image Interpretation. Intravascular Imaging: Current Applications and Research Developments. IGI Global. 2011(2): 10–35.

[14] Gupta R, Kaur H, Tiwari N. Denoising of Intravascular Ultrasound Images: A Comparative Study. International Journal of Emerging Technology and Advanced Engineering. 2014;4(4): 437–41.

[15] Michailovich OV, Tannenbaum A. Despeckling of medical ultrasound images. IEEE Transactions on Ultrasonics, Ferroelectrics, and Frequency Control. 2006;53(1): 64–78.

[16] Loizou CP, Pattichis CS, Christodoulou CI, Istepanian RSH, Pantziaris M, Nicolaides A. Comparative evaluation of despeckle filtering in ultrasound imaging of the carotid artery. IEEE Transactions on Ultrasonics, Ferroelectrics, and Frequency Control. 2005;52(10): 1653–69.

[17] Narayanan SK, Wahidabanu R. A View on Despeckling in Ultrasound Imaging. International Journal of Signal Processing, Image Processing and Pattern Recognition. 2009;2(3): 85–98.

[18] Loizou CP, Theofanous C, Pantziaris M, Kasparis T. Despeckle filtering software toolbox for ultrasound imaging of the common carotid artery. Computer Methods and Programs in Biomedicine. 2014;114(1): 109–24.

[19] Koga T, Uchino E, Suetake N, Hashimoto G, Hiro T, Matsuzaki M. Speckle noise reduction and edge-enhancement of coronary plaque tissue in intravascular ultrasound image by using anisotropic diffusion filter. International Journal of Circuits, System and Signal Processing. 2008;4(2): 239–48.

[20] Perona P, Malik J. Scale-space and edge detection using anisotropic diffusion. IEEE Transactions on Pattern Analysis and Machine Intelligence. 1990;12(7): 629–39.

[21] Gunjan. Despeckling of ultrasound images. IPASJ International Journal of Computer Science (IIJCS). 2013;1(2): 29–35.

[22] Vinita AC, Shrikant L. A review on image denoising techniques using wavelet transform methods. International Journal of Recent Development in Engineering and Technology. 2014;3(4):37–41.

[23] Katouzian A, Angelini E, Lorsakul A, Sturm B, Laine AF. Lumen Border Detection of Intravascular Ultrasound via Denoising of Directional Wavelet Representations. In: Ayache N, Delingette H, Sermesant M, editors. Functional Imaging and Modeling of the Heart: 5th International Conference, FIMH 2009, Nice, France, June 3–5, 2009 Proceedings. Berlin, Heidelberg: Springer Berlin Heidelberg; 2009. p. 104–13.

[24] Meyer FG, Coifman RR. Brushlets: a tool for directional image analysis and image compression. Applied and Computational Harmonic Analysis. 1997;4 (2): 147–87.

[25] Candès E, Demanet L, Donoho D, Ying L. Fast discrete curvelet transforms. Multiscale Modeling & Simulation. 2006;5(3): 861–99.

[26] Jean-Luc S, Candes EJ, Donoho DL. The curvelet transform for image denoising. IEEE Transactions on Image Processing. 2002;11(6): 670–84.

[27] Rizi FY, Setarehdan SK, editors. Noise reduction in intravascular ultrasound images using curvelet transform and adaptive complex diffusion filter: a comparative study. 20th Iranian Conference on Electrical Engineering (ICEE 2012); 2012 15–17 May 2012.

[28] Papadogiorgaki M, Mezaris V, Chatzizisis YS, Giannoglou GD, Kompatsiaris I. Image analysis techniques for automated IVUS contour detection. Ultrasound in Medicine & Biology. 2008;34(9): 1482–98.

[29] Herrington DM, Johnson T, Santago P, Snyder WE, editors. Semi-automated boundary detection for intravascular ultrasound. Computers in Cardiology 1992, Proceedings of; 1992: IEEE.

[30] Sonka M, Xiangmin Z, Siebes M, *et al.* Segmentation of intravascular ultrasound images: a knowledge-based approach. IEEE Transactions on Medical Imaging. 1995;14(4): 719–32.

[31] Li W, Birgelen CV, Mario CD, *et al.*, editors. Semi-automatic contour detection for volumetric quantification of intracoronary ultrasound. Computers in Cardiology 1994;1994: 25–28.

[32] von Birgelen C, Di Mario C, Li W, *et al.* Morphometric analysis in three-dimensional intracoronary ultrasound: an in vitro and in vivo study performed with a novel system for the contour detection of lumen and plaque. American Heart Journal. 1996;132(3): 516–27.

[33] Meier DS, Cothren RM, Vince DG, Cornhill JF. Automated morphometry of coronary arteries with digital image analysis of intravascular ultrasound. American Heart Journal. 1997;133(6): 681–90.

[34] Zhongchi L, Yuanyuan W, Weiqi W. Estimating coronary artery lumen area with optimization-based contour detection. IEEE Transactions on Medical Imaging. 2003;22(4): 564–6.

[35] Kass M, Witkin A, Terzopoulos D. Snakes: active contour models. International Journal of Computer Vision. 1988;1(4): 321–31.

[36] Lobregt S, Viergever MA. A discrete dynamic contour model. IEEE Transactions on Medical Imaging. 1995;14(1): 12–24.

[37] Kovalski G, Beyar R, Shofti R, Azhari H. Three-dimensional automatic quantitative analysis of intravascular ultrasound images. Ultrasound in Medicine & Biology. 2000;26(4): 527–37.

[38] Cohen LD. On active contour models and balloons. CVGIP: Image Underst. 1991;53(2): 211–8.

[39] Shekhar R, Cothren RM, Vince DG, Chandra S, Thomas JD, Cornhill JF. Three-dimensional segmentation of luminal and adventitial borders in serial intravascular ultrasound images. Computerized Medical Imaging and Graphics. 1999;23(6): 299–309.

[40] Klingensmith JD, Shekhar R, Vince DG. Evaluation of three-dimensional segmentation algorithms for the identification of luminal and medial-adventitial borders in intravascular ultrasound images. IEEE Transactions on Medical Imaging. 2000;19(10): 996–1011.

[41] Plissiti ME, Fotiadis DI, Michalis LK, Bozios GE. An automated method for lumen and media-adventitia border detection in a sequence of IVUS frames. IEEE Transactions on Information Technology in Biomedicine: A Publication of the IEEE Engineering in Medicine and Biology Society. 2004;8(2): 131–41.

[42] Gil D, Radeva P, Saludes J, Mauri J, editors. Automatic segmentation of artery wall in coronary IVUS images: a probabilistic approach. Computers in Cardiology 2000;2000: 2000.

[43] Taki A, Najafi Z, Roodaki A, *et al.* Automatic segmentation of calcified plaques and vessel borders in IVUS images. International Journal of Computer Assisted Radiology and Surgery. 2008;3(3): 347–54.

[44] Haas C, Ermert H, Holt S, Grewe P, Machraoui A, Barmeyer J. Segmentation of 3D intravascular ultrasonic images based on a random field model. Ultrasound in Medicine and Biology. 2000;26(2): 297–306.

[45] Brusseau E, Korte CLd, Mastik F, Schaar J, Steen AFWvd. Fully automatic luminal contour segmentation in intracoronary ultrasound imaging-a statistical approach. IEEE Transactions on Medical Imaging. 2004;23(5): 554–66.

[46] Cardinal MHR, Meunier J, Soulez G, Maurice RL, Therasse E, Cloutier G. Intravascular ultrasound image segmentation: a three-dimensional fast-marching method based on gray level distributions. IEEE Transactions on Medical Imaging. 2006;25(5): 590–601.

[47] Unal G, Bucher S, Carlier S, Slabaugh G, Fang T, Tanaka K. Shape-driven segmentation of the arterial wall in intravascular ultrasound images. IEEE Transactions on Information Technology in Biomedicine:

A Publication of the IEEE Engineering in Medicine and Biology Society. 2008;12(3): 335–47.

[48] Katouzian A, Baseri B, Konofagou EE, Laine AF. Automatic Detection of Blood Versus Non-Blood Regions on Intravascular Ultrasound (IVUS) Images Using Wavelet Packet Signatures. Proceedings of SPIE 6920, Medical Imaging; 2008.

[49] Garcia-Garcia HM, Costa MA, Serruys PW. Imaging of coronary atherosclerosis: intravascular ultrasound. European Heart Journal. 2010;31 (20): 2456–69.

[50] Zhang X, McKay CR, Sonka M. Tissue characterization in intravascular ultrasound images. IEEE Transactions on Medical Imaging. 1998;17(6): 889–99.

[51] Brunenberg E, Pujol O, ter Haar Romeny B, Radeva P. Automatic IVUS Segmentation of Atherosclerotic Plaque with Stop & Go Snake. In: Larsen R, Nielsen M, Sporring J, editors. Medical Image Computing and Computer-Assisted Intervention – MICCAI 2006: 9th International Conference, Copenhagen, Denmark, October 1–6, 2006 Proceedings, Part II. Berlin, Heidelberg: Springer Berlin Heidelberg; 2006. p. 9–16.

[52] Santos Filho E, Saijo Y, Tanaka A, Yoshizawa M. Detection and quantification of calcifications in intravascular ultrasound images by automatic thresholding. Ultrasound in Medicine & Biology. 2008;34(1): 160–5.

[53] Moghaddam RF, Cheriet M. AdOtsu: an adaptive and parameterless generalization of Otsu's method for document image binarization. Pattern Recognition. 2012;45(6): 2419–31.

[54] Zhang Q, Wang Y, Wang W, Ma J, Qian J, Ge J. Automatic segmentation of calcifications in intravascular ultrasound images using snakes and the contourlet transform. Ultrasound in Medicine & Biology. 2010;36(1): 111–29.

[55] Athanasiou LS, Karvelis PS, Tsakanikas VD, *et al.* A Novel semiautomated atherosclerotic plaque characterization method using grayscale intravascular ultrasound images: comparison with virtual histology. IEEE Transactions on Information Technology in Biomedicine. 2012;16(3): 391–400.

[56] König A, Klauss V. Virtual histology. Heart. 2007;93(8): 977–82.

[57] Athanasiou LS, Karvelis PS, Sakellarios AI, *et al.* A hybrid plaque characterization method using intravascular ultrasound images. Technology and Health Care. 2013;21(3): 199–216.

[58] Nair A, Kuban BD, Tuzcu EM, Schoenhagen P, Nissen SE, Vince DG. Coronary plaque classification with intravascular ultrasound radiofrequency data analysis. Circulation. 2002;106(17): 2200–6.

[59] Kawasaki M, Takatsu H, Noda T, *et al.* In vivo quantitative tissue characterization of human coronary arterial plaques by use of integrated backscatter intravascular ultrasound and comparison with angioscopic findings. Circulation. 2002;105(21): 2487–92.

[60] Sano K, Kawasaki M, Ishihara Y, *et al.* Assessment of vulnerable plaques causing acute coronary syndrome using integrated backscatter intravascular ultrasound. Journal of the American College of Cardiology. 2006;47(4): 734–41.

[61] Sathyanarayana S, Carlier S, Li W, Thomas L. Characterisation of atherosclerotic plaque by spectral similarity of radiofrequency intravascular ultrasound signals. EuroIntervention. 2009;5(1): 133–9.

[62] Okubo M, Kawasaki M, Ishihara Y, *et al.* Tissue characterization of coronary plaques comparison of integrated backscatter intravascular ultrasound with virtual histology intravascular ultrasound. Circulation Journal. 2008;72(10): 1631–9.

[63] Wahle A, Prause GPM, DeJong SC, Sonka M. 3-D Fusion of Biplane Angiography and Intravascular Ultrasound for Accurate Visualization and Volumetry. Proceedings of the First International Conference on Medical Image Computing and Computer-Assisted Intervention. 709600: Springer-Verlag; 1998. p. 146–55.

[64] Slager CJ, Wentzel JJ, Schuurbiers JCH, *et al.* True 3-dimensional reconstruction of coronary arteries in patients by fusion of angiography and IVUS (ANGUS) and its quantitative validation. Circulation. 2000; 102(5): 511–6.

[65] Bourantas CV, Kourtis IC, Plissiti ME, *et al.* A method for 3D reconstruction of coronary arteries using biplane angiography and intravascular ultrasound images. Computerized Medical Imaging and Graphics. 2005;29(8): 597–606.

[66] Wahle A, Olszewski ME, Sonka M. Interactive virtual endoscopy in coronary arteries based on multimodality fusion. IEEE Transactions on Medical Imaging. 2004;23(11): 1391–403.

[67] van der Giessen AG, Schaap M, Gijsen FJH, *et al.* 3D fusion of intravascular ultrasound and coronary computed tomography for in-vivo wall shear stress analysis: a feasibility study. The International Journal of Cardiovascular Imaging. 2010;26(7): 781–96.

[68] Ziada KM, Kapadia SR, Tuzcu EM, Nissen SE. The current status of intravascular ultrasound imaging. Current Problems in Cardiology. 1999;24(9): 541–616.

[69] Nakatani S, Proniewska K, Pociask E, *et al.* How clinically effective is intravascular ultrasound in interventional cardiology? Present and future perspectives. Expert Review of Medical Devices. 2013;10(6): 735–49.

[70] Bourantas CV, Garcia-Garcia HM, Naka KK, *et al.* Hybrid intravascular imaging current applications and prospective potential in the study of coronary atherosclerosis. Journal of the American College of Cardiology. 2013;61(13): 1369–78.

[71] Giannoglou GD, Antoniadis AP. Future Trends in 3D Intravascular Ultrasound (IVUS) Reconstruction. Intravascular Imaging: Current Applications and Research Developments. IGI Global. 2011.

[72] Carlier S, Didday R, Slots T, *et al.* A new method for real-time co-registration of 3D coronary angiography and intravascular ultrasound or optical coherence tomography. Cardiovascular Revascularization Medicine. 2014;15(4): 226–32.

[73] Li X, Wu W, Chung Y, *et al.* 80-MHz intravascular ultrasound transducer using PMN-PT free-standing film. IEEE Transactions on Ultrasonics, Ferroelectrics, and Frequency Control. 2011;58(11): 2281–8.

[74] Gurun G, Tekes C, Zahorian J, *et al.* Single-chip CMUT-on-CMOS front-end system for real-time volumetric IVUS and ICE imaging. IEEE Transactions on Ultrasonics, Ferroelectrics, and Frequency Control. 2014;61(2): 239–50.

Chapter 26

Introduction to speckle tracking in cardiac ultrasound imaging

Damien Garcia[1], Pierre Lantelme[1,2] and Éric Saloux[3]

In this chapter, we will first recall some basic principles of speckle tracking. The fundamentals of speckle tracking in a wider context are essentially described in Chapter 13. We will then treat speckle-tracking echocardiography and echocardiographic particle image velocimetry (echo-PIV) and indicate a number of clinical applications in the context of evaluation of cardiac function. We will then briefly introduce color Doppler approaches complementary to speckle tracking. We will finally present how speckle-tracking techniques could benefit from high-frame-rate echocardiography (also called "ultrafast echocardiography"). We will conclude with the expected contribution of high-frame-rate ultrasound for speckle tracking in three-dimensional (3-D) echocardiography.

26.1 Speckle formation and speckle tracking

The word "speckle" refers to the granular appearance of an image generated by a coherent imaging system, such as laser, optical coherence tomography, and ultrasound. As explained in detail in Chapter 2, speckles appear when a random collection of scatterers is illuminated by waves whose wavelength is larger than the size of the individual scatterers. The grainy aspect of a speckle pattern is produced by the multiple backscattered signals of similar frequency that interfere constructively and destructively, depending on their relative phases and amplitudes (Figure 26.1). In medical ultrasound imaging, as soft tissues contain many scatterers, the ultrasound waveforms detected by the transducer are the combination (interference) of the different wave reflections induced by the distinct scatterers. The resulting speckles are visible in the unfiltered gray-level (B-mode) images as dark and bright specks.

[1]INSERM. CREATIS, UMR 5220, U1206, Université de Lyon, INSA-Lyon, Université Claude Bernard Lyon 1, UJM-Saint Étienne, France
[2]Fédération de Cardiologie Croix-Rousse, Lyon-Sud, Hospices Civils de Lyon, Université de Lyon, France
[3]Department of Cardiology, CHU de Caen. EA 4650, SEILIRM, Université de Normandie, France

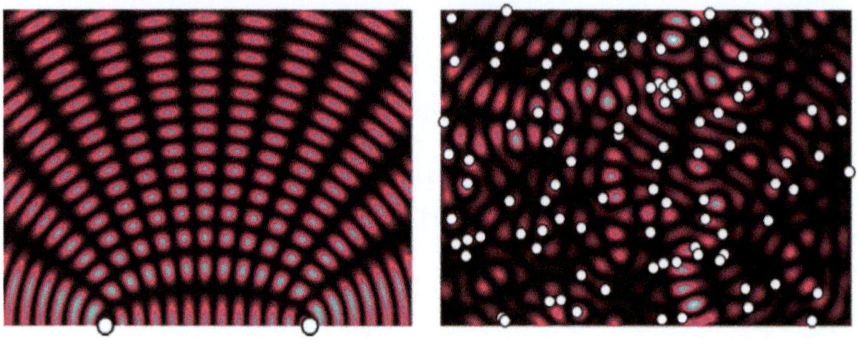

Figure 26.1 Speckle formation. Left: interferences produced by two scatterers. Right: speckles produced by the interference of backscattered waves generated by randomly distributed scatterers (white dots)

When the individual contributions of the scatterers are independent, the speckle patterns can be accurately modeled by various statistical distributions whose physical meanings have been thoroughly discussed in [1]. Chapter 3 also provides an overview of the statistical models introduced since the pioneering work of Burckhardt in 1978 [2]. Because medical ultrasound images are made exclusively of speckles, they can significantly affect visualization quality or postprocessing tasks, and in turn negatively impact the diagnostic potential of medical ultrasound [3]. Despeckling can thus be a necessary task in some specific imaging situations. This angle is a main theme of this handbook and is largely addressed in the chapters devoted to speckle filtering (i.e., part II). On the contrary, in the present chapter, we consider the speckle patterns as intrinsic signatures of the insonated medium. In such a case, these distinctive imprints must be sufficiently preserved from one frame to the next one to allow analysis of tissue dynamics through *speckle tracking*.

Speckle tracking for ultrasound imaging has been introduced by Trahey *et al.* [4], from Duke University, North Carolina, United States, to produce a blood flow velocity vector field in a human vein (Figure 26.2, left). Although it does not appear in the paper's references, it is likely that Trahey *et al.*'s approach has been influenced by two-dimensional (2-D) speckle velocimetry, a former speckle photography technique to measure 2-D velocity fields in unsteady flows [6]. Since then, speckle tracking in medical ultrasound imaging has been the subject of a yearly increasing number of investigations (Figure 26.3), mainly in the field of myocardial strain imaging (deformation imaging of the cardiac muscle). Another strong interest for speckle tracking later emerged in contrast echocardiography (cardiac ultrasound imaging with contrast agents) to display 2-D blood velocity vector fields in the cardiac left ventricular cavity, a technique often called "echocardiographic particle image velocimetry" (or echo-PIV). The following paragraphs will describe these two common applications of speckle tracking in cardiac ultrasound imaging. Although strain imaging and echo-PIV are also of interest in ultrasound vascular imaging, the vascular field will not be discussed in the present chapter. We invite the

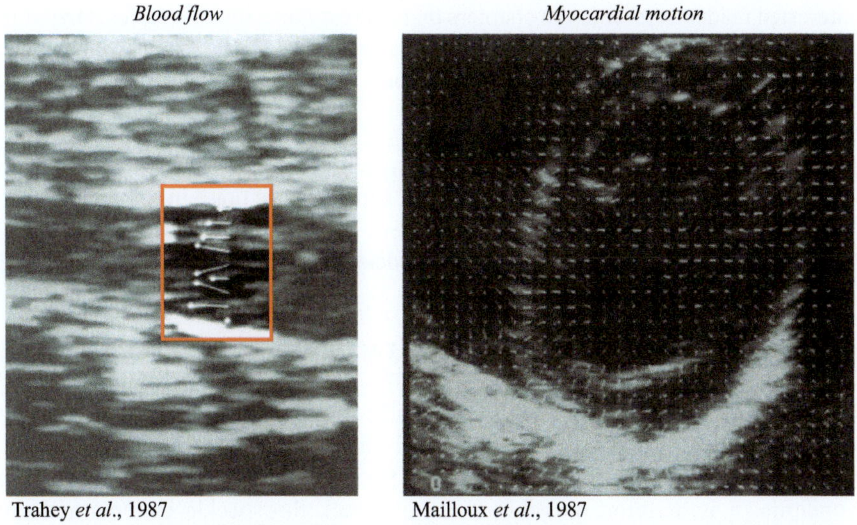

Figure 26.2 First applications of speckle tracking. Left: Venous blood velocity profile obtained with a cross-correlation-based block-matching approach [4]. Right: Myocardial motion from a global Horn–Schunck optical flow method [5]

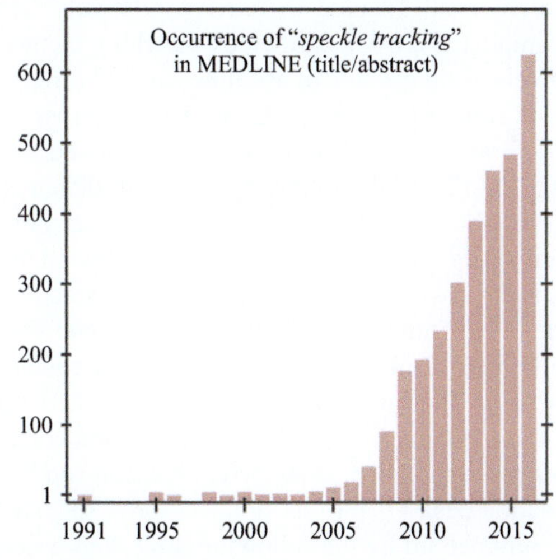

Figure 26.3 Yearly occurrence of "speckle tracking" in abstracts and/or titles of MEDLINE-referred papers. The first occurrence of "speckle tracking" is in [7]

interested reader to refer to the chapters that address these specific topics. One of the reasons for focusing on cardiac imaging is that speckle tracking is mostly used clinically in the context of cardiac evaluation.

In summary—Speckles are issued from the interference of the wave reflections induced by the tissue scatterers. Although considered as noise in some imaging applications, speckle patterns also represent local signatures of the insonified tissues. These speckles can be tracked to determine frame-to-frame motion.

26.2 Basic principles of speckle tracking

As explained earlier, speckles can be considered as acoustic markers of the insonified tissues. In a time series of ultrasound images, these markers are sufficiently preserved from one frame to the next if the frame rate is high enough. In this latter condition, it is therefore possible to locally track the speckle patterns and thus deduce the local tissue displacements with a frame-wise approach as explained in detail in Part III. For example, in the current clinical practice, a frame rate of 50–80 frames/s is recommended to obtain optimal conditions for speckle tracking in the resting heart [8]. Ultrasound speckles can be tracked frame to frame by various approaches, such as differential optical-flow methods [9,10] or block-matching algorithms [10–12]. A block-matching algorithm is a method used to estimate motion in a video sequence by locating similar blocks between two successive images. It is generally well adapted to retrieve relatively large frame-to-frame displacements. A simple though standard block-matching method is to compare the intensities of the pixels using the sum of absolute/squared differences measure [13]. Among a number of similarity criteria, the normalized cross-correlation was historically the first [7], and is still one of the most applied methods, in medical ultrasound imaging [14–17]. In the following, although different similarity criteria can be used, we thus focus on the normalized cross-correlation without loss of generality. The normalized cross-correlation can be evaluated directly in the spatial domain by using small subwindows in one frame, and search areas of larger size in a subsequent frame [18]. Another possibility is to calculate the normalized cross-correlation in the Fourier domain (Figure 26.4), a consequence of the Wiener–Khinchin theorem [19]. The latter approach is often called "phase correlation" [20]. The peak location of the normalized cross-correlation corresponds to the local displacement with a pixel precision. A subpixel precision can be returned from 2-D fitting of the correlation peak [19]. In its simplest form, speckle tracking by cross-correlation can be summed up by the following three-step process: (1) division of two successive B-mode images into small subwindows, (2) normalized cross-correlation of the subwindow pairs, and (3) peak fitting and estimation of the displacements. In the Fourier domain (phase correlation), it boils down to the following steps (see also Figure 26.4):

Let I_1 and I_2 represent two successive gray-level B-mode images. These two images are both subdivided into evenly-spaced subwindows of size $(m \times n)$, w_1^k and

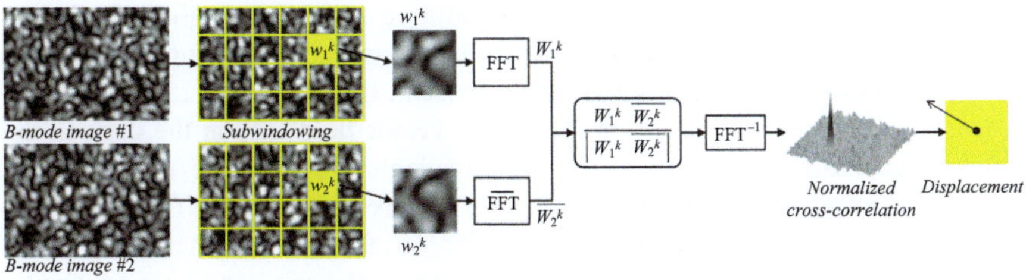

Figure 26.4 Speckle tracking using the normalized cross-correlation implemented in the Fourier domain. This block-matching scheme can be generalized with other similarity criteria, such as the SAD or SSD (sum of absolute/squared differences)

w_2^k, with $k = 1 \ldots M$, M denoting the total number of subwindows. Size and overlap of the subwindows must be adapted to adjust the precision/accuracy compromise, as well as the resolution of the output displacement field. Let $\boldsymbol{W}_1^k = \mathscr{F}\left(w_1^k\right)$ and $\boldsymbol{W}_1^k = \mathscr{F}\left(w_1^k\right)$ be the 2-D Fourier transforms of two paired subwindows. The Fast Fourier Transform (FFT)-based normalized cross-correlation for each subwindow k is given by

$$\mathrm{NCC}^k = \mathscr{F}^{-1}\left(\frac{\boldsymbol{w}_1^k \overline{\boldsymbol{w}_2^k}}{\left|\boldsymbol{w}_1^k \overline{\boldsymbol{w}_2^k}\right|}\right).$$

The inverse Fourier transform is denoted by $\mathscr{F}^{-1}$, and the overbar denotes the complex conjugate. The divisions and multiplications are elementwise. The relative translation (Δi^k, Δj^k) between the two subwindows w_1^k and w_2^k is given by the location of the peak in NCC^k:

$$\left(\Delta i^k, \Delta j^k\right) = \arg\max_{(i,j)}\left(\mathrm{NCC}^k\right)$$

To determine the translation with subpixel accuracy, a simple and robust method is to fit the correlation peak to some function, such as a paraboloid or Gaussian surface [19]. The displacement vectors in standard units are finally deduced by knowing the pixel size.

The phase correlation is only one approach for speckle tracking among a large variety of template-matching methods; it was here described in its most basic form. Part III provides a broader overview of the principles of speckle tracking. More advanced numerical methods exist in the technical literature devoted to image registration or optical PIV. Just to name a few for cross-correlation, these methods include ensemble cross-correlation, coarse-to-fine analysis, and interrogation subwindow deformations [19]. Other algorithms can also be found, for example, in the families of differential optical flow [9,21,22], nonrigid transformation [23,24], and point matching [25–27]. Yet, speckle tracking in medical ultrasound imaging is traditionally associated with cross-correlation, likely for historical and expedient reasons. On a final note, regardless of the approach used to track the speckles, robust postprocessing of the raw displacements is essential if differential quantities must be derived (e.g., strains, shears), as required in strain imaging. Such post-processing can include replacement of incorrect data and smoothing of the vector field. To this effect, advanced algorithms exist in the literature [28,29,16]. Post-processing has a major impact on the output vector field and on the derived differential quantities. In the commercially available workstations for ultrasound speckle tracking, postprocessing is hidden in "black boxes" and differs from vendor to vendor. As discussed later, intervendor variability is the main reason why global longitudinal strain (GLS) is the only myocardial strain parameter which may be used in routine clinical practice [30].

In summary—Numerous algorithms have been derived for speckle tracking in ultrasound imaging. Both local and global techniques have been introduced. One of the most used approaches is local block matching based on the measure of the normalized cross-correlation.

26.3 Speckle-tracking echocardiography

The vast majority of the "speckle tracking" references included in the MEDLINE database (Medical Literature Analysis and Retrieval System Online, National Library of Medicine—National Institutes of Health) are devoted to the motion analysis of the left ventricular myocardium (Figure 26.5). This trend has emerged naturally since echocardiography is the main clinical imaging modality for the evaluation of cardiac function. As the temporal resolution of echocardiography became satisfactory through the 1980s, there was an increasing interest in the quantitative analysis of the myocardium movement, since its visual evaluation was subjective and thus highly operator-dependent. In particular, the first thorough

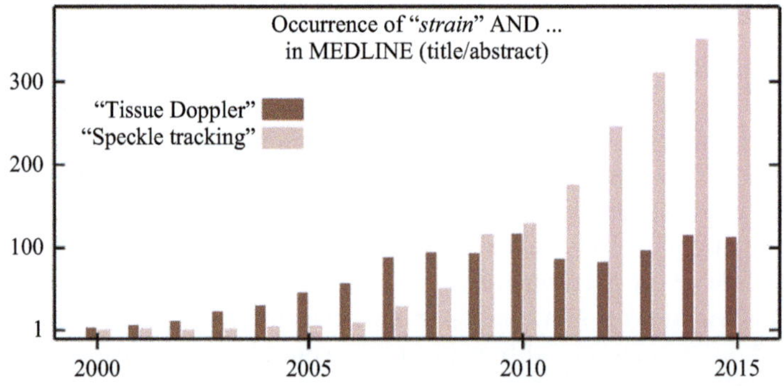

Figure 26.5 "Tissue Doppler" vs. "speckle tracking" for strain imaging. Yearly occurrence of [("tissue Doppler " or "speckle tracking") and "strain"] in abstracts and/or titles of MEDLINE-referred papers

investigations worth mentioning are those of Mailloux *et al.*, from École Polytechnique de Montréal, Canada [5,9]. In their studies, the authors estimated the cardiac motion field in a short-axis view (i.e., a cross-sectional slice of the heart, see right picture in Figure 26.2) by tracking the speckle patterns automatically using the Horn–Schunck's global optical flow method [31]. Later on, block-matching schemes have been preferred and are now parts of commercial software [32,33]. Speckle tracking, in and of itself, returns local displacements and/or velocities and thus truly characterizes wall motion. To distinguish active myocardial motion from passive translational or tethering movements, physicians have preferably examined the regional deformations, mostly by estimating regional strains and strain rates. This echocardiographic modality for regional deformation imaging is referred to as "strain imaging." Strain (deformation) and strain rates (rate of deformation) can be derived from the spatial derivatives of the displacements and velocities, respectively. Strain (rate) imaging originated from tissue Doppler [34–36], an echocardiographic technique that uses the Doppler mode to measure the velocities of the cardiac muscle (myocardium). Although tissue Doppler was the first modality of choice for cardiac strain imaging, speckle tracking in gray-scale 2-D images has then become the standard procedure since 2010 (Figure 26.5). In particular, a strong interest in cardiac speckle tracking has been demonstrated in cardiac resynchronization therapy [37]. When speckle tracking is used in cardiac imaging, strain imaging is commonly referred to as "speckle-tracking echocardiography." The advantages of speckle tracking over tissue Doppler for myocardial strain imaging have been the subject of key handbooks and review papers [38–40]. To enumerate a few: speckle tracking is angle independent, offers better spatial and temporal resolutions, and is less sensitive to noise. In this chapter, we do not dwell upon this particular point.

Over the last 10 years, a number of clinical software tools and algorithms have been marketed by different vendors for speckle-tracking echocardiography. The access of speckle-tracking echocardiography presented a new opportunity for a better evaluation of the heart function. Numerous clinical studies show that speckle-tracking echocardiography can provide complementary quantification of regional and global cardiac function. More specifically, speckle-tracking echocardiography offers a unique insight into the impairment of the left ventricular function. Some of its main areas of clinical application are [41]: detection of subclinical myocardial dysfunction, diagnosis of ischemia and location of myocardial infarction, risk stratification in cardiomyopathy, prediction of the response to cardiac resynchronization therapy, assessment of the systolic and diastolic dysfunctions, evaluation of myocardial mechanics in heart failure, follow-up after heart valve surgery. Readers interested in a detailed portrayal of the clinical applications of speckle-tracking echocardiography are referred to recent clinical review papers [41–43]. Despite its broad clinical appeal over the last decade (Figure 26.5) and the numerous studies described in high-impact journals, no clear consensus has yet been reached to standardize left ventricular strain imaging [8]. The main reason for this reluctance has been the significant variability in regional strains, which is observed among the software packages. Intervendor inconsistencies stem from different causes: (1) speckle tracking is dependent upon the image characteristics, which differ across ultrasound scanners; (2) divergences in the terminology describing the myocardial mechanics are also noted; and (3) finally, and it is likely the primary source of discordances, the software packages use proprietary algorithms for pre- and postprocessing, speckle tracking, and data regularization. To complicate matters, whether the whole process is more or less unsupervised can also affect interoperator reproducibility [8,30]. As a consequence, the current echocardiographic guidelines do not recommend quantitative measures of regional deformation, despite the strong clinical interest of strain imaging. Conceding the critical necessity for consistencies in speckle-tracking echocardiography, leaders of the European Association of Cardiovascular Imaging and the American Society of Echocardiography have invited technical representatives from several industrial partners to cooperate with a view to reducing intervendor variability in strain imaging [8,44]. The main conclusion from this task force is that global longitudinal strain (GLS) is the most robust deformation parameter and is presently the only myocardial strain parameter which may be safely used in routine clinical practice [30]. GLS is a diagnostic and prognostic marker of the global left ventricular systolic function, which can be measured clinically by speckle-tracking echocardiography [45]. It reflects the relative longitudinal contraction (in %) of the left ventricular myocardium (Figure 26.6). The instantaneous GLS (in %) can be written as $\mathrm{GLS}(t) = 100\ [L(t) - L(\mathrm{ED})]/L(\mathrm{ED})$, where $L(t)$ is the longitudinal myocardial length at time t, and $L(\mathrm{ED})$ is the length at end-diastole. The GLS peak is around −20% in normal subjects [46]. Speckle-tracking echocardiography will receive a renewed resurgence of interest if manufacturers can match their regional strains. A plan of action will consist in comparing echo-derived strains with local strains determined by sonomicrometry in an *in vitro* phantom [47] which reproduces myocardial shortening, torsion, and contraction (lengthening, untwisting, and dilation) during systole (diastole).

In summary—Speckle-tracking echocardiography has supplanted tissue Doppler for strain (rate) imaging. Although speckle-tracking echocardiography was first designed to determine regional deformations, it was found that substantial intervendor variability prevents its use in routine clinical practice. It followed that the GLS is presently the only myocardial strain parameter which may be safely used. Speckle-tracking echocardiography, which is a local tool, is thus constrained to limit itself to global assessment.

26.4 Clinical utility of global longitudinal strain in speckle-tracking echocardiography

Assessment of global left ventricular systolic function plays a key role in the prognosis of cardiac diseases. The most widely used parameter is the left ventricular ejection fraction, commonly determined by echocardiography.

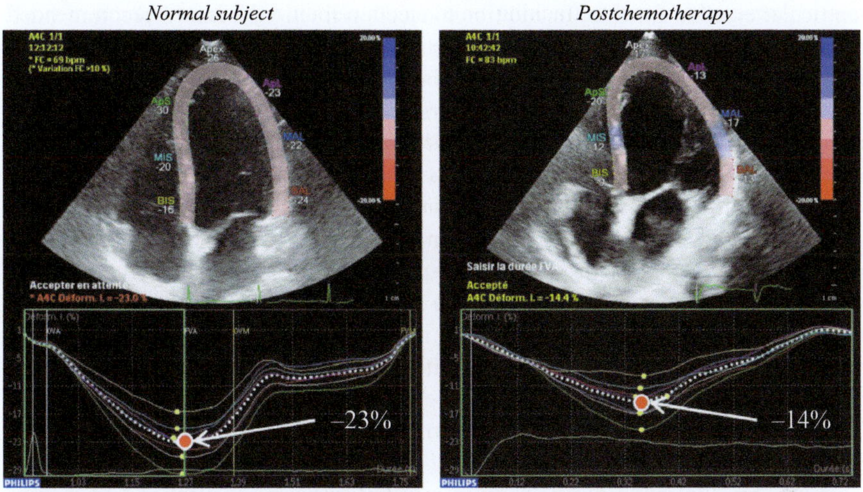

Figure 26.6 *Global longitudinal strain. The global longitudinal strains (GLS) are represented by the white dotted curves. The colored ribbons represent the regional longitudinal strains, here in the four-chamber view. In the normal subject, the peak GLS is −23%, which reflects a normal systolic function. In the patient after chemotherapy, the peak GLS is −14%, which denotes a reduced systolic function due to cardiotoxicity*

Left ventricular ejection fraction represents the amount of blood leaving the left ventricle each time it contracts. An ejection fraction of 60% means that 60% of the total amount of blood within the left ventricle is pumped out with each heartbeat. A normal ejection fraction is between 50% and 70%. It can be calculated by delineating the endocardium in 2-D echo images, at both end diastole and end systole [48]. Although widely used, left ventricular ejection fraction has a number of important limitations in assessing systolic function and can offer a poor prognosis in many situations. In comparison, the prognostic value of the abovementioned GLS is recognized to be superior [45] since GLS is more sensitive to detect subtle changes in myocardial function (Figure 26.6). In addition, some cardiomyopathies can be marked by a reduced GLS although the ejection fraction is preserved. We here briefly describe the clinical utility of GLS in a few clinical contexts.

Cardiotoxicity in chemotherapy—Breast cancer is the principal type of cancer in women. Chemotherapeutic treatments (administration of anticancer drugs) increase rate of cure and reduce relapse significantly. Chemotherapy, however, is limited by the risk of cardiotoxicity, which can appear early in the treatment and may induce irreversible heart failure if not detected subclinically. Treatment must be promptly discontinued or modified before the onset of observable symptoms related to cardiotoxicity. Cardiac dysfunction induced by chemotherapy is commonly diagnosed through echocardiographic examination, primarily on the basis of the left ventricular ejection fraction. In addition to ejection fraction, it is now recommended to measure GLS [49], as an early reduction in GLS (Figure 26.6) may help to diagnose subclinical systolic dysfunction before a drop in ejection fraction [50,51].

Aortic stenosis—Aortic stenosis refers to narrowing of the aortic valve opening, which restricts blood ejection [52]. The most common cause is senile calcification of the valve cusps, making the valve stiff and obstructive. If the stenosis is severe, the aortic valve must be replaced surgically or transcutaneously. Timing for replacement is decided through the presence of symptoms, the severity of the stenosis, and its impact on the left ventricular volume. A substantial reduction in ejection fraction may denote irreversible damage of the myocardium. Left ventricular GLS has been shown to provide incremental prognosis in aortic stenosis and to predict mortality in patients with preserved ejection fraction [53,54]. Incorporation of GLS into the echocardiographic parameters for the assessment of aortic stenosis may thus improve the determination of the optimal timing for aortic valve replacement [55].

Coronary artery disease and myocardial infarction—Peak GLS is significantly impaired in patients with myocardial infarction and correlates with infarct size [56,57]. A significantly reduced GLS (<15%; the normal value being 20%) has also been shown to be an independent predictor of sudden cardiac death after acute myocardial infarction, even if left ventricular ejection fraction is preserved [58,59]. GLS impairment can also be effectively used to detect non-obstructive coronary heart disease [60], and subclinical left ventricular systolic dysfunction in patients with obstructive coronary heart disease [61].

Left ventricular GLS derived by speckle tracking has also been shown to be clinically relevant in terms of prognosis in patients with hypertrophic cardiomyopathy [62], mitral valve regurgitation [63], and aortic regurgitation [64]. On one final note, the GLS is also of clinical value in evaluation of right ventricular function [65].

In summary—Left ventricular ejection fraction has long been the most essential parameter for global assessment of left ventricular function. However, GLS might have a better prognostic value in a variety of cardiac conditions. Left ventricular ejection fraction and GLS are thus complementary clinical indices of cardiac function. Because GLS has been shown to be reproducible despite intervendor variability in strain imaging, it is likely that GLS will be soon part of the routinely measured parameters during an echocardiographic examination.

26.5 Echocardiographic particle image velocimetry (Echo-PIV)

When speckle tracking is applied to contrast-enhanced blood images, the technique is generally called "echo-PIV," the short name for "echocardiographic particle image velocimetry" [66]. Echo-PIV is an adaptation of optical PIV, a commonly used indirect technique for measuring two or three velocity components in experimental fluid dynamics [67]. In some way, echo-PIV is a resurgence of speckle velocimetry [6], from which optical PIV emerged. In optical PIV, two sequential laser pulses illuminate a slice or volume of a flow seeded with microscopic light-scattering particles. The scattered light is recorded in two successive images by digital camera(s). These images are subdivided into small areas for calculating the mean particle displacement between two corresponding subareas using block-matching techniques (as in Figure 26.4). Knowing the lag between two laser pulses, the particle velocities can be thus determined [68]. Since visible laser lights are used, optical PIV requires transparent experimental setups. With the objective of obtaining velocity vector fields in the blood circulation, optical PIV was adapted to ultrasound imaging [7,69,70] to become echo-PIV. In echo-PIV, well-established speckle-tracking methods (such as block matching through normalized cross-correlation, see Section 26.2) are applied on contrast-enhanced B-mode images obtained during intravenous administration of gas-filled microbubbles (contrast agents). Ultrasound contrast agents are made of gas encapsulated in a hydrophilic shell. Their mean size (<6 μm) is less than the diameter of the pulmonary and systemic capillaries they must transit when delivered intravenously [71]. In contrast to optical PIV where Mie scattering dominates, Rayleigh scattering governs echo-PIV. In other words, while optical PIV generates images of the particles, echo-PIV does not produce images of the microbubbles but images of the interferences (speckles). Echo-PIV has been successfully used to investigate the carotid blood flow [72,73]. As with strain imaging, however, echo-PIV has spread clinically in transthoracic echocardiography, the most common application being the quantitative analysis of the main intraventricular vortex (Figure 26.7) for a better evaluation of left ventricular cardiac function [74–76], as clarified in the next section.

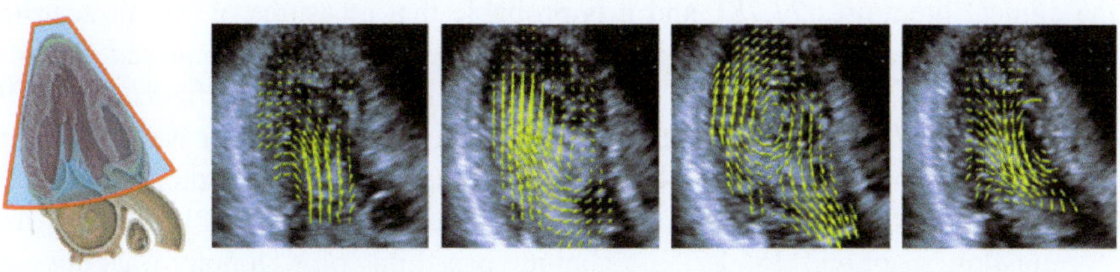

Figure 26.7 Echo-PIV in the left ventricle. Echo-PIV makes it possible to decipher and quantify the dynamics of the vortex that forms in the left ventricle during left ventricular filling. Tracking of the intraventricular microbubbles were here carried out in a three-chamber view. Dynamical properties of this vortex are potential biomarkers of the diastolic function. Courtesy of Pr. Y.J. Moon, School of Mechanical Engineering, Korea University

In summary—Echo-PIV is a promising tool to decipher the blood flow dynamics within the left ventricle. It requires administration of gas-filled microbubbles to enhance the blood signal for blood speckle tracking, which may prevent its routine clinical applicability.

26.6 Potential clinical utility of vortex flow imaging in echo-PIV

Left ventricular diastole refers to blood filling of the left ventricle. An accurate assessment of left ventricular diastolic function is of utmost clinical importance in patients with dyspnea (shortness of breath) or heart failure. Heart failure occurs when the heart muscle is weakened and is unable to pump enough blood to meet the body's needs for metabolites and oxygen. Among these patients, about half of them have normal or nearly normal left ventricular ejection fraction. Diagnosis of diastolic dysfunction can be ambiguous since patient's history, physical examination, electrocardiogram, or chest X-ray is frequently unhelpful. The wide accessibility of echocardiography, as well as its ability to provide real-time information, makes ultrasound the prerequisite technique for evaluating left ventricular diastolic function. However, current echocardiographic indices of diastolic function have major limitations that may hinder accurate diagnosis. Recent studies suggest that a deeper look at the intraventricular flow during filling can improve diastology (assessment of diastolic function) by echocardiography [77,78]. The intraventricular flow dynamics is indeed much richer during diastole (filling phase) than during ejection. Diastole of the left ventricle is featured by the formation of a wide whirling motion (vortex) which originates during early filling [79]. In the normal heart, most of the left ventricular intracavitary blood volume is involved in the vortical pattern [80]. Clinical observations in patients and normal subjects indicate that the diastolic intraventricular blood vortices have particular shapes and locations, which can be biomarkers of the cardiac function [74,80,81–83]. Characterization of the intraventricular vortex flow by echocardiography is becoming increasingly popular in the clinical literature [77,78], and it is probable that measures of the intracardiac vortex hemodynamics can play a key role in the assessment of cardiac function (Figure 26.7). Vortex formation in the normal left ventricle was first outlined by Rodevand *et al.* who interpreted intraventricular color Doppler velocities and pulsed-wave Doppler spectra [84]. The two predominant echocardiographic tools for vector flow imaging within the left ventricle are now echo-PIV [85,76] and "vector flow mapping" [86,87], a technique based on color Doppler imaging (see Section 26.7). Figure 26.7 shows how echo-PIV can disclose the vortex formation in the left ventricle.

Since vortex flow imaging by ultrasound imaging is a very recent technique, no clear clinical conclusion has yet been reached on the vortical parameters that must be preferably determined (size, vorticity, circulation, energy, elongation, time, location ...) to improve the assessment of cardiac function. *In vivo* research on this topic is exploratory, and the pathophysiological relevance of intraventricular fluid dynamics still needs to be demonstrated in large cohorts. In addition, only a very few teams have investigated the potential clinical relevance of vortex flow imaging by echo-PIV, so that intergroup reproducibility has not yet been explored. However, it appears that diastole has to be more than a mere passive suction: the dynamics of the diastolic vortex has a key physiological impact on left ventricular filling. Blood flow keeps swirling in late diastole and maintains momentum during the isovolumetric contraction phase [88]. This avoids any period of blood flow stasis and helps coupling filling phase to ejection phase. Broadly speaking, the diastolic vortex can be seen as a primer of the cardiac pump. This diastole-to-systole dynamical coupling has been shown to be suboptimal in patients with heart failure and reduced left ventricular ejection fraction [89]. In line with these observations, echo-PIV investigation in patients with acute myocardial infarction revealed a progressive decline in vortex flow dynamics as left ventricular dysfunction develops [90]. Vortex geometry and dynamics, as well as intraventricular blood transport, have also been shown to be modified after left ventricular remodeling, i.e., after changes in cardiac size and shape [74,76,91]. We invite the reader to consult recent review papers for a clinical survey of intraventricular flow imaging by echocardiography [76–78,92]. The principal clinical limitation of echo-PIV is the requirement of intravenous administration of microbubbles. Although no major side effect has been noticed, this procedure is time and staff consuming and thus cannot be recommended in routine clinical practice. To put an end to this obstacle, Fadnes *et al.* introduced a contrast-free procedure to track the native speckles of blood [93]. This speckle-tracking tool was shown to offer better visualization and quantification of septal defect—a congenital heart disease in which there is an opening in the septum—in neonates [94]. It has been proposed in the context of high-frame-rate echocardiography (see Section 26.8) and adapted for transthoracic echocardiographic in the adults (Figure 26.8).

In summary—The physiological and pathophysiological implications of intraventricular fluid dynamics are still being prospected. Its analysis by echo-PIV can bring additional insights into the echocardiographic evaluation of diastolic function. As was (and still is) the case for speckle-tracking echocardiography, large-scale clinical trials are required to demonstrate the significance of echo-PIV in terms of cost effectiveness and clinical outcomes before being accepted as a standard echocardiographic examination.

26.7 Color Doppler as an alternative or complementary to speckle tracking

As shown in Figure 26.5, tissue Doppler had been the most frequent method for strain and strain rate imaging before 2010. One key advantage of tissue Doppler is

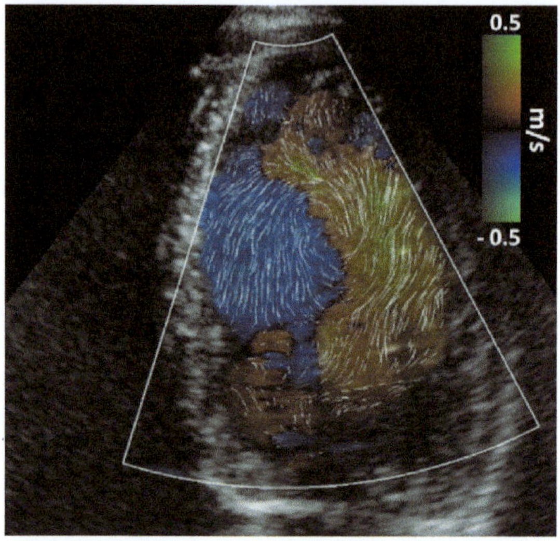

Figure 26.8 Contrast-agent-free echo-PIV overlaid on color Doppler. Intraventricular vortex revealed by speckle tracking without administration of contrast agent. It was overlaid on color Doppler to make the flow visualization easier (red ¼ towards the probe, blue ¼ away from the probe). Courtesy of Pr. Lasse Løvstakken, Norwegian University of Science and Technology

that it directly yields Eulerian velocities of myocardial or blood tissues. One main drawback is its angle dependency since Doppler modes return the axial velocity components, i.e., the components parallel to the ultrasound beam axes [40]. Speckle tracking thus logically imposed itself as the superior method for motion analysis of the left ventricle. Likewise, as discussed in the previous section, speckle tracking has become the most accepted technique for investigation of the intraventricular blood flow. To work around the one-dimensional issue of color Doppler, multi-Doppler approaches have been developed. By registering two series of color Doppler images acquired with significantly different steering angles, Arigovindan *et al.* produced long-axis motion fields of the left ventricular myocardium [95]. Gomez *et al.* then generalized this method [96,97] and proposed a time-resolved volumetric reconstruction of the intraventricular flow from volumetric color Doppler images (Figure 26.9, left picture). Postprocessing of conventional color Doppler images has also been proposed to retrieve 2-D intraventricular vector fields in apical long-axis views [86,98]. The vector flow mapping technique introduced by Garcia *et al.* (Figure 26.9, right picture) is now implemented in a commercially available ultrasound machine [99] and has been the basic tool for a number of clinical pilot studies [87,100]. Another very promising strategy consists in combining the better of the two worlds in an optimization problem [101–103]. Since this approach requires both color/tissue Doppler and B-mode, it will be best suited for high-frame-rate ultrasound imaging. With the advent of high-frame-rate echocardiography

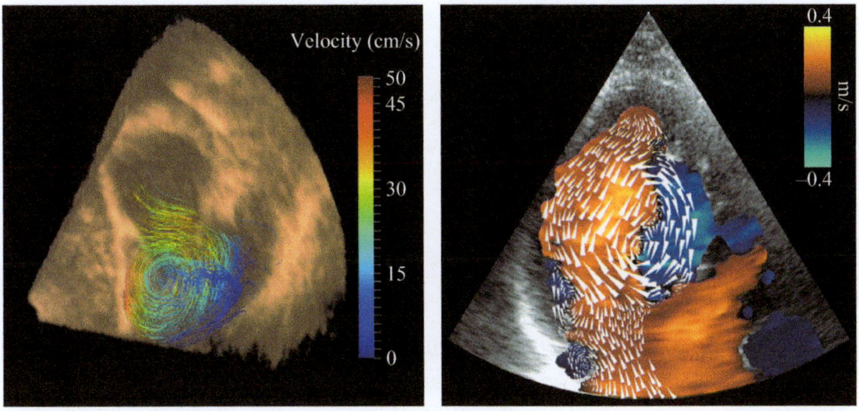

Figure 26.9 Intraventricular flow dynamics from color Doppler. Formation of a wide vortex in the left ventricle. Left: Intraventricular volumetric blood flow obtained by registration of several volumetric color Doppler images. Courtesy of Alberto Gomez, King's College of London, UK [96]. Right: Intraventricular vector flow mapping obtained by postprocessing conventional color Doppler images (single steering) using a regularized least-squares method. Adapted from [86]

(see Section 26.8), improvements in motion detection can be expected by getting both color/tissue Doppler and B-mode images in a single heart beat at high frame rates [104]. By using advanced and robust algorithms, the inter-software variability may ultimately become small enough to allow accurate estimation of regional deformations.

In summary—Color Doppler can be combined to speckle tracking to improve motion tracking. Although this assertion remains speculative, some evidence of such potential improvement has been reported in the recent literature.

26.8 Potential benefits of high-frame-rate echocardiography

Conventional echocardiography consists in scanning the heart using a series of successive focused beams (typically 64 to 128) that cover the sector of interest (see Figure 26.10, leftmost picture). The resulting scanlines are then stacked together to reconstruct a single image. The time required to build one frame is thus proportional to the number of gathered lines. Since the acoustic waves must travel down to the maximal depth then come back to the probe at the speed of ~1,540 m/s, wave travel time is roughly 0.2 ms in adult echocardiography (when considering a maximal range of 15 cm). For a wide sector containing 100 scanlines, the frame

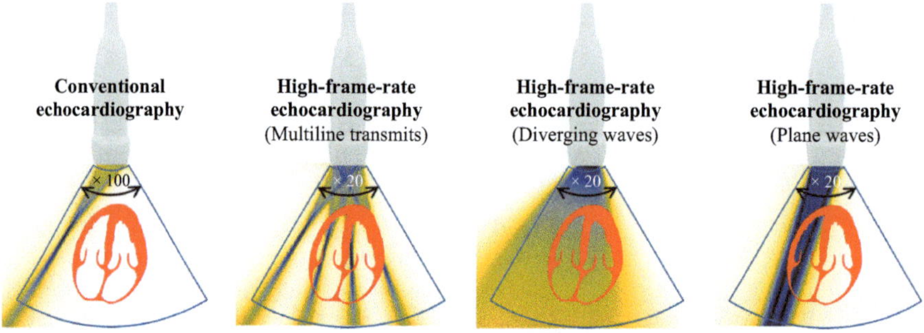

Figure 26.10 Conventional vs. High-frame-rate echocardiography. Conventional echocardiography requires ∼100 scanlines to produce a wide-sector cardiac image. High-frame-rate echocardiography can provide a 5-fold increase in frame rate without deteriorating image quality significantly. See also [105]

rate is thus around 50. Parallel computing, high-performance data transfer and high-speed processors have recently changed ultrasound imaging drastically [105–107]. Instead of transmitting a series of successive focused emissions (Figure 26.10, leftmost picture), large planar or circular wavefronts (Figure 26.10, third and fourth pictures) can be emitted to insonify wide regions. Alternatively, several focused beams can be transmitted simultaneously (Figure 26.10, second picture). The radiofrequency echoes are acquired all together by each element to reconstruct an image in postprocessing, which offers high-frame-rate (or ultrafast) ultrasound imaging. In comparison with conventional echocardiography, it has been shown in normal subjects that high-frame-rate echocardiography can provide a 5-fold increase in frame rate without deteriorating image quality significantly [108,104].

In the current clinical practice, a useful rule of thumb is that the frame rate must be roughly equal to the heart rate to yield optimal conditions for speckle-tracking echocardiography. In some echocardiographic examinations, such as during the evaluation and management of coronary artery disease, it can be clinically relevant to increase the heart rate, a technique called "stress echocardiography." It consists in scanning a patient during a cardiac stress induced by exercise (treadmill or bicycle) or by administration of a pharmacological stressor. The images acquired before and after stress are compared to detect the presence of regions with abnormal wall motion [109]. Dobutamine is a widely available stressor which increases heart rate up to 120–140 beats per minute. In a stressed myocardium, the mechanical events become shorter; the acquisition frame rate thus should be increased proportionally with the heart rate (>100 frames per second) according to the abovementioned rule of thumb. Acquiring the whole left ventricular myocardium at such high frame rates can be very challenging with the conventional imaging systems [110]. The physicians have several stratagems to increase the frame rate, decrease imaging depth, narrow sector size, and reduce line density. However, this is obviously at the expense of image quality, which can make speckle tracking difficult or impossible. Speckle-tracking echocardiography under dobutamine-induced stress could thus benefit from high-frame-rate ultrasound imaging, where frame rates greater than 250 with well-preserved speckles have been reported in the left ventricle [104]. Up to now, most of the speckle-tracking echocardiography studies have been devoted to single cardiac chamber (mostly the left ventricle), for several practical reasons. A recent study performed in normal subjects, however, illustrates that simultaneous measurement of longitudinal strains in all four cardiac chambers could provide new insights into inter-chamber functional relationships [111]. Since simultaneous 4-chamber strain requires both large depth and width, it is very likely that high-frame-rate echocardiography can also enlarge the spectrum of its applications. Note finally that the frame-rate limitation is also especially true with echo-PIV, even in the resting heart, since greater displacements (intraventricular blood flow) must be measured. In conventional echo-PIV, the frame rate can be increased through decreasing depth and narrowing sector. Echo-PIV could thus take advantage of high-frame-rate echocardiography. An example to this effect is given in Figure 26.8.

In summary—High-frame-rate echocardiography is an emerging modality in clinical imaging. It can provide very high frame rates without degrading image quality significantly. Dobutamine stress echocardiography or full-heart strain imaging may profit from this innovative imaging method.

26.9 Toward volumetric speckle-tracking echocardiography

3-D echocardiography is a recent and major innovation in cardiac ultrasound. It is a volumetric method of visualizing the dynamic anatomy and function of the heart. Over the last years, there has been a steady stream of fundamental and clinical publications on 3-D echocardiography [112]. One can safely advance that 3-D transthoracic echocardiography would not have had the rise in popularity that we observe today if it had not benefited from 3-D transesophageal echocardiography. 3-D transesophageal echocardiography has made it possible to see the previously invisible, in particular, the mitral valve. It marked the beginning of modern catheter-based interventions [113] such as mitral valve repair, left atrial appendage occlusion, closure of paravalvular leaks and septal defects, and transcutaneous aortic valve implantation. In this interventional context, 3-D transesophageal echocardiography allows visualizing the entire percutaneous procedures in a single volumetric view. 3-D transthoracic echocardiography was first left behind for two main reasons: (1) 2-D transthoracic echocardiography is fast and good enough and (2) the off-line analysis was laborious due to limited software packages. Owing to the recent progress of user interfaces and the related postprocessing analysis, the advent of 3-D transthoracic echocardiography has significantly impacted the clinical management of cardiac diseases. Clinicians now agree that 3-D echo imaging

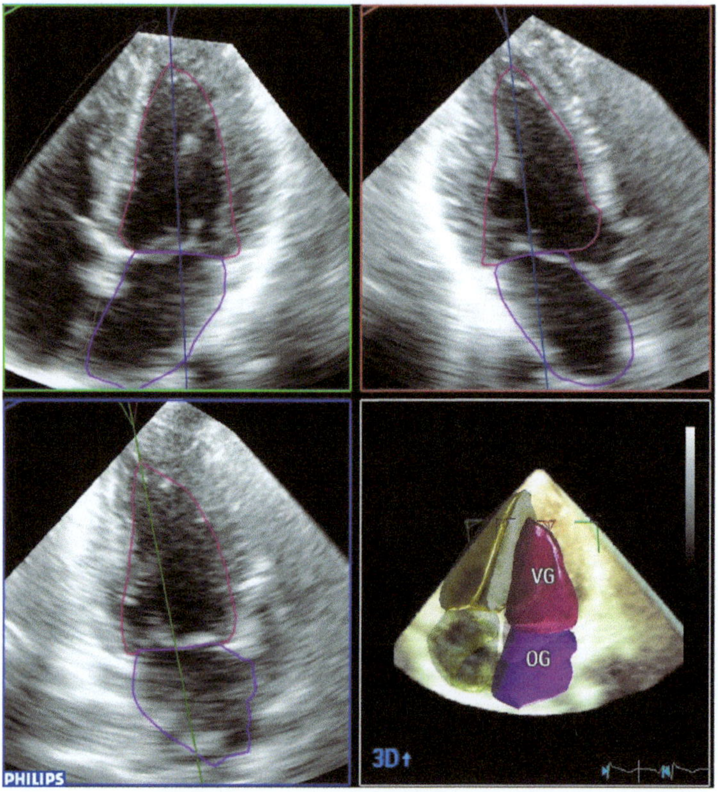

Figure 26.11 Three-dimensional echocardiography. 3-D echocardiography makes it possible to get an accurate estimate of the cardiac chamber volumes. Volumetric speckle-tracking echocardiography, however, is far from being readily available

can be both complementary and supplementary to 2-D echocardiography. A comprehensive description of practical applications of real-time 3-D echocardiography can be found in the recent book of Buck *et al.* [114]. For example, 3-D transthoracic echocardiography can allow the physician to obtain accurate estimates of the cardiac chamber volumes (Figure 26.11). This imaging modality, however, is still rarely used at patient bedside. With up-to-date clinical scanners, it is indeed not possible to perform volumetric sequences at adequate temporal and spatial resolutions in a single heartbeat. To obtain volume images at acceptable spatial resolution, they must be captured by stacking several narrow volumes acquired during successive heart cycles, typically 5 for a left ventricle. This technique requires electrocardiogram (ECG) gating, patient's breath-holding, and negligible beat-to-beat variability. On the other hand, single-beat 3-D imaging can be achieved in specific situations, but at the expense of spatial resolution. Clinical benefits of 3-D transthoracic echocardiography have been demonstrated in the evaluation of (1) cardiac chamber volumes and masses, (2) regional left ventricular wall motion, and (3) cardiac shunts and heart valve regurgitations. Due to its technical limitations, however, 3-D echocardiography is very challenging, if not infeasible, in patients with cardiac arrhythmias and/or breath-holding difficulty. To become a standard echo examination procedure, 3-D echocardiography must offer high spatial and temporal resolution, preferably in a single heartbeat. It is thus obvious that the path toward reproducible volumetric speckle-tracking echocardiography is still strewn with major, but surmountable, obstacles. Efforts were already made with a synthetic database of volumetric and realistic B-mode image sequences in the perspective of developing appropriate tracking techniques [115]. In addition, ongoing studies on transthoracic high-frame-rate echocardiography could change the situation [104,106,116–119] in a near future. However, although the *in vivo* feasibility of high-volume-rate 3-D echocardiography has been demonstrated by Provost *et al.* [117], we are only in the very early stages of this promising imaging modality.

In summary—Volumetric speckle-tracking echocardiography is presently not feasible with the conventional ultrasound scanners. High-frame-rate 3-D echocardiography could potentially change the situation. Extensive technical and software developments, however, are still required.

26.10 Historical and clinical conclusion

A complete echocardiographic examination must ideally allow quantification of the regional cardiac function, in particular for detecting regional myocardial anomalies under stress. Developed in the 1990s, the first way to quantify regional left ventricular wall motion was through endocardial (inner wall) tracking, a technique called "*color kinesis.*" This technique enabled endocardium tracking by identifying pixel transitions from blood (cavity) to tissue (wall) on a frame-wise basis [120]. However, it soon became apparent that it was difficult to distinguish active from passive motion with this approach. *Tissue Doppler imaging* thus emerged at the end of the 1990s (Figure 26.5). This new method was supposed to strongly improve physicians' ability to detect regional dysfunctions through the measurement of the local deformations. But, as mentioned earlier, tissue Doppler imaging is angle dependent [40]. It was thus gradually replaced then supplanted by *speckle tracking* (see Figure 26.5). The sequel has been discussed in this chapter: speckle-tracking echocardiography is now struggling to demonstrate its clinical utility, due to a lack of robustness and complexity of use. With time, the initially desired regional aspects have disappeared in favor of the global aspect. Fortunately, speckle-tracking echocardiography seems to find an honorable output as the GLS has been shown to be an early and reproducible marker of left ventricular dysfunction. We expect that the ongoing advances in medical ultrasound imaging will enable speckle tracking to return to the true source of its founding principles: detect regional myocardial dysfunctions.

References

[1] Destrempes F, Cloutier G. A critical review and uniformized representation of statistical distributions modeling the ultrasound echo envelope. Ultrasound Med Biol. 2010;36(7): 1037–51.

[2] Burckhardt CB. Speckle in ultrasound B-mode scans. IEEE Trans Sonics Ultrason. 1978;25(1): 1–6.

[3] Michailovich OV, Tannenbaum A. Despeckling of medical ultrasound images. IEEE Trans Ultrason Ferroelectr Freq Control. 2006;53(1): 64–78.

[4] Trahey GE, Allison JW, von Ramm OT. Angle independent ultrasonic detection of blood flow. IEEE Trans Biomed Eng. 1987;BME-34(12): 965–7.

[5] Mailloux GE, Bleau A, Bertrand M, Petitclerc R. Computer analysis of heart motion from two-dimensional echocardiograms. IEEE Trans Biomed Eng. 1987;BME-34(5): 356–64.

[6] Meynart R. Instantaneous velocity field measurements in unsteady gas flow by speckle velocimetry. Appl Opt. 1983;22(4): 535–40.

[7] Bohs LN, Trahey GE. A novel method for angle independent ultrasonic imaging of blood flow and tissue motion. IEEE Trans Biomed Eng. 1991;38(3): 280–6.

[8] Voigt J-U, Pedrizzetti G, Lysyansky P, *et al.* Definitions for a common standard for 2D speckle tracking echocardiography: consensus document of the EACVI/ASE/Industry Task Force to standardize deformation imaging. Eur Heart J—Cardiovasc Imaging. 2015;16(1): 1–11.

[9] Mailloux GE, Langlois F, Simard PY, Bertrand M. Restoration of the velocity field of the heart from two-dimensional echocardiograms. IEEE Trans Med Imaging. 1989;8(2): 143–53.

[10] Hein IA, O'Brien WD. Current time-domain methods for assessing tissue motion by analysis from reflected ultrasound echoes—a review. IEEE Trans Ultrason Ferroelectr Freq Control. 1993;40(2): 84–102.

[11] Friemel BH, Bohs LN, Trahey GE. Relative performance of two-dimensional speckle-tracking techniques: normalized correlation, non-normalized correlation and sum-absolute-difference. In: Proceedings of the IEEE Ultrasonics Symposium. 1995. p. 1481–1484.

[12] Yeung F, Levinson SF, Parker KJ. Multilevel and motion model-based ultrasonic speckle tracking algorithms. Ultrasound Med Biol. 1998;24(3): 427–41.

[13] Langeland S, D'hooge J, Torp H, Bijnens B, Suetens P. Comparison of time-domain displacement estimators for two-dimensional RF tracking. Ultrasound Med Biol. 2003;29(8): 1177–86.

[14] Luo J, Konofagou EE. A fast normalized cross-correlation calculation method for motion estimation. IEEE Trans Ultrason Ferroelectr Freq Control. 2010;57(6): 1347–57.

[15] Kolias TJ, Hagan PG, Chetcuti SJ, et al. New universal strain software accurately assesses cardiac systolic and diastolic function using speckle tracking echocardiography. Echocardiography. 2014;31(8): 947–55.

[16] Gao H, Bijnens N, Coisne D, Lugiez M, Rutten M, D'hooge J. 2-D left ventricular flow estimation by combining speckle tracking with Navier–Stokes-based regularization: an in silico, in vitro and in vivo study. Ultrasound Med Biol. 2015;41(1): 99–113.

[17] Curiale AH, Vegas-Sánchez-Ferrero G, Aja-Fernández S. Influence of ultrasound speckle tracking strategies for motion and strain estimation. Med Image Anal. 2016;32: 184–200.

[18] Barnea DI, Silverman HF. A class of algorithms for fast digital image registration. IEEE Trans Comput. 1972;C-21(2): 179–86.

[19] Raffel M, Willert CE, Wereley S, Kompenhans J. Image evaluation methods for PIV. In: Particle image velocimetry: a practical guide. 2nd edition. Heidelberg?; New York: Springer; 2007. p. 122–176.

[20] Reddy BS, Chatterji BN. An FFT-based technique for translation, rotation, and scale-invariant image registration. IEEE Trans Image Process. 1996;5(8): 1266–71.

[21] Baraldi P, Sarti A, Lamberti C, Prandini A, Sgallari F. Evaluation of differential optical flow techniques on synthesized echo images. IEEE Trans Biomed Eng. 1996;43(3): 259–72.

[22] Suhling M, Arigovindan M, Jansen C, Hunziker P, Unser M. Myocardial motion analysis from B-mode echocardiograms. IEEE Trans Image Process. 2005;14(4): 525–36.

[23] Yeung F, Levinson SF, Fu D, Parker KJ. Feature-adaptive motion tracking of ultrasound image sequences using a deformable mesh. IEEE Trans Med Imaging. 1998;17(6): 945–56.

[24] Ledesma-Carbayo MJ, Kybic J, Desco M, *et al.* Spatio-temporal nonrigid registration for ultra-sound cardiac motion estimation. IEEE Trans Med Imaging. 2005;24(9): 1113–26.

[25] Bashford GR, von Ramm OT. Ultrasound three-dimensional velocity measurements by feature tracking. IEEE Trans Ultrason Ferroelectr Freq Control. 1996;43(3): 376–84.

[26] Yu W, Yan P, Sinusas AJ, Thiele K, Duncan JS. Towards pointwise motion tracking in echocardio-graphic image sequences – comparing the reliability of different features for speckle tracking. Med Image Anal. 2006;10(4): 495–508.

[27] Widynski N, Géraud T, Garcia D. Speckle spot detection in ultrasound images: application to speckle reduction and speckle tracking. In: 2014 IEEE International Ultrasonics Symposium. 2014. p. 1734–1737.

[28] Garcia D. A fast all-in-one method for automated post-processing of PIV data. Exp Fluids. 2011;50(5): 1247–59.

[29] Vlasenko A, Schnorr C. Physically consistent and efficient variational denoising of image fluid flow estimates. IEEE Trans Image Process. 2010;19(3): 586–95.

[30] Farsalinos KE, Daraban AM, Ünlü S, Thomas JD, Badano LP, Voigt J-U. Head-to-head comparison of global longitudinal strain measurements among nine different vendors: the EACVI/ASE inter-vendor comparison study. J Am Soc Echocardiogr. 2015;28(10): 1171–1181.

[31] Le Tarnec L, Destrempes F, Cloutier G, Garcia D. A proof of convergence of the Horn–Schunck optical flow algorithm in arbitrary dimension. SIAM J Imaging Sci. 2014;7(1): 277–93.

[32] Leitman M, Lysyansky P, Sidenko S, *et al.* Two-dimensional strain—a novel software for real-time quantitative echocardiographic assessment of myocardial function. J Am Soc Echocardiogr. 2004;17(10): 1021–9.

[33] Lysyansky P, Rappaport D. Method and apparatus for quantitative myocardial assessment. US6994673 B2, 2006. Available from: http://www.google.com/patents/US6994673.

[34] Fleming AD, Xia X, McDicken WN, Sutherland GR, Fenn L. Myocardial velocity gradients detected by Doppler imaging. Br J Radiol. 1994;67(799): 679–88.

[35] Uematsu M, Miyatake K, Tanaka N, *et al.* Myocardial velocity gradient as a new indicator of regional left ventricular contraction: detection by a two-dimensional tissue doppler imaging technique. J Am Coll Cardiol. 1995;26 (1): 217–23.

[36] Heimdal A, Støylen A, Torp H, Skjærpe T. Real-time strain rate imaging of the left ventricle by ultrasound. J Am Soc Echocardiogr. 1998;11(11): 1013–9.

[37] Tanaka H, Nesser H-J, Buck T, *et al.* Dyssynchrony by speckle-tracking echocardiography and response to cardiac resynchronization therapy: results of the Speckle Tracking and Resynchronization (STAR) study. Eur Heart J. 2010;31(14): 1690–700.

[38] Heimdal A. Technical principles of tissue velocity and strain imaging methods. In: TH Marwick, CM Yu, JP Sun, editors. Myocardial Imaging: Tissue Doppler and Speckle Tracking. Blackwell Publishing Ltd; 2007. p. 1–16.

[39] D'hooge J. Principles and different techniques for speckle tracking. In: T Marwick, C-M Yu, JP Sun, editors. Myocardial Imaging: Tissue Doppler and Speckle Tracking. Blackwell Publishing Ltd; 2007. p. 17–25. Available from: http://onlinelibrary.wiley.com/doi/10.1002/9780470692448.ch2/summary.

[40] Gorcsan III J, Tanaka H. Echocardiographic assessment of myocardial strain. J Am Coll Cardiol. 2011;58(14): 1401–13.

[41] Claus P, Omar AMS, Pedrizzetti G, Sengupta PP, Nagel E. Tissue tracking technology for assessing cardiac mechanics: principles, normal values, and clinical applications. JACC Cardiovasc Imaging. 2015;8(12): 1444–60.

[42] Smiseth OA, Torp H, Opdahl A, Haugaa KH, Urheim S. Myocardial strain imaging: how useful is it in clinical decision making? Eur Heart J. 2016;37(15): 1196–207.

[43] Collier P, Phelan D, Klein A. A test in context: myocardial strain measured by speckle-tracking echocardiography. J Am Coll Cardiol. 2017;69(8): 1043–56.

[44] Thomas JD, Badano LP. EACVI-ASE-industry initiative to standardize deformation imaging: a brief update from the co-chairs. Eur Heart J—Cardiovasc Imaging. 2013;14(11): 1039–40.

[45] Kalam K, Otahal P, Marwick TH. Prognostic implications of global LV dysfunction: a systematic review and meta-analysis of global longitudinal strain and ejection fraction. Heart. 2014;100(21): 1673–80.

[46] Yingchoncharoen T, Agarwal S, Popović ZB, Marwick TH. Normal ranges of left ventricular strain: a meta-analysis. J Am Soc Echocardiogr. 2013;26(2): 185–91.

[47] Saloux E, Tournoux F. Heart phantom assembly. WO/2014/201571, 2014. Available from: https://patentscope.wipo.int/search/en/detail.jsf?docId=WO2014201571.

[48] Otterstad JE, Froeland G, St John Sutton M, Holme I. Accuracy and reproducibility of biplane two-dimensional echocardiographic measurements of left ventricular dimensions and function. Eur Heart J. 1997;18(3): 507–13.

[49] Plana JC, Galderisi M, Barac A, *et al.* Expert consensus for multimodality imaging evaluation of adult patients during and after cancer therapy: a report from the American Society of Echocardiography and the European Association of Cardiovascular Imaging. J Am Soc Echocardiogr. 2014;27(9): 911–39.

[50] Thavendiranathan P, Poulin F, Lim K-D, Plana JC, Woo A, Marwick TH. Use of myocardial strain imaging by echocardiography for the early detection of cardiotoxicity in patients during and after cancer chemotherapy: a systematic review. J Am Coll Cardiol. 2014;63(25, Part A): 2751–68.

[51] Nolan MT, Plana JC, Thavendiranathan P, Shaw L, Si L, Marwick TH. Cost-effectiveness of strain-targeted cardioprotection for prevention of chemotherapy-induced cardiotoxicity. Int J Cardiol. 2016;212: 336–45.

[52] Pibarot P, Garcia D, Dumesnil JG. Energy loss index in aortic stenosis. From fluid mechanics concept to clinical application. Circulation. 2013;127(10): 1101–4.

[53] Kearney LG, Lu K, Ord M, *et al.* Global longitudinal strain is a strong independent predictor of all-cause mortality in patients with aortic stenosis. Eur Heart J—Cardiovasc Imaging. 2012;13(10): 827–33.

[54] Kusunose K, Goodman A, Parikh R, *et al.* Incremental prognostic value of left ventricular global longitudinal strain in patients with aortic stenosis and preserved ejection fraction. Circ Cardiovasc Imaging. 2014;7(6): 938–945.

[55] Dulgheru R, Pibarot P, Sengupta PP, *et al.* Multimodality imaging strategies for the assessment of aortic stenosis. Circ Cardiovasc Imaging. 2016;9(2): e004352.

[56] Gjesdal O, Helle-Valle T, Hopp E, *et al.* Noninvasive separation of large, medium, and small myocardial infarcts in survivors of reperfused

ST-elevation myocardial infarction. A comprehensive tissue Doppler and speckle-tracking echocardiography study. Circ Cardiovasc Imaging. 2008;1(3): 189–96.
[57] Hoit BD. Strain and strain rate echocardiography and coronary artery disease. Circ Cardiovasc Imaging. 2011;4(2): 179–90.
[58] Ersbøll M, Valeur N, Andersen MJ, *et al.* Early echocardiographic deformation analysis for the prediction of sudden cardiac death and life-threatening arrhythmias after myocardial infarction. JACC Cardiovasc Imaging. 2013;6(8): 851–60.
[59] Ersbøll M, Valeur N, Mogensen UM, *et al.* Prediction of all-cause mortality and heart failure admissions from global left ventricular longitudinal strain in patients with acute myocardial infarction and preserved left ventricular ejection fraction. J Am Coll Cardiol. 2013;61(23): 2365–73.
[60] Montgomery DE, Puthumana JJ, Fox JM, Ogunyankin KO. Global longitudinal strain aids the detection of non-obstructive coronary artery disease in the resting echocardiogram. Eur J Echocardiogr. 2012;13(7): 579–87.
[61] Nucifora G, Schuijf JD, Delgado V, *et al.* Incremental value of subclinical left ventricular systolic dysfunction for the identification of patients with obstructive coronary artery disease. Am Heart J. 2010;159(1): 148–57.
[62] Reant P, Mirabel M, Lloyd G, *et al.* Global longitudinal strain is associated with heart failure outcomes in hypertrophic cardiomyopathy. Heart. 2016;102(10): 741–7.
[63] Witkowski TG, Thomas JD, Debonnaire PJMR, *et al.* Global longitudinal strain predicts left ventricular dysfunction after mitral valve repair. Eur Heart J—Cardiovasc Imaging. 2013;14(1): 69–76.
[64] Smedsrud MK, Pettersen E, Gjesdal O, *et al.* Detection of left ventricular dysfunction by global longitudinal systolic strain in patients with chronic aortic regurgitation. J Am Soc Echocardiogr. 2011;24(11): 1253–9.
[65] Park SJ, Park J-H, Lee HS, *et al.* Impaired RV global longitudinal strain is associated with poor long-term clinical outcomes in patients with acute inferior STEMI. JACC Cardiovasc Imaging. 2015;8(2): 161–9.
[66] Poelma C. Ultrasound imaging velocimetry: a review. Exp Fluids. 2017;58(1): 3.
[67] Raffel M, Willert CE, Wereley S, Kompenhans J. Particle image velocimetry: a practical guide. 2nd edition. Heidelberg?; New York: Springer; 2007. 448 p.
[68] Willert CE, Gharib M. Digital particle image velocimetry. Exp Fluids. 1991;10(4): 181–93.
[69] Crapper M, Bruce T, Gouble C. Flow field visualization of sediment-laden flow using ultrasonic imaging. Dyn Atmos Oceans. 2000;31(1–4): 233–45.
[70] Kim HB, Hertzberg JR, Shandas R. Development and validation of echo PIV. Exp Fluids. 2003;36(3): 455–62.
[71] Lindner JR. Microbubbles in medical imaging: current applications and future directions. Nat Rev Drug Discovery. 2004;3(6): 527–33.

[72] Kim HB, Hertzberg JR, Shandas R. Echo PIV for flow field measurements in vivo. Biomed Sci Instrum. 2004;40: 357–63.

[73] Zhang F, Lanning C, Mazzaro L, *et al.* In vitro and preliminary in vivo validation of echo particle image velocimetry in carotid vascular imaging. Ultrasound Med Biol. 2011;37(3): 450–64.

[74] Hong G-R, Pedrizzetti G, Tonti G, *et al.* Characterization and quantification of vortex flow in the human left ventricle by contrast echocardiography using vector particle image velocimetry. JACC Cardiovasc Imaging. 2008; 1(6): 705–17.

[75] Kheradvar A, Houle H, Pedrizzetti G, *et al.* Echocardiographic particle image velocimetry: a novel technique for quantification of left ventricular blood vorticity pattern. J Am Soc Echocardiogr. 2010;23(1): 86–94.

[76] Pedrizzetti G, La Canna G, Alfieri O, Tonti G. The vortex, an early predictor of cardiovascular outcome? Nat Rev Cardiol. 2014;11(9): 545–53.

[77] Sengupta PP, Pedrizzetti G, Kilner PJ, *et al.* Emerging trends in CV flow visualization. JACC Cardiovasc Imaging. 2012;5(3): 305–16.

[78] Bermejo J, Martínez-Legazpi P, del Álamo JC. The clinical assessment of intraventricular flows. Annu Rev Fluid Mech. 2015;47(1): 315–42.

[79] Kilner PJ, Yang G-Z, Wilkes AJ, Mohiaddin RH, Firmin DN, Yacoub MH. Asymmetric redirection of flow through the heart. Nature. 2000;404(6779): 759–61.

[80] Arvidsson PM, Kovács SJ, Töger J, *et al.* Vortex ring behavior provides the epigenetic blueprint for the human heart. Sci Rep. 2016;6: 22021.

[81] Nogami Y, Ishizu T, Atsumi A, *et al.* Abnormal early diastolic intraventricular flow "kinetic energy index" assessed by vector flow mapping in patients with elevated filling pressure. Eur Heart J—Cardiovasc Imaging. 2013;14(3): 253–60.

[82] Bermejo J, Benito Y, Alhama M, *et al.* Intraventricular vortex properties in nonischemic dilated cardiomyopathy. Am J Physiol—Heart Circ Physiol. 2014;306(5): H718–29.

[83] Martínez-Legazpi P, Bermejo J, Benito Y, *et al.* Contribution of the diastolic vortex ring to left ventricular filling. J Am Coll Cardiol. 2014;64(16): 1711–21.

[84] Rodevand O, Bjornerheim R, Edvardsen T, Smiseth OA, Ihlen H. Diastolic flow pattern in the normal left ventricle. J Am Soc Echocardiogr. 1999;12(6): 500–7.

[85] Sengupta PP, Khandheria BK, Korinek J, *et al.* Left ventricular isovolumic flow sequence during sinus and paced rhythms: new insights from use of high-resolution Doppler and ultrasonic digital particle imaging velocimetry. J Am Coll Cardiol. 2007;49(8): 899–908.

[86] Garcia D, del Álamo JC, Tanné D, *et al.* Two-dimensional intraventricular flow mapping by digital processing conventional color-Doppler echocardiography images. IEEE Trans Med Imaging. 2010;29(10): 1701–13.

[87] Stugaard M, Koriyama H, Katsuki K, *et al.* Energy loss in the left ventricle obtained by vector flow mapping as a new quantitative measure of severity

of aortic regurgitation: a combined experimental and clinical study. Eur Heart J Cardiovasc Imaging. 2015;16(7): 723–30.
[88] Cimino S, Pedrizzetti G, Tonti G, *et al.* In vivo analysis of intraventricular fluid dynamics in healthy hearts. Eur J Mech—B/Fluids. 2012;35: 40–6.
[89] Abe H, Caracciolo G, Kheradvar A, *et al.* Contrast echocardiography for assessing left ventricular vortex strength in heart failure: a prospective cohort study. Eur Heart J—Cardiovasc Imaging. 2013;14(11): 1049–60.
[90] Agati L, Cimino S, Tonti G, *et al.* Quantitative analysis of intraventricular blood flow dynamics by echocardiographic particle image velocimetry in patients with acute myocardial infarction at different stages of left ventricular dysfunction. Eur Heart J Cardiovasc Imaging. 2014;15(11): 1203–12.
[91] Hendabadi S, Bermejo J, Benito Y, *et al.* Topology of blood transport in the human left ventricle by novel processing of Doppler echocardiography. Ann Biomed Eng. 2013;41(12): 2603–16.
[92] Hong G-R, Kim M, Pedrizzetti G, Vannan MA. Current clinical application of intracardiac flow analysis using echocardiography. J Cardiovasc Ultrasound. 2013;21(4): 155–62.
[93] Fadnes S, Nyrnes SA, Torp H, Lovstakken L. Shunt flow evaluation in congenital heart disease based on two-dimensional speckle tracking. Ultrasound Med Biol. 2014;40(10): 2379–91.
[94] Angelelli P, Snare SR, Nyrnes SA, Bruckner S, Hauser H, Løvstakken L. Live ultrasound-based particle visualization of blood flow in the heart. In: Proceedings of the 30th Spring Conference on Computer Graphics. New York, NY: ACM; 2014. p. 13–20. (SCCG '14).
[95] Arigovindan M, Suhling M, Jansen C, Hunziker P, Unser M. Full motion and flow field recovery from echo Doppler data. IEEE Trans Med Imaging. 2007;26(1): 31–45.
[96] Gomez A, de Vecchi A, Jantsch M, *et al.* 4D blood flow reconstruction over the entire ventricle from wall motion and blood velocity derived from ultrasound data. IEEE Trans Med Imaging. 2015;34(11): 2298–308.
[97] Gomez A, Pushparajah K, Simpson JM, Giese D, Schaeffter T, Penney G. A sensitivity analysis on 3D velocity reconstruction from multiple registered echo Doppler views. Med Image Anal. 2013;17(6): 616–31.
[98] Uejima T, Koike A, Sawada H, *et al.* A new echocardiographic method for identifying vortex flow in the left ventricle: numerical validation. Ultrasound Med Biol. 2010;36(5): 772–88.
[99] Tanaka T, Asami R, Kawabata K, *et al.* Intracardiac VFM technique using diagnostic ultrasound system. Hitachi Rev. 2015;64(8): 489.
[100] Ro R, Halpern D, Sahn DJ, *et al.* Vector flow mapping in obstructive hypertrophic cardiomyopathy to assess the relationship of early systolic left ventricular flow and the mitral valve. J Am Coll Cardiol. 2014;64(19): 1984–95.

[101] Suhling M, Arigovindan M, Jansen C, Hunziker P, Unser M. Bimodal myocardial motion analysis from B-mode and tissue Doppler ultrasound. Proc IEEE Int Symp Biomed Imaging. 2004;1: 308–11.

[102] Tavakoli V, Bhatia N, Longaker RA, Stoddard MF, Amini AA. Tissue Doppler imaging optical flow (TDIOF): a combined B-mode and tissue Doppler approach for cardiac motion estimation in echocardiographic images. IEEE Trans Biomed Eng. 2014;61(8): 2264–77.

[103] Porras AR, Alessandrini M, Mirea O, D'hooge J, Frangi AF, Piella G. Integration of multi-plane tissue Doppler and B-Mode echocardiographic images for left ventricular motion estimation. IEEE Trans Med Imaging. 2016;35(1): 89–97.

[104] Porée J, Posada D, Hodzic A, Tournoux F, Cloutier G, Garcia D. High-frame-rate echocardiography using coherent compounding with Doppler-based motion-compensation. IEEE Trans Med Imaging. 2016;35(7): 1647–57.

[105] Cikes M, Tong L, Sutherland GR, D'hooge J. Ultrafast cardiac ultrasound imaging: technical principles, applications, and clinical benefits. JACC Cardiovasc Imaging. 2014;7(8): 812–23.

[106] Papadacci C, Pernot M, Couade M, Fink M, Tanter M. High-contrast ultrafast imaging of the heart. IEEE Trans Ultrason Ferroelectr Freq Control. 2014;61(2): 288–301.

[107] Tanter M, Fink M. Ultrafast imaging in biomedical ultrasound. IEEE Trans Ultrason Ferroelectr Freq Control. 2014;61(1): 102–19.

[108] Tong L, Ramalli A, Jasaityte R, Tortoli P, D'hooge J. Multi-transmit beam forming for fast cardiac imaging—experimental validation and in vivo application. IEEE Trans Med Imaging. 2014;33(6): 1205–19.

[109] Joyce E, Delgado V, Bax JJ, Marsan NA. Advanced techniques in dobutamine stress echo-cardiography: focus on myocardial deformation analysis. Heart. 2015;101(1): 72–81.

[110] Caballero L, Lancelotti P. Exercise 2D strain echocardiography: is it feasible? Argent J Cardiol. 2014;82(2): 89–90.

[111] Addetia K, Takeuchi M, Maffessanti F, *et al.* Simultaneous longitudinal strain in all 4 cardiac chambers. A novel method for comprehensive functional assessment of the heart. Circ Cardiovasc Imaging. 2016;9(3):e003895.

[112] Lang RM, Badano LP, Tsang W, *et al.* EAE/ASE recommendations for image acquisition and display using three-dimensional echocardiography. J Am Soc Echocardiogr. 2012;25(1): 3–46.

[113] Faletra FF, Pedrazzini G, Pasotti E, *et al.* 3D TEE during catheter-based interventions. JACC Cardiovasc Imaging. 2014;7(3): 292–308.

[114] Buck T, Franke A, Monaghan MJ. Three-dimensional echocardiography. Berlin, Heidelberg: Springer Verlag, 2014. 313 p.

[115] De Craene MD, Marchesseau S, Heyde B, *et al.* 3D strain assessment in ultrasound (Straus): a synthetic comparison of five tracking methodologies. IEEE Trans Med Imaging. 2013;32(9): 1632–46.

[116] Osmanski BF, Maresca D, Messas E, Tanter M, Pernot M. Transthoracic ultrafast Doppler imaging of human left ventricular hemodynamic function. IEEE Trans Ultrason Ferroelectr Freq Control. 2014;61(8): 1268–75.

[117] Provost J, Papadacci C, Arango JE, *et al.* 3D ultrafast ultrasound imaging in vivo. Phys Med Biol. 2014;59(19): L1.

[118] Posada D, Poree J, Pellissier A, *et al.* Staggered multiple-PRF ultrafast color Doppler. IEEE Trans Med Imaging. 2016;35: 1510–1521.

[119] Tong L, Ramalli A, Tortoli P, *et al.* Wide-angle tissue Doppler imaging at high frame rate using multi-line transmit beamforming: an experimental validation in-vivo. IEEE Trans Med Imaging. 2016;35(299): 521–8.

[120] Lang RM, Vignon P, Weinert L, *et al.* Echocardiographic quantification of regional left ventricular wall motion with color kinesis. Circulation. 1996;93(10): 1877–85.

Chapter 27

Assessment of systolic and diastolic heart failure

Alan G Fraser[1,2], Carmen C Beladan[3] and Bogdan A Popescu[3]

Abstract

Heart failure is becoming more common in western societies as their populations age. In the Rotterdam community study of nearly 8,000 people, the lifetime risk of developing heart failure from the age of 55 years was 33 per cent for men and 29 per cent for women, and its prevalence in those aged more than 85 years was 17 per cent [1]. Since heart failure is a severe disease with a poor prognosis, imaging is important for early detection, accurate diagnosis, estimating prognosis, and planning and monitoring responses to treatment. Many diagnostic targets can be studied to establish the particular phenotype in a person who is suspected of having heart failure (Table 27.1), and most invasive and non-invasive diagnostic techniques have been used to study them. In this chapter, we concentrate on evidence relating to the use of speckle tracking to study left ventricular, left atrial, and right ventricular function in heart failure. We review its technical strengths and limitations from a clinical perspective and describe how it is applied to determine the pathophysiological mechanisms of heart failure, to identify the underlying aetiology and to estimate prognosis. We also suggest some technical developments that if feasible might assist clinicians in improving treatment and outcomes for patients with heart failure.

27.1 Clinical phenotypes

Heart failure is a clinical syndrome in which the heart is unable to meet the demands of the circulation, whether at rest or on exercise. Traditionally, diagnosis has been based on measurement of the ejection fraction (EF) of the left ventricle (LV) – that is, the percentage of its volume that is ejected with each beat [2]. The normal EF has been quoted almost arbitrarily as >50 per cent, but a recent

[1]Emeritus Professor of Cardiology, School of Medicine, Cardiff University, UK
[2]Cardiovascular Imaging and Dynamics, Department of Cardiovascular Sciences, KU Leuven, Belgium
[3]Carol Davila University of Medicine and Pharmacy, Romania

Table 27.1 Targets for non-invasive imaging in heart failure

Phenotyping by measurements of myocardial function and global function:

- Preclinical effects of risk factors such as ageing, hypertension, and diabetes; and of myocardial toxicity from factors such as chemotherapy
- LV volumes (end-diastolic volume, end-systolic volume) and global function (stroke volume, ejection fraction)
- Regional function of the LV (longitudinal shortening and lengthening, radial thickening and thinning, circumferential fibre shortening)
- Rotation, torsion, twisting, and untwisting of the LV
- Segmental function, related to left ventricular shape and load, regional wall thickness, and by coronary arterial territory; for example distribution and extent of post-systolic shortening as a marker of ischaemia or scar
- Transmurality of scar in patients who have had a myocardial infarction
- Synchrony of contraction and relaxation between the ventricles (interventricular dyssynchrony), within the left ventricle (intraventricular dyssynchrony), between the atria and ventricles (atrioventricular dyssynchrony), and between the atria (interatrial dyssynchrony)
- Functional reserve of the left ventricle (e.g. exercise-induced changes in long-axis function, stroke volume, end-systolic volume, and ejection fraction)
- Left atrial volumes and function
- Right ventricular volumes, shape, and function; both global (such as RV volume), regional (such as tricuspid annular longitudinal excursion), and segmental (such as deformation of the RV free wall)

Haemodynamic variables estimated by Doppler echocardiography include:

- Left atrial pressure
- Left ventricular suction and diastolic filling pressures
- Intracavitary gradients and flow within the cardiac chambers
- Stroke volume and cardiac output
- Pulmonary arterial pressure
- Right atrial pressure
- Pulmonary and systemic vascular resistances
- Severity of any valve stenosis or regurgitation

individual-subject meta-analysis of more than 23,000 healthy recruits to population studies has refined the normal ranges. In European men and women aged over 50 years, the lower limit (fifth centile) of EF is 47 per cent [3]. Patients with a large LV and a reduced stroke volume (the volume of blood ejected with each beat, normally about 50–70 ml in an adult at rest) have a low EF; that is described as heart failure with reduced ejection fraction (HFrEF; previously known as systolic heart failure). Other patients may have a normal LV EF and cardiac output (stroke volume × heart rate) at rest, but be unable to increase cardiac output on exercise sufficiently to maintain normal perfusion to exercising skeletal muscles.

Those patients have heart failure with preserved ejection fraction (HFpEF; previously called diastolic heart failure).

The severity of symptoms can be summarised using functional class, as proposed by the New York Heart Association (NYHA). NYHA class I means breathlessness only on marked exertion, while at the other end of the spectrum NYHA class 4 means that the patient is breathless even at rest. In classes 2a, 2b, and 3, respectively, subjects are breathless on moderate, mild, and minimal exertion. After excluding respiratory disease or other non-cardiac causes of breathlessness such as anaemia, then heart failure may be diagnosed in a breathless subject when there is echocardiographic evidence of abnormal LV function and/or indirect evidence of increased LV filling pressures [4,5]. Imaging may show a specific cause, such as extensive scar or LV aneurysm from myocardial infarction, or else more diffuse disease such as a dilated or hypertrophic cardiomyopathy (HCM).

When LV end-diastolic wall stress is elevated, patients develop high blood levels of a circulating hormone, brain natriuretic peptide (BNP); this is released from cells in the sub-endocardium of the LV as a compensatory response [6], that is beneficial because it promotes salt and water excretion by the kidney. Elevation of BNP, or of its N-terminal propeptide (NTpro-BNP), is a very useful confirmatory diagnostic test for heart failure. Limitations include that it is more elevated in patients with atrial fibrillation than in those with normal sinus rhythm, and that it is less elevated in HFpEF than in HFrEF. When there is doubt, the definitive test to quantify the severity of heart failure is a cardiopulmonary exercise stress test (known as CPEX) with measurement of expired gases. Peak oxygen consumption (VO_2 max) is the accepted reference criterion, and in addition, the ventilatory cost of carbon dioxide excretion (VE/VCO_2 slope) provides an objective test of the efficiency of gas exchange in the lungs (with an increased slope implying an increased alveolar–capillary distance and possible pulmonary congestion).

Diagnosis that relies on EF is illogical. Symptoms may be caused by ‘forward failure’, in which the cardiac output response to exercise is poor, there is insufficient oxygen delivery to exercising skeletal muscles, and the resulting metabolic acidosis leads to reflex hyperventilation triggered by activation of chemoreceptors in the carotid bodies – and/or by ‘backward failure’, in which the diastolic filling pressure of the LV and in the left atrium is so elevated that there is pulmonary venous congestion with breathlessness due to stiff lungs or pulmonary oedema. Heart size and EF are not the key discriminants of cardiac function in heart failure; those are stroke volume, functional reserve, and the haemodynamic settings at which the heart is performing, particularly the LV end-diastolic pressure. Since it is a ratio, EF as a single measurement indicates neither the stroke volume nor the cardiac output; it should always be reported together with its components which are the LV end-diastolic volume (EDV) and end-systolic volume (indexed for body size).

Classification by EF has been confused further by the recent consensus recommendation that HFrEF should be diagnosed when EF is <40 per cent, HFpEF when it is >50 per cent, and a ‘new’ entity – heart failure with mid-range ejection fraction (HFmrEF) – when the EF is between 40 per cent and 50 per cent [4].

This is irrational when EF is a physiological variable that is normally distributed [7], that has considerable measurement variability, and that correlates poorly with symptoms and prognosis. Repeated measurements of EF during follow-up show that reclassification is common. It was reported that 39 per cent of patients who had been diagnosed initially as HFrEF had an EF >50 per cent at some time afterwards and also 39 per cent of patients with HFpEF developed an EF <50 per cent [8]. In a more recent study, >50 per cent of patients diagnosed as HFmrEF had transitioned to one of the other diagnostic categories within 1 year [9]. We need to implement more useful indices than EF.

27.2 Applying basic principles of myocardial deformation

The systolic shortening of individual myocardial cells results from diastolic stretch. Within limits, the greater their end-diastolic length, the greater the shortening; this is Starling's Law and it is reflected in the Frank–Starling curve. When myocardial velocity imaging was developed to allow post-processing of regional strain, it was confirmed in experimental animal models that strain similarly reflects LV volume, or stretch of the myocardium [10]. In other words, strain is 'preload dependent', and changes in strain may not inform about regional contractile function of the myocardium but instead about the response to local stretch. Comparisons of strain are more informative if the values are adjusted for preload (strain/LVEDV), as reported in volume overload from mitral regurgitation [11]. In a patient with heart failure, changes in strain might be accounted for in part by simultaneous changes in LVEDV.

Load-independent indices would be most informative about the intrinsic properties of the myocardium. In life, the heart is never completely unloaded, but myocardial contractility can be estimated non-invasively using the rate of change of deformation, which is strain rate [12], that can also be normalised for LVEDV [11]. This correlates with inotropic status, not preload [10,13]. The least load-sensitive, or the most load-insensitive, index of regional myocardial contractile function that has been reported may be the rate of change of the LV longitudinal velocity or strain rate during isovolumic contraction, termed isovolumic acceleration (or IVA); it reflects the change in shape of the LV cavity at the onset of systole, which can be measured from velocity signals of long-axis motion recorded before the aortic valve opens. IVA is a useful index but it has suboptimal reproducibility [14] so it should be obtained by imaging with high temporal resolution. It can be used to assess the intrinsic contractile function of the LV when measuring the force–frequency relationship, which is another basic property of myocardium: in a normal heart, the force of contraction increases as the heart rate increases. This is usually measured by recording IVA while the heart rate is changed using a pacing wire in the right atrium. It has also been studied using speckle tracking and deformation [15]. More advanced diagnostic information about myocardial function can be obtained using strain if it is combined with simultaneously acquired pressures to derive local pressure–strain relationships as an index of regional myocardial work [16].

Patients with coronary artery disease typically develop angina only during exercise, so it is widely accepted that stress testing is essential to confirm a diagnosis of myocardial ischaemia. Symptoms of heart failure may also be present only during exercise but, surprisingly, diagnosis has usually been made at rest. Now, stress echocardiography is being used more often to diagnose heart failure, especially if global systolic function appears normal, and here the preload dependence of myocardial strain is again relevant. At peak stress, there is a fall in left ventricular EDV and systolic volume, which explains why a biphasic response of strain has been shown during all stress protocols including semi-supine exercise, bicycle exercise, and dobutamine infusion [17]. Strain values increase at a submaximal workload but then fall at peak workload. Unfortunately, this finding has been ignored in some recent studies that have proposed using global longitudinal strain (GLS) to quantify maximal responses to stress [18]. Changes in strain at submaximal exercise can be used, if the workload is standardised [19], but otherwise post-systolic strain is a better indicator for identifying regional myocardial ischaemia than is systolic strain derived from speckle tracking [20]. It represents the recoil of myocardium that has been stretched by the contraction of adjacent segments during systole. Post-systolic shortening can be a passive phenomenon, whereas the development of strain rate in an affected segment indicates active contraction.

Speckle tracking is used to measure myocardial velocity and motion (displacement) as well as deformation (strain) and rate of change of deformation (strain rate). All these measurements can of course also be obtained using myocardial velocity imaging with phase correlation. Both techniques acquire the same basic measurement – local tissue velocity – but they are not interchangeable. In order to resolve and accurately measure physiological events that are very transient, images need to be acquired at high frame rates. This is possible with myocardial velocity imaging, whereas speckle tracking is limited to 60–80 frames per second. That is adequate for assessing strain but it becomes a problem when measuring strain rate. At low temporal resolution, undersampling means that peak amplitudes are underestimated, and transient events during isovolumic periods may not be detected at all. Most vendors do still derive strain rate from speckle tracking but it must be interpreted with great caution, especially if imaging is being used to measure dyssynchrony. Conversely, because of its lower frame rate, there is less variability and artefact in strain signals derived from speckle tracking, which means that its reproducibility is better.

27.3 Accuracy, reproducibility, and normal values

For reliable clinical diagnosis, echocardiographic tools should be accurate, so any new method for quantifying regional myocardial function should be validated against independent reference criteria. This is possible with *in vitro* testing against imaging phantoms but there is no universal industry standard for calibrating strain.

Another option would be *in vivo* comparisons against changes in the length of a myocardial segment between implanted microsonic crystals, in an animal model [21], but that is not routinely reported by manufacturers. A third option that has been used in recent comparisons of 2-D-strain diagnostic software is an *in silico* evaluation of artificial data sets and images that are indistinguishable by the human eye from real images but for which ground truth is known [22].

Measurements obtained using different echocardiographic systems or vendor-independent platforms should be similar. During signal processing of speckle tracking, however, each manufacturer applies its own analytical algorithms and software and uses its own choices to define regions of interest and to average and smooth the data by fitting splines. Perhaps unsurprisingly, inter-vendor differences have been detected both *in silico* [22] and in clinical comparisons when subjects were studied at the same time using different systems [23,24]. Inter-vendor differences were greater when measuring segmental than regional strain values [25,26]. These consistent differences mean that strain and strain rate measurements obtained using systems made by different manufacturers are not interchangeable, and regional quantification is problematic. For reliable serial measurements, patients with heart failure should be examined using the same machine and software.

The clinical utility of speckle tracking depends on the measurements being reproducible. Ideally, studies should compare repeated acquisitions of images from the same patients made by independent observers, and not just repeated measurements made by reanalysis of the same digitally stored images by different observers or by a single observer. For inter- and intra-observer reproducibility, respectively, the coefficients of variation for longitudinal 2-D strain were 15.4 per cent and 8.3 per cent compared with 21 per cent and 11 per cent for strain derived from myocardial velocity imaging [27]. Reproducibility of GLS is almost as good when measured during stress and by novice readers as by experts [28], but less good for post-systolic shortening [29]. These and other similar studies may explain why GLS is now popular as a clinical diagnostic tool, but it should be borne in mind during clinical studies that a coefficient of variation of 10 per cent implies that variations between consecutive measurements of <28 per cent could be explained by chance. The reproducibility of radial strain is insufficient for it to be useful; coefficients of variation of 30 per cent or more have been reported.

Consensus recommendations have been published in order to minimise variations between systems, techniques, and measurements [30]. Applying these standards for obtaining images has approximately halved the inter-vendor variability of strain [31,32].

Finally, any new diagnostic tool should be evaluated in a very large number of healthy people in order to define reference ranges. A meta-analysis of 2,597 subjects aged 47 ± 11 years who had been recruited to 28 studies gave an average normal value for GLS of -19.7 per cent (with 95 per cent confidence intervals 18.9–20.4 per cent) [33]. GLS declines with age [34], however, so those values may not be applicable as comparators for older subjects with suspected heart failure.

27.4 Pathophysiology of heart failure

The muscle bundles in the wall of the LV are not aligned uniformly. Instead they have a spiral arrangement that gradually changes across the wall in a smooth transition from a sub-epicardial 'left-handed' helix to a sub-endocardial 'right-handed' helix. During systole, their contraction twists the myocardium in a wringing motion. Since the bundles are attached at the base of the heart to the mitral annulus, this results in shortening of the long axis of the LV. In the midwall of the LV, the orientation of the muscle bundles is circumferential. Because myocardium is incompressible, long-axis and circumferential fibre shortening produce radial thickening of the wall with inward motion of the endocardium, although of course no muscle fibres are aligned from the epicardial to the endocardial surface of the heart. This geometrical configuration allows muscle cells that individually shorten by 10–20 per cent, collectively to eject 50–70 per cent of the volume of the LV. The wringing motion also leads to deformation of the fibrous interstitial matrix of the heart, and at the end of systole, the energy that has been stored is released with the onset of elastic recoil. These 'restoring forces' and rapid untwisting reduce LV diastolic pressure and generate suction in the LV cavity and in the coronary arteries [35]. Once the pressure in the LV falls below the pressure in the aorta, the aortic valve closes, and when the pressure falls further below the pressure in the left atrium, the mitral valve opens.

Patterns of regional contraction and relaxation of both ventricles can be observed using magnetic resonance imaging with tissue tagging, but amongst non-invasive echocardiographic methods, the angle-independence of speckle tracking makes it the best technique to measure thickening, thinning, and motion of the myocardium in longitudinal, circumferential, and radial directions in all cardiac chambers. In the context of heart failure, it is particularly useful for measuring long-axis shortening of the LV, which is a sensitive marker of early disease, and for assessing rotation (Figure 27.1). Shortening of the longitudinally oriented muscle bundles results in clockwise and counter-clockwise rotation at the base and apex of the LV. Using speckle tracking in healthy humans, apical rotation is about -10.9 degrees and basal rotation about 4.6 degrees [36]. Systolic twist is reduced in enlarged hearts with increased sphericity, for example in severe dilated cardiomyopathy, while untwisting is delayed and reduced in pathological left ventricular hypertrophy and HFpEF [37].

LV EF is the net result of long-axis shortening and radial thickening of the wall, but speckle tracking gives more detailed and specific measurements of regional function. When combined with intracardiac pressures, it can be used to construct pressure-volume loops that are very informative about ventricular and atrial function [38,39]. Combined with estimated LV pressures, it can give detailed insights into regional function and pathology [40]. Currently, these are research methods but they could be implemented in clinical practice if more user-friendly software was developed and incorporated into reporting systems. Apical rotation is easier to

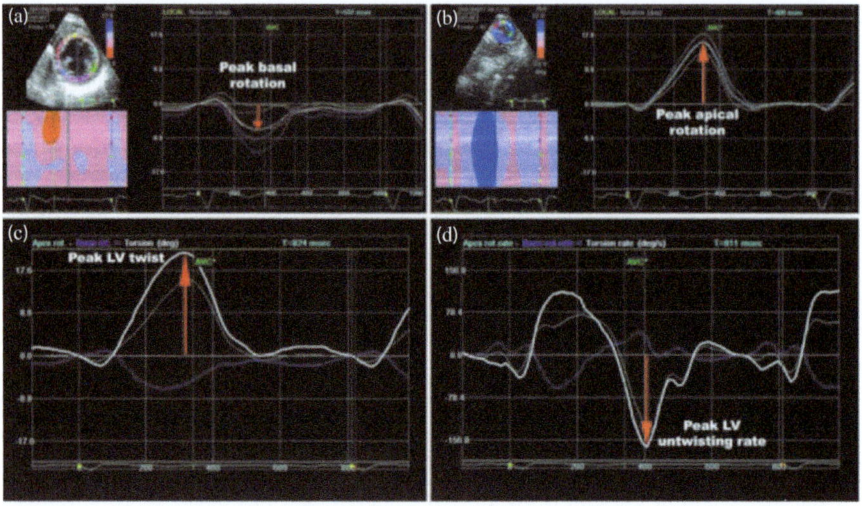

Figure 27.1 Myocardial rotation and twist. Strain curves derived from speckle tracking in a normal subject, showing rotation at the base (a) and apex (b), in short-axis images of the LV, and the derived traces for systolic twist (c) and early diastolic untwisting (d). Reproduced, with permission, from [37]

measure than basal rotation, and it contributes more to LV torsion, so measurement of apical rotation alone has been proposed as a simple bedside test [41].

27.5 Early diagnosis

With ageing, and in pathological LV hypertrophy, there is an increase in the interstitial collagen content of the heart. This is most marked in the sub-endocardial layer of the LV where the process starts at the base of the ventricular septum. That is the site where the radius of curvature of the LV cavity is greatest so it is also the site of the highest regional wall stress, which triggers the earliest pathophysiological changes. The extent of interstitial fibrosis correlates with sub-endocardial dysfunction and with reduced long-axis function. This was reconfirmed in a recent study that compared GLS measured in diseased hearts before transplantation with pathological studies of the explanted hearts; the C statistic for GLS as an indicator of collagen deposition was 0.92 [42]. Extensive fibrosis also leads to reduced end-diastolic compliance of the myocardium, an increase in the LV stiffness constant, an upward shift of the end-diastolic pressure–volume relationship, and increased diastolic filling pressures. Left ventricular hypertrophy and diastolic dysfunction are related to increased stiffness of central conduit arteries; analysis of ventricular–arterial coupling has shown that it is the mid- to end-systolic load that is most important for triggering these changes [43].

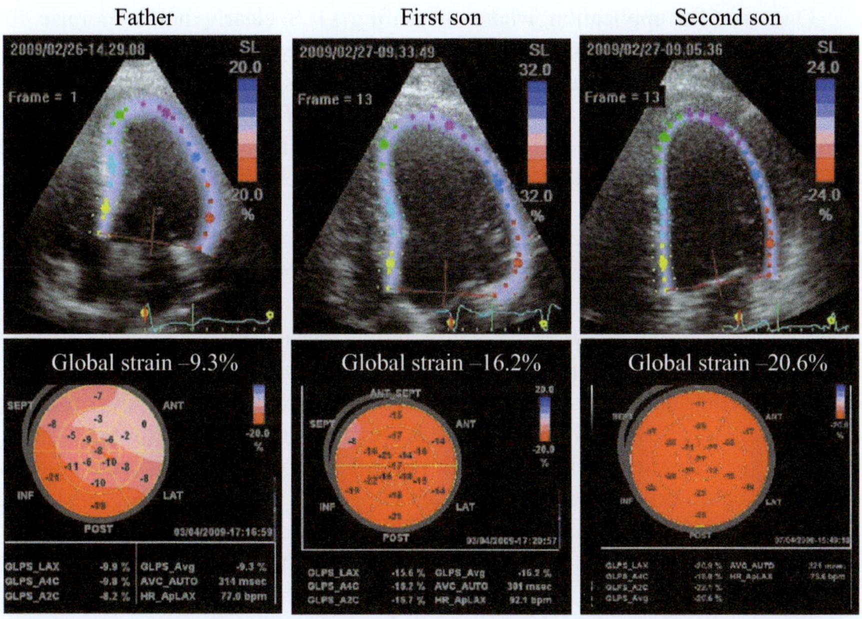

Figure 27.2 *Utility of 2-D strain for early diagnosis. Upper panels: apical four-chamber views of the LV in a patient with hypertrophic cardiomyopathy (HCM) (father) and in two asymptomatic sons. All have normal ejection fraction. Lower panels: in the patient, the bull's eye plot of strain shows that the apical lateral wall is affected more than the septum, and global longitudinal strain was only −9.3 per cent. In the second son, GLS was normal (−20.6 per cent) confirming that he was unaffected, whereas in the first son, the GLS measurement of −16.2 per cent strongly suggests that he has inherited the condition from his father*

Subclinical long-axis dysfunction of the LV correlates with the number of cardiovascular risk factors [44]. The pathophysiological link may be that increased central aortic stiffness, endothelial dysfunction, and microvascular ischaemia are all related to an inflammatory state [45]; all these phenomena occur in subjects who have major risk factors for HPpEF including age, type 2 diabetes, obesity, and hypertension. A large population study confirmed that cumulative risk factors are associated with reduced GLS [46] just as they were previously shown to be associated with reduced longitudinal myocardial velocities. Long-axis dysfunction has not yet been proved to be reversible, however, so the utility of preclinical diagnosis in subjects at risk of developing HFpEF has yet to be established. Detecting early changes is definitely possible, using GLS amongst other measurements as a surrogate marker (Figure 27.2), but the trend to early diagnosis will only be justified if the results can be translated into better outcomes.

One specific application where measuring GLS clearly holds promise for reducing the risk of subsequent heart failure is the early detection of cardiotoxicity during and after cancer chemotherapy. A meta-analysis has confirmed that an early reduction of GLS by 10–15 per cent is the most useful parameter for predicting cardiotoxicity [47]. Trials are in progress to test if applying this knowledge can reduce the incidence of heart failure without compromising the benefits of the chemotherapy.

27.6 Aetiology

Heart failure is a clinical syndrome with multiple causes and mechanisms. Both of the classical phenotypes (HFpEF and HFrEF) may result from many contributory causes or aetiologies. These include respectively chronic pressure overload, for example in hypertensive heart disease or aortic stenosis, and chronic volume overload, for example in severe aortic or mitral valve regurgitation – although that distinction is artificial since the LV dilates in patients with end-stage heart failure from aortic stenosis, and patients with chronic volume overload also have some LV hypertrophy. Other common causes include ischaemic heart disease with damage to LV myocardium from scar caused by myocardial infarction or from the cumulative impact of recurrent ischaemia (myocardial stunning), and cardiomyopathy or specific heart muscle diseases due to genetic or acquired causes.

Speckle tracking with measurement of GLS has become a common method for quantifying long-axis function in patients with suspected or known heart failure. In hypertensive heart disease, the basal part of the septum becomes hypertrophied first, and then concentric hypertrophy may develop over time. Interstitial fibrosis and reduced myocardial deformation are most abnormal in the basal septum. A typical septal bulge that narrows the LV outflow tract in an elderly patient is more likely to be caused by central arterial hypertension than by HCM. These conditions can be distinguished by speckle tracking since HCM typically affects all walls and also the right ventricle (Figure 27.3), whereas in HFpEF secondary to hypertension, the changes will most likely be confined to the LV. Other patterns of abnormal deformation in a hypertrophied LV suggest different causes such as amyloidosis or Anderson–Fabry disease (see also Figure 27.3) [48].

In any pathologically hypertrophied LV (but not in athlete's heart), there will be reduced long-axis systolic contraction; this was recognised first as reduced systolic velocities [49] but now is most easily detected using GLS [50]. In breathless patients with aortic stenosis or hypertensive heart disease and in HFpEF, early diastolic untwisting is delayed and reduced, which reduces LV suction and contributes to increased filling pressures [51].

In dilated cardiomyopathy, GLS is reduced and there is reduced torsion. Reversed apical rotation may be a marker of severity [52]. The detection of post-systolic shortening may suggest myocardial ischaemia. Recurrent ischaemia causes stunning which can be detected from reduced early diastolic strain [53]. Changes will probably correspond to a particular coronary arterial territory, unless there has been a stress-induced ischaemic injury (also called Tako Tsubo

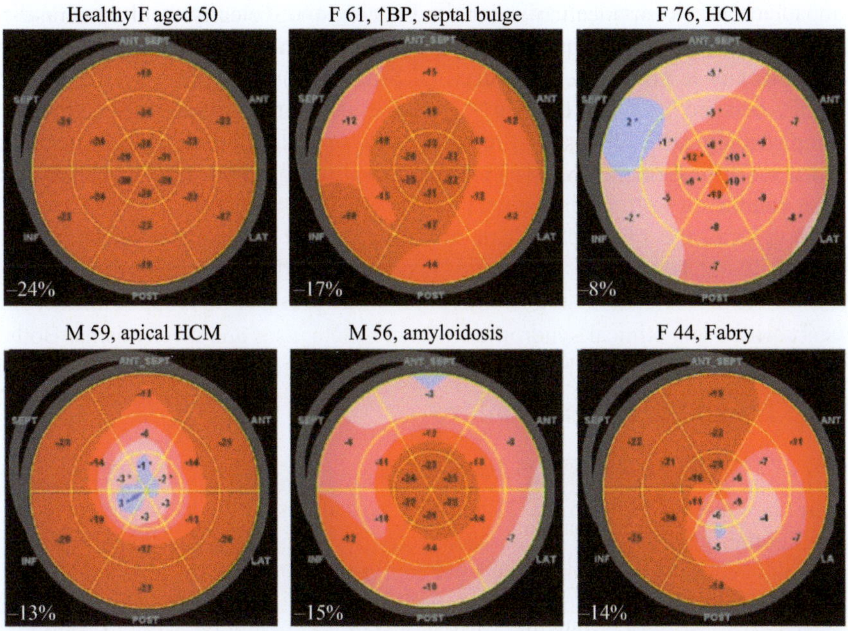

Figure 27.3 Segmental patterns of deformation in diseases causing heart failure. In a healthy subject, longitudinal strain shows very little variation between segments. With ageing, hypertension, or increased conduit arterial stiffness, there is hypertrophy and reduced deformation in the basal septum. In classical hypertrophic cardiomyopathy, there is severely reduced longitudinal deformation in the septum and also some reduction of strain in the free walls of the LV and RV; in apical hypertrophic cardiomyopathy, however, the hypertrophy and deformation is most prominent in apical segments in all walls. In contrast, with interstitial deposition of amyloid, there is an opposite pattern, since the apical segments are relatively spared while basal segments show greatly reduced strain. With a metabolic condition such as Anderson–Fabry disease, accumulation of glycolipids is greatest in the basal lateral segments so these have the least deformation. The number in the bottom left corner of each plot is the average value for global longitudinal strain in each subject. BP = blood pressure; HCM = hypertrophic cardiomyopathy. Redrawn, with permission, from [48]

cardiomyopathy); in which case, a patient may present in acute left heart failure with markedly impaired or absent deformation of apical segments in all coronary arterial territories.

When the cause of breathlessness is unclear, stress echocardiography can identify the origins of the patient's symptoms [54]. In a healthy heart, exercise and sympathetic stress increase early systolic twisting and diastolic recoil, so LV diastolic suction and rapid filling are enhanced [55]. In heart failure, impaired functional capacity is predicted by reduced GLS more accurately than by EF [56]. In HFpEF, delayed and reduced early diastolic untwisting may be an important pathophysiological mechanism of reduced exercise capacity since it leads to failure to increase filling on exercise [57]. This is confirmed by the lack of increase in stroke volume on exercise in patients with severe HFpEF [58].

In general, speckle tracking can only give clues to a particular cause of heart failure, without being pathognomonic. It can give little direct information about the haemodynamic state of the heart, which is the preserve of Doppler ultrasound (see Table 27.1).

27.7 Prognosis of heart failure

Measurement of GLS is a useful tool for estimating prognosis in patients with heart failure. In a meta-analysis of 5,721 adults, it was almost twice as predictive of all-cause mortality as EF [59]. In another study of 1,065 patients with HFrEF who were followed for 40 months, every 1 per cent decrease in GLS was associated with a hazard ratio of 1.2 for increased mortality, while no other echocardiographic measurement was independently predictive [60]. In 569 patients with previous myocardial infarction, mechanical dispersion was estimated using 2-D strain as the standard deviation of the times from the electrocardiographic R-wave to peak negative strain in 16 segments; both GLS and mechanical dispersion predicted arrhythmias (although only with a positive predictive value of 21 per cent), whereas LV EF did not [61]. In subjects with HFpEF, and after adjustment for LV strain, left atrial (LA) reservoir strain predicted subsequent events with a hazard ratio of 1.54; the utilities of other indices of LA strain were similar [62].

27.8 Left atrial and right ventricular function

Speckle tracking was developed to assess LV function and then reproduced by all manufacturers. Their software has also been applied to measurements of atrial function and right ventricular function, without special adaptation. Longitudinal strain profiles measured in atrial and ventricular muscle are virtual mirror images since the chambers are interconnected at the mitral annulus (Figure 27.4) [63]. Its systolic excursion towards the apex and diastolic displacement towards the base of the heart cause simultaneous and opposite shortening and lengthening of ventricular and atrial myocardial segments. The exception to this occurs during atrial contraction when the LV is relaxed, and atrial mechanical properties may reflect LV end-diastolic compliance. There is a large literature on LA strain measured by speckle tracking in heart failure, but many studies have not assessed if it has incremental value over that which is obtained by measuring LV strain.

Left atrial filling during ventricular systole when the mitral valve is closed (reservoir function) is influenced primarily by LV contraction, which affects the

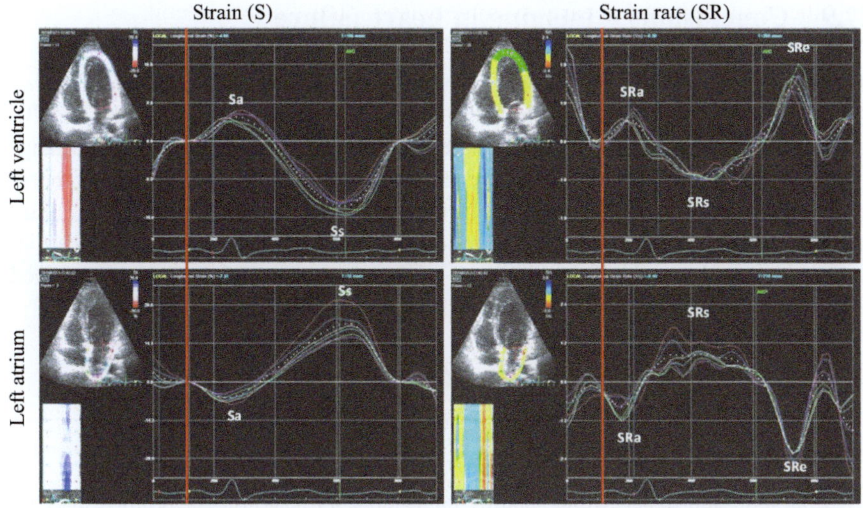

Figure 27.4 Symmetry of left atrial and left ventricular deformation. Left atrial and left ventricular strain and strain rate measured by speckle tracking in the same apical four-chamber loop from the onset of atrial contraction; the vertical red lines indicate the beginning of the P wave of the electrocardiogram. Peak strain rate in the left atrium during atrial contraction precedes the corresponding peak in the left ventricle, but otherwise the aligned traces are virtual mirror images. Note that the temporal resolution of strain rate derived from speckle tracking means that no deformation signals are detected during the isovolumic periods. Reproduced with permission from [63]

ascent of the mitral annulus, and to a lesser degree by LA myocardial relaxation and stiffness [64]. LA reservoir strain has been reported as a correlate of LV filling pressure [65] and peak LA strain as a good correlate of pulmonary capillary wedge pressure [66]. These were relatively small studies, however, so the utility for patients with heart failure of measuring LA strain during reservoir and conduit phases remains uncertain; it is likely that LA strain during booster pump function is more informative [67].

Right ventricular function and tricuspid annular plane systolic excursion have been demonstrated in many studies to have a significant prognostic impact in patients with heart failure. Studies using speckle tracking have shown similar results. For example, RV strain provided incremental prognostic information in patients with HFrEF, after adjusting for measurements of LV function [68]. A more recent study in 657 patients with HFrEF or HFpEF and matched healthy controls demonstrated that the magnitude of reduction of RV longitudinal strain, after adjusting for pulmonary arterial pressure, was independently related to a composite endpoint of all-cause death and HF hospitalisation, with a hazard ratio of 3.1 in both HFrEF and HFpEF [69].

27.9 Conclusions – imaging in heart failure

A 'big data' analysis of 3.6 million hospitalisations in the USA demonstrated that patients who had echocardiography during their admission for heart failure, had 20-per-cent lower mortality [70]. The implication is that accurate and detailed diagnosis may have guided more effective treatment. There is no doubt that comprehensive echocardiography is extremely informative in patients with heart failure and that it is now an essential investigation. In this context, measuring myocardial deformation with speckle tracking is a useful investigation that must be combined

Table 27.2 Technical developments of help for diagnosing heart failure

- Routine reporting of the performance of new software against standard *in silico* and *in vitro* phantoms
- Consensus agreements within industry on methods for measuring myocardial function (e.g. sub-endocardial deformation as an index of LV long-axis function)
- Adjustable region of interest so that its width matches segmental myocardial thickness
- Increased spatial resolution of speckle (especially for 3-D acquisitions) and higher temporal resolution (including applications for stress imaging)
- New tools for averaging global deformation when some LV segments cannot be imaged; standard methods for interpolation or for omitting segments
- Technical solutions for averaging 2-D strain in patients with an irregular rhythm such as atrial fibrillation, or with high beat-to-beat variability
- Automated methods for measuring LV strain, strain rate, volumes, and ejection fraction – that are accurate and reproducible
- Dedicated software for measuring deformation in the left atrium, and in the right ventricle
- Transparent quality indices for assessing adequacy of data used to calculate deformation
- Algorithms implemented within the reporting software on the machine, and in offline analysis workstations, that allow for age and other risk factors to be taken in account when determining normal values in comparison with normative databases – so that each measurement in an individual patient can be reported as a *Z* score adjusted for pretest probability
- More user-friendly tools for measuring torsion and untwisting
- Easier tools for quantifying early diastolic relaxation and time-to-maximal or time-to-peak early diastolic filling
- Tools to measure left ventricular shape, and regional load (when combined with estimates of pressure), to derive stress–strain relationships
- Tools for producing LV pressure–volume loops
- Tools for measuring the curvature of the ventricular septum, to allow diagnosis of ventricular interaction (e.g. when a dilated and failing right ventricle makes the septum bulge towards the left, which impedes diastolic filling of the left ventricle)
- Simple tools for timing cardiac events, such as the ability to acquire or import two simultaneous signals, which would make it easier to quantify post-systolic deformation
- Tools for simultaneous acquisition of an arterial pressure waveform and LV strain, to assess ventricular–arterial coupling

with other methods. It is most informative for measuring GLS and less reliable when used to assess segmental function. It is used especially for early diagnosis, for identifying aetiological clues from the pattern of abnormal deformation, and for estimating prognosis.

In Table 27.2, we list some technical developments that in our opinion would increase the value of speckle tracking in subjects with heart failure. Its clinical utility would be greater if the technique had higher temporal and spatial resolution and reproducibility, and if analytical software and diagnostic decision aids were available that could be integrated into routine reporting systems. For example, it would be important to include tools that allow for missing segments, as may occur due to rib artefact or failure of tracking at the base of the heart. Also, if vendors apply algorithms to indicate the quality and adequacy of tracking, then it would be helpful if the bases for these decisions are disclosed.

References

[1] Bleumink GS, Knetsch AM, Sturkenboom MC, *et al.* Quantifying the heart failure epidemic: prevalence, incidence rate, lifetime risk and prognosis of heart failure The Rotterdam Study. European Heart Journal 2004;25:1614–9.

[2] Folse R, Braunwald E. Determination of fraction of left ventricular volume ejected per beat and of ventricular end-diastolic and residual volumes. Experimental and clinical observations with a precordial dilution technic. Circulation 1962;25:674–85.

[3] Echocardiographic Normal Ranges Meta-Analysis of the Left Heart Collaboration. Ethnic-specific normative reference values for echocardiographic LA and LV size, LV mass, and systolic function: the EchoNoRMAL Study. JACC Cardiovascular Imaging 2015;8:656–65.

[4] Ponikowski P, Voors AA, Anker SD, *et al.*; Authors/Task Force Members. 2016 ESC Guidelines for the diagnosis and treatment of acute and chronic heart failure: the Task Force for the diagnosis and treatment of acute and chronic heart failure of the European Society of Cardiology (ESC). European Heart Journal 2016;37:2129–200.

[5] Paulus WJ, Tschöpe C, Sanderson JE, *et al.* How to diagnose diastolic heart failure: a consensus statement on the diagnosis of heart failure with normal left ventricular ejection fraction by the Heart Failure and Echocardiography Associations of the European Society of Cardiology. European Heart Journal 2007;28:2539–50.

[6] Iwanaga Y, Nishi I, Furuichi S, *et al.* B-type natriuretic peptide strongly reflects diastolic wall stress in patients with chronic heart failure: comparison between systolic and diastolic heart failure. Journal of the American College of Cardiology 2006;47:742–8.

[7] Brutsaert DL. Diastolic heart failure: perception of the syndrome and scope of the problem. Progress in Cardiovascular Disease 2006;49:153–6.

[8] Dunlay SM, Roger VL, Weston SA, Jiang R, Redfield MM. Longitudinal changes in ejection fraction in heart failure patients with preserved and reduced ejection fraction. Circulation Heart Failure 2012;5:720–6.

[9] Tsuji K, Sakata Y, Nochioka K, *et al.*; CHART-2 Investigators. Characterization of heart failure patients with mid-range left ventricular ejection fraction – a report from the CHART-2 Study. European Journal of Heart Failure 2017 Mar 31. [Epub ahead of print]. doi: 10.1002/ejhf.807.

[10] Weidemann F, Jamal F, Kowalski M, *et al.* Can strain rate and strain quantify changes in regional systolic function during dobutamine infusion, B-blockade, and atrial pacing – implications for quantitative stress echocardiography. Journal of the American Society of Echocardiography 2002;15:416–24.

[11] Marciniak A, Claus P, Sutherland GR, *et al.* Changes in systolic left ventricular function in isolated mitral regurgitation. A strain rate imaging study. European Heart Journal 2007;28:2627–36.

[12] Greenberg NL, Firstenberg MS, Castro PL, *et al.* Doppler-derived myocardial systolic strain rate is a strong index of left ventricular contractility. Circulation 2002;105:99–105.

[13] Urheim S, Edvardsen T, Torp H, Angelsen B, Smiseth OA. Myocardial strain by Doppler echocardiography. Validation of a new method to quantify regional myocardial function. Circulation 2000;102:1158–64.

[14] Margulescu AD, Thomas DE, Ingram TE, *et al.* Can isovolumic acceleration be used in clinical practice to estimate ventricular contractile function? Reproducibility and regional variation of a new noninvasive index. Journal of the American Society of Echocardiography 2010; 23:423–31.

[15] Mak S, Van Spall HG, Wainstein RV, Sasson Z. Strain, strain rate, and the force frequency relationship in patients with and without heart failure. Journal of the American Society of Echocardiography 2012;25:341–8.

[16] Urheim S, Rabben SI, Skulstad H, Lyseggen E, Ihlen H, Smiseth OA. Regional myocardial work by strain Doppler echocardiography and LV pressure: a new method for quantifying myocardial function. American Journal of Physiology Heart and Circulatory Physiology 2005;288: H2375–80.

[17] Davidavicius G, Kowalski M, Williams RI, *et al.* Can regional strain and strain rate measurement be performed during both dobutamine and exercise echocardiography, and do regional deformation responses differ with different forms of stress testing? Journal of the American Society of Echocardiography 2003;16:299–308.

[18] Ng AC, Sitges M, Pham PN, *et al.* Incremental value of 2-dimensional speckle tracking strain imaging to wall motion analysis for detection of coronary artery disease in patients undergoing dobutamine stress echocardiography. American Heart Journal 2009;158:836–44.

[19] Erdei T, Smiseth OA, Marino P, Fraser AG. A systematic review of diastolic stress tests in heart failure with preserved ejection fraction, with proposals

from the EU-FP7 MEDIA study group. European Journal of Heart Failure 2014;16:1345–61.
[20] Uusitalo V, Luotolahti M, Pietilä M, *et al.* Two-dimensional speckle-tracking during dobutamine stress echocardiography in the detection of myocardial ischemia in patients with suspected coronary artery disease. Journal of the American Society of Echocardiography 2016;29:470–9.
[21] Amundsen BH, Helle-Valle T, Edvardsen T, *et al.* Noninvasive myocardial strain measurement by speckle tracking echocardiography: validation against sonomicrometry and tagged magnetic resonance imaging. Journal of the American College of Cardiology 2006;47:789–93.
[22] D'hooge J, Barbosa D, Gao H, *et al.*; EACVI/ASE/Industry Task Force to Standardize Deformation Imaging. Two-dimensional speckle tracking echocardiography: standardization efforts based on synthetic ultrasound data. European Heart Journal Cardiovascular Imaging 2016;17:693–701.
[23] Nagata Y, Takeuchi M, Mizukoshi K, *et al.* Intervendor variability of two-dimensional strain using vendor-specific and vendor-independent software. Journal of the American Society of Echocardiography 2015;28:630–41.
[24] Farsalinos KE, Daraban AM, Ünlü S, Thomas JD, Badano LP, Voigt JU. Head-to-head comparison of global longitudinal strain measurements among nine different vendors: The EACVI/ASE Inter-Vendor Comparison Study. Journal of the American Society of Echocardiography 2015;28:1171–81.
[25] Mirea O, Pagourelias ED, Duchenne J, *et al.*; EACVI-ASE-Industry Standardization Task Force. Intervendor differences in the accuracy of detecting regional functional abnormalities: a report from the EACVI-ASE Strain Standardization Task Force. JACC Cardiovascular Imaging 2017 May 11. doi: 10.1016/j.jcmg.2017.02.014. [Epub ahead of print].
[26] Mirea O, Pagourelias ED, Duchenne J, *et al.*; EACVI-ASE-Industry Standardization Task Force. Variability and reproducibility of segmental longitudinal strain measurement: a report from the EACVI-ASE Strain Standardization Task Force. JACC Cardiovascular Imaging 2017 May 12. doi: 10.1016/j.jcmg.2017.01.027. [Epub ahead of print].
[27] Cho GY, Chan J, Leano R, Strudwick M, Marwick TH. Comparison of two-dimensional speckle and tissue velocity based strain and validation with harmonic phase magnetic resonance imaging. American Journal of Cardiology 2006;97:1661–6.
[28] Yamada A, Luis SA, Sathianathan D, *et al.* Reproducibility of regional and global longitudinal strains derived from two-dimensional speckle-tracking and Doppler tissue imaging between expert and novice readers during quantitative dobutamine stress echocardiography. Journal of the American Society of Echocardiography 2014;27:880–7.
[29] Coiro S, Huttin O, Bozec E, *et al.* Reproducibility of echocardiographic assessment of 2D-derived longitudinal strain parameters in a population-based study (the STANISLAS Cohort study). International Journal of Cardiovascular Imaging 2017 Mar 31. doi: 10.1007/s10554-017-1117-z. [Epub ahead of print].

[30] Voigt JU, Pedrizzetti G, Lysyansky P, *et al.* Definitions for a common standard for 2D speckle tracking echocardiography: consensus document of the EACVI/ASE/Industry Task Force to standardize deformation imaging. European Heart Journal Cardiovascular Imaging 2015;16:1–11.
[31] Yang H, Marwick TH, Fukuda N, *et al.* Improvement in strain concordance between two major vendors after the strain standardization initiative. Journal of the American Society of Echocardiography 2015;28:642–8.
[32] Shiino K, Yamada A, Ischenko M, *et al.* Intervendor consistency and reproducibility of left ventricular 2D global and regional strain with two different high-end ultrasound systems. European Heart Journal Cardiovascular Imaging 2017;18:707–16.
[33] Yingchoncharoen T, Agarwal S, Popovic ZB, Marwick TH. Normal ranges of left ventricular strain: a meta-analysis. Journal of the American Society of Echocardiography 2013;26:185–91.
[34] Dalen H, Thorstensen A, Aase SA, *et al.* Segmental and global longitudinal strain and strain rate based on echocardiography of 1266 healthy individuals: the HUNT study in Norway. European Journal of Echocardiography 2010; 11:176–83.
[35] Opdahl A, Remme EW, Helle-Valle T, Edvardsen T, Smiseth OA. Myocardial relaxation, restoring forces, and early-diastolic load are independent determinants of left ventricular untwisting rate. Circulation 2012; 126:1441–51.
[36] Helle-Valle T, Crosby J, Edvardsen T, *et al.* New noninvasive method for assessment of left ventricular rotation: speckle tracking echocardiography. Circulation 2005;112:3149–56.
[37] Beladan CC, Călin A, Roşca M, Ginghină C, Popescu BA. Left ventricular twist dynamics: principles and applications. Heart 2014;100:731–40.
[38] Hioki A, Masuda K, Asanuma T, Goto Y, Nakatani S. Application of three-dimensional speckle tracking echocardiography to assess left ventricular regional work using wall tension-regional area loop. American Journal of Physiology Heart and Circulatory Physiology 2015;308:H1258–64.
[39] Marino PN, Degiovanni A, Baduena L, *et al.*; Novara Atrial Fibrillation (NAIF) Study Group. Non-invasively estimated left atrial stiffness is associated with short-term recurrence of atrial fibrillation after electrical cardioversion. Journal of Cardiology 2017;69:731–8.
[40] Russell K, Eriksen M, Aaberge L, *et al.* A novel clinical method for quantification of regional left ventricular pressure-strain loop area: a non-invasive index of myocardial work. European Heart Journal 2012;33:724–33.
[41] Opdahl A, Helle-Valle T, Remme EW, *et al.* Apical rotation by speckle tracking echocardiography: a simplified bedside index of left ventricular twist. Journal of the American Society of Echocardiography. 2008;21:1121–8.
[42] Cameli M, Mondillo S, Righini FM, *et al.* Left ventricular deformation and myocardial fibrosis in patients with advanced heart failure requiring transplantation. Journal of Cardiac Failure 2016;22:901–7.

[43] Fraser AG, Gillebert TC, Leite-Moreira AF. Ventricular–arterial coupling in heart failure with preserved ejection fraction – the devil is in the details. Cardiovascular Research 2017;113:844–6.

[44] Vinereanu D, Mädler CF, Gherghinescu C, Ciobanu AO, Fraser AG. Cumulative impact of cardiovascular risk factors on regional left ventricular function and reserve: progressive long-axis dysfunction with compensatory radial changes. Echocardiography 2011;28:813–20.

[45] Paulus WJ, Tschöpe C. A novel paradigm for heart failure with preserved ejection fraction: comorbidities drive myocardial dysfunction and remodeling through coronary microvascular endothelial inflammation. Journal of the American College of Cardiology 2013;62:263–71.

[46] Selvaraj S, Aguilar FG, Martinez EE, *et al.* Association of comorbidity burden with abnormal cardiac mechanics: findings from the HyperGEN study. Journal of the American Heart Association 2014;3:e000631.

[47] Thavendiranathan P, Poulin F, Lim KD, Plana JC, Woo A, Marwick TH. Use of myocardial strain imaging by echocardiography for the early detection of cardiotoxicity in patients during and after cancer chemotherapy: a systematic review. Journal of the American College of Cardiology 2014;63:2751–68.

[48] Liu D, Hu K, Nordbeck P, Ertl G, Störk S, Weidemann F. Longitudinal strain bull's eye plot patterns in patients with cardiomyopathy and concentric left ventricular hypertrophy. European Journal of Medical Research 2016; 21:21.

[49] Vinereanu D, Nicolaides E, Tweddel AC, Fraser AG. "Pure" diastolic dysfunction is associated with long-axis systolic dysfunction. Implications for the diagnosis and classification of heart failure. European Journal of Heart Failure 2005;7:820–8.

[50] Kraigher-Krainer E, Shah AM, Gupta DK, *et al.*; for the PARAMOUNT Investigators. Impaired systolic function by strain imaging in heart failure with preserved ejection fraction. Journal of the American College of Cardiology 2014;63:447–56.

[51] Popescu BA, Calin A, Beladan CC, *et al.* Left ventricular torsional dynamics in aortic stenosis: relationship between left ventricular untwisting and filling pressures. A two-dimensional speckle tracking study. European Journal of Echocardiography 2010;11:406–13.

[52] Popescu BA, Beladan CC, Calin A, *et al.* Left ventricular remodelling and torsional dynamics in dilated cardiomyopathy: reversed apical rotation as a marker of disease severity. European Journal of Heart Failure 2009; 11:945–51.

[53] Williams RI, Payne N, Phillips T, D'hooge J, Fraser AG. Strain rate imaging after dynamic stress provides objective evidence of persistent regional myocardial dysfunction in ischaemic myocardium: regional stunning identified? Heart 2005;91:152–60.

[54] Erdei T, Aakhus S, Marino P, Paulus WJ, Smiseth OA, Fraser AG. Pathophysiological rationale and diagnostic targets for diastolic stress testing. Heart 2015;101:1355–60.

[55] Esch BT, Warburton DE. Left ventricular torsion and recoil: implications for exercise performance and cardiovascular disease. Journal of Applied Physiology (1985) 2009;106:362–9.

[56] Hasselberg NE, Haugaa KH, Sarvari SI, *et al.* Left ventricular global longitudinal strain is associated with exercise capacity in failing hearts with preserved and reduced ejection fraction. European Heart Journal Cardiovascular Imaging 2015;16:217–24.

[57] Tan YT, Wenzelburger F, Lee E, *et al.* The pathophysiology of heart failure with normal ejection fraction: exercise echocardiography reveals complex abnormalities of both systolic and diastolic ventricular function involving torsion, untwist, and longitudinal motion. Journal of the American College of Cardiology 2009;54:36–46.

[58] Kasner M, Sinning D, Lober J, *et al.* Heterogeneous responses of systolic and diastolic left ventricular function to exercise in patients with heart failure and preserved ejection fraction. ESC Heart Failure 2015;2:121–32.

[59] Kalam K, Otahal P, Marwick TH. Prognostic implications of global LV dysfunction: a systematic review and meta-analysis of global longitudinal strain and ejection fraction. Heart 2014;100:1673–80.

[60] Sengeløv M, Jørgensen PG, Jensen JS, *et al.* Global longitudinal strain is a superior predictor of all-cause mortality in heart failure with reduced ejection fraction. JACC Cardiovascular Imaging 2015;8:1351–9.

[61] Haugaa KH, Grenne BL, Eek CH, *et al.* Strain echocardiography improves risk prediction of ventricular arrhythmias after myocardial infarction. JACC Cardiovascular Imaging 2013;6:841–50.

[62] Freed BH, Daruwalla V, Cheng JY, *et al.* Prognostic utility and clinical significance of cardiac mechanics in heart failure with preserved ejection fraction: importance of left atrial strain. Circulation Cardiovascular Imaging 2016 Mar;9(3). pii: e003754.

[63] Margulescu AD, Rees E, Coulson RM, Rees AD, Vinereanu D, Fraser AG. Do left atrial strain and strain rate reflect intrinsic atrial function or are they determined by left ventricular function? Kardiologia Polska 2015; 73:539–48.

[64] Barbier P, Solomon SB, Schiller NB, Glantz SA. Left atrial relaxation and left ventricular systolic function determine left atrial reservoir function. Circulation 1999;100:427–36.

[65] Singh A, Addetia K, Maffessanti F, Mor-Avi V, Lang RM. LA strain for categorization of LV diastolic dysfunction. JACC Cardiovascular Imaging 2017;10:735–43.

[66] Cameli M, Lisi M, Mondillo S, *et al.* Left atrial longitudinal strain by speckle tracking echocardiography correlates well with left ventricular filling pressures in patients with heart failure. Cardiovascular Ultrasound 2010;8:14.

[67] Sanchis L, Andrea R, Falces C, *et al.* Prognostic value of left atrial strain in outpatients with de novo heart failure. Journal of the American Society of Echocardiography 2016;29:1035–42.

[68] Motoki H, Borowski AG, Shrestha K, *et al.* Right ventricular global longitudinal strain provides prognostic value incremental to left ventricular ejection fraction in patients with heart failure. Journal of the American Society of Echocardiography 2014;27:726–32.

[69] Bosch L, Lam CSP, Gong L, *et al.* Right ventricular dysfunction in left-sided heart failure with preserved versus reduced ejection fraction. European Journal of Heart Failure 2017 Jun 8. doi: 10.1002/ejhf.873 [Epub ahead of print].

[70] Papolos A, Narula J, Bavishi C, Chaudhry FA, Sengupta PP. U.S. Hospital use of echocardiography: insights from the Nationwide Inpatient Sample. Journal of the American College of Cardiology 2016;67:502–11.

Chapter 28

Myocardial elastography and electromechanical wave imaging

Elisa E. Konofagou[1]

Abstract

Cardiovascular diseases remain America's primary killer by a large margin, claiming the lives of more Americans than the next two main causes of death combined (cancer and pulmonary complications). In particular, coronary artery disease (CAD) is by far the most lethal, causing 17% of all (cardiac related or not) deaths every year. One of the main reasons for this high death toll is the severe lack of effective and accessible imaging tools upon anomaly detected on the electrocardiogram, especially at the early stages when CAD can be stabilized with appropriate pharmacological regimen. On the other hand, arrhythmias refer to the disruption of the natural heart rhythm. Cardiac arrhythmias lead to a significant number of cardiovascular morbidity and mortality. This irregular heart rhythm causes the heart to suddenly stop pumping blood. Atrial pathologies are the most common arrhythmias with atrial fibrillation and atrial flutter being the most prevalent.

28.1 Myocardial elastography

28.1.1 Introduction

According to the latest report on heart disease and stroke statistics by the American Heart Association [1], more than 2,150 Americans die of cardiovascular disease each day, an average of one death every 40 s. Cardiovascular disease currently claims more lives each year in both men and women than the next two most deadly diseases combined, i.e., cancer and chronic lower respiratory disease. Among the cardiovascular diseases, coronary artery disease (CAD) is by far the most deadly causing approximately one of every six deaths in the United States in 2010. Approximately, in every 34 s, one American has a coronary event, and approximately in every 1 min 23 s, an American will die of one. It is estimated that an additional 150,000 silent first myocardial infarctions occur each year [1].

[1]Department of Biomedical Engineering, Columbia University, USA

However, there are currently no screening or early detection imaging techniques that can identify abnormalities prior to any symptoms or fatalities. Clinically available imaging techniques such as echocardiography or nuclear perfusion (radionuclide imaging) are typically used after a cardiac event has already occurred to determine the extent of damage. Despite the fact that over the past few years, therapeutic techniques, such as angioplasty, heart valve surgery and pacemakers, have experienced exponential growth in new procedures; the progress in the development of novel diagnostic techniques has stalled by comparison.

28.1.2 Mechanical deformation of normal and ischemic or infarcted myocardium

Detection of cardiac dysfunction through assessment of the mechanical properties of the heart, and more specifically, the left-ventricular muscle, has been a long-term goal in diagnostic cardiology. This is because both ischemia [2], i.e., the reduced oxygenation of the muscle necessary for its contraction, and infarction [3], i.e., the complete loss of blood supply inducing myocyte death, alter the mechanical properties and contractility of the myocardium. In the ischemic heart, the diastolic left-ventricular pressure–volume or pressure–length curve slope is typically increased, suggesting increased chamber stiffness [4]. Regional myocardial stiffness has also been reported to increase as a result of ischemia [5–8]. The increased stiffness could be due to myocardial remodeling, including elevated collagen and desmin expression as well as the titin isoform switch [4]. Acute myocardial infarction caused by partial or total blockage of one or more coronary arteries can cause complex structural alterations of the left-ventricular muscle [9]. These alterations may lead to collagen synthesis and scar formation, which can cause the myocardium to irreversibly change its mechanical properties. Holmes *et al.* [10] reported that this myocardial stiffening can be measured within the first 5 min following ischemic onset. As reported by Gupta *et al.* [9], in vitro mechanical testing showed that the stiffness of the infarcted region increases within the first 4 h and continues to rise by up to 20 times, peaking 1–2 weeks following the infarct and decreasing 4 weeks later (down to 1–10 times the noninfarcted value). The fact that the mechanical properties induced by the ischemia change right at the onset, continue changing thereafter and peak 2 weeks later, indicate the potential for a mechanically based imaging technique to detect the ischemia and infarct extent early. Regarding its conduction pattern, ischemia or infarction will alter the normal pattern and result into reduced and complete lack of conduction, respectively, at the region of abnormality since the myocytes no longer properly conduct the action potential.

28.1.3 Myocardial elastography

Myocardial elastography (i.e., strain imaging—see the section on terminology in Chapter 14) has been developing for more than a decade [11–18]. This technique encompasses imaging of mechanical (cumulative or systolic; Figure 28.1) strain to highlight the mechanical function of the myocardium. Myocardial elastography

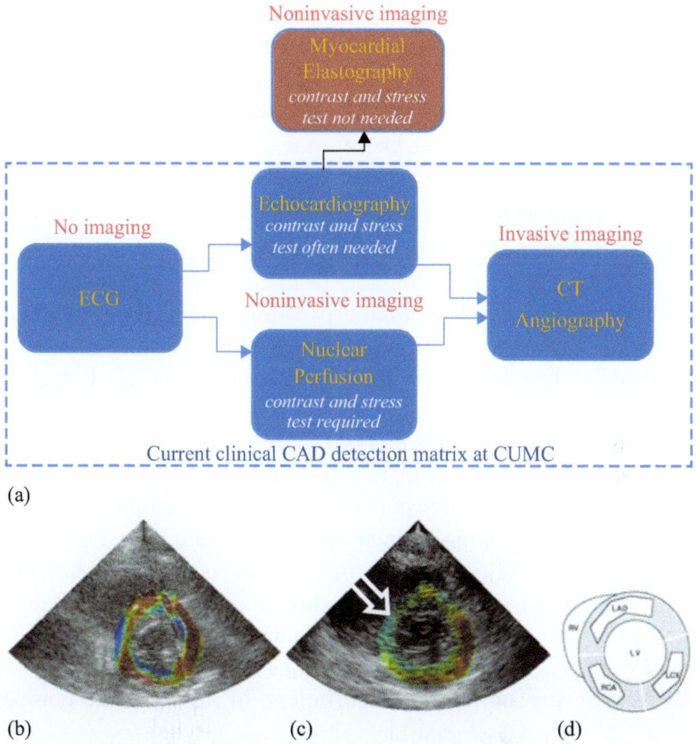

Figure 28.1 *(a) Envisioned role and (b) and (c) initial findings of myocardial elastography in the current clinical routine to avoid false positives and/or thus unnecessary invasive procedures and false negatives by the currently used techniques; (b) Normal short-axis radial strain image [largely red (thickening) myocardium] in an echocardiography false positive case where CT angiography was administered only to confirm normal function; (c) abnormal short-axis radial strain image containing an ischemic region (in blue or thinning; arrow) in a nuclear perfusion and subsequently CT angiography confirmed myocardial elastography findings regarding two occluded territories (64-year-old female, 40% LAD and 30% RCA occlusion); (d) coronary territories given for reference. CUMC, Columbia University Medical Center; LAD, Left anterior descending artery; LCx, Left-circumflex artery; RCA, right coronary artery. Myocardial elastography was capable of detecting normal function and identifying both compromised territories*

benefits from the development of techniques be used for high-precision 2D-time-shift-based strain estimation [19] and high frame rates available in echocardiography scanners [14] to obtain a detailed map of the transmural strain in normal [18,20,21], ischemic [20] and infarcted [22] cases in vivo. These strain imaging techniques aim at achieving high precision estimates through recorrelation techniques [19] and customized cross-correlation methods [23] and are thus successful in mapping the full 2D and 3D strain tensors [18,24,25]. Please refer to Chapter 14 for a more detailed explanation of radiofrequency (RF)-based block-matching strategies.

28.1.3.1 2D strain estimation and imaging

For the studies referred to in this chapter, a fast, normalized cross-correlation function will first be used on RF signals from consecutive frames reconstructed using parallel beamforming to compute two-dimensional motion and deformation [19,26]. The technique is namely Parallel Beamforming Myocardial Elastography (PBME). The cross-correlation function uses a 1D kernel (length = 5.85 mm, overlap = 90%) in a 2D (or 3D) search to estimate both axial and lateral (and elevational) displacements [(28.1); Figures 28.1 and 28.2]. The correlation kernel size is approximately ten wavelengths, which has been found to be the optimal length using cross-correlation [27]. It should also be noted that the elastographic resolution has been shown to depend mainly on the kernel shift (not the kernel size) [28], which in our studies is 10%, or 0.6 mm. When searching in the lateral (or elevational) direction, the RF signals are linearly interpolated by a factor of 10 in order to improve lateral (or elevational) displacement [19,20,29]. Recorrelation techniques are applied in two iterations that aim at increasing the correlation coefficient of each strain component by

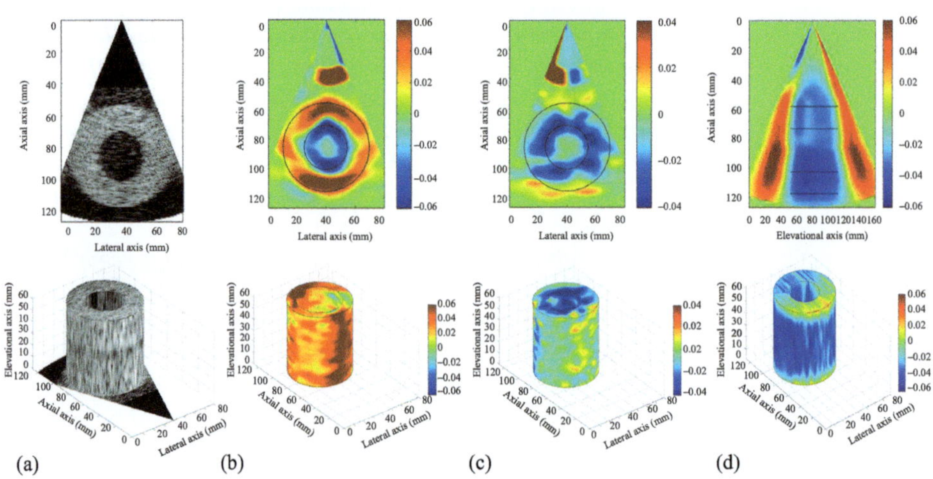

Figure 28.2 (a) B-mode, (b) radial, (c) circumferential and (d) longitudinal strain images of a cylindrical model undergoing radial deformation using PBME in phased array configuration in FIELD II for 2D (top panel) and 3D (bottom panel) myocardial elastography

correction or shifting the RF signals by the displacements estimated in the other (two) orthogonal direction(s) [19,29]. A least-squares kernel [30] is finally applied to compute the axial and lateral strains in 2D-PBME and axial, lateral and elevational strains in 3D-PBME. The estimated displacements use a reference point of the first frame in each estimation pair, yielding incremental (interframe) strains that are then accumulated over the entire systolic phase. Radial, circumferential and longitudinal strains will then be calculated. For **2D**, radial and circumferential strains are estimated in a short-axis view (Figure 28.2 (b) and (c)). In 2D-PBME, a rotation matrix, **R**, for each material point within the myocardium in a 2D short-axis view is written as

$$\mathbf{R} = \begin{bmatrix} \cos\theta & \sin\theta \\ -\sin\theta & \cos\theta \end{bmatrix} \tag{28.1}$$

where θ is the angle relative to the origin of the Cartesian coordinates in the finite-element models. Strains in cardiac coordinates are therefore obtained by

$$\hat{\mathbf{E}} = \mathbf{R}\mathbf{E}\mathbf{R}^T \tag{28.2}$$

where E is the 2D Lagrangian finite strain tensor and $\hat{\mathbf{E}}$ is the 2D radial–circumferential strain tensor. The diagonal components of $\hat{\mathbf{E}}$ are radial ($\mathbf{E}_{rr}$) and circumferential ($\mathbf{E}_{cc}$) strains. Positive and negative radial strains indicate myocardial thickening and thinning, respectively, while myocardial stretching and shortening are represented by positive and negative circumferential strains, respectively. A standard B-mode image (Figure 28.2(a)) is reconstructed from the RF data, allowing for manually initialized segmentation of the myocardial border which are subsequently automatically tracked throughout the cardiac cycle based on the estimated displacements [26].

28.1.3.2 3D strain estimation and imaging

3D will include the estimation of longitudinal strains. The MATLAB® function interp3 is used to interpolate all three orthogonal components (axial, lateral, radial and circumferential) between each of the 16 slices. The interpolated data set is depicted in 3D, on two surfaces: one located near the endocardium, the other located near the epicardium. The framerates are lower by a 16-fold compared to 2D, i.e., 344 frames/s (fps) in 3D (from 5,500 fps in 2D), but are tested whether it can be sufficient to estimate strain at high signal-to-noise ratio (SNR) as predicted by preliminary findings (Figure 28.3).

28.1.3.3 PBME performance assessment

A probabilistic framework has been developed in order to compare the strain estimation quality between conventional and parallel beamforming [22,31]. The elastographic SNR (SNR_e) is calculated for each sequence over the phase of systole. SNR_e is computed for every point in an image using

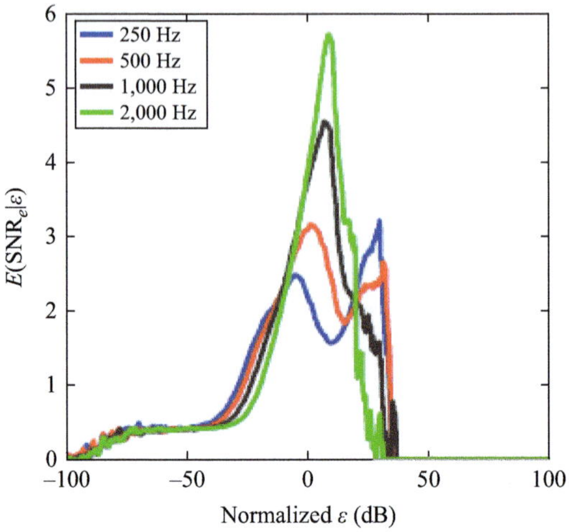

Figure 28.3 E(SNR$_e$/ε) transverse strain curves increase with frame rate

$$\mathrm{SNR}_e = \frac{\mu(\varepsilon)}{\sigma(\varepsilon)} \tag{28.3}$$

where $\mu(\varepsilon)$ and $\sigma(\varepsilon)$ refer to the mean and standard deviation of the strain (ε) magnitude within a small 2D region of interest (ROI) (3.0 × 3.2 mm). Since both strain and SNR$_e$ are computed for each point in the myocardium throughout systole, a large number (>600,000) of strain-SNR$_e$ pairs is generated for each sequence [22]. The conditional expected value of SNR$_e$ for each strain is calculated using [22,31]

$$E(\mathrm{SNR}_e|\varepsilon) = \int_0^{+\infty} \mathrm{SNR}_e \frac{f(\mathrm{SNR}_e, \varepsilon)}{f(\varepsilon)} d\mathrm{SNR}_e \tag{28.4}$$

$E(\mathrm{SNR}_e|\varepsilon)$ curves are generated for each sequence, which allows for a relatively easy comparison to be performed between different sequences for a wide range of strain values. Example of $E(\mathrm{SNR}_e|\varepsilon)$ curves for radial strain estimation is provided in Figure 28.3. The SNR$_e$ of both 2DPBME and 3D-PBME are computed with respect to the strain (equivalent to frame rate) and compared to focused (standard 2D and 3D myocardial elastography) to perform a quality comparison with parallel beamforming techniques.

28.1.3.4 Compounding

A compounding technique is applied to determine increase in SNR when parallel beamforming is applied. Plane waves are electronically steered and transmitted at three different angles separated by 20° (−20°,0°,20°), and the resulting RF frames are combined into a compounded image. The received RF frames are reconstructed by applying a delay-and-sum method on Graphics Processing Unit (GPU)-based parallel computing to accelerate reconstruction processing [31]. In preliminary studies, we have found that compounding in human hearts in vivo decreases the frame rate from 5,500 to 1,375 fps, which is sufficiently high for myocardial elastography (Figure 28.3) while SNR increases by a 4-fold.

28.1.4 Simulations

Field II, an established and publicly available ultrasound field simulation program [32,33], is used to simulate the RF signals of the myocardium. The simulated mesh including the myocardium, cavity and background are loaded into Field II [34,35]. Instead of a focused wave, a diverging wave sequence is employed for transmit by placing the focus 6.75 mm (half the size of the aperture) behind the array surface to achieve a 90° angle insonification [31]. For 2D-PBME, the RF signals are obtained from 192 elements and 3.5-MHz center frequency with 60% bandwidth (at −6 dB) phased array similar to what are used in the canine study. Hanning apodization is applied both during transmit and receive to reduce grating lobes. The width and height of the phased array are 43 and 7 mm, respectively. The RF signals are reconstructed by coherent summation of the signals received by all the elements using a delay-and sum algorithm. For 3D-PBME, RF signals are obtained from a 2D array with 16×16, 32×32 and 64×64 elements and 3-MHz center frequency, similar to what are used in experiments.

28.1.5 Phantoms

As in our previous studies [36], polyacrylamide (Acros Organics, Geel, Belgium) gel phantoms containing agar powder that produces full speckle are used to model the left ventricle of the human heart. The cylindrical phantom (Figure 28.4) is molded as a thick-walled, hollow cylinder in order to mimic the geometry of the left ventricle in the short-axis view, and the center is left hollow to allow water to flow through the phantom and cause wall motion and deformation. Two phantoms are prepared for this study: one of uniform wall stiffness (noninclusion; 25 kPa; [36]) and one containing a stiff inclusion representing a region of reduced compliance (50 kPa). A combination of rotation and deformation is studied to better mimic the cardiac function using an existing setup. The pumping frequency is 1 pulse/s, and the motor inducing rotation is synchronized for clockwise rotation to start with the pump stroke. One motor will rotate for 30° clockwise at a speed of 112°/s (268 ms) while the other is fixed.

28.1.6 Myocardial ischemia and infarction detection in canines in vivo

28.1.6.1 Ischemic model

In order to test myocardial elastography, in the assessment of ischemia by depicting the change in both mechanical and electrical properties, 12 ($n = 12$) adult male dogs (20–25 kg) are used within 2–3 years according to well-established anesthetized canine models. The flow in that artery was continuously controlled via pressure–flow curves: *Step 1 (control)*: Mongrel dogs with normal/healthy

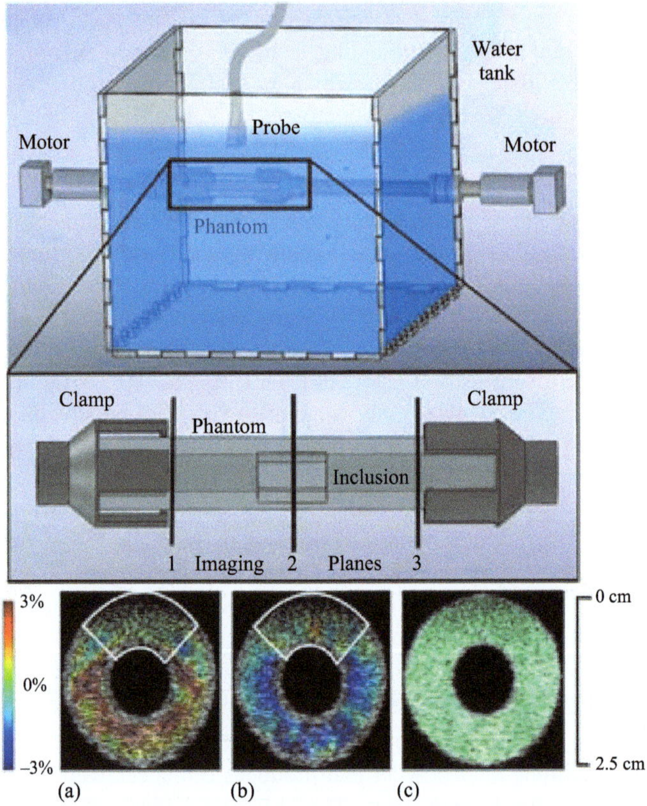

Figure 28.4 Top: experimental setup used to impose motion schemes on a phantom. Bottom: peak cumulative (a) radial and (b) circumferential strain and (c) peak rotation during relaxation in an inclusion phantom. The inclusion is outlined in white. Note the regions of reduced strains within the region of the inclusion (ROI shown; Okrasinski et al. [36])

myocardium, as verified using standard echocardiography, are used for control measurements. Channel data with both 2D- and 3D-PBME are continuously acquired during 5 min in sets of three cardiac cycles each taken 20 s apart, i.e., approximately 15 sets total. This established the strain baseline. *Step 2 (mild-to-acute ischemia)*: The dogs underwent a left thoracotomy followed by gradual constriction of the midproximal left anterior descending (LAD) coronary artery using the ameroid constrictor by 0%–100% of baseline, at intervals of 20% for 15 min each. Strain images are shown in Figure 28.5(a). The slope of the coronary pressure–flow curves (using Millar catheters and sonomicrometry) is used to monitor the ischemic onset at each occlusion step. RF data in the same views as in Step 1 were continuously acquired during the full 15 min in sets of three cardiac cycles (10 s apart), i.e., approximately 70 sets total.

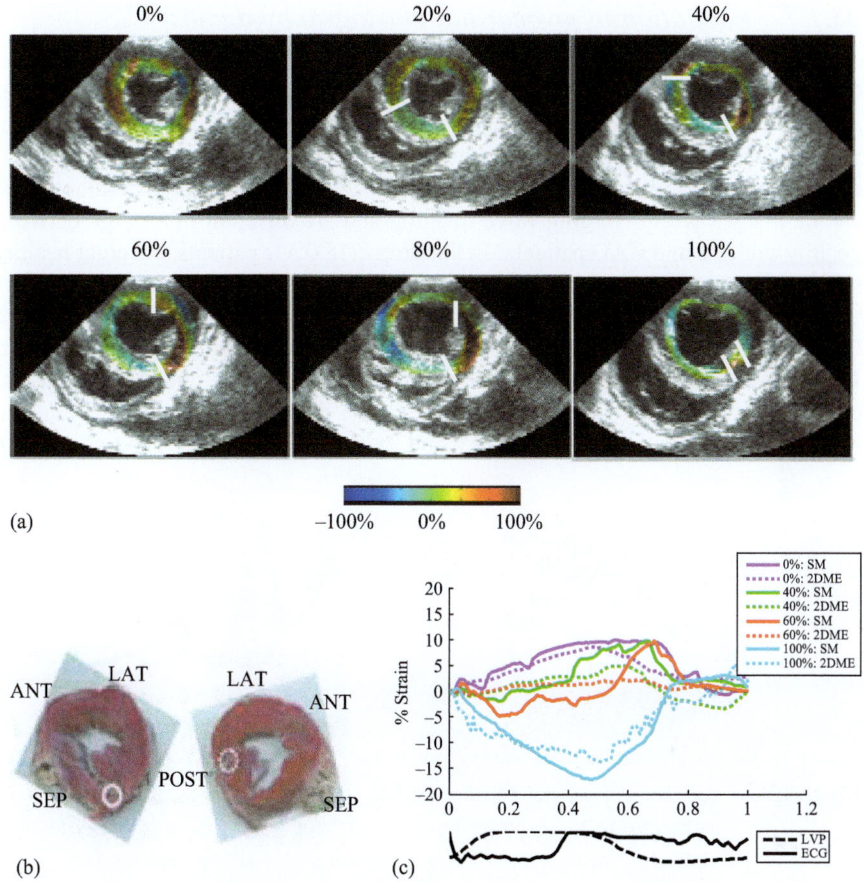

Figure 28.5 *(a) Progression of ischemia [in "blue" or thinning systolic strain as indicated compared to the surrounding "red" or nonischemic (thickening) strain] from 0% to 100% occlusion in the same dog using 2D-PBME and identifying the region and extent of ischemia in each case (shown with the ROI); (b) TTC pathology showing pale (unstained by TTC; ischemic) vs. red (stained by TTC; normal) myocardium. (c) Temporal radial strain profiles in the anterior wall region of 3×3 mm^2 at 0%, 40%, 60% and 100% occlusion levels with sonomicrometry (SM) and 2DME (Lee et al. [20])*

28.1.6.2 Infarct model

Mongrel dogs underwent similar surgical procedure as in the ischemia model but survived for 4 days after complete ligation only in order to develop a fully developed infarct.

28.1.7 Validation of myocardial elastography against CT angiography

Computed tomography (CT) angiography is an established technique used for reliable detection of a coronary occlusion and was used to confirm the occlusion and validate the location of the ischemia or infarct as detected by myocardial elastography. The objectives of this study were to show that 2D myocardial strains can be imaged with diverging wave imaging and are different in average between healthy subjects and CAD patients. In this study, 15 CAD patients and eight healthy subjects were imaged with Myocardial Elastography. Patients with more than 50% occlusion in one of the main coronary arteries were considered to have obstructive CAD. Incremental axial and lateral displacements were estimated using normalized 1D cross-correlation and then accumulated during systole. Axial and lateral cumulative strains were then estimated from the displacements and converted to radial cumulative strains (Figures 28.7 and 28.8). The end-systolic radial strain in

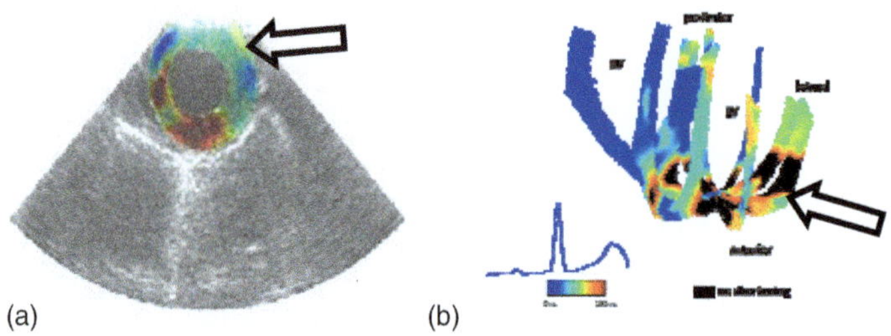

Figure 28.6 (a) Transthoracic systolic radial strain image of a canine left ventricle in vivo. Thinning (blue) strain region clearly indicates the extent of infarction. (b) Electromechanical isochrones in 3D identifying spatial extent of MI. Arrow denotes MI region

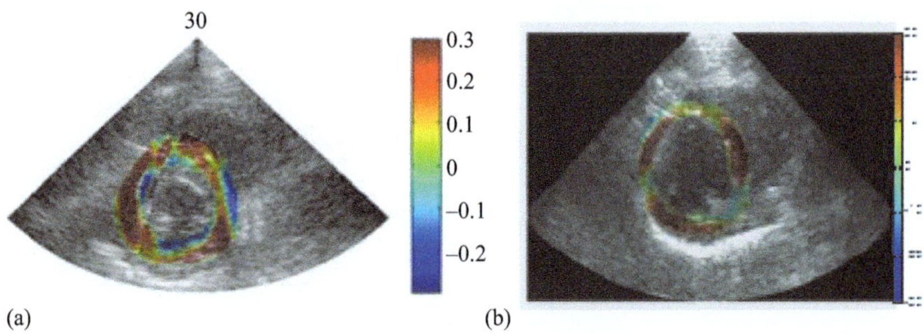

Figure 28.7 Comparison between (a) 2DME [conventional (focused) beamforming] using ECG gating and (b) 2D-PBME (parallel beamforming) systolic radial strain image in a normal patient. The quality is comparable without the artifacts from sector matching and ECG gating in the former (a)

the total cross section of the myocardium in healthy subjects (14.9±8.2%) was significantly higher than obstructive CAD patients (−0.9±7.4%, $p < 0.001$) and in nonobstructive CAD patients (3.7±5.7%, $p < 0.05$). Endsystolic radial strain in the LAD territory was found to be significantly higher in healthy subjects (16.9±12.9%) than in patients with obstructed LAD (2.2±7.0%, $p < 0.05$) and patients with non-obstructed LAD (1.7±10.3%, $p < 0.05$) (Figure 28.9). These preliminary findings indicate that end-systolic radial strain measured with

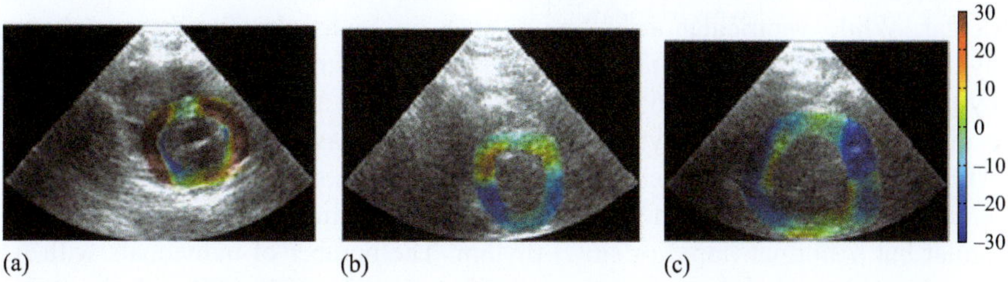

Figure 28.8 2D-PBME showing progression of coronary disease in three different patients: (a) normal, (b) (RCA: 90%; LAD: 20%; LCX: 20%) occlusions and (c) (RCA: 99%; LAD: 100%; LCX: 100%) occlusions. Figure 28.1(d) can be used for reference of coronaries

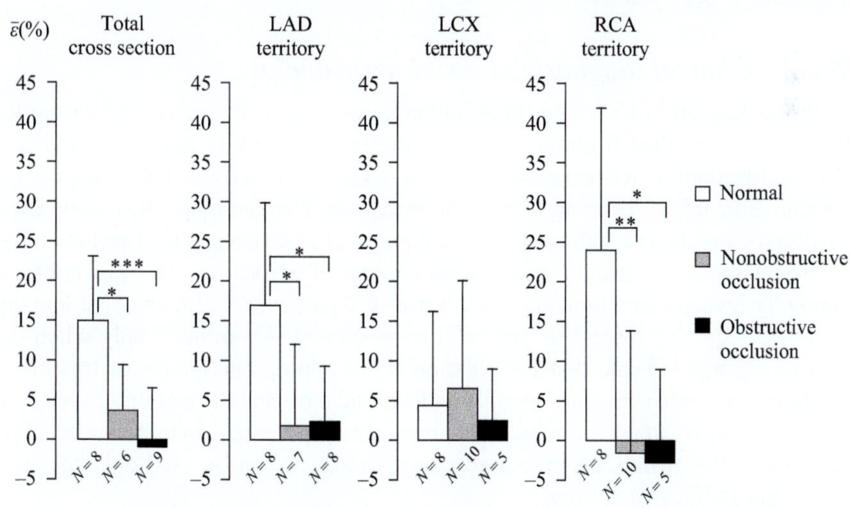

Figure 28.9 Preliminary findings in 25 human subjects (19 patients and 6 normals) using PBME. Nonsevere CAD (stenosis <50%) and severe (>50% stenosis). LAD, left anterior descending artery; LCx, left-circumflex artery; RCA, right coronary artery; Total, all territories. In all territories except LCx PBME was capable of differentiating normal from nonsevere and from severe CAD

myocardial elastography is higher on average in healthy subjects compared to CAD patients and indicate that myocardial elastography has the potential to be used for noninvasive, radiation free early detection of CAD.

28.2 Electromechanical wave imaging

28.2.1 Cardiac arrhythmias

Cardiac arrhythmias can be separated into atrial (or supraventricular) and ventricular. While ventricular arrhythmias, such as ventricular fibrillation (chaotic rhythm), ventricular tachycardia (rapid rhythm) and ventricular bradycardia (slow rhythm), incur the most episodes of sudden death, they are less common and easier to diagnose than atrial arrhythmias. Atrial arrhythmias include atrial fibrillation (Afib or AF) and atrial flutter (AFL) which are the most common. Similar to the ventricular definition, AF denotes the chaotic rhythm, while AFL denotes the regular but abnormal (rapid or slow) rhythm. The number of individuals with AF in the United States is expected to reach 12 million by 2050 [37] with the AFLs, often a result of treatment, also expected to rise as more of these treatments are administered. One of the main objectives of Electromechanical Wave Imaging is to aid in both enhancing the diagnosis and treatment planning and guidance of arrhythmias that are the most common and most difficult to diagnose, i.e., the atrial arrhythmias. A short overview of the state-of-the-art diagnostic and treatment techniques is provided below.

28.2.2 Clinical diagnosis of atrial arrhythmias

Electrocardiogram (ECG) recordings and no imaging modality is typically used for the noninvasive identification of atrial arrhythmias. If ECG recordings indicate AFL or fibrillation, RF ablation (see next section) is warranted that allows for catheterized cardiac mapping during its procedure. Cardiac mapping involves the insertion of a catheter containing a small number of electrodes in the heart chamber to contact the endocardium and measure times of activation. The procedure is minimally invasive and ionizing since it uses CT guidance, but it can be a lengthy procedure requiring topical or general anesthesia and is warranted only when the ECG recordings indicate that RF ablation is the appropriate course of treatment. Limitations include some inaccessible endocardial sites and the inability to map the midmyocardium and epicardium. More importantly, potentials in only one or a few locations in the atrium are measured per heartbeat, it can be used only to study stable, repeatable arrhythmias.

28.2.3 Treatment of atrial arrhythmias

RF ablation is a minimally invasive technique rapidly emerging as the most commonly used therapeutic modality for AFL and AF. For this treatment, a catheter, whose tip carries an electrode, is inserted through the femoral vein and the tip of the electrode is positioned at the arrhythmic origin. The tip causes a frictional heat generated by intracellular ions moving in response to an alternating current. The electrode is connected to a function generator, and the electrical current flows and raises the local temperature up to 95 °C maintaining it for about 15 min, generating thermal lesions in the vicinity of the ablating catheter. The treatment consists thus in modifying or in blocking the circuits of electrical conduction in heart. Current surgical procedures are invasive and have a moderate efficiency in the persistent forms of AF. AF in some patients may be due to focal activity originating in the pulmonary veins, and 70% of these patients can be successfully treated by RF ablation of the focus inside the pulmonary veins [38]. However, the treatment of AF using RF ablation can often lead to the development of other arrhythmias. For example, a sizeable increase of atypical flutter is due to catheter ablation of AF.

28.2.4 Electromechanical wave imaging

28.2.4.1 The cardiac electromechanics

The heart will not adequately contract unless it is electrically activated via a very specific route (Figure 28.10; arrows). In sinus rhythm (or natural contraction), the path of activation originates at the sinoatrial node (right before the ECG's P-wave), from which the electrical signal in the form of an action potential spreads to both right and left atria causing their contraction (during the P-wave). The wave then propagates to the atrioventricular node (right after the P-wave), through the bundle of His and along the left and right bundles on the interventricular septum (during the Q–R segment) to the Purkinje fibers (S-wave) finally causing both ventricles to synchronously contract, starting at the apex toward their lateral and

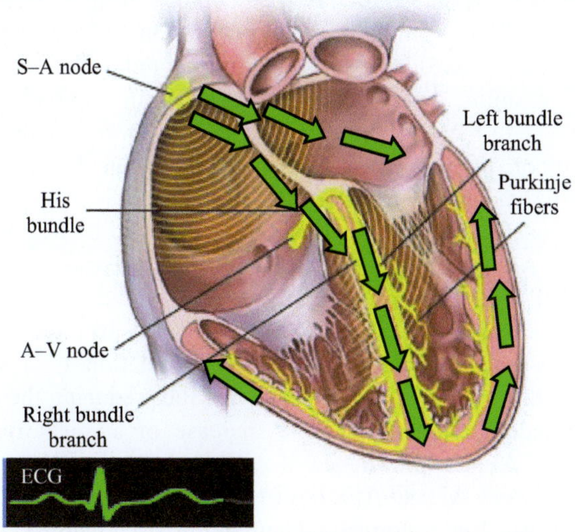

Figure 28.10 Illustration of the cardiac conduction system of the heart. The green arrows indicate the path of activation as the action potential propagates along the Purkinje fiber network (in yellow)

posterior walls (Figure 28.10). The heart is thus an electromechanical pump that requires to first be electrically activated in order to contract. Propagating electrical waves of excitation result into localized contractions. Each electrical activation in Figure 28.10 is followed by an electromechanical one, i.e., the depolarization of a cardiac muscle cell, or myocyte, is followed by an uptake of calcium, which triggers contraction [39] after a certain electromechanical delay of a few milliseconds [40,41]. In the presence of arrhythmia, electrical and electromechanical patterns are disrupted.

28.2.4.2 Electromechanical wave imaging

Our group has pioneered a unique noninvasive and direct (as opposed to inverse problem) imaging technique that could reliably map the conduction wave in the heart in all of its four cardiac chambers. Electromechanical wave imaging (EWI) [15,42–46] has been shown capable of noninvasively mapping the conduction wave during propagation. We identified that high frame rate (>500 fps) and precise 2D imaging of the cardiac deformation is feasible so that the transient cardiac motion resulting from the fast electromechanical wave (EW) can be mapped in murine [15,43,47,48], canine [15] and human [15,45,49] hearts in vivo. We were also capable of demonstrating that EWI is angle independent [46], has excellent correlation with electrical activation measurements in canines in vivo ([49]; slope of 0.99 and r^2=0.88; Figures 28.11 and 28.12) and is in excellent agreement with electromechanical simulations [49,50]. More importantly, our group was capable of recently showing that EWI was feasible in the atria of human hearts in vivo undergoing sinus rhythm [49]. There is simply no other modality that can directly map the conduction of the atria under sinus rhythm noninvasively in the clinic. An important additional advantage of this methodology is that it can be routinely applied in the clinic through straightforward integration with any echocardiography system. It could thus be used both at the diagnostic and at the treatment guidance levels, either off- or online. Despite the fact that EWI can map both the atria and the ventricles, we chose to focus on the atrial arrhythmias in this study given that they are far more common, more salvageable and completely lacking of any noninvasive imaging modality that can map their conduction properties.

EWI can be useful in a number of diseases that can be treated with ablation therapy e.g., AF, AFL, ventricular tachycardia, Wolff–Parkinson–White (WPW) syndrome, etc. WPW is a heart condition where an additional electrical pathway links the atria to the ventricles. It is the most common heart rate disorder in infants and children and is preferably treated using catheter ablation. EWI could be used in predicting the location of the accessory pathway, thus reducing the overall time of the ablation procedure. Since a sizeable increase of atypical flutter is due to catheter ablation of AF, the prevalence of AFL is also expected to rise. However, the relationship between AF and AFL is still not fully understood [51]. AFL, a type of atrial tachycardia, has historically been defined exclusively from the ECG recordings. More specifically, differentiation between flutter and other tachycardias was based on the atrial rate and the presence or absence of isoelectric baselines between atrial deflections. Since then, electrophysiological studies and RF ablation

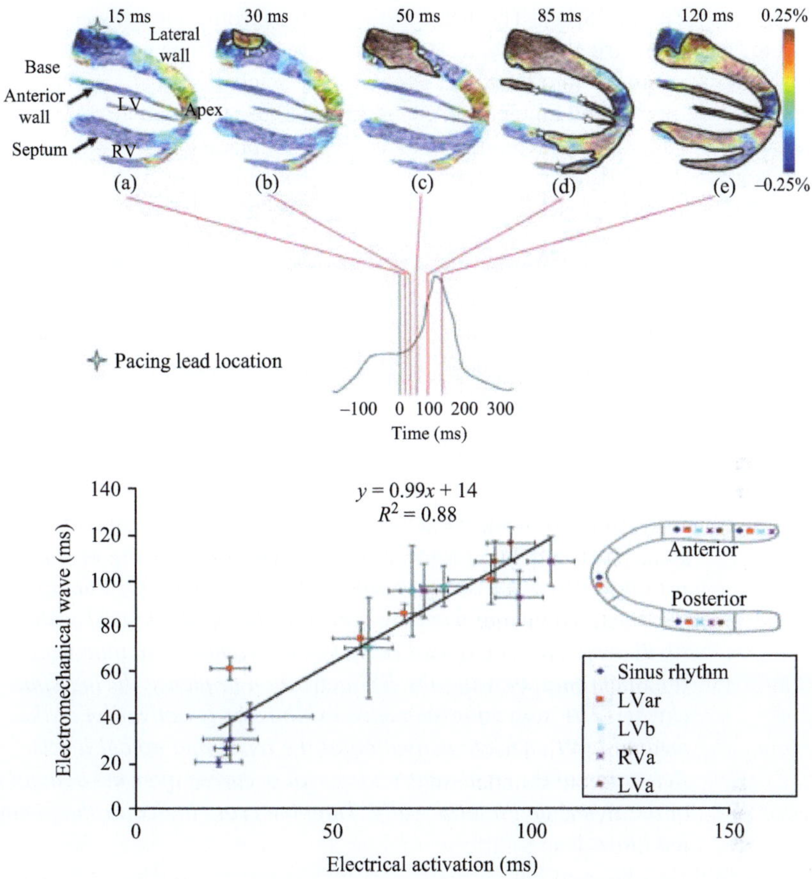

Figure 28.11 *Top: propagation of the electromechanical wave when paced from the lateral wall, near the base. Activation in this view corresponds to thickening of the tissue (red). Activated regions are traced at (a) 15, (b) 30, (c) 50, (d) 85 and (e) 120 ms and indicated on the (f) electrocardiogram. 0 ms corresponds to the pacing stimulus. (a–c) The EW propagates from the basal part of the lateral wall toward the apex. (d) Note that in the apical region, a transition from lengthening to shortening is observed rather than a transition from thinning to thickening. (d and e) In the anterior wall, the EW propagates from both the base and apex. The scale shows interframe strains. Bottom: electrical and electromechanical activation times during the four pacing protocols and sinus rhythm in four different heart segments in the posterior and anterior walls*

brought new understanding into the atrial tachycardia mechanisms, which did not correlate well with these ECG-based definitions [52]. In other words, ECG recordings offer only a limited value in the determination of specific atrial

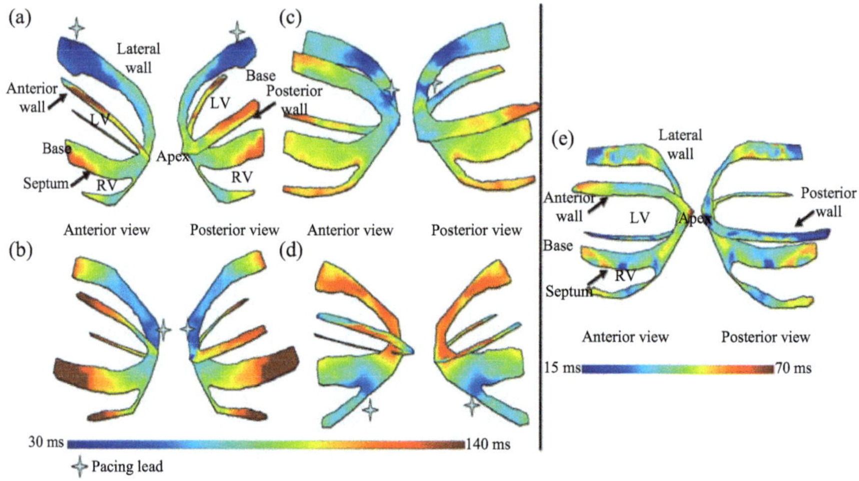

Figure 28.12 Isochrones showing the activation sequence under different pacing protocols as shown. Arrow indicates the pacing origin. (a) Pacing from the basal region of the lateral wall. (b) Pacing from the apex. (c) Pacing from the apical region of the lateral wall. (d) Pacing from the apical region of the right-ventricular wall. (e) Isochrones showing the EW activation sequence during sinus rhythm. The activation sequence exhibits early activation at the median level and late activation at the basal and apical levels. Activation of the right-ventricular wall occurred after the activation of the septal and lateral walls. The blue cross indicates the pacing lead location

tachycardia mechanisms, and, ultimately, for the selection of the appropriate course of treatment. Cardiac mapping allowed different mechanisms of macroreentrant atrial tachycardia to be identified, such as typical flutter, reverse typical flutter, left AFL, etc., although a significant number of atypical flutters is still poorly understood [52,53]. While mapping the right atrium is routinely undertaken successfully using this procedure, mapping the left atrium is riskier since it requires a transseptal puncture. However, as it currently stands in the clinic, right-atrium arrhythmia cannot be distinguished from left-atrium one prior to treatment and only the latter warrants transseptal puncture, which is a riskier procedure. In some cases, the left-atrium arrhythmia is not diagnosed until the entire right atrium is ablated (which may involve several unproductive hours of intervention), posing further risk to the patient. Consequently, left-atrial activation sequences are not well characterized in many atrial tachycardia cases [52]. Moreover, the surface ECG is insufficiently specific to distinguish left from right AFLs [51,53]. EWI could thus offer an important step for the localization of the right vs. left-atrial arrhythmia as well as localize the origin(s) at the treatment planning stage, i.e., prior to the catheterization of the patient rendering the treatment to be more efficient, much shorter in duration with unnecessary ablations in the wrong chamber or avoiding unnecessary transseptal punctures.

28.2.4.3 Treatment guidance capability of EWI

Currently, there is simply no noninvasive electrical conduction mapping techniques of the heart that can be used in the clinic. In addition, apart from being currently available, clinical electrical mapping methods are all catheter based and limited to mapping the endocardial or epicardial activation sequence; they are also time consuming and costly. Even in a laboratory setting, mapping the 3D electrical activation sequence of the heart can be a daunting task [54]. Studies of transmural electrical activation usually require usage of a large number of plunge electrodes to attain sufficient resolution [55–57] or are applied to small regions of interest in vivo [40]. Noncontact methods to map the electrical activation sequence have also emerged but are not used in the clinic. Optical imaging techniques use voltage-sensitive dyes that bind to cardiac cell membranes and, following illumination, fluoresce if the cell undergoes electrical activation. Optical imaging methods can map the activation sequence of ex vivo tissue on the endo—an epicardial surfaces [58–60] and transmurally [61–63] but cannot be applied in the clinic since they require the use of an electromechanical decoupler that inhibits cardiac contraction during imaging. Other newly developed methods to map the local electrical activity of the heart based on inverse problems are available: electrocardiographic imaging [64–66] and noncontact mapping [67–69]. The former is based on body surface potentials and Computed Tomography or Magnetic Resonance Imaging (MRI) scans and provides reconstructed epicardial action potentials, including the atria [70]. The latter consists in reconstructing the transmural potentials from potentials measured in the heart chamber based on specific assumptions that may be susceptible to inverse problem errors [71–73].

28.2.5 Imaging the electromechanics of the heart

As of today, no imaging method currently used in the clinic has been capable of mapping the electromechanics of the heart. Initial measurements to determine the correlation between the electrical and electromechanical activities have been reported [74,75]. These results suggest that the electrical activation sequence could be deduced from the electromechanics. Clinically available imaging modalities such as standard echocardiography or MRI cannot adequately detect the EW since they are too slow, i.e., the time required to acquire a single image is similar to the duration of the entire ventricular depolarization. The electrical activation lasts approximately 60 to 100 ms and requires a resolution of a few milliseconds (e.g., 2–5 ms) to generate precise activation maps. Moreover, the regional interframe deformation to be measured at these frame rates is very small (~0.25% at a 2-ms temporal resolution) and requires a highly accurate strain estimator [44,46,49]. We have shown that EWI is capable of reaching high frame rates (up to 2,000 fps) as well attain the precision of the incurred strains (up to 0.25%) which result from an electromechanical activation and therefore fulfill the requirements of both high temporal and spatial resolution unique to this technology.

28.2.6 EWI sequences

A block diagram of EWI is shown in Figure 28.13. Two imaging sequences, the automated composite technique (ACT) [45] and the temporally unequispaced acquisition sequences (TUAS) [46], have been developed and implemented [46,76–78] as well as the single-heartbeat sequence [31,79–81].

28.2.6.1 The ACT sequence

An Ultrasonix RP or MDP system with a 3.3-MHz phased array was used to acquire RF frames from 390 to 520 fps using an ACT [45]. Briefly, to increase the resulting frame rate, the image is divided into partially overlapping sectors corresponding to separate cardiac cycles (Figure 28.13(a)). The axial incremental displacements are obtained with a RF-based cross-correlation method (Figure 28.13(b)) (window size: 4.6 mm, 80% overlap). This method consists in dividing every ultrasound beam in a large number of overlapping, one-dimensional, 4.6-mm-long windows. Then, the following process is applied to each window and each sampled time t. A reference window at time t_1 is compared with all the windows contained in the same beam at sampled time t_2. The axial location of the window providing the highest correlation determines the axial displacement between two consecutive sampled times. After repeating this process for every available window and every available sampled time, we obtain axial displacements at multiple locations along the ultrasound beam and for every sampled time. The full-view image is then reconstructed using the motion-matching technique (Figure 28.13(c)) [49]. Briefly, this method consists of comparing, through a cross-correlation method, the incremental displacements measured in the overlapping line of two sectors obtained at different heartbeats to synchronize the sectors. More specifically, the acquisition sequence is designed such that each sector contains at least one ultrasound beam that is also part of the following sector. Therefore, this overlapping beam is expected to result in identical (or highly similar) axial displacements whether they corresponds to heartbeat h that occurred when sector s was acquired or to heartbeat $h+1$ that occurred when sector $s+1$ was acquired. By comparing, over time, the displacements obtained in the overlapping beams, the time delay corresponding to the maximum cross-correlation coefficient are obtained to synchronize each set of neighboring sectors. The procedure is repeated for each pair of sectors, allowing the reconstruction of the full view of the heart, hence ensuring the continuity of the transition incremental displacements across sectors. This method does not rely on the ECG. Therefore, it is especially useful in cases where the ECG may be unavailable or too irregular to perform ECG gating [49]. The axial incremental strains were then obtained by taking the spatial derivative of incremental strains in the axial direction using a least square estimator [30] with a kernel equal to 6.75 mm (Figure 28.13(d)). The myocardium was segmented using an automated contour tracking technique [34], and displacement and strain maps were then overlaid onto the corresponding B-mode images (Figure 28.13(e)). Isochrones were generated by mapping the first time occurrence at which the incremental strains crossed zero following the Q-wave. More specifically, the absolute value of the incremental

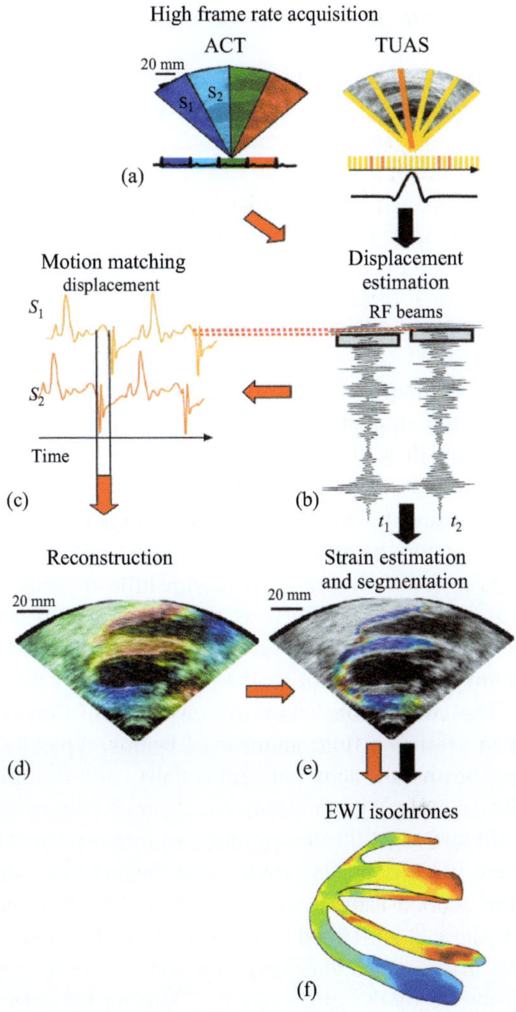

Figure 28.13 Block diagram of the EWI technique. (a) High frame rate acquisition is first performed using either ACT (follow red arrows) or TUAS (black arrows). (b) High precision displacement estimation between two consecutively acquired RF beams (t_1, t_2) is then performed using very high frame rate RF speckle tracking. (c) In ACT only, a region of the heart muscle, common to two neighboring sectors, is then selected. By comparing the temporally varying displacements measured in neighboring sectors (s_1, s_2) via a cross-correlation technique, the delay between them is estimated. (d) In ACT only, a full view ciné-loop of the displacement overlaid onto the B-mode can then be reconstructed with all the sectors in the composite image synchronized. (e) In ACT and TUAS, the heart walls are then segmented, and incremental strains are computed to depict the EW. (f) By tracking the onset of the EW, isochrones of the sequence of activation are generated

strains was minimized in a temporal window following the Q-wave in up to a hundred manually selected regions. Noisy data were excluded. Subsample resolution was obtained through spline interpolation, and Delaunay interpolation was used to construct continuous isochronal maps. Two echocardiographic planes, identical to the planes imaged in the standard apical four- and two-chamber views, were imaged across the long axis of the heart. These two views were temporally coregistered using the ECG signals, spatially coregistered by an echocardiography expert, and displayed in a three-dimensional biplane view in Amira 4.1 (Visage Imaging, Chelmsford, MA) (Figures 28.2 and 28.13(f)).

28.2.6.2 The TUAS sequence

We have developed and implemented in an Ultrasonix MDP system, a TUAS (Figure 28.14) [31], which is a sector-based sequence [82], adapted to optimally estimate cardiac deformations. In TUAS, it is possible to simultaneously achieve a wide range of frame rates for motion estimation, large beam density and a large field of view in a single heartbeat, thus avoiding the motion-matching and reconstruction steps in EWI (Figure 28.10), with little dependence on depth and beam density. Consequently, for a given set of imaging parameters, motion can be estimated at frame rates varying from a few Hz to kHz. The prior knowledge, in this case, is the minimum sampling rate, i.e., the Nyquist rate, of the motion over time at a given pixel. The conventional way to construct an ultrasound image using a phased array is to acquire a finite number of beams, typically 64 or 128, over a 90° angle. These beams are acquired sequentially, and the process is repeated for each frame. For example, a given beam, e.g., beam 3 (Figure 28.14), is acquired at a fixed rate (Figure 28.14, conventional sequence). In TUAS, the beam acquisition sequence is reordered to provide two distinct rates, defined as follows (Figure 28.14): the motion-estimation rate and the motion-sampling rate. The motion-estimation rate r_{me} is defined as the inverse of the time, i.e., T_{me}, lapsing between the two RF frames used to estimate motion. The motion-sampling rate r_{ms} is defined as the inverse of the time, i.e., T_{ms}, lapsing between two consecutive displacement maps. In conventional imaging sequences, these two rates are equal, because a given frame is typically used for two motion estimations (u_n and u_{n+1} in Figure 28.14). In TUAS, the operator can adjust the motion-estimation rate. As shown in Figure 28.14, a frame in the TUAS case is used only once for motion estimation, thus halving the motion-sampling rate relative to the conventional method. For example, an acquisition performed at a 12-cm depth with 64 beams with a conventional sequence will correspond to a frame rate of 100 Hz. However, while 100 Hz may suffice to satisfy the Nyquist sampling criterion of cardiac motion, it is usually insufficient for accurate motion tracking using RF cross-correlation. Therefore, to reach a higher frame rate of, e.g., 400 Hz typically used for EWI, the conventional sequence requires to divide the number of beams by four and thus reduces either the beam density, the field of view or both. At the same depth and beam density, TUAS provides a motion-sampling rate of 50 Hz and a motion-estimation rate that can be varied, as shown in the following section, within the following group: {6,416, 3,208, 1,604, 802, 401, 201, 100} Hz. This has

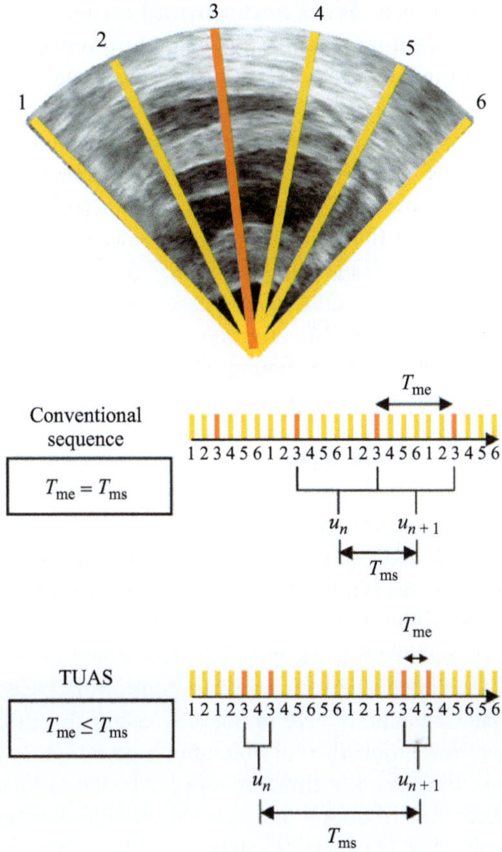

Figure 28.14 Illustration of an acquisition sequences in a simple case where only six lines form an image with each sector using two lines. In a conventional acquisition sequence, the time separating two acquisitions of the same line is the same. In TUAS, the time separating two acquisitions of the same line are modulated to optimize motion estimation

numerous advantages. For example, both the beam density and the field of view can be maintained while estimating the cardiac motion with an optimal frame rate, which could be, e.g., either 401 or 802 Hz, depending on the amplitude of the cardiac motion. This results into halving of the motion-sampling rate; however, the motion-sampling rate has only little effect on the motion-estimation accuracy. Theoretically, if this rate remains above the Nyquist rate of the estimated cardiac motion, it will have no effect. We estimated that, at a motion-sampling rate above 120 Hz, the effect of the motion-sampling rate became negligible compared to the effect of the motion-estimation rate [31].

28.2.6.3 Single-heartbeat EWI and optimal strain estimation

In TUAS, a wide range of frame rates can be achieved, including very high frame rates, independently of other imaging parameters. Therefore, by maintaining a set of imaging parameters (e.g., field of view, imaging depth), and varying the frame rate, it is possible to identify an optimal frame rate by studying the link between the strain SNR_e and the EW. Previous report [83] on the strain filter indicates that the SNR_e will depend mostly on the value of the strains to be measured, when the imaging parameters are fixed. This theoretical framework allows the construction of an upper limit on the SNR_e as a function of the strain amplitude (a.k.a. the strain filter). The strain filter corresponds, in this case, to the Ziv–Zakai lower bound (ZZLB) on the variance. The ZZLB is a combination of the Cramér–Rao lower bound (CRLB) and the Barankin bound (BB). The ZZLB transitions from the CRLB to the BB when decorrelation becomes important to the point that only the envelope of the signal contains information on the motion [84]. In the correlation model used here [85], this transition occurs only at very large strains. Since the amplitudes of strains to be measured are directly related to the motion-estimation rate (a large motion-estimation rate will result in small interframe strains), finding an optimal strain value is equivalent to finding an optimal motion-estimation rate. The strain filter was calculated with the imaging parameters used in this study as a reference; however, it was developed for the analysis of strains occurring in static elastography and is not adapted to the more complex motion of the heart. We have therefore developed a new probabilistic framework based on experimental data acquired in a paced canine in vivo to not only establish an upper bound on the SNR_e but to estimate the probability of obtaining a given SNR_e for a given strain amplitude [31]. Since the motion-estimation rate can be used as a means to translate and narrow the strain distribution, the optimal motion-estimation rate can be found by studying the link between the strains and the SNR_e. More specifically, a conditional probability density function spanning a large range of strains values was constructed (Figure 28.15) and was found in agreement with the strain-filter theory, which provides a higher bound on the SNR_e. The ZZLB predicts a sharp transition between the CRLB and BB when decorrelation becomes important to the point that the phase of the signal does not contain information about motion. Figure 28.15 shows that the conditional probability density function is comprised within the CRLB up to approximately 4% before it becomes comprised within the BB. A sharp decrease in the expected value of the SNR_e is also observed at 4% strain, underlining the importance of using the phase information of the RF signal for accurate strain measurements. A distortion in the strain distribution may indicate that while a high SNR_e can be maintained, the accuracy of the strain estimator is strongly impaired at low motion-estimation rates, i.e., less than 350 Hz in this case (Figure 28.15(b)). Finally, we showed that TUAS is capable of accurately depicting nonperiodic events at high temporal resolution. Therefore, the optimal frame rate will need to be between 389 and 3,891 Hz according to the strains estimated (Figure 28.15). Strain patterns expected during such a phenomenon were depicted, such as a disorganized contraction, leading to little to

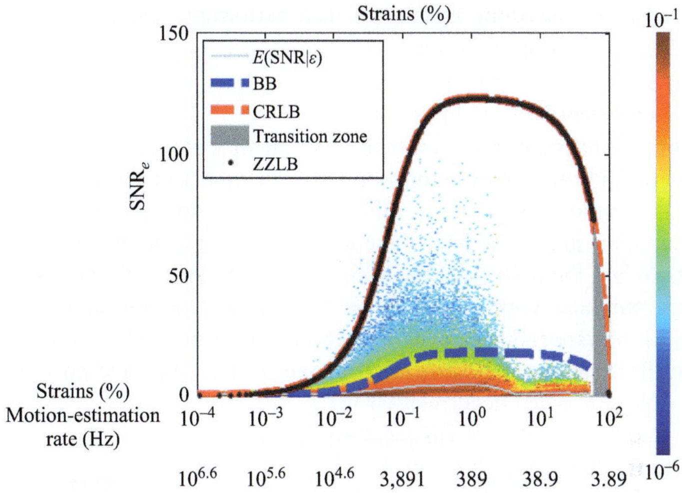

Figure 28.15 Conditional probability density function of the SNR_e knowing the strain value (and the corresponding motion-estimation rate). The conditional expectation value of SNR_e, the ZZLB, BB and CRLB are also displayed

no large scale motion of the heart. Regions of the myocardium were oscillating rapidly from thinning to thickening and thickening to thinning over time. Studying the frequencies of these oscillations could be useful in understanding the mechanisms of fibrillation [86], and such as Fourier-based analysis and principal component analysis in order to identify those components in fibrillation and better identify the arrhythmic origin(s).

28.2.7 Characterization of atrial arrhythmias in canines in vivo

28.2.7.1 Electrical mapping

Data from the St. Jude EnSite system was exported to a workstation for coregistration with EWI isochrones. Comma-separated-value files containing the coordinates of the 3D mesh as well as the data from each acquired point (activation time and spatial coordinates) were retrieved. The 3D mesh was recreated in Maya (Maya 2016, Autodesk, San Rafael, CA, USA) and the open-source software MeshLab (Visual Computing Lab—ISTI, CNR, meshlab.sourceforge.net). 3D coregistration was performed by aligning the isochrones with the 3D mesh using anatomical landmarks such as the location of the apex, the mitral valve annulus, the lateral wall or the septum. Once both the isochrones and the mesh were aligned, positions of the acquired points on the EnSite system were projected onto the isochrones and times of activation were compared. This process provided pairs of electrical and electromechanical activation times which were then plotted against each other. Linear regression was then performed, and slope, intercept and R^2 values were obtained.

28.2.7.2 Validation

The objective of this study was to validate EWI against electrical mapping using an electroanatomical mapping system, in all four chambers of the heart. Six ($n = 6$) normal adult canines were used in this study. The electrical activation sequence was mapped in all four chambers of the heart, both endocardially and epicardially using a St. Jude EnSite mapping system (St. Jude Medical, Secaucus, NJ). EWI acquisitions were performed during normal sinus rhythm and pacing, and isochrones of the electromechanical activation were generated. Electromechanical and electrical activation times were plotted against each other, and linear regression

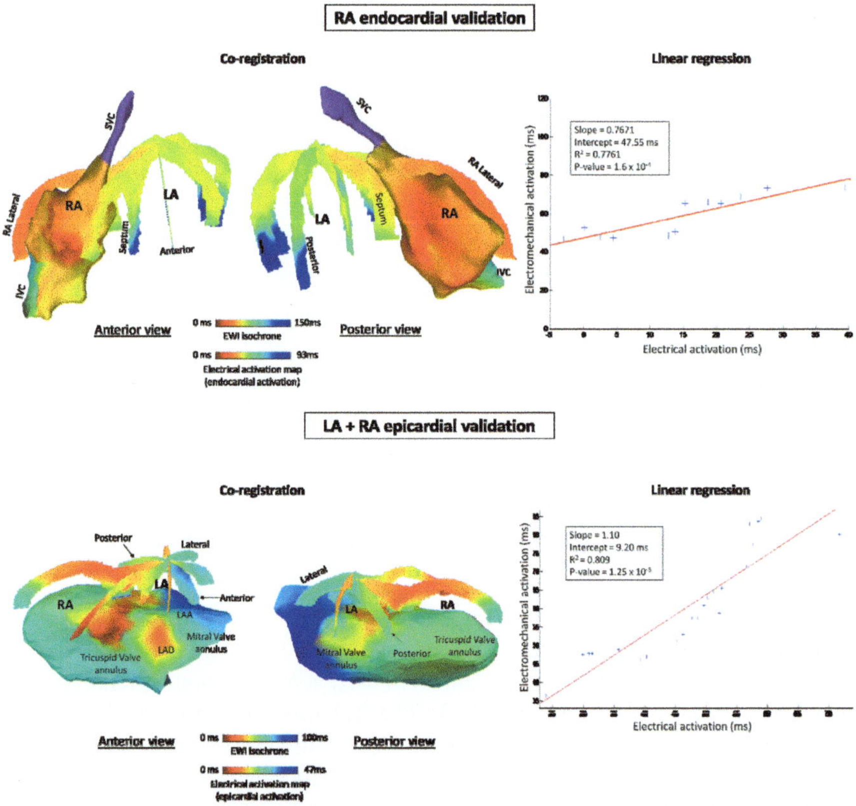

Figure 28.16 Endocardial RA and epicardial RA+LA EWI validation in two canines during normal sinus rhythm. Both endocardial and epicardial maps were acquired using a bipolar catheter. IVC, inferior vena cava; LA, left atrium; LAD, left anterior descending artery; LV, left ventricle; RA, right atrium; RV, right ventricle; SVC, superior vena cava

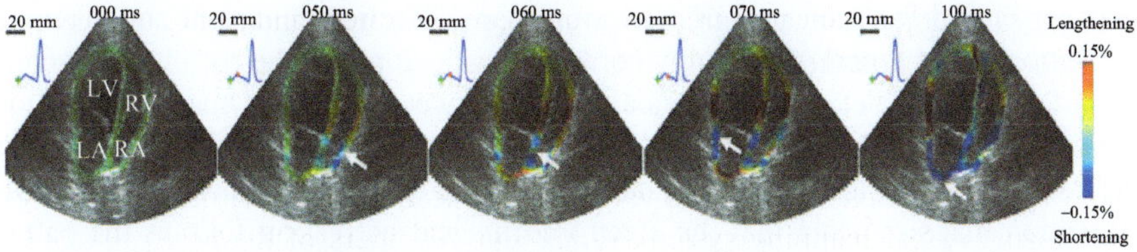

Figure 28.17 EWI using a flash sequence for motion estimation (motion sampling rate: 2,000 Hz, motion-estimation rate: 500 Hz) overlaid on a standard 128-beam, 30-fps B-mode. All four chambers are mapped but only atrial activation is shown here. Activation (shortening, in blue) was initiated in the right atrium (RA) (50 ms) and propagated toward the atrial septum (60 ms), the left atrium (LA) (70 ms) until complete activation of both atria (100 ms). RV, right ventricle; LV, left ventricle

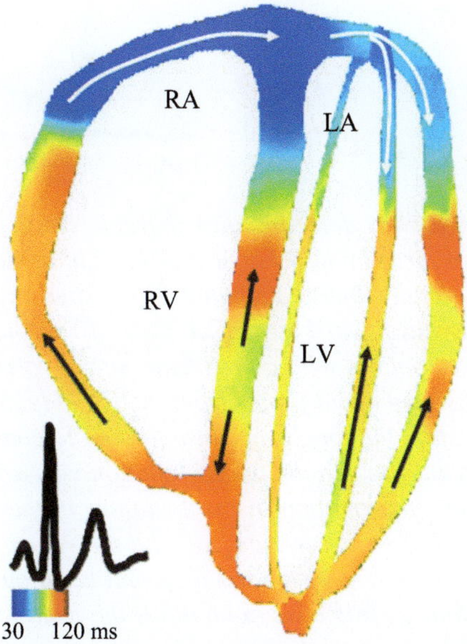

Figure 28.18 EWI isochrone in all four chambers in a healthy, 23-year-old male subject. Activation in this view corresponds to shortening of the tissue (blue). Activation is initiated in the right atrium and propagates in the left atrium. After the atrioventricular delay, activation is initiated in the ventricles from multiple origins, which are possibly correlated with the Purkinje terminals locations. Arrows (both white and black) indicate the direction of propagation

was performed for each pair of activation maps. Electromechanical and electrical activations were found to be highly correlated with slopes of the correlation ranging from 0.77 to 1.83, electromechanical delays between 9 and 58 ms and R^2 values from 0.71 to 0.92 (Figure 28.16). The excellent linear correlation between electromechanical and electrical activation and good agreement between the activation maps indicate that the electromechanical activation follows the pattern of propagation of the electrical activation. This suggests that EWI could be used to accurately characterize arrhythmias and localize its source.

28.2.8 EWI in normal human subjects and with arrhythmias

The objectives of the clinical studies [22,31,44,81] were (1) to determine the potential for clinical role of EWI, by predicting activation patterns in normal subjects, (2) to determine the feasibility of EWI to identify the site of origin in subjects with tachyarrhythmia and (3) to identify the myocardial activation sequence in patients undergoing Cardiac Resynchronization Therapy. In normal subjects (Figures 28.17 and 28.18), the EW propagated, in both the atria and the ventricles, in accordance with the expected electrical activation sequences based on

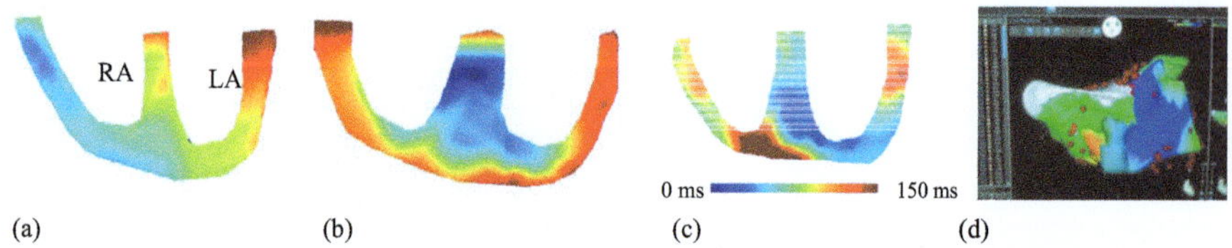

Figure 28.19 Noninvasively detecting and characterizing atrial flutter with EWI in three human subjects (RA, right atrium; LA, left atrium). (a) Normal subject (activation is initiated in the right atrium and propagates toward the left atrium); (b) unknown atrial flutter in a flutter patient with a prosthetic mitral valve, which was believed to cause the atrial flutter from the left side. Since the patient could not sustain the long procedure needed to construct a full activation map using cardiac mapping, ablation was attempted without complete information in two locations in the left atrium, which did not lead to cardioversion, i.e., did not return to sinus rhythm. The patient was sent home and a second ablation is scheduled in the near future. This case exemplifies the need for a faster mapping method, which could have led to the proper identification of the ablation site and potentially limit the number of ablation procedures needed to treat this patient. Indeed the EWI isochrones shown here display the initial activation in the left atrium, close to the septum; (c) atypical left atrial flutter patient confirmed by cardiac mapping. EWI isochrones also show early activation is initiated in the left atrium. See Appendix 1 for the corresponding EWI cine-loops. (d) CARTO map of a left-sided flutter case

reports in the literature. In subjects with CRT, EWI successfully characterized two different pacing schemes, i.e., left-ventricular epicardial pacing and right-ventricular endocardial pacing vs. sinus rhythm with conducted complexes. In two subjects with AFL (Figures 28.4–28.7), the propagation patterns obtained with EWI were in agreement with results obtained from invasive intracardiac mapping studies, indicating that EWI may be capable of distinguishing left-atrial from right-atrial flutters transthoracically. Finally, we have shown the feasibility of EWI to describe the activation sequence during a single heartbeat in a patient with AFL and right bundle branch block ([31]; Figure 28.19). The results presented demonstrate for the first time that mapping the transient strains occurring in response to the electrical activation, i.e., the EW propagation, can be used to characterize both normal rhythm and arrhythmias in humans, in all four cardiac chambers transthoracically using multiple and single-heartbeat methodologies. EWI has the potential to noninvasively assist in clinical decision-making prior to invasive treatment, and to aid in optimizing and monitoring response to CRT.

Acknowledgments

The results presented herein were produced by current and previous members of the Ultrasound and Elasticity Imaging Laboratory: Ethan Bunting, PhD, Alexandre Costet, PhD, Julien Grondin, PhD, Wei-Ning Lee, PhD and Jean Provost, PhD. The studies were in part supported by R01 EB006042 and R01 HL 114358.

References

[1] A. S. Go, D. Mozaffarian, V. L. Roger, *et al.*, "Heart disease and stroke statistics—2014 update: a report from the American Heart Association," *Circulation*, vol. 129, pp. e28–292, Jan 2014.

[2] J. H. Haga, A. J. Beaudoin, J. G. White, and J. Strony, "Quantification of the passive mechanical properties of the resting platelet," *Ann Biomed Eng*, vol. 26, pp. 268–77, Mar–Apr 1998.

[3] M. E. Bertrand, M. F. Rousseau, J. M. Lefebvre, *et al.*, "Left ventricular compliance in acute transmural myocardial infarction in man," *Eur J Cardiol*, vol. 7 Suppl, pp. 179–93, Jun 1978.

[4] C. Neagoe, M. Kulke, F. del Monte, *et al.*, "Titin isoform switch in ischemic human heart disease," *Circulation*, vol. 106, pp. 1333–41, Sep 2002.

[5] J. Amano, J. X. Thomas, Jr., M. Lavallee, *et al.*, "Effects of myocardial ischemia on regional function and stiffness in conscious dogs," *Am J Physiol*, vol. 252, pp. H110–7, Jan 1987.

[6] C. H. Edwards, 2nd, J. S. Rankin, P. A. McHale, D. Ling, and R. W. Anderson, "Effects of ischemia on left ventricular regional function in the conscious dog," *Am J Physiol*, vol. 240, pp. H413–20, Mar 1981.

[7] N. Varma, F. R. Eberli, and C. S. Apstein, "Increased diastolic chamber stiffness during demand ischemia: response to quick length change

differentiates rigor-activated from calcium-activated tension," *Circulation*, vol. 101, pp. 2185–92, May 2000.

[8] N. Varma, F. R. Eberli, and C. S. Apstein, "Left ventricular diastolic dysfunction during demand ischemia: rigor underlies increased stiffness without calcium-mediated tension. Amelioration by glycolytic substrate," *J Am Coll Cardiol*, vol. 37, pp. 2144–53, Jun 2001.

[9] K. B. Gupta, M. B. Ratcliffe, M. A. Fallert, L. H. Edmunds, Jr., and D. K. Bogen, "Changes in passive mechanical stiffness of myocardial tissue with aneurysm formation," *Circulation*, vol. 89, pp. 2315–26, May 1994.

[10] J. W. Holmes, T. K. Borg, and J. W. Covell, "Structure and mechanics of healing myocardial infarcts," *Annu Rev Biomed Eng*, vol. 7, pp. 223–53, 2005.

[11] E. Konofagou, J. D'hooge, and J. Ophir, "Cardiac elastography—a feasibility study," in *2000 IEEE Ultrasonics Symposium Proceedings, Vols 1 and 2*, pp. 1273–6, 2000.

[12] E. Konofagou, W. N. Lee, and J. Luo, "Cardiovascular elasticity imaging," in *Biomedical Applications of Vibration and Acoustics in Imaging and Characterizations*, M. Fatim and A. Al-Jumaily, Eds., New York, NY: ASME, 2008.

[13] E. Konofagou, J. Luo, K. Fujikura, D. Cervantes, and J. Coromilas, "Imaging the electromechanical wave activation of the left ventricle in vivo," in *IEEE Ultrasonics Symposium*, Vancouver, Canada, 2006, pp. 985–8.

[14] E. E. Konofagou, J. D'Hooge, and J. Ophir, "Myocardial elastography—a feasibility study in vivo," *Ultrasound Med Biol*, vol. 28, pp. 475–82, Apr 2002.

[15] E. E. Konofagou, S. Fung-Kee-Fung, J. Luo, and M. Pernot, "Imaging the mechanics and electromechanics of the heart," *Conf Proc IEEE Eng Med Biol Soc*, vol. Suppl, pp. 6648–51, 2006.

[16] E. E. Konofagou, T. Harrigan, and S. Solomon, "Assessment of regional myocardial strain using cardiac elastography: distinguishing infarcted from non-infarcted myocardium," in *2001 IEEE Ultrasonics Symposium Proceedings, Vols 1 and 2*, pp. 1589–92, 2001.

[17] E. E. Konofagou, W. Manning, K. Kissinger, and S. D. Solomon, "Myocardial elastography— comparison to results using MR cardiac tagging," in *2003 IEEE Ultrasonics Symposium Proceedings, Vols 1 and 2*, pp. 130–3, 2003.

[18] E. E. Konofagou and J. Provost, "Electromechanical wave imaging for noninvasive mapping of the 3D electrical activation sequence in canines and humans in vivo," *J Biomech*, vol. 45, pp. 856–64, Mar 2012.

[19] E. Konofagou and J. Ophir, "A new elastographic method for estimation and imaging of lateral displacements, lateral strains, corrected axial strains and Poisson's ratios in tissues," *Ultrasound Med Biol*, vol. 24, pp. 1183–99, Oct 1998.

[20] W. N. Lee, J. Provost, K. Fujikura, J. Wang, and E. E. Konofagou, "In vivo study of myocardial elastography under graded ischemia conditions," *Phys Med Biol*, vol. 56, pp. 1155–72, Feb 2011.

[21] J. Provost, W. N. Lee, K. Fujikura, and E. E. Konofagou, "Electromechanical wave imaging of normal and ischemic hearts in vivo," *IEEE Trans Med Imaging*, vol. 29, pp. 625–35, Mar 2010.

[22] E. A. Bunting, J. Provost, and E. E. Konofagou, "Stochastic precision analysis of 2D cardiac strain estimation in vivo," *Phys Med Biol*, vol. 59, pp. 6841–58, Nov 2014.

[23] E. E. Konofagou, "Estimation and Imaging of Three-dimensional Motion and Poisson's Ratio in Elastography," Houston, Texas: University of Houston, 1999.

[24] W. N. Lee and E. E. Konofagou, "Angle-independent and multi-dimensional myocardial elastography— from theory to clinical validation," *Ultrasonics*, vol. 48, pp. 563–7, Nov 2008.

[25] I. K. Zervantonakis, S. D. Fung-Kee-Fung, W. N. Lee, and E. E. Konofagou, "A novel, view-independent method for strain mapping in myocardial elastography: eliminating angle and centroid dependence," *Phys Med Biol*, vol. 52, pp. 4063–80, Jul 2007.

[26] J. Luo and E. Konofagou, "A fast normalized cross-correlation calculation method for motion estimation," *IEEE Trans Ultrason Ferroelectr Freq Control*, vol. 57, pp. 1347–57, Jun 2010.

[27] J. Luo and E. E. Konofagou, "Effects of various parameters on lateral displacement estimation in ultrasound elastography," *Ultrasound Med Biol*, vol. 35, pp. 1352–66, Aug 2009.

[28] R. Righetti, J. Ophir, and P. Ktonas, "Axial resolution in elastography," *Ultrasound Med Biol*, vol. 28, pp. 101–13, Jan 2002.

[29] W. N. Lee, C. M. Ingrassia, S. D. Fung-Kee-Fung, K. D. Costa, J. W. Holmes, and E. E. Konofagou, "Theoretical quality assessment of myocardial elastography with in vivo validation," *IEEE Trans Ultrason Ferroelectr Freq Control*, vol. 54, pp. 2233–45, Nov 2007.

[30] F. Kallel and J. Ophir, "A least-squares strain estimator for elastography," *Ultrason Imaging*, vol. 19, pp. 195–208, Jul 1997.

[31] J. Provost, S. Thiebaut, J. Luo, and E. E. Konofagou, "Single-heartbeat electromechanical wave imaging with optimal strain estimation using temporally unequispaced acquisition sequences," *Phys Med Biol*, vol. 57, pp. 1095–112, Feb 2012.

[32] J. A. Jansen, "Field: a program for simulating ultrasound systems," *Med Biol Eng Comput*, vol. 34, pp. 351–3, 1996.

[33] J. A. Jensen and N. B. Svendsen, "Calculation of pressure fields from arbitrarily shaped, apodized, and excited ultrasound transducers," *IEEE Trans Ultrason Ferroelectr Freq Control*, vol. 39, pp. 262–7, 1992.

[34] J. Luo and E. E. Konofagou, "High-frame rate, full-view myocardial elastography with automated contour tracking in murine left ventricles in vivo," *IEEE Trans Ultrason Ferroelectr Freq Control*, vol. 55, pp. 240–8, Jan 2008.

[35] J. Luo, W. N. Lee, and E. E. Konofagou, "Fundamental performance assessment of 2-D myocardial elastography in a phased-array configuration," *IEEE Trans Ultrason Ferroelectr Freq Control*, vol. 56, pp. 2320–7, Oct 2009.

[36] S. J. Okrasinski, B. Ramachandran, and E. E. Konofagou, "Assessment of myocardial elastography performance in phantoms under combined physiologic motion configurations with preliminary in vivo feasibility," *Phys Med Biol*, vol. 57, pp. 5633–50, Sep 2012.

[37] D. Lloyd-Jones, R. Adams, M. Carnethon, *et al.*, "Heart disease and stroke statistics—2009 update: a report from the American Heart Association Statistics Committee and Stroke Statistics Subcommittee," *Circulation*, vol. 119, pp. e21–181, Jan 2009.

[38] M. Haissaguerre, P. Jais, D. C. Shah, *et al.*, "Spontaneous initiation of atrial fibrillation by ectopic beats originating in the pulmonary veins," *N Engl J Med*, vol. 339, pp. 659–66, Sep 1998.

[39] D. M. Bers, "Cardiac excitation-contraction coupling," *Nature*, vol. 415, pp. 198–205, Jan 2002.

[40] H. Ashikaga, B. A. Coppola, B. Hopenfeld, E. S. Leifer, E. R. McVeigh, and J. H. Omens, "Transmural dispersion of myofiber mechanics: implications for electrical heterogeneity in vivo," *J Am Coll Cardiol*, vol. 49, pp. 909–16, Feb 2007.

[41] J. M. Cordeiro, L. Greene, C. Heilmann, D. Antzelevitch, and C. Antzelevitch, "Transmural heterogeneity of calcium activity and mechanical function in the canine left ventricle," *Am J Physiol Heart Circ Physiol*, vol. 286, pp. H1471–9, Apr 2004.

[42] E. E. Konofagou, W. N. Lee, and S. Fung-Kee-Fung, "Angle-independent myocardial elastography: theoretical analysis and clinical validation," in *SPIE*, San Diego, CA, 2007, pp. 65130G-1–10.

[43] M. Pernot and E. E. Konofagou, "Electromechanical imaging of the canine myocardium in normal and pathological states," in *IEEE Proc. Symp. Ultras., Ferr. and Freq. Control*, Rotterdam, Netherlands, pp. 1091–4, 2005.

[44] J. Provost, V. Gurev, N. Trayanova, and E. E. Konofagou, "Mapping of cardiac electrical activation with electromechanical wave imaging: an in silico–in vivo reciprocity study," *Heart Rhythm*, vol. 8, pp. 752–9, May 2011.

[45] S. Wang, W. N. Lee, J. Provost, J. Luo, and E. E. Konofagou, "A composite high-frame-rate system for clinical cardiovascular imaging," *IEEE Trans Ultrason Ferroelectr Freq Control*, vol. 55, pp. 2221–33, Oct 2008.

[46] J. Provost, W. N. Lee, K. Fujikura, and E. E. Konofagou, "Imaging the electromechanical activity of the heart in vivo," *Proc Natl Acad Sci USA*, vol. 108, pp. 8565–70, May 2011.

[47] E. Konofagou, J. Luo, D. Saluja, K. Fujikura, D. Cervantes, and J. Coromilas, "Noninvasive electromechanical wave imaging and conduction velocity estimation in vivo," in *IEEE International Ultrasonics Symposium*, New York, NY, 2007, pp. 969–72.

[48] E. E. Konofagou, J. Luo, D. Saluja, D. O. Cervantes, J. Coromilas, and K. Fujikura, "Noninvasive electromechanical wave imaging and conduction-relevant velocity estimation in vivo," *Ultrasonics*, vol. 50, pp. 208–15, Feb 2010.

[49] J. Provost, V. T. Nguyen, D. Legrand, *et al.*, "Electromechanical wave imaging for arrhythmias," *Phys Med Biol*, vol. 56, pp. L1–11, Nov 2011.

[50] V. Gurev, J. Provost, E. E. Konofagou, and N. Trayanova, "In silico characterization of ventricular activation pattern by electromechanical wave imaging," *Heart Rhythm*, vol. Suppl, p. S357, 2009.

[51] H. Garan, "Atypical atrial flutter," *Heart Rhythm*, vol. 5, pp. 618–21, Apr 2008.

[52] N. Saoudi, F. Cosio, A. Waldo, *et al.*, "A classification of atrial flutter and regular atrial tachycardia according to electrophysiological mechanisms and anatomical bases; a Statement from a Joint Expert Group from The Working Group of Arrhythmias of the European Society of Cardiology and the North American Society of Pacing and Electrophysiology," *Eur Heart J*, vol. 22, pp. 1162–82, Jul 2001.

[53] A. Bochoeyer, Y. Yang, J. Cheng, *et al.*, "Surface electrocardiographic characteristics of right and left atrial flutter," *Circulation*, vol. 108, pp. 60–6, Jul 2003.

[54] M. P. Nash and A. J. Pullan, "Challenges facing validation of noninvasive electrical imaging of the heart," *Ann Noninvasive Electrocardiol*, vol. 10, pp. 73–82, Jan 2005.

[55] N. Chattipakorn and R. E. Ideker, "The vortex at the apex of the left ventricle: a new twist to the story of the electrical induction of rotors?" *J Cardiovasc Electrophysiol*, vol. 14, pp. 303–5, Mar 2003.

[56] D. Durrer, R. T. van Dam, G. E. Freud, M. J. Janse, F. L. Meijler, and R. C. Arzbaecher, "Total excitation of the isolated human heart," *Circulation*, vol. 41, pp. 899–912, Jun 1970.

[57] D. R. Sutherland, Q. Ni, R. S. MacLeod, R. L. Lux, and B. B. Punske, "Experimental measures of ventricular activation and synchrony," *Pacing Clin Electrophysiol*, vol. 31, pp. 1560–70, Dec 2008.

[58] M. W. Kay, P. M. Amison, and J. M. Rogers, "Three-dimensional surface reconstruction and panoramic optical mapping of large hearts," *IEEE Trans Biomed Eng*, vol. 51, pp. 1219–29, Jul 2004.

[59] F. Qu, C. M. Ripplinger, V. P. Nikolski, C. Grimm, and I. R. Efimov, "Three-dimensional panoramic imaging of cardiac arrhythmias in rabbit heart," *J Biomed Opt*, vol. 12, p. 044019, Jul–Aug 2007.

[60] C. M. Ripplinger, Q. Lou, W. Li, J. Hadley, and I. R. Efimov, "Panoramic imaging reveals basic mechanisms of induction and termination of ventricular tachycardia in rabbit heart with chronic infarction: implications for low-voltage cardioversion," *Heart Rhythm*, vol. 6, pp. 87–97, Jan 2009.

[61] E. M. Hillman, O. Bernus, E. Pease, M. B. Bouchard, and A. Pertsov, "Depth-resolved optical imaging of transmural electrical propagation in perfused heart," *Opt Express*, vol. 15, pp. 17827–41, Dec 2007.

[62] D. A. Hooks, I. J. LeGrice, J. D. Harvey, and B. H. Smaill, "Intramural multisite recording of transmembrane potential in the heart," *Biophys J*, vol. 81, pp. 2671–80, Nov 2001.

[63] W. Kong, R. E. Ideker, and V. G. Fast, "Transmural optical measurements of Vm dynamics during long-duration ventricular fibrillation in canine hearts," *Heart Rhythm*, vol. 6, pp. 796–802, Jun 2009.

[64] C. Ramanathan, R. N. Ghanem, P. Jia, K. Ryu, and Y. Rudy, "Noninvasive electrocardiographic imaging for cardiac electrophysiology and arrhythmia," *Nat Med*, vol. 10, pp. 422–8, Apr 2004.

[65] C. Ramanathan, P. Jia, R. Ghanem, K. Ryu, and Y. Rudy, "Activation and repolarization of the normal human heart under complete physiological conditions," *Proc Natl Acad Sci U S A*, vol. 103, pp. 6309–14, Apr 2006.

[66] X. Zhang, R. R. Kinnick, M. Fatemi, and J. F. Greenleaf, "Noninvasive method for estimation of complex elastic modulus of arterial vessels," *IEEE Trans Ultrason Ferroelectr Freq Control*, vol. 52, pp. 642–52, Apr 2005.

[67] R. J. Schilling, N. S. Peters, and D. W. Davies, "Simultaneous endocardial mapping in the human left ventricle using a noncontact catheter: comparison of contact and reconstructed electrograms during sinus rhythm," *Circulation*, vol. 98, pp. 887–98, Sep 1998.

[68] B. Taccardi, G. Arisi, E. Macchi, S. Baruffi, and S. Spaggiari, "A new intracavitary probe for detecting the site of origin of ectopic ventricular beats during one cardiac cycle," *Circulation*, vol. 75, pp. 272–81, Jan 1987.

[69] C. T. Tai, T. Y. Liu, P. C. Lee, Y. J. Lin, M. S. Chang, and S. A. Chen, "Non-contact mapping to guide radiofrequency ablation of atypical right atrial flutter," *J Am Coll Cardiol*, vol. 44, pp. 1080–6, Sep 2004.

[70] Y. Wang, R. B. Schuessler, R. J. Damiano, P. K. Woodard, and Y. Rudy, "Noninvasive electrocardiographic imaging (ECGI) of scar-related atypical atrial flutter," *Heart Rhythm*, vol. 4, pp. 1565–7, Dec 2007.

[71] F. B. Belgacem, "Why is the Cauchy problem severely ill-posed?" *Inverse Probl*, vol. 23, pp. 823–36, 2007.

[72] R. L. Lux, "Noninvasive assessment of cardiac electrophysiology for predicting arrhythmogenic risk: are we getting closer?" *Circulation*, vol. 118, pp. 899–900, Aug 2008.

[73] B. Olshansky, "Electrocardiographic imaging: back to the drawing board?" *Heart Rhythm*, vol. 8, pp. 700–1.

[74] F. R. Badke, P. Boinay, and J. W. Covell, "Effects of ventricular pacing on regional left ventricular performance in the dog," *Am J Physiol*, vol. 238, pp. H858–67, Jun 1980.

[75] B. T. Wyman, W. C. Hunter, F. W. Prinzen, and E. R. McVeigh, "Mapping propagation of mechanical activation in the paced heart with MRI tagging," *Am J Physiol*, vol. 276, pp. H881–91, Mar 1999.

[76] J. Provost, W. N. Lee, K. Fujikura, and E. E. Konofagou, "Electromechanical wave propagation in the normal and ischemic canine myocardium in vivo," in *International Tissue Elasticity Conference*, Lake Travis, Austin, Texas, 2008.

[77] J. Provost, W. N. Lee, K. Fujikura, and E. E. Konofagou, "Electromechanical wave imaging for noninvasive localization and quantification of partially ischemic regions in vivo," in *Proceedings of the 2010*

IEEE 36th Annual Northeast Bioengineering Conference (NEBEC), Roma, Italy, 2010, pp. 1–2.

[78] J. Provost, S. Okrasinski, W. N. Lee, and E. E. Konofagou, "Abstract AB15-6: a noninvasive, direct method for cardiac mapping: electromechanical wave imaging," in *Hearth Rhythm*, Denver, Colorado, 2010, p. S32.

[79] A. Costet, E. Bunting, J. Grondin, A. Gambhir, and E. E. Konofagou, "Atrial electromechanical cycle length mapping in paced canine hearts in vivo," *IEEE Trans Ultrason Ferroelectr Freq Control*, vol. 62, pp. 1277–87, Jul 2015.

[80] A. Costet, J. Provost, A. Gambhir, *et al.*, "Electromechanical wave imaging of biologically and electrically paced canine hearts in vivo," *Ultrasound Med Biol*, vol. 40, pp. 177–87, Jan 2014.

[81] J. Provost, A. Costet, E. Wan, *et al.*, "Assessing the atrial electromechanical coupling during atrial focal tachycardia, flutter, and fibrillation using electromechanical wave imaging in humans," *Comput Biol Med*, vol. 65, pp. 161–7, Oct 2015.

[82] A. Baghani, A. Brant, S. Salcudean, and R. Rohling, "A high-frame-rate ultrasound system for the study of tissue motions," *IEEE Trans Ultrason Ferroelectr Freq Control*, vol. 57, pp. 1535–47, Jul 2010.

[83] T. Varghese and J. Ophir, "A theoretical framework for performance characterization of elastography: the strain filter," *IEEE Trans Ultrason Ferroelectr Freq Control*, vol. 44, pp. 164–72, 1997.

[84] E. Weinstein and A. Weiss, "Fundamental limitations in passive time-delay estimation—Part II: Wideband systems," *IEEE Trans Acoust Speech Signal Process*, vol. 31, pp. 1064–78, 1984.

[85] J. Meunier and M. Bertrand, "Echographic image mean gray level changes with tissue dynamics: a system-based model study," *IEEE Trans Biomed Eng*, vol. 42, pp. 403–10, Apr 1995.

[86] J. Chen, R. Mandapati, O. Berenfeld, A. C. Skanes, and J. Jalife, "High-frequency periodic sources underlie ventricular fibrillation in the isolated rabbit heart," *Circ Res*, vol. 86, pp. 86–93, Jan 2000.

[87] E. J. Ciaccio, A. B. Biviano, W. Whang, J. Coromilas, and H. Garan, "A new transform for the analysis of complex fractionated atrial electrograms," *Biomed Eng Online*, vol. 10, p. 35, May 2011.

Chapter 29

Summary and future directions

Christos P. Loizou[1]

In this final chapter of Part IV, we present the summary findings on selected applications of speckle filtering and speckle tracking, presented in Part IV. Furthermore, areas of future research directions on speckle filtering and tracking will be briefly discussed.

29.1 Summary on selected applications

Despeckle filtering (see Part II) and speckle tracking (see Part III) are important operations in the enhancement, tracking and segmentation of ultrasound images and videos of the carotid artery. There are a lot of application areas ranging from filtering, histogram normalization, segmentation, texture analysis, quality evaluation, visual evaluation by the experts, speckle tracking, and in image and video encoding as also presented in Parts III and IV. It should be furthermore noted that the combination of despeckle filtering and speckle tracking applications as document in this book, still remains too little explored and further investigation is required on the above subjects.

Chapter 19 discussed intima-media thickness (IMT) segmentation techniques in ultrasound imaging. Ultrasound imaging is a human-dependent scanning technique and therefore different operators may render the same object in different manners. Speckle is another obstacle to overcome when developing segmentation methods for ultrasound images. Another complication in automatic carotid IMT segmentation techniques is given by the high variability in normal vessel morphology and in vessel appearance under pathology. These challenges justify why, currently, the IMT segmentation in ultrasound images is often still an open problem. Because of the variability caused by physiology and by pathological conditions, it is not possible to pick an "ideal" technique for the IMT segmentation of all carotid artery ultrasound images. However, robustness is certainly a key point for all techniques. When facing the problem of carotid IMT segmentation, it is important to remember that carotid arteries are different for several parameters, including shape, size, orientation and composition.

[1]Department of Electrical Engineering, Computer Engineering and Informatics, Cyprus University of Technology, Cyprus

In Chapter 20, ultrasound video plaque segmentation of the common carotid artery (CCA) was discussed and an integrated system for the segmentation of atherosclerotic carotid plaque in longitudinal ultrasound image sequences was presented and evaluated. The method integrates video frames normalization, despeckling and accurate segmentation using active contours. Such a system can reduce the time required for the video analysis, and also the subjectivity that accompanies manual delineations and measurements. The proposed segmentation method may be used as an automated system for the early diagnosis and the assessment of the risk of stroke or to measure the transversal as well as the longitudinal movements at the two arterial sides of the CCA (left and right CCA) in order to find differences between the two sides. The proposed integrated plaque video segmentation method will greatly facilitate the automated plaque motion analysis providing close to real-time video processing.

Chapter 21 demonstrated how image texture and morphology analysis algorithms are used in order to classify ultrasound images of carotid plaques. Until now, the results using different classifiers are very promising and have the potential for computer-assisted identification of patients with asymptomatic carotid stenosis at increased risk of stroke. Additionally, morphological features help us understand the interrelations among different intensity regions. Morphological results from dark, midrange and high intensity regions were examined and found that there was significant overlap between the pattern spectra coming from symptomatic and asymptomatic plaques.

Chapter 22 provided a review on 3D US-based methods for the segmentation of carotid plaques and their use in quantifying plaque composition using image texture metrics. Specifically, the chapter reviewed algorithms used to segment the carotid media-adventitia) and lumen–intima of CCA, internal carotid artery and external carotid artery. Some review methods, which have used these segmented boundaries to provide information on plaque composition using image texture metrics, were finally presented and discussed.

In Chapter 23, the mechanical behavior of carotid arteries which is mainly determined by the fibers in the vessel wall was discussed. Elastin and collagen fibers are found, both with different orientation and acting in different pressure ranges, resulting in nonlinear mechanical behavior. The deformation of an artery is the result or response of its loading and its mechanical properties. The chapter explores loading and deformation and introduces typical parameters and relations between loading and deformation.

In Chapter 24, a number of speckle-tracking-based methodologies were outlined, suitable for the estimation of motion and strain of the carotid artery from ultrasound images. Various versions of intensity- and phase-based techniques were suggested and validated mostly in phantoms, in in silico and in vitro data. Waveforms showing displacements, velocities and accelerations can be obtained from these methods, and a number of indices can be calculated. Spatial mapping (imaging) of tissue strains is achieved with elastography, a major application of motion analysis. Through their application in real data, these methods are promising for revealing valuable quantitative in vivo information about arterial mechanics. Compared to other ultrasound-based indices, a major advantage of motion-derived indices is that they provide functional, rather than mere anatomical information, which is more sensitive to early wall changes. Their full potential in predicting, diagnosing and monitoring carotid-related disorders, such as cerebrovascular events, as well as in characterizing the burden of other diseases, remains to be confirmed in large clinical trials, toward an integrated personalized approach for disease management and increased patient safety.

Chapter 25 presented intravascular ultrasound (IVUS) as an invasive coronary imaging modality, which provides insights in the diagnosis and therapy of CAD. The main advantage of IVUS compared to other coronary imaging techniques such as traditional invasive angiography, is that it allows the tomographic assessment of: the lumen area, the external elastic membrane area, the plaque size, the distribution and the composition of the plaque. It can safely detect and characterize the following types of plaques: necrotic core, fibrous plaque and calcified plaque. One other aspect worth mentioning is that it also provides accurate measurement of the luminal dimensions of the artery of interest. With IVUS, lipid-laden lesions appear hypoechoic, fibromuscular lesions generate low-intensity echoes and fibrous or calcified tissues are echogenic. However, IVUS suffers from a few drawbacks directly connected to its innate image quality. For example, calcium obscures the underlying wall, a phenomenon called acoustic shadowing. One other major image quality issue that emerges from the use of IVUS is the so-called speckle noise, which is the main reason for the grainy texture of IVUS images. This results to poor quality images, which makes their interpretation and processing nontrivial for computed-based diagnostic systems.

In Chapter 26, some basic principles of speckle tracking are first introduced and the fundamentals of speckle tracking in a wider context are described. Speckle tracking echocardiography and echocardiographic particle image velocimetry was then introduced and several clinical applications in the context of evaluation of cardiac function were proposed. Color Doppler approaches, complementary to speckle tracking, were furthermore introduced, and finally, it was shown how speckle tracking techniques could be benefited from high-frame-rate echocardiography (also called "ultrafast echocardiography"). The chapter concluded with the expected contribution of high-framerate ultrasound for speckle tracking in three-dimensional echocardiography.

In Chapter 27, assessment of systolic and diastolic heart failure is presented. Heart failure is becoming more common in western societies as their populations age. Since heart failure is a severe disease with a poor prognosis, imaging is important for early detection, accurate diagnosis, estimating prognosis, and planning and monitoring responses to treatment. Many diagnostic targets can be studied to establish the particular phenotype in a person who is suspected of having heart failure, and most invasive and non-invasive diagnostic techniques have been used to study them. Chapter 27 concentrated on evidence relating to the use of speckle tracking to study left ventricular, left atrial, and right ventricular function in heart failure. Its technical strengths and limitations from a clinical perspective were reviewed and it was described how it is applied to determine the pathophysiological mechanisms of heart failure, to identify the underlying aetiology and to estimate prognosis. The authors furthermore suggested some technical developments that if feasible might assist clinicians in improving treatment and outcomes for patients with heart failure.

In Chapter 28, myocardial elastography and electromechanical wave imaging was discussed. Cardiovascular diseases remain America's primary killer by a large margin, claiming the lives of more Americans than the next two main causes of death combined (cancer and pulmonary complications). In particular, coronary artery disease (CAD) is by far the most lethal, causing 17% of all (cardiac related or not) deaths every year. One of the main reasons for this high death toll is the severe lack of effective and accessible imaging tools upon anomaly detected on the electrocardiogram, especially at the early stages when CAD can be stabilized with appropriate pharmacological regimen. Arrhythmias refer to the disruption of the natural heart rhythm. Cardiac arrhythmias lead to a significant number of cardiovascular morbidity and mortality. This irregular heart rhythm causes the heart to suddenly stop pumping blood. Atrial pathologies are the most common arrhythmias with atrial fibrillation and atrial flutter being the most prevalent.

29.2 Future directions

As it has already been documented in the corresponding section on the future directions in Chapters 11 and 18, the despeckle filtering algorithms, speckle tracking techniques, segmentation techniques, measures for evaluating them and the measures for image quality evaluation introduced in this book can also be generalized and applied to other image and video processing applications. Only a small number of filtering, segmentation and tracking algorithms, evaluation metrics and image quality evaluation metrics were investigated in this book, and numerous extensions and improvements can be envisaged. Most importantly, more comparative studies of despeckle filtering, speckle tracking and segmentation in image and video are necessary, where different filters and techniques with parameter optimization, could be evaluated by multiple experts as well as based on image quality and evaluation metrics as also proposed in this book.

Additionally, the issue of video despeckling and segmentation is still in its infancy and this area of research work will receive significant attention in the following years. Although it is noted that the proposed methodology and filtering, segmentation and tracking algorithms documented in this book may be also investigated in video sequences (by frame filtering or segmentation). There are many issues related to video despeckle filtering and segmentation that remain to be solved. In general, the development of a multiplicative model based on video sequences is required, since most of the models developed for video filtering were for additive noise [1–4].

Despeckle filtering, segmentation and tracking may be also applied for other organs, including the detection of hyperechoic or hypoechoic lesions in the kidney, liver, spleen, thyroid, kidney, echocardiographic images, mammography and other. It may be particularly effective when despeckle filtering is combined with harmonic imaging, since both can increase tissue contrast. Speckle reduction can also be extremely valuable when attempting to fuse ultrasound with computed tomography (CT), MRI, positron emission tomography or optical coherence tomography images. It would be furthermore interesting to investigate the effect of despeckle filtering on segmentation and tracking in these areas. For example, when a lesion is suspected on a CT scan but it is not clearly visible, ultrasound despeckle filtering can be applied in order to accentuate subtle borders that may be masked by speckle and thus segmentation and tracking may be improved.

Great efforts are also currently made in optimizing despeckle filtering [5–7], segmentation [9–11] and tracking algorithms [12,13] in order to achieve better performance [6]. It is foreseen that optimization of a despeckling segmentation and tracking algorithms, would be dependent on transducer geometry, operating frequency, focal point(s), distribution of pixel values due to speckle, subject being scanned, etc. Automatic selection of optimal despeckling, segmentation and tracking algorithm's parameters would provide a useful tool for research and clinical applications.

Ultrasound imaging instrumentation, linked with imaging hardware and software technology have been rapidly advancing in the last two decades. Although these advanced imaging devices produce higher quality images and video, the need still exists for better image and video processing techniques including despeckle filtering, segmentation and tracking. Toward this direction, it is anticipated that the effective use of despeckle filtering, segmentation and tracking (by exploiting the algorithms documented in this book) will greatly help in producing images and videos with higher quality, accurate segmentation of structures and reliable border tracking. These images and videos that would be not only easier to visualize, segment and track and to extract useful information, but would also enable the development of more robust minimizing routine manual image analysis and facilitating more accurate automated measurements of both industrially and clinically relevant parameters.

References

[1] S. Winkler, "Digital video quality," Vision models and metrics, Chichester, West Sussex: John Wiley & Sons Ltd., 2005.

[2] J.-H. Jung, K. Hong, S. Yang, "Noise reduction using variance characteristics in noisy image sequence," Int. Conf. on Consumer Electronics, pp. 213–214, 8–12 Jan. 2005.

[3] M. Bertalmio, V. Caselles, A. Pardo, "Movie denoising by average of warped lines," IEEE Trans. Image Process., vol. 16, no. 9, pp. 2333–2347, 2007.

[4] B. Alp, P. Haavisto, T. Jarske, K. Oestaemoe, Y. Neuro, "Median based algorithms for image sequence processing," SPIE Visual Communications and Image Processing, pp. 122–133, 1990.

[5] J. M. Bioucas-Dias, M. A. T. Figueiredo, "Multiplicative noise removal using variable splitting and constrained optimization, "IEEE Trans. Image Process., vol. 9, no. 10, pp. 1720–1730, 2010.
[6] C. Kotropoulos, I. Pitas, "Optimum nonlinear signal detection and estimation in the presence of ultrasonic speckle," Ultrason. Imaging, vol. 14, pp. 249–275, 1992.
[7] C. Debono, B. Micallef, N. Philip, A. Alinejad, R. Istepanian, N. Amso, "Cross layer design for optimised region of interest of ultrasound video data over mobile WiMAX," IEEE Trans. Inf. Technol. Biomed., vol. 16, no. 6, pp. 1007–1014, Nov. 2012.
[8] M. Rahman, A. Aziz, M. Kukar, *et al.*, "An optimized speckle noise reduction filter for ultrasound images using anisotropic diffusion technique", Int. J. Imaging Robotics, vol. 8, no. 2, pp. 55–60, 2012.
[9] S. Rosati, G. Balestra, F. Molinari, U. Rajendra Acharya, J. S. Suri, "A selection and reduction approach for the optimization of ultrasound carotid artery images segmentation", Mach. Learn. Healthc. Inf., vol. 56, pp. 309–332, 2013.
[10] J. Rouco, A. Camilho, "Robust common carotid artery lumen detection in B-mode ultrasound images using local phase symmetry", Int. Conf. on Acoustics, Speech and Signal Processing (ICASSP), 26–31 May 2013.
[11] R. Hemalatha, N. Santhiyakumari, M. Madheswaran, S. Suresh, "Segmentation of 2D and 3D images of carotid artery on unified technology learning platform", Procedia Technol., vol. 25, pp. 12–19, 2016.
[12] E. Y. Yang, G. Brunner, H. Dokainish, *et al.*, "Application of speckle tracking in the evaluation of carotid artery function in subjects with hypertension and diabetes", J. Am. Soc. Echogardiogr. vol. 26, no. 8, pp. 901–909, 2013.
[13] C. H. Leow, E. Bazigou, R. J. Eckersley, *et al.*, "Flow velocity mapping using contrast enchanced high-frame-rate plane wave ultrasound and image tracking: methods and initial in vitro and in vivo evaluation", Ultrasound Med. Biol., vol. 4, no. 11, pp. 2913–2925, 2015.

Index